DECISION-MAKING IN

Dermatology

DECISION-MAKING IN

Dermatology

JENNIFER L. HSIAO, MD
Associate Professor
Department of Dermatology
Keck School of Medicine
University of Southern California
Los Angeles, California

VIVIAN Y. SHI, MD
Professor
Department of Dermatology
University of Washington
Seattle, Washington

SCOTT D. WORSWICK, MD
Clinical Professor
Department of Dermatology
Keck School of Medicine
University of Southern California
Los Angeles, California

RAVEENA GHANSHANI, MS
Managing Editor
Keck School of Medicine
University of Southern California
Los Angeles, California

ELSEVIER

Elsevier
1600 John F. Kennedy Blvd.
Ste 1800
Philadelphia, PA 19103-2899

DECISION-MAKING IN DERMATOLOGY ISBN: 978-0-443-10723-8

For accessibility purposes, images in electronic versions of this book are accompanied by alt text descriptions provided by Elsevier. For more information, see https://www.elsevier.com/about/accessibility.

Publisher's note: Elsevier takes a neutral position with respect to territorial disputes or jurisdictional claims in its published content, including in maps and institutional affiliations.

Notice

Practitioners and researchers must always rely on their own experience and knowledge in evaluating and using any information, methods, compounds or experiments described herein. Because of rapid advances in the medical sciences, in particular, independent verification of diagnoses and drug dosages should be made. To the fullest extent of the law, no responsibility is assumed by Elsevier, authors, editors or contributors for any injury and/or damage to persons or property as a matter of products liability, negligence or otherwise, or from any use or operation of any methods, products, instructions, or ideas contained in the material herein.

Executive Content Strategist: Charlotta Kryhl
Senior Content Development Specialist: Vasowati Shome
Publishing Services Manager: Deepthi Unni
Project Manager: Prasanna Kalyanaraman
Design Direction: Renee Duenow

Printed in India at Replika Press Pvt. Ltd.
Plot No. 310-311, EPIP, HSIIDC, Kundli Industrial Park,
Sonipat, Haryana – 131028.

Last digit is the print number: 9 8 7 6 5 4 3 2 1

Contributors

JENNIFER ADAMS, MD
Associate Professor
Department of Dermatology
University of Nebraska Medical Center
Omaha, Nebraska

BRANDON L. ADLER, MD
Clinical Associate Professor
Department of Dermatology
Keck School of Medicine
University of Southern California
Los Angeles, California

HANA AHMED, MD
Dermatopathology Fellow
Dermatology
Department of Dermatology, University of Alabama at Birmingham
Birmingham, Alabama

MARIA ALESHIN, MD
Clinical Associate Professor
Dermatology
Stanford Medicine
Redwood City, California

EMILY MICHELLE ALTMAN, MD
Associate Professor
Dermatology
University of New Mexico
Albuquerque, New Mexico

SANMEET ATWAL, BS, MD
Resident Physician
Dermatology
Keck School of Medicine of USC
Los Angeles, California

LIAT BAINVOLL, BS
Medical Student
Dermatology
Keck School of Medicine of USC
Los Angeles, California

MARIA C. BELL, MD
Dermatology Resident
Department of Dermatology
Indiana University School of Medicine
Indianapolis, Indiana

FRANKLIN R. BLUM, MD, BS
Resident Physician
Dermatology
University of North Carolina at Chapel Hill School of Medicine
Chapel Hill, North Carolina

AMBER Y. BO, BS, MD
Resident Physician
Anesthesiology
University of Michigan
Ann Arbor, Michigan

ROBERT BORUCKI, JR., MD
Resident Physician
Department of Dermatology
University of Nebraska Medical Center
Omaha, Nebraska

ALISON J. BRUCE, MB, CHB
Professor
Dermatology
Mayo Clinic Florida
Jacksonville, Florida

ANGEL S. BYRD, MD, PHD
Associate Professor
Department of Dermatology
Howard University College of Medicine
Washington, District of Columbia
Adjunct Assistant Professor
Department of Dermatology
Johns Hopkins University School of Medicine
Baltimore, Maryland

DAVID Y. CAO, MS
Medical Student
School of Medicine
Medical College of Wisconsin
Milwaukee, Wisconsin

ALEXANDRA PHILIPPA CHARROW, MD, MBE
Assistant Professor
Dermatology
Brigham and Women's Hospital
Quincy, Massachusetts

EVAN ALEXANDER CHOATE, MD
Dermatology Resident
Department of Dermatology
University of New Mexico School of Medicine
Albuquerque, New Mexico

ASHLEY B. CREW, MD
Clinical Professor of Dermatology
Dermatology
University of Southern California
Los Angeles, California

DAVID CROITORU, MD, MSC, FRCPC, FAAD
Associate Professor
Dermatology
University Health Network
Toronto, Canada
Clinical Associate
Wound Care
Women's College Hospital
Toronto, Canada

STEVEN DAVELUY, MD
Professor
Dermatology
Wayne State University
Detroit, Michigan

SAPANA DESAI, MD, MPH
Research Fellow
Department of Dermatology
George Washington University School of Medicine and Health Sciences
Washington, District of Columbia

GABRIELLE E. DUPRAT, MD
Assistant Professor
Dermatology
Dartmouth Health
Lebanon, New Hampshire

NADA ELBULUK, MD, MSC
Associate Professor
Director, Skin of Color and Pigmentary Disorders Program
Director, Diversity and Inclusion Program
Dermatology
University of Southern California
Los Angeles, California

MEGAN S. EVANS, MD
Assistant Professor
Dermatology
University of Arkansas for Medical Sciences
Little Rock, Arkansas

CRISTINA M. FOSCHI, MD
Resident Physician
Department of Dermatology
Medical College of Wisconsin
Milwaukee, Wisconsin

LINDY FOX, MD
Professor
Dermatology
UCSF
San Francisco, California

NATALIE M. FRAGOSO, MD
Assistant Professor
Department of Dermatology
Dartmouth Health
Lebanon, New Hampshire

ADAM J. FRIEDMAN, MD
Professor and Chair of Dermatology, Residency Program Director, Director of Translational Research
Department of Dermatology
George Washington School of Medicine and Health Sciences
Washington, District of Columbia

HANNAH Y. GANTZ, BS
Medical Student
Department of Dermatology
Wake Forest University School of Medicine
Winston-Salem, North Carolina

RAVEENA GHANSHANI, MS
Medical Student
Keck School of Medicine
University of Southern California
Los Angeles, California

NOAH GOLDFARB, MD
Associate Professor
Dermatology and Internal Medicine
University of Minnesota
Minneapolis, Minnesota
Staff Physician
Dermatology and Internal Medicine
Minneapolis VA Health Care System
Minneapolis, Minnesota

NATHANIEL GOLDMAN, MD
Research Fellow
Dermatology
Brigham and Women's Hospital
Boston, Massachusetts
Resident
Dermatology
Larkin Community Hospital
South Miami, Florida
Resident
Medicine
Lincoln Medical Center
Bronx, New York

SARAH GONZALEZ, BS
Dermatology Research Fellow
Department of Dermatology
Keck Medicine of USC
Los Angeles, California
Medical Student
Wayne State University School of Medicine
Detroit, Michigan

XOCHITL A. GREEN, BS
Medical Student
UC Davis School of Medicine, UC Davis
Sacramento, California

JANA S. GUENTHER, MD
Dermatology Resident
Department of Dermatology
University of Southern California
Los Angeles, California

AUDREY HAO, BS
Medical Student
Dermatology
University of Southern California
Los Angeles, California

JASON E. HAWKES, MD, MS
Associate Professor
Dermatology
University of California, Davis
Sacramento, California

MARCIA HOGELING, MD, FAAP, FAAD
Associate Professor
Division of Dermatology, Department of Medicine
University of California, Los Angeles
Los Angeles, California

JENNIFER L. HSIAO, MD
Associate Professor
Department of Dermatology
Keck School of Medicine
University of Southern California
Los Angeles, California

SYLVIA HSU, MD
Professor and Chair
Dermatology
Temple University Lewis Katz School of Medicine
Philadelphia, Pennsylvania

JENNY C. HU, MD, MPH
Clinical Professor
Dermatology
Keck School of Medicine of University of Southern California
Los Angeles, California

VICTOR HUANG, MD
Associate Professor
Dermatology
UC Davis Health
University of California
Davis, Sacramento
California

HENNA HUNDAL, MPP
Medical Student
School of Medicine
Stanford University
Stanford, California

AMEIJE ISMAILI, DO
Resident Physician
Dermatology
HCA Florida Largo Hospital
Largo, Florida

TERESA JU, MD
Doctor
Department of Dermatology
University of Miami
Miami, Florida

KANIKA KAMAL, BA
Medical Student
Department of Dermatology
Harvard Medical School
Boston, Massachusetts

JESSE J. KELLER, MD, MCR
Associate Professor
Department of Dermatology
Oregon Health & Science University
Portland, Oregon

CHRISTINA NICOLE KRAUS, MD
Assistant Professor
Dermatology
University of California, Irvine
Irvine, California

DANIELA KROSHINSKY, MD, MPH
Associate Professor of Dermatology
Dermatology
Harvard Medical School/MGH
Boston, Massachusetts

ANGELINA LABIB, MD
Doctor
Department of Dermatology
University of Miami
Miami, Florida

KATRINA H. LEE, MD
Clinical Assistant Professor
Department of Dermatology
USC Keck School of Medicine
Los Angeles, California

BRANDON ANDREW LEVIAN, BA, MD CANDIDATE
Medical Student
Dermatology
USC Keck School of Medicine
Los Angeles, California

WILLIAM LEWIS, MD
Resident Physician
Department of Dermatology
University of Pennsylvania
Philadelphia, Pennsylvania

HENRY W. LIM, MD
Former Chair
Dermatology
Henry Ford Health
Detroit, Michigan

PETER A. LIO, MD
Assistant Clinical Professor
Dermatology & Pediatrics
Northwestern University Feinberg School of Medicine
Chicago, Illinois
Founding Partner
Medical Dermatology Associates of Chicago
Chicago, Illinois

CHAOCHENG LIU, MD
Dermatology Resident
Department of Dermatology and Skin Science
University of British Columbia
Vancouver, Canada

SARAH LONOWSKI, MD, MBA
Assistant Professor of Dermatology
Dermatology
University of Nebraska
Omaha, Nebraska

KAREN M. LY, MD
Resident Physician
Department of Dermatology
Dartmouth-Hitchcock Medical Center
Lebanon, New Hampshire

SOPHIA LY, BA
Medical Student
Department of Dermatology
University of Arkansas for Medical Sciences College of Medicine
Little Rock, Arkansas

ELAINE J. MA, BA
Medical Student
Dermatology
USC Keck School of Medicine
Los Angeles, California

SHAE MARGULIES, MD
Medical Resident
Department of Internal Medicine
University of Florida College of Medicine
Gainesville, Florida

RAHUL MASSON, MD
Dermatology Resident
Keck School of Medicine of USC
University of Southern California
Los Angeles, California

TIFFANY MAYO, MS, MD
Associate Professor
Dermatology
The University of Alabama at Birmingham
Birmingham, Alabama

ERIKA T. MCCORMICK, BS
Research Fellow, MD Candidate
Department of Dermatology
George Washington University School of Medicine and Health Sciences
Washington, District of Columbia

AMY MCMICHAEL, MD
Professor
Dermatology
Wake Forest University School of Medicine
Winston-Salem, North Carolina

ROBERT G. MICHELETTI, MD
Associate Professor
Dermatology and Medicine
University of Pennsylvania
Philadelphia, Pennsylvania

KIRAN MOTAPARTHI, MD
Clinical Professor
Department of Dermatology
University of Florida College of Medicine
Gainesville, Florida

MOHAMMED MOUMEN, MD
Resident
Department of Dermatology
MedStar Health—Georgetown University
Washington, District of Columbia

NIKHIL NAIR, BA
Medical Student
College of Medicine
University of Arkansas for Medical Sciences
Little Rock, Arkansas

EDITA M. NEWTON, MD, PHD
Assistant Professor
Dermatology
Indiana University
Indianapolis, Indiana

THOMAS E. NORMAN, MD
Dermatology Resident
Department of Dermatology
Henry Ford
Detroit, MI

DANIELLE E. NOVACK, BA
Medical Student
Icahn School of Medicine at Mount Sinai
New York, New York

MARGARET A. O'BRIEN, MD
Resident Physician
Department of Dermatology
Temple University Hospital
Philadelphia, Pennsylvania

CHIDUBEM A.V. OKEKE, MD
Research Fellow
Department of Dermatology
Howard University College of Medicine
Washington, District of Columbia

ALEX G. ORTEGA-LOAYZA, MD, MCR
Associate Professor
Department of Dermatology
Oregon Health & Science University
Portland, Oregon

KATHERINE ELIZABETH PARK, MD
Resident
Department of Dermatology
University of New Mexico
Albuquerque, New Mexico

SARAH E. PARK, BA
Medical Student
David Geffen School of Medicine
UCLA
Los Angeles, California

NEHA PARVATHALA, BS
Medical Student
Dermatology
Keck Hospital of USC
Los Angeles, California

MCKAYLA J. POPPENS, MD
Resident Physician
David Geffen School of Medicine
University of California Los Angeles
Los Angeles, California

MARTINA PORTER, MD
Vice Chair of Research
Dermatology
Beth Israel Deaconess Medical Center
Boston, Massachusetts

SMRITI PRASAD, MD, MPH
Resident
Dermatology
OHSU
Portland, Oregon

CLAUDIA QUARSHIE, MD, MPH
Dermatology Resident
Department of Dermatology
University of Miami Miller School of Medicine
Miami, FL

MEGANA RAO, BS
Medical Student
Dermatology
Indiana University School of Medicine
Indianapolis, Indiana

MADISON H. READ, BS
Medical Student
Wake Forest University School of Medicine
Winston-Salem, North Carolina

JONATHAN RICK, MD
Assistant Clinical Professor
Dermatology
University of California, Davis
Sacramento, California

CALLIE M. ROBERTS, MS BIOMEDICAL, BS BIOLOGY
MD Candidate
Dermatology
UC Davis School of Medicine
Sacramento, California

NATHAN ROJEK, MD
Associate Professor
Department of Dermatology
University of California, Irvine
Irvine, California

KATELYN J. RYPKA, MD
Clinical Research Fellow
Department of Dermatology
University of Minnesota
Minneapolis, Minnesota

RACHEL L. SADOWSKY, MD
Resident Physician
Dermatology
Rush University Medical Center
Chicago, Illinois

LINA SAEED, MD
Resident Physician
Dermatology
UC Irvine
Irvine, California

ISABELLA INEZ SANCHEZ, PHD
Medical Student
School of Medicine
University of California, Irvine
Irvine, California

KATHYANA PAOLA SANTIAGO MANGUAL, BA
Medical Student
David Geffen School of Medicine
University of California, Los Angeles
Los Angeles, California

REBECCA SARAC, MD, FAAD
Physician
Dermatology
University Hospitals
Cleveland, Connecticut
Dermatologist
Schweiger Dermatology
Stamford, Connecticut

CHRISTOPHER SAYED, MD
Professor
Dermatology
UNC Department of Dermatology
Chapel Hil, North Carolina

JANYLA A. SELTZER, MD
Resident Physician
Dermatology
Howard University Hospital
Washington, District of Columbia

NEDA SHAHRIARI, MD
Associate Physician
Dermatology
Brigham and Women's Hospital, Harvard Medical School
Boston, Massachusetts

TIMMIE R. SHARMA, MD
Assistant Professor
Department of Dermatology
University Hospitals Cleveland Medical Center
Cleveland, Ohio

NAYHA SHETTY, MD
Resident Physician
Department of Dermatology
Henry Ford Health
Detroit, Michigan

CATHRYN SIBBALD, MD, MSC, FRCPC FAAD
Assistant Professor
Dermatology
University of Toronto
Toronto, Ontario
Canada
Staff Physician
Dermatology
Unity Health
Toronto, Ontario
Canada
Staff Physician
Dermatology
The Hospital for Sick Children
Toronto, Ontario
Canada

JAN M. SMOGORZEWSKI, MD
Chief of Dermatology
Los Angeles General Medical Center
Los Angeles, California
Associate Program Director
Harbor-UCLA Dermatology
Torrance, California

COREY L. SNYDER, MD
Research Fellow
Dermatology
Beth Israel Deaconess Medical Center
Boston, Massachusetts

OLAYEMI SOKUMBI, MD
Associate Professor
Department of Dermatology
Department of Laboratory Medicine & Pathology
Mayo Clinic
Jacksonville, Florida

SAMUEL A. STETKEVICH, MD
Resident Physician
Department of Medicine
UCLA- Olive View Medical Center
Sylmar, California

LINDSAY C. STROWD, MD
Professor
Dermatology
Wake Forest University School of Medicine
Winston Salem, North Carolina

ALICE J. TAN, BS
Medical Student
Dermatology
Massachusetts General Hospital
Boston, Massachusetts

MILAD TORABI, MD
Medical Student
Department of Dermatology
Stanford University School of Medicine
Palo Alto, California

ASHLEY VANDER DOES, MD
Resident Physician
Department of Dermatology
University of Colorado School of Medicine
Aurora, CO

NATALIA VECEREK, MD
Clinical Assistant Professor
Department of Dermatology
Keck School of Medicine of USC
Los Angeles, California

RUTH ANN VLEUGELS, MD, MPH, MBA
Professor of Dermatology
Dermatology
Brigham and Women's Hospital
Boston, Massachusetts
Heidi and Scott C. Schuster Distinguished Chair, Dermatology
Dermatology
Brigham and Women's Hospital
Boston, Massachusetts
Vice-Chair of Academic Affairs
Dermatology
Brigham and Women's Hospital
Boston, Massachusetts
Autoimmune Skin Disease Program Director
Dermatology
Brigham and Women's Hospital
Boston, Massachusetts

KAROLYN A. WANAT, MD
Professor
Dermatology and Pathology
Medical College of Wisconsin
Milwaukee, Wisconsin

KATHERINE L. WANG, BS
Medical Student
Mayo Clinic Alix School of Medicine
Mayo Clinic
Jacksonville, Florida

ZACHARY D. WENDLAND, MD, MPH
Dermatology Research Fellow
Department of Dermatology
University of Minnesota
Minneapolis, Minnesota
Dermatology Research Fellow
Department of Dermatology
Minneapolis VA Medical Center
Minneapolis, Minnesota

LINNEA WESTERKAM, MD
Resident
School of Medicine
University of North Carolina
Chapel Hill, North Carolina

KIRK WILLIAMS, II, MEDICAL DOCTOR
Physican
Alumni
Wayne State School Medicine
Detroit, Michigan

MAKANA D. WILLIAMS, MD
Resident Physician
Division of Dermatology, Department of Medicine
University of California
Los Angeles, California

HENRY K. WONG, MD, PHD
Professor
Dermatology
University of Arkansas for Medical Sciences
Little Rock, Arkansas
Staff Dermatologist
Dermatology Service
San Diego Veterans Heatth System
San Diego, California

SCOTT D. WORSWICK, MD
Clinical Professor
Department of Dermatology
Keck School of Medicine
University of Southern California
Los Angeles, California

JOYCE XIA, MD
Research Fellow
Dermatology
Massachusetts General Hospital
Boston, Massachusetts

CHEN YAO, MD
Clinical Fellow
Dermatology
University of California, San Francisco
San Francisco, California

GIL YOSIPOVITCH, MD
Professor and Stiefel Chair of Medical Dermatology and Director of Miami Itch Center
Dr. Phillip Frost Department of Dermatology and Cutaneous Surgery
Miller School of Medicine University of Miami
Miami, Florida

SUHA ZAWAWI, MD
Resident Physician
Internal Medicine
UHS
Las Vegas, Nevada

AMINA ZIAD, BA
Research Fellow
Department of Dermatology
Brigham and Women's Hospital
Boston, Massachusetts
Medical Student
Harvard Medical School
Boston, Massachusetts

Acknowledgments

The editors would like to thank all of the contributors to this immense undertaking in designing, refining, and generously sharing their expert clinical decision-making algorithms. We hope that this textbook serves as a helpful guide for all clinicians who care for patients with dermatologic conditions.

JENNIFER L. HSIAO, VIVIAN Y. SHI, SCOTT D. WORSWICK

Contents

PART I
Erythema Without Scale

1 Facial Erythema

Nathaniel Goldman and Sarah Lonowski

Facial erythema is a common presenting symptom for patients seeking dermatologic care. Facial erythema may be due to a primary skin condition, may occur as a reaction to an internal or external stimulus, or may represent a cutaneous manifestation of an underlying systemic disease.

Initial evaluation should include a detailed history and full skin examination, including the examination of nonfacial skin. It is important to assess whether the facial erythema is constant or intermittent and whether there are associated symptoms, such as burning, itching, or pain. The provider should also ask about potential triggers and obtain a list of current and recent medications. When suspected, a targeted review of systems can also be useful in revealing an underlying rheumatologic disease.

On physical examination, it is important to note the distribution of the erythema and whether part of or all of the face is involved. Other features to assess include the presence of edema, associated papules, pustules or scaling, and the sparing or involvement of certain parts of the face (i.e. nasolabial fold, central face). Close examination of nearby structures (i.e. eyes, eyelids, scalp) can also provide useful diagnostic clues.

A. **Rosacea** is a chronic inflammatory skin condition that is a common cause of facial erythema. Rosacea exists in four subtypes: (1) erythematotelangiectatic, (2) papulopustular, (3) phymatous, and (4) ocular. Patients often experience a relapsing-remitting course and often report flaring with certain triggers, such as heat, alcohol, and spicy foods. This condition classically presents with inflammatory papules and pustules overlying persistent central facial erythema and telangiectasias. Patients may also report transient facial flushing without papules or pustules.

B. **Acne vulgaris** can present as facial erythema, particularly when inflammatory papules, pustules, and nodules are present. In contrast to rosacea, acne is characterized by the presence of comedones and will generally not result in diffuse midfacial erythema or telangiectasias.

C. **Perioral/periorificial dermatitis** is likely to cause erythema localized around the mouth and nose. Lesions will appear acneiform or eczematous with potential scaling and characteristically spare the vermillion border. Patients with this condition may also report focal stinging or burning.

D. In patients presenting with chronic erythema and greasy scaling overlying hair-covered (seborrheic) regions of the face, clinicians should suspect a diagnosis of **seborrheic dermatitis**. This condition is most likely to affect the scalp, face, eyebrows, and nasolabial folds.

E. Contact dermatitis can present anywhere on the body and occurs when a patient is exposed to an exogenous trigger, causing either a direct toxic effect (**irritant contact dermatitis**) or an immunologic inflammatory reaction (**allergic contact dermatitis**). Patients are likely to experience burning when irritant in nature and pruritis when allergic. Examination reveals erythematous papules or plaques with sharp, often geometric demarcation. Intrinsic atopic dermatitis can also affect the face.

F. Patients taking systemic or topical medications reporting a photosensitive, erythematous facial rash may have a **phototoxic** or **photoallergic drug eruption**. Various drugs have been implicated, although tetracyclines, antihypertensives, and nonsteroidal anti-inflammatory drugs are common triggers. Patients will often display a sunburn-like rash on the face and other photosensitive areas, which may become pruritic or blister. Temporal relationship with an offending medication is key to a diagnosis.

G. **Cellulitis** and **erysipelas** are bacterial infections that can affect adults and children, causing an erythematous, warm facial plaque (and if erysipelas, typically with well-defined borders). Fever and other systemic symptoms may be present.

H. **Flushing** is a transient cause of facial erythema due to cutaneous vasodilation, leading to a feeling of warmth and heat. Causes range from benign/physiological (i.e. emotional distress, menopause) to systemic/pathological (i.e. neuroendocrine tumors). Flushing can also be secondary to external triggers, such as alcohol or food. Patients may report associated symptoms of autonomic hyperactivation, including sweating and gastrointestinal discomfort.

I. **Acute cutaneous lupus erythematosus (ACLE)** and **dermatomyositis (DM)** are rare, systemic autoimmune diseases that frequently present with facial erythema. ACLE occurs in patients with systemic lupus erythematosus and classically presents as a malar "butterfly" rash on the cheeks and central face, which spares the nasolabial folds. Symptoms will often be transient and brought on by sun exposure. Patients may also report erythema in other photosensitive areas, including the hands, arms, and chest. Facial erythema in DM is also midfacial but will also involve the nasolabial folds, which can help to differentiate it from ACLE. Patients with DM may also have papules on the dorsal hands/knuckles (Gottron papules), an erythematous to violaceous rash on the upper eyelids (heliotrope rash), or a poikilodermatous rash on the upper trunk (shawl sign) or lateral thighs (holster sign).

J. **Drug reaction with eosinophilia and systemic symptoms (DRESS)** syndrome is a potentially life-threatening hypersensitivity reaction that classically occurs 2 to 6 weeks after drug initiation. Anticonvulsants are commonly implicated, although many other medications may also cause this condition. The rash is typically morbilliform, and patients will often develop fever and facial edema with the risk of end organ involvement and autoimmune sequelae.

See Appendix 1 for Further Reading and Image References.

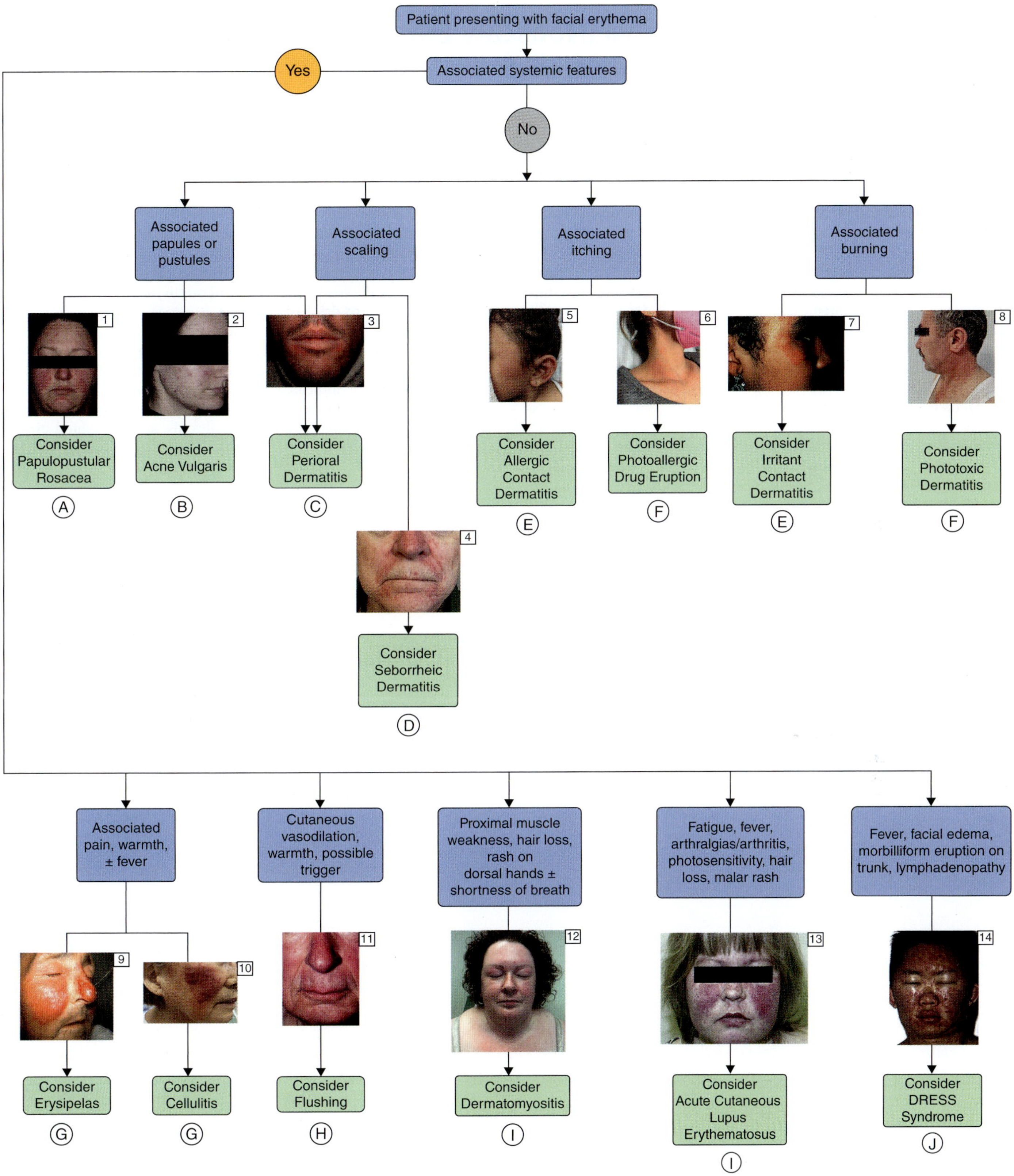
Patient presenting with facial erythema
Associated systemic features
Yes
No
Associated papules or pustules
Associated scaling
Associated itching
Associated burning
1
2
3
4
5
6
7
8
Consider Papulopustular Rosacea
A
Consider Acne Vulgaris
B
Consider Perioral Dermatitis
C
Consider Seborrheic Dermatitis
D
Consider Allergic Contact Dermatitis
E
Consider Photoallergic Drug Eruption
F
Consider Irritant Contact Dermatitis
E
Consider Phototoxic Dermatitis
F
Associated pain, warmth, ± fever
Cutaneous vasodilation, warmth, possible trigger
Proximal muscle weakness, hair loss, rash on dorsal hands ± shortness of breath
Fatigue, fever, arthralgias/arthritis, photosensitivity, hair loss, malar rash
Fever, facial edema, morbilliform eruption on trunk, lymphadenopathy
9
10
11
12
13
14
Consider Erysipelas
G
Consider Cellulitis
G
Consider Flushing
H
Consider Dermatomyositis
I
Consider Acute Cutaneous Lupus Erythematosus
I
Consider DRESS Syndrome
J

2 Red Scrotum/Vulva (Nonscaly Entities)

Alexandra Philippa Charrow and Kanika Kamal

A red scrotum/vulva is a common, often distressing condition for patients. Genital dermatoses may be difficult to identify by both the patient and dermatologist because of the limitations of self-examination and the diverse skin textures and colors considered normal for this area. A thorough history and physical examination can help differentiate the various etiologies of a red scrotum/vulva.

A. The initial evaluation of a patient presenting with a red scrotum/vulva includes inquiring about onset, duration, and associated symptoms and gathering a medical history (history of dermatosis, medication and personal product history, and sexual history). Inspect and palpate the skin as well as the lymph nodes and mucosal surfaces. The patient may benefit from further workup with bacterial, fungal, or viral swabs and cultures, urine tests, and skin biopsies per clinical judgement.

B. Nonscaling causes of a red scrotum/vulva can first be divided into two broad categories: vesiculobullous/ulcerative versus nonulcerative. We will first explore the vesiculobullous/ulcerative causes of red scrotum/vulva. If the patient presents with acute onset of grouped vesicles on an erythematous base with punched out ulcers, inguinal lymphadenopathy, and/or a prodrome of fever or malaise, consider ***Herpesviridae*** **infection** (herpes simplex virus I, II, varicella zoster virus). If the patient presents with chronic, waxing and waning vesicles and bullae that ulcerate in intertriginous areas, particularly if there is a family history of similar lesions, consider **Hailey-Hailey disease**. Finally, if a child presents with nonpruritic vesicles in skin folds with a history of multisystem involvement, consider **Langerhans cell histiocytosis**.

Pyoderma gangrenosum may present as a vulvar/scrotal ulceration with a violaceous and undermined border. In decompensating, immunocompromised patients, an ulcer with a central black necrotic eschar may indicate **ecthyma gangrenosum**. Finally, consider **Crohn's disease** in patients with genital swelling, linear ulcers symmetrically distributed in the inguinal folds, and associated diarrhea and abdominal pain.

Patient presenting with red, nonscaling scrotum/vulva

↓

Obtain detailed history and physical examination of the skin, nails, lymph nodes, and mucosa to differentiate underlying etiology

(A) → Management generally involves treating underlying etiology (infectious vs. inflammatory vs. iatrogenic vs. neoplastic) with oral anti-infectives (fungal, bacterial, viral) or topical steroids applied to the scrotum/vulva

↓

Predominant morphology

(B) → Nonulcerative/nonbullous → *continued on next page*

→ Ulcerative/Vesiculobullous

- **Vesiculobullous**
  - Begins as small, flaccid vesicles to bullae that rupture, leaving moist ulceration in intertriginous areas. Serpiginous plaques may form. Family history of similar lesions; chronic, but waxes and wanes. Heat, humidity, ultraviolet exposure exacerbate disease.

    16 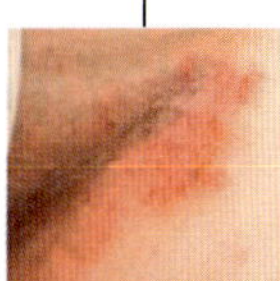

    → Consider Hailey-Hailey Disease
  - Grouped vesicles, punched out ulcers, crusting on an erythematous base. Dermatomal distribution. Prodrome of fever, malaise, lymphadenopathy; recent sexual contact with an infected individual, stress, immunosuppressed.

    17 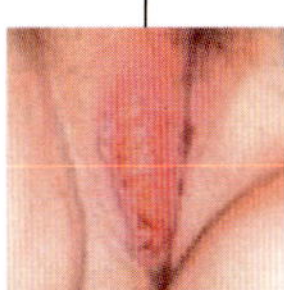

    → Consider Herpesviridae (HSV I, II, VZV)
  - Painful, nonpruritic vesicles or nodules that may ulcerate, weep, and develop hemorrhagic crust. Often in skin folds. Typically white male child age 1-4, but can present in adulthood. History of multiple infections, lymphadenopathy, Possible multi-system (i.e. gastrointestinal, lung, central nervous system) involvement, failure to thrive.

    18 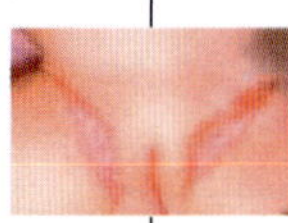

    → Consider Langerhans Cell Histiocytosis
- **Ulcerative**
  - Begins as extremely painful deep-seated nodule that forms a deep ulcer with violaceous and undermined border. Purulent coating may form over center of ulcer. May have foul odor or become infected. Often in middle-aged adult. Can be acute or chronic. 50% associated with systemic disease (inflammatory bowel disease, hematogenous disorders, autoimmune disorders). Self-limited condition.

    19 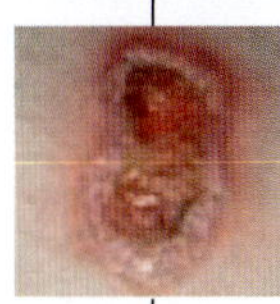

    → Consider Pyoderma Gangrenosum
  - Initially painless erythematous macule that becomes a painful bulla in 12-24 hours. Evolves into an ulcer with central black necrotic eschar. Immunocompromised patients predominantly infected with *pseudomonas aeruginosa*. May have osteomyelitis, shock, disseminated intravascular coagulation or Gram-negative sepsis. Life-threatening condition.

    20 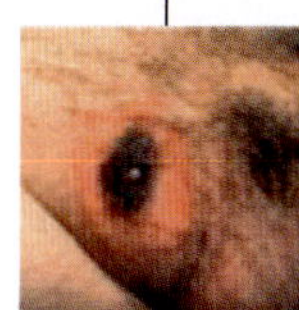

    → Consider Ecthyma Gangrenosum
  - Aphthous/"knife cut" ulcers (linear in folds) with a symmetrically swollen, red, labia majora. May have fistulas/sinuses. More common in females of Ashkenazi Jewish or Northern European descent. Patient often presents with abdominal pain, diarrhea, weight loss, malnutrition, fistulas, abscesses (often perianal), and other extraintestinal manifestations.

    21 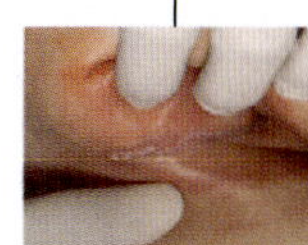

    → Consider Crohn's Disease

Continued

C. The majority of groin rashes are nonulcerative/nonbullous. For the rest of this chapter, we will discuss the nonulcerative/nonbullous causes of red scrotum/vulva. Morphological differences (i.e., papules vs. nodules vs. plaques) can help further elucidate diagnosis.

D. If a patient presents with a red vulva (specifically, red labia) and painful nodules or abscesses, especially with extensive scars or draining tunnels, consider **hidradenitis suppurativa**.

E. Papular causes of red scrotum/vulva include scabies and candidiasis. The **scabies** rash presents as extremely pruritic papules and burrows with terminal black specks (the mites). Patients on long-term antibiotics/steroids or oral contraceptive pills presenting with shiny, erythematous, discrete patches or plaques and satellite papules may have **Candida intertrigo/vulvovaginal candidiasis**.

F. To differentiate the numerous etiologies of red plaques on the scrotum/vulva, consider inquiring about dermatologic history, personal care products, and recent medication exposures. Consider **lichen planus** in a patient who presents with pruritic, flat-topped polygonal plaques with lacy white striae.

In patients with a history of psoriasis and a new red scrotum/vulva (most often, a red labia majora) with a well-demarcated, smooth, moist pink plaque, consider **inverse psoriasis**. Finally, patients may present with vulvar redness, sclerosis of the vaginal introitus, and papules/plaques or masses contributing to obliteration of vulvar anatomy and involving the perianal skin. A biopsy is necessary to differentiate between **intraepithelial neoplasia** and [G] **vulvar cancer**.

H. The majority of nonulcerative groin rashes present as erythematous patches. The presence of geometric shapes, additional color, or systemic symptoms can help further narrow the diagnosis.

I. In patients with systemic symptoms, consider **testicular torsion** when a red scrotum is preceded by recent trauma, intense exercise, or an absent cremasteric reflex, but there are no urinary symptoms. Consider **epididymo-orchitis** with the above symptoms plus dysuria, dysorgasmia, and a history of high-risk sexual behavior or recent genitourinary tract instrumentation. Rapid onset (<5 days) of fever, accompanied by erythema, pain, and genital swelling in a patient with recent barrier disruption, Methicillin-resistant Staphylococcus aureus (MRSA) history, or immunocompromised status, may indicate **cellulitis/necrotizing fasciitis**. Children presenting with more than 5 days of fever, cervical lymphadenopathy (>1.5 cm), conjunctival injection without exudate, strawberry tongue, and a viral exanthem may indicate **Kawasaki disease**.

J. Some patients may present with geometric lesions overlying erythematous patches due to scratching. In patients with eczematous and lichenified labia majora/scrotum, **allergic contact dermatitis** must be ruled out along with a careful review of personal care products. Leathery thickened skin, especially in older patients, should prompt consideration of **lichen simplex chronicus**.

K. For patients with erythematous patches and additional colors, **lichen sclerosus** may range from flat white patches to atrophied, porcelain lesions. Patients taking new medications (e.g., sulfonamides, tetracyclines) or Nonsteroidal Anti-Inflammatory Drugs presenting with well-demarcated violaceous genital plaques or erythematous circular patches may have **fixed drug eruption**. These plaques often recur in the same spot with each drug reexposure.

L. Finally, consider **red scrotum syndrome** in older males with burning scrotal pain in the absence of swelling, atrophy, and telangiectasias. This presentation often occurs secondary to abrupt cessation of topical steroid after long term use (>27 months).

See Appendix 1 for Further Reading and Image References.

Patient presenting with red, nonscaling scrotum/vulva

→ Obtain detailed history and physical examination of the skin, nails, lymph nodes, and mucosa to differentiate underlying etiology (A)

→ Management generally involves treating underlying etiology (infectious vs. inflammatory vs. iatrogenic vs. neoplastic) with appropriate therapy such as oral anti-infectives (fungal, bacterial, viral) or topical steroids applied to the scrotum/vulva

→ Predominant morphology (B)

- Ulcerative/vesiculobullous continued on previous page
- Non-ulcerative/Non-bullous (C)

Nodules (D)

Firm, tender, erythematous to dark brown nodules, abscesses, scar, and tunnels. Associated with obesity, cigarette smoking, inflammatory bowel disease (IBD).

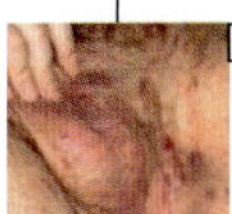

1

→ Consider Hidradenitis Suppurativa

Papules (E)

Erythematous papular rash that can crust or form sores; burrow (fine, threadlike line) often seen. Direct contact with infested fomites. Common among kids, sexually active adults, immuno-suppressed, those in long-term care facilities.

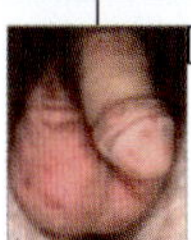

2

→ Consider Scabies

Moist, shiny, erythematous, discrete patches or plaques and satellite papules with overlying soft, caseous crust. Immuno-compromised (diabetes, HIV, autoimmune disease, chemotherapy) patients, recent antibiotic, steroid, OCP, immuno-suppressant use.

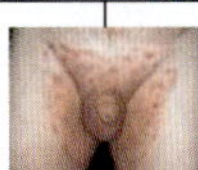

3

→ Consider Candida/ Intertrigo

Plaques (F)

Pruritic, flat-topped purple polygonal plaques evolve to diffuse ulceration of vulva/ vaginal canal +/- lacy Wickham striae. Adults 40-60; exhibits Koebner phenomenon; pruritus, dyspareunia.

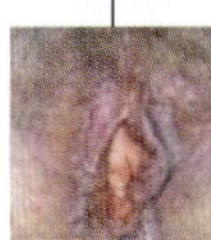

4

→ Consider Lichen Planus

Smooth, moist, macerated pink irregular plaque with sharply demarcated edge. Lacks silver scale. Affects up to 30% patients with plaque psoriasis. Pruritic, irritated, may have secondary infection. Exacerbated by friction.

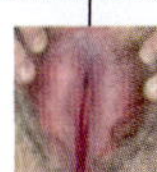

5

→ Consider Inverse Psoriasis

May see plaques on non-hair bearing parts of vulva/scrotum that change color from red to white. Premalignant condition progressed from lichen sclerosus. Patients in their 50s, associated with HPV infection, tobacco, immuno-suppression.

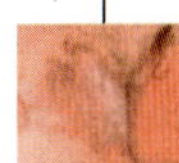

6

→ Consider Vulvar/Penile Intraepithelial Neoplasia

Masses (G)

Hyperkeratotic firm mass with colors including red, pink, and skin colored. May scale, crust, erode. Preceded by lichen sclerosus or VIN. Associated with HPV, prior melanoma, Paget, or immuno-compromised state.

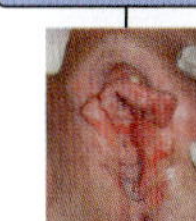

7

→ Consider Vulvar Cancer

Predominantly erythematous patches (H)

With systemic symptoms (I)

Scrotal edema, tenderness, uniform erythema in patients with recent instrumentation of GU tracts or those who are at high risk of STIs (new sexual partners, high risk behavior). Associated with inflammation from bacterial infection (chlamydia/ gonorrhea in young patients) or *E. coli* from UTI or prostatic infection in older patients.

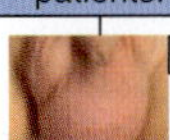

8

→ Consider Epididymo-orchitis

Diffuse blanching erythema with desquamation in groin (in week 2 of illness) with lymphadenopathy (LAD) and/or joint involvement. Fever >5 days, conjunctival injection without exudate, strawberry tongue, extremity edema, viral exanthem, cervical LAD >1.5 cm.

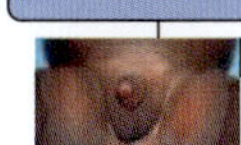

9

→ Consider Kawasaki Disease

Poorly defined border, erythema, swelling, warmth. May form vesicles, bullae, pustules, or necrosis with red streaking (lymphangitis) or LAD. Risks: barrier disruption, prior cellulitis, MRSA risk factor. Direct bacterial seeding in immune-competent patients; hematogenous spread in immuno-compromised patients.

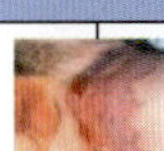

10

→ Consider Cellulitis/ Necrotizing Fasciitis

Unilateral erythematous/ darkened swollen scrotum with raised testicle and absent cremasteric reflex. Typically patients <20 years old. Rapid-onset pain, dysuria, fever. Preceded by minor trauma or intense physical activity. Can spontaneously resolve and may recur.

→ Consider Testicular Torsion

With geometric shapes/ linear lesions (J)

Isolated pruritic patch on scrotum, not base of penis. Leathery, thickened, with lichenified skin. Chronic disorder affecting older patients. Associated with itching often due to unknown cause, or atopic dermatitis. Pruritus may be localized or generalized.

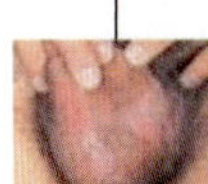

11

→ Consider Lichen Simplex Chronicus/ Friction or Rubbing

Erythema with round erosions or crusts. May present with lichenification or fissures if chronic. 24-48 hr delayed reaction to topical, ingested, implanted, or airborne agent. Requires repeated exposure. Review personal care products (e.g., menstrual products).

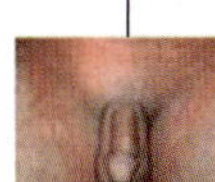

12

→ Consider Allergic Contact Dermatitis

With additional color (white, purple) (K)

Flat, white patches with red, purple, violet borders. Sclerosis, atrophy, loss of normal vulva architecture. Prepubertal and postmenopausal females. Associated with autoimmune disease. Dry, tender, severely pruritic.

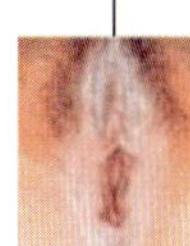

13

→ Consider Lichen Sclerosus

One or more well-demarcated erythematous or violaceous round plaques. Recurs in same area. Recent exposure to antibiotics (e.g., sulfa, tetracyclines) or NSAIDs. Usually asymptomatic, may be pruritic.

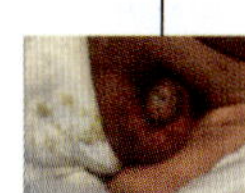

14

→ Consider Fixed Drug Eruption

Other (L)

Well-demarcated bright red erythema on anterior scrotum/vulva. Atrophy and telangiectasias may be present along with localized erythromelalgia. Common in white males 50+. Rebound vasodilation after long-term (~27 months) topical steroid use. Neurogenic inflammation.

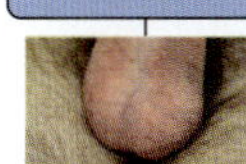

15

→ Consider Red Scrotum/Vulva Syndrome

3 Intertriginous Erythema

David Y. Cao and Karolyn A. Wanat

Intertriginous erythema is a superficial skin eruption localized to skin folds and flexures that contact each other at rest or experience frictional rubbing, including the axillae, inframammary skin, groin, abdominal folds, and gluteal cleft. There are a variety of morphologies that can be present in these areas. Many diseases can present with intertriginous erythema, although the majority of causes of this pattern fall into the inflammatory and infectious categories.

Intertriginous erythema that presents predominantly without scale will be discussed in this chapter. Intertriginous erythema with scale has an additional set of potential differential diagnoses and is discussed in other chapters.

Due to the diversity of morphological presentations, a comprehensive patient history should include the onset, duration, and clinical course of the erythema; current medications and response to prior therapies; comorbidities; and family history. Any concomitant physical findings of nails and nonintertriginous skin should also be noted.

A. **Symmetrical drug-related intertriginous and flexural exanthema (SDRIFE)** appears as sharply demarcated symmetrical erythema in the inguinal/genital or gluteal/perianal region following exposure to systemic drugs, most commonly β-lactam antibiotics (amoxicillin) or antimicrobial drugs (clindamycin or erythromycin). It resolves after discontinuing the systemic medication. In SDRIFE, systemic symptoms are absent.

B. **Toxic erythema of chemotherapy** affects patients receiving chemotherapy drugs (doxorubicin, cytarabine, etc.) with symmetric, deep red, painful erythema primarily of the hands and feet, although it can extend to intertriginous sites on the body (resembling SDRIFE). Symptoms usually resolve within a few days to weeks of chemotherapy discontinuation.

C. **Acute generalized exanthematous pustulosis** presents as an acute erythema, often first in the axillae and/or groin, that quickly becomes studded with numerous nonfollicular pustules. Fever is often present, and antimicrobial drugs are a common cause.

D. **Dermatitis (contact or atopic)** can appear in intertriginous areas (e.g., the axilla, gluteal fold, or groin). Contact dermatitis is an irritant-dependent erythema with geometric or linear shapes and patterns present, with possible edema, bullae, or vesicles. Atopic dermatitis (eczema) is most commonly found in flexural areas (neck, wrists and ankles, antecubital and popliteal fossae, etc.) as intensely pruritic erythematous papules and vesicles.

E. **Hailey-Hailey disease**, also known as benign familial pemphigus, is present during childhood or after puberty with deep red, macerated, painful intraepidermal blisters and erosions. Lesions may appear in many intertriginous areas and even extend beyond the axillae, groin, and inframammary creases.

F. **Langerhans cell histiocytosis** rarely occurs in adults and presents with red-orange plaques and erosions in the groin and other intertriginous areas. These intertriginous areas can also be associated with yellow-brown or red-orange plaques and erosions all over the body, along with multisystem diseases (lytic bone lesions, endocrinopathies, etc.).

G. **Intertrigo** (irritant dermatitis) can occur at any age (particularly in people with obesity, diabetes, or who are immunocompromised); rash occurs within skin folds due to a combination of friction and moisture. Intertrigo is a broad term that encompasses noninfectious and infectious etiologies. **Candida intertrigo** (commonly caused by *Candida albicans*) appears with delicate satellite pustules surrounding deep red plaques, which can evolve into superficial erosions.

H. **Granular parakeratosis** appears in females (and sometimes in males and children) as pruritic, pink-brown hyperkeratotic papules that most commonly present in the axillae but may appear in inframammary folds or inguinal and genital creases. Papules can coalesce to form plaques with satellite papules.

I. **Intertrigo secondary to bacteria** (such as *beta-hemolytic streptococcus*) presents as areas of bright red erythema. A bacterial culture can confirm the diagnosis of streptococcal intertrigo. Erythrasma due to *Corynebacterium spp*. infection can present as pink plaques with coral-red fluorescence under Wood's lamp.

J. **Unilateral laterothoracic exanthem (ULE)** is most common in young children, although it has been occasionally reported in adults with recent viral infection. ULE presents as unilateral, morbilliform pruritic exanthema near the groin or one axilla and may progress to the other axilla.

K. **Inverse psoriasis** should be considered in patients with well-demarcated erythematous patches in the axillae, groin, and inframammary creases that can be macerated. These patients often have a family history of psoriasis or other classic concomitant features of psoriasis (nail abnormalities, silvery-scaled erythematous plaques elsewhere).

L. **Extramammary Paget disease** is typically present in elderly adults with pruritic red plaques with pale dots on dermoscopy on genital, perianal, or perineal skin. There can also be crusting, erosions, lichenification, or verrucae on those skin areas.

M. **Noninfectious intertrigo** secondary to irritation and chronic friction should be considered in patients who are less mobile (infants or debilitated adults) or obese, presenting with moist, dull red to red-brown pruritic patches. Diagnosis of noninfectious intertrigo is made based on the distribution of lesions during physical examination since culture and KOH skin preparation would be negative.

See Appendix 1 for Further Reading and Image References.

Patient presenting with erythematous patches or plaques WITHOUT SCALE

→ Detailed history and physical exam of skin and nails

→ Does the history reveal the patient developed skin changes following exposure to a new medication?

Yes →

- Symmetrical erythema following exposure to systemic drugs

  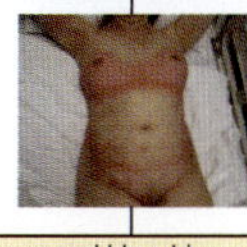
  1

  Erythema and blanching papules coalescing into plaques with vesicles on the abdomen, bilateral inframammary, and inguinal folds

  (A) Consider Symmetrical Drug-Related Intertriginous and Flexural Exanthema (SDRIFE)

- Deep red, painful erythema primarily on the hands and feet, extending to intertriginous areas

  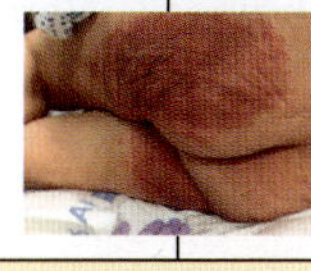
  2

  Marked eruption involving intertriginous areas of the gluteal and inner thigh folds with erythema and erosions

  (B) Consider Toxic Erythema of Chemotherapy (TEC)

- Febrile patient with acute eruption of nonfollicular pustules

  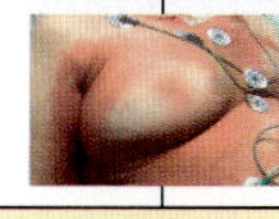
  3

  Widespread erythematous eruption favoring intertriginous areas with sheets of nonfollicular pustules

  (C) Consider Acute Generalized Exanthematous Pustulosis (AGEP)

No → Are there erosions or vesicles/bullae present on exam?

Yes →

- Erythema dependent on irritants (with patterns or shapes) or allergens (pruritic vesicles and papules)

  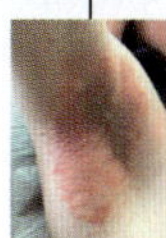
  4

  Plaque-like erythema with papules in the right axilla after application of antiperspirant

  (D) Consider Dermatitis (Contact or Atopic)

- Red, macerated erythematous areas, with painful blisters and erosions

  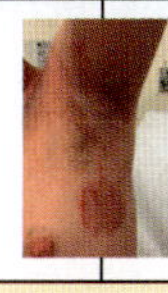
  5

  Extensive, erythematous macerated plaques with some satellite papules within the left axilla that extend inferiorly

  (E) Consider Hailey-Hailey Disease

- Young child (or uncommonly adult) with red-orange patches or plaques in intertriginous areas

  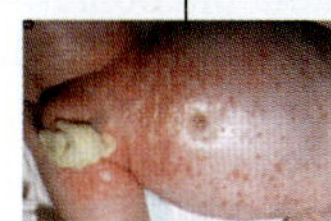
  6

  Macerated, eroded pink papules localized to the suprapubic, inguinal, and genital areas

  (F) Consider Langerhans Cell Histiocytosis

No → Are there satellite papules and pustules present on exam?

Yes →

- Red plaques with satellite papules or pustules, and positive KOH skin preparation

  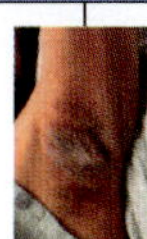
  7

  Well-demarcated, large plaque in the left axilla with satellite papules and pustules

  (G) Consider Candida Intertrigo

- Pink-brown hyperkeratotic papules in the axillae and intertriginous areas

  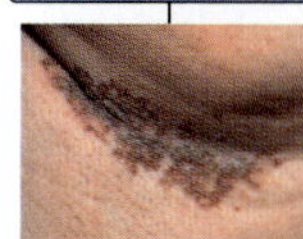
  8

  Coalescing brown papules localized to the axilla with hyperkeratosis and maceration

  (H) Consider Granular Parakeratosis

No → Is the erythematous eruption mostly unilateral?

Yes →

- Bright red erythema (if pus present consider swabbing), with positive bacterial culture

  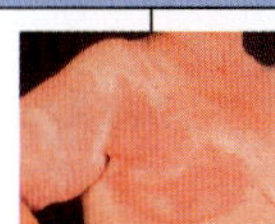
  9

  Cutaneous streptococcal infection showing sharply demarcated erythema on the chest, upper arm, and axillary areas

  (I) Consider Bacterial Intertrigo

- Young child (or uncommonly adult) with unilateral, morbilliform exanthema near the groin or one axilla—may progress to the other axilla

  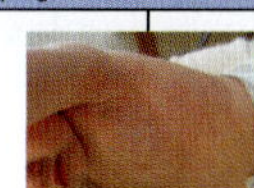
  10

  Lacy erythematous macules and papules localized to the left lateral trunk, axilla, and proximal inner arm

  (J) Consider Unilateral Laterothoracic Exanthem (ULE)

No → Is the rash well-demarcated?

Yes →

- Well-demarcated erythematous patches or plaques that can be macerated (smooth and shiny)

  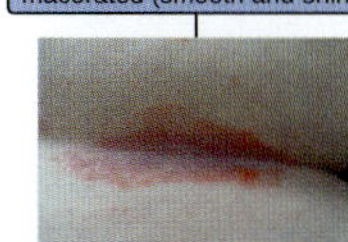
  11

  Pink, well-demarcated erythematous plaque in the inframammary fold with minimal scale

  (K) Consider Inverse Psoriasis

- Well-demarcated plaques on genital, perianal, or perineal skin

  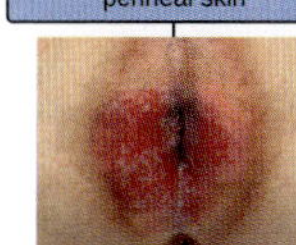
  12

  Erythematous plaque of the vulva with pale white dots within erosions demonstrating a "strawberries and cream" morphology

  (L) Consider Extramammary Paget Disease

No →

- Less mobile patient with moist, dull red to red-brown pruritic patches or thin plaques with negative culture or KOH skin preparation

  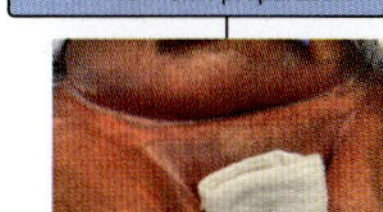
  13

  Diffuse, deep red erythema and maceration in the subpannicular and groin fold regions

  (M) Consider Noninfectious Intertrigo

4 Acral Erythema

Scott D. Worswick and Thomas E. Norman

Acral erythema is defined as a diffuse red or pink color of the skin that principally affects distal parts of the body (e.g., hands, feet, ears, or nose).[1] Although many conditions may affect one acral surface, only conditions affecting more than one site (e.g., bilateral ears) are included in this chapter.

A. Initial evaluation begins with history and physical examination, with particular attention given to unique features of the erythema, associated symptoms, and potential inciting factors.

B. When erythema is caused by exposure to cold temperature, **frostbite, Raynaud phenomenon (RP), acrocyanosis, perniosis, and resolving cold urticaria** should be considered. Frostbite and RP begin with pallor that becomes erythematous on rewarming. In contrast, acrocyanosis and perniosis present as red to violet without preceding pallor. Since primary RP and acrocyanosis are usually painless and bilateral, the presence of pain, asymmetry, or necrosis should raise concern for secondary causes, such as connective tissue disease. Perniosis presents with painful or pruritic erythrocyanotic macules, papules, or nodules that can ulcerate. Type 1 cryoglobulinemia and chilblain lupus may present similarly. A history of wheals should prompt consideration of cold urticaria.

C. When erythema is warm and painful, worsened by heat, and improved with cooling, **erythromelalgia** should be considered. While erythromelalgia usually affects both feet and is episodic, it can affect any acral site and be constant. Erythromelalgia can be hereditary or secondary to systemic conditions, such as myeloproliferative disorders, other malignancies, connective tissue diseases, and neuropathy.

D. **Relapsing polychondritis** and **red ear syndrome (RES)** should be considered when patients have episodes of painful erythema limited to the ears. Relapsing polychondritis usually affects the pinna and has concurrent edema and disfiguration. Since it is due to immune-mediated cartilage destruction, the condition may also present with a collapsed nasal bridge, tracheobronchomalacia, and joint pain. RES most often affects the earlobe and may be triggered by touch, temperature changes, or neck movement. RES has been associated with neurological disorders, including headaches, trigeminal neuralgia, and cervical nerve injury.

E. When erythema is constant and unrelated to temperature, distinctive rash morphologies can narrow the differential. For instance, in patients with painful red to violaceous nodules on the hands or feet, ***Pseudomonas aeruginosa* eccrine hidradenitis (PEH)** and **neutrophilic eccrine hidradenitis (NEH)** should be considered. PEH typically affects the feet of children or adolescents after swimming in water with a high *Pseudomonas aeruginosa* concentration. In contrast, NEH is mostly observed in patients with malignancies, particularly acute myeloid leukemia, receiving chemotherapy. More rarely, NEH occurs following nonchemotherapeutic medications, in immunosuppressed patients, and idiopathically. **Papular-purpuric gloves and socks syndrome (PPGSS)** should be considered in patients with confluent red to purpuric papules on their hands and feet. Edema, pain, and pruritus may be present. PPGSS may be triggered by a variety of infections but is predominantly observed in children and adolescents with parvovirus B19 infection. **Acrodynia**, a manifestation of chronic mercury poisoning, should be considered in patients with edema, erythema, superficial desquamation, and numbness of acral sites. Mood changes, impaired concentration, muscle weakness, and gastrointestinal symptoms may also be present.

F. If the previously discussed features are absent and a new medication was started, consider **chemotherapy-induced acral erythema** and **fixed drug eruption**. In contrast to fixed drug eruptions, chemotherapy-induced erythema is often extremely painful and may desquamate, blister, and ulcerate.[2,3]

G. In patients with painless constant erythema limited to the hands, **systemic diseases** should be considered. These include hepatobiliary disease (most commonly cirrhosis), thyrotoxicosis, rheumatoid arthritis, diabetes, and malignancy. Erythema due to **natural physiologic variation** is also possible. Pregnancy is the most common example, but senile, hereditary, and idiopathic palmar erythema have also been observed.

See Appendix 1 for Further Reading and Image References.

[1]This chapter focuses on the differential for acral erythema without scaling. While not covered in this chapter, the differential from acral erythema with overlying scale includes contact dermatitis, psoriasis, seborrheic dermatitis, and acrokeratosis paraneoplastica.

[2]*Toxic epidermal necrolysis* (TEN) and *graft-versus-host disease* (GVHD) could initially present similarly to chemotherapy-induced acral erythema and fixed drug eruption. Importantly, though, TEN and GVHD will likely progress beyond acral surfaces (see Chapters 6 and 42).

[3]The appearance of *necrolytic acral erythema* might be similar to that of chemotherapy-induced acral erythema that ulcerates and becomes necrotic. However, necrolytic acral erythema is not associated with chemotherapy but rather chronic infections, such as hepatitis C viral infection. Moreover, necrolytic acral erythema is often more psoriasiform and hyperkeratotic in appearance.

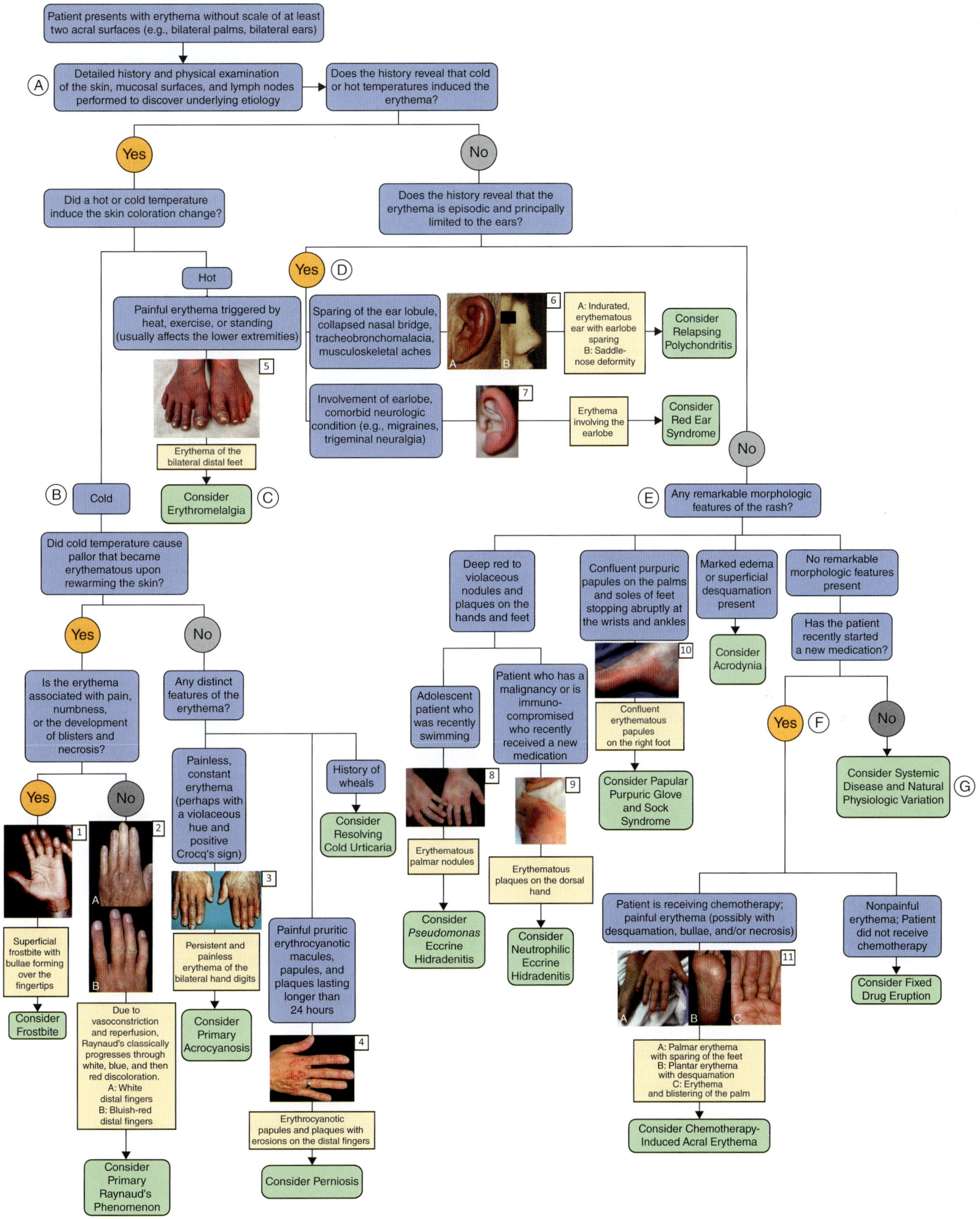
Patient presents with erythema without scale of at least two acral surfaces (e.g., bilateral palms, bilateral ears)
A
Detailed history and physical examination of the skin, mucosal surfaces, and lymph nodes performed to discover underlying etiology
Does the history reveal that cold or hot temperatures induced the erythema?
Yes
Did a hot or cold temperature induce the skin coloration change?
Hot
Painful erythema triggered by heat, exercise, or standing (usually affects the lower extremities)
5
Erythema of the bilateral distal feet
Consider Erythromelalgia
C
B
Cold
Did cold temperature cause pallor that became erythematous upon rewarming the skin?
Yes
Is the erythema associated with pain, numbness, or the development of blisters and necrosis?
Yes
1
Superficial frostbite with bullae forming over the fingertips
Consider Frostbite
No
2
A
B
Due to vasoconstriction and reperfusion, Raynaud's classically progresses through white, blue, and then red discoloration. A: White distal fingers B: Bluish-red distal fingers
Consider Primary Raynaud's Phenomenon
No
Any distinct features of the erythema?
Painless, constant erythema (perhaps with a violaceous hue and positive Crocq's sign)
3
Persistent and painless erythema of the bilateral hand digits
Consider Primary Acrocyanosis
History of wheals
Consider Resolving Cold Urticaria
Painful pruritic erythrocyanotic macules, papules, and plaques lasting longer than 24 hours
4
Erythrocyanotic papules and plaques with erosions on the distal fingers
Consider Perniosis
No
Does the history reveal that the erythema is episodic and principally limited to the ears?
Yes
D
Sparing of the ear lobule, collapsed nasal bridge, tracheobronchomalacia, musculoskeletal aches
6
A
B
A: Indurated, erythematous ear with earlobe sparing B: Saddle-nose deformity
Consider Relapsing Polychondritis
Involvement of earlobe, comorbid neurologic condition (e.g., migraines, trigeminal neuralgia)
7
Erythema involving the earlobe
Consider Red Ear Syndrome
No
E
Any remarkable morphologic features of the rash?
Deep red to violaceous nodules and plaques on the hands and feet
Adolescent patient who was recently swimming
8
Erythematous palmar nodules
Consider Pseudomonas Eccrine Hidradenitis
Patient who has a malignancy or is immuno-compromised who recently received a new medication
9
Erythematous plaques on the dorsal hand
Consider Neutrophilic Eccrine Hidradenitis
Confluent purpuric papules on the palms and soles of feet stopping abruptly at the wrists and ankles
10
Confluent erythematous papules on the right foot
Consider Papular Purpuric Glove and Sock Syndrome
Marked edema or superficial desquamation present
Consider Acrodynia
No remarkable morphologic features present
Has the patient recently started a new medication?
Yes
F
Patient is receiving chemotherapy; painful erythema (possibly with desquamation, bullae, and/or necrosis)
11
A
B
C
A: Palmar erythema with sparing of the feet B: Plantar erythema with desquamation C: Erythema and blistering of the palm
Consider Chemotherapy-Induced Acral Erythema
Nonpainful erythema; Patient did not receive chemotherapy
Consider Fixed Drug Eruption
No
Consider Systemic Disease and Natural Physiologic Variation
G

5 Isolated Erythema

Joyce Xia and Daniela Kroshinsky

The differential for isolated erythema of the skin is broad, with etiologies including infectious, inflammatory, vascular, and neoplastic. Initial evaluation should take place in a well-lit environment and include a detailed history and physical, with special attention paid to exposures, onset, location, and time course of erythema.

Distribution of erythema can provide an initial clue to etiology. Erythema presenting multifocally or broadly may be indicative of **acute inflammatory erythema**, **stasis dermatitis**, **contact dermatitis**, or **erythema nodosum**.

A. Critically ill patients with risk factors such as obesity, fluid overloaded status, and impaired lymphatic return may develop **acute inflammatory erythema**. Skin examination should focus on areas of increased pressure to detect sparing, including skin folds, areas in contact with external devices, sacrum, and back.

B. **Stasis dermatitis** is a localized eczematous disorder which occurs due to venous insufficiency of the lower extremities, which presents with intense pruritus, erythema, and scale. Lesions may go on to ulcerate.

C. Acute **contact dermatitis** may present with erythema and vesiculation. Patients with irritant contact dermatitis usually experience pain, burning, or stinging, while pruritus is more prominent in allergic contact dermatitis. Geometric, linear, or other nonorganic patterns of dermatosis are frequently the most important clue to diagnosis.

D. Diagnosis of **erythema nodosum** is supported by the identification of a deep palpable component in addition to localized erythema. Associated symptoms may include fever, malaise, weight loss, arthralgias, and lymphadenopathy. Although many cases are idiopathic, providers should rule out any possible contributing underlying disease. Other less common forms of panniculitis can be found in Chapter 16 and may be considered in patients with erythematous patches and deep nodules. Erythema that is localized in nature but also associated with systemic symptoms, including fever, malaise, or laboratory abnormalities, should prompt consideration of infectious or inflammatory etiologies.

E. **Erysipelas** is a cutaneous infection affecting the superficial dermis and lymphatics, usually affecting the extremities and face, with clearly defined borders of inflammation. For a skin infection without distinct borders, consider **cellulitis**, which involves subcutaneous tissue. Patients should be evaluated to identify the source of infection.

F. Patients with **Wells syndrome (eosinophilic cellulitis)**, an inflammatory reaction to arthropod bites, develop prodromal itching/burning, followed by cellulitis-like plaques. These plaques are initially edematous and then become indurated. Additional features may include violaceous borders, vesicles or bullae, and an annular configuration. Plaques usually occur on the extremities and resolve within 4 to 8 weeks. Wells syndrome is commonly associated with malaise and eosinophilia.

G. **Erythema migrans**, due to *Borrelia burgdorferi*, typically occurs in the New England, Middle Atlantic, and North Central regions of the United States during the late spring/summer. Well-demarcated erythema (often annular or targetoid) develops 1 to 2 weeks following inoculation and may present with malaise, headache, fevers, chills, myalgias, or arthralgias. There is a high false-negative rate when testing is performed in the 4 to 6 weeks following exposure. Detailed history and risk factors may help narrow the differential for isolated localized erythema without obvious systemic features.

H. Elderly or immunocompromised patients may develop reactivation of varicella zoster virus, leading to **herpes zoster (shingles)**. Isolated erythema may occur during a preeruptive phase characterized by intense pain, pruritus, tingling, or hyperesthesia, followed by the development of a dermatomal rash with grouped vesicles on an erythematous base.

I. **Gout** should be considered in middle-aged and older men presenting with joint pain, warmth, and swelling. Tophaceous gout may present with subcutaneous nodules. Risk factors include obesity, alcohol intake, renal insufficiency, and diuretic medications.

J. **Superficial thrombophlebitis** presents with tenderness and erythema at a vein with an occasionally palpable cord-like structure. Varicose veins, underlying malignancy, or other hypercoagulable states may predispose patients to the condition.

K. The most common plaque variant of **morphea** presents early on as multiple asymmetric erythematous/edematous plaques on the trunk, which undergo centrifugal expansion. Early lesions are typically asymptomatic and progress for 3 to 5 years becoming indurated and sclerotic before resolving spontaneously.

L. **Carcinoma erysipeloides**, a rare cutaneous metastasis with a poor prognosis, has a similar presentation to cellulitis or erysipelas. Patients may additionally experience edema secondary to lymphatic obstruction.

M. **Fixed drug eruption** presents following exposure to an inciting drug with one or several round/oval, sharply demarcated, erythematous/edematous plaques anywhere on the body (including mucous membranes). Plaques may have a dusky violaceous hue and vesiculate. Symptoms develop days to weeks following initial exposure but will subsequently reappear in the same areas within 24 hours following additional exposures. Patch testing at the involved site may be useful in diagnosing sensitivity, although it may be negative in the refractory period following an exacerbation.

N. **Thermal injury** occurs following damage to the skin from an external heat source. Superficial burns may present with erythema, pain, and tenderness. Partial-thickness burns will additionally present with bullae, erosions, or exudate. Full-thickness burns are typically hypesthetic due to epidermal and dermal destruction.

O. **Vaccination site reaction** may cause self-limited erythema, swelling, and tenderness at the injection site.

See Appendix 1 for Further Reading and Image References.

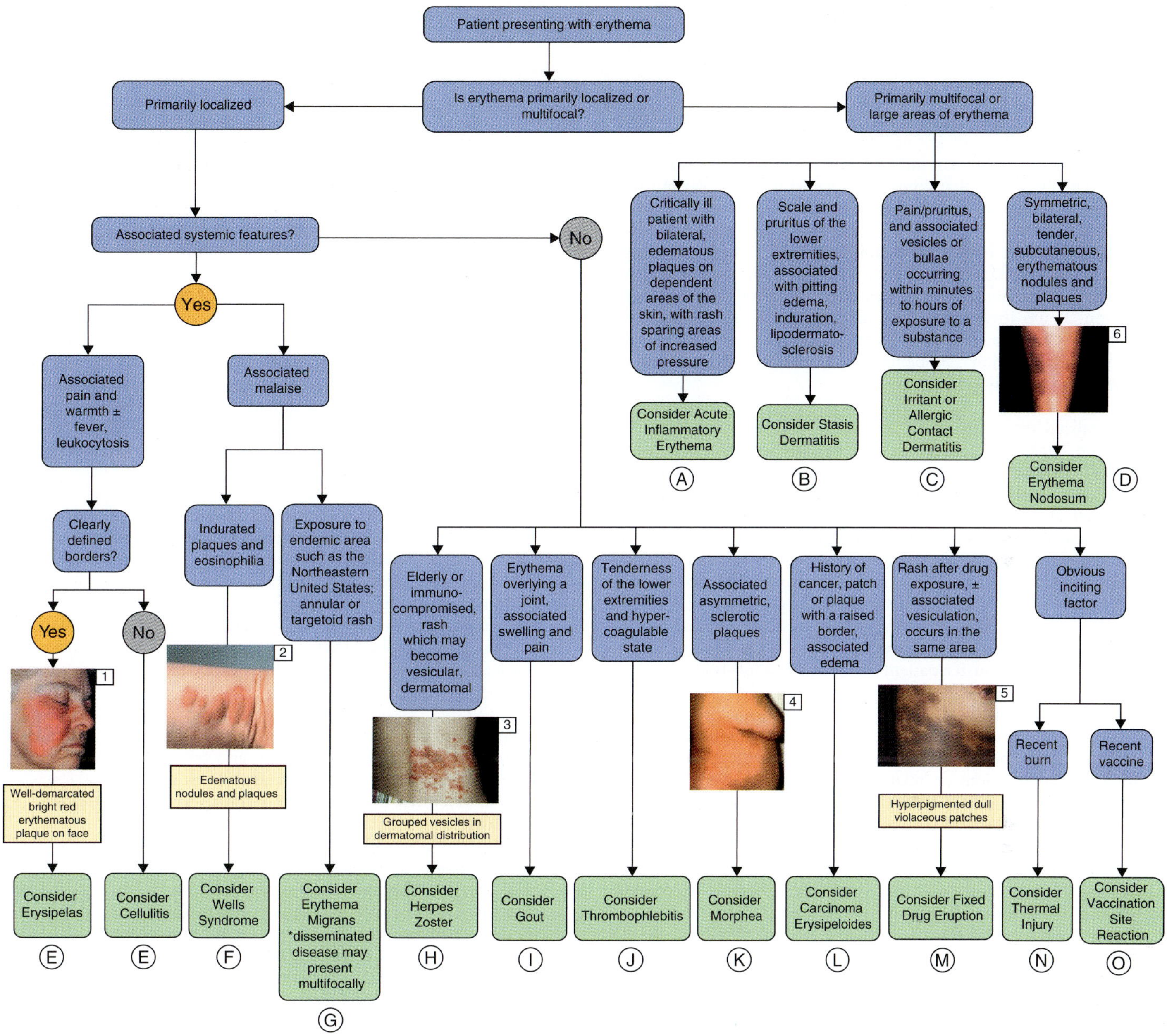
Patient presenting with erythema
Is erythema primarily localized or multifocal?
Primarily localized
Primarily multifocal or large areas of erythema
Associated systemic features?
No
Yes
Associated pain and warmth ± fever, leukocytosis
Associated malaise
Clearly defined borders?
Yes
No
1
Well-demarcated bright red erythematous plaque on face
Consider Erysipelas
E
Consider Cellulitis
E
Indurated plaques and eosinophilia
2
Edematous nodules and plaques
Consider Wells Syndrome
F
Exposure to endemic area such as the Northeastern United States; annular or targetoid rash
Consider Erythema Migrans *disseminated disease may present multifocally
G
Elderly or immuno-compromised, rash which may become vesicular, dermatomal
3
Grouped vesicles in dermatomal distribution
Consider Herpes Zoster
H
Erythema overlying a joint, associated swelling and pain
Consider Gout
I
Tenderness of the lower extremities and hyper-coagulable state
Consider Thrombophlebitis
J
Associated asymmetric, sclerotic plaques
4
Consider Morphea
K
History of cancer, patch or plaque with a raised border, associated edema
Consider Carcinoma Erysipeloides
L
Rash after drug exposure, ± associated vesiculation, occurs in the same area
5
Hyperpigmented dull violaceous patches
Consider Fixed Drug Eruption
M
Obvious inciting factor
Recent burn
Consider Thermal Injury
N
Recent vaccine
Consider Vaccination Site Reaction
O
Critically ill patient with bilateral, edematous plaques on dependent areas of the skin, with rash sparing areas of increased pressure
Consider Acute Inflammatory Erythema
A
Scale and pruritus of the lower extremities, associated with pitting edema, induration, lipodermato-sclerosis
Consider Stasis Dermatitis
B
Pain/pruritus, and associated vesicles or bullae occurring within minutes to hours of exposure to a substance
Consider Irritant or Allergic Contact Dermatitis
C
Symmetric, bilateral, tender, subcutaneous, erythematous nodules and plaques
6
Consider Erythema Nodosum
D

6 Generalized Erythema

Scott D. Worswick and Thomas E. Norman

Generalized erythema is defined as a diffuse red or pink color of the skin without scaling, involving at least 90% of the body surface area. Because this presentation can indicate a life-threatening disease, initial management should involve supportive care while efficiently but thoroughly investigating the underlying etiology.

A. Initial evaluation begins with monitoring the patient's vital signs and eliciting a thorough history, with particular attention given to whether a new medication was recently started. Physical examination should involve the skin, nails, lymph nodes, and mucosal surfaces. Obtaining previous photographs and performing serial physical examinations can be helpful to develop a thorough understanding of the rash's evolution.

B. Generalized erythema could be due to a drug-induced flushing reaction, such as that observed with **vancomycin**. However, generalized erythema can also be the initial presentation of serious drug reactions, including **toxic epidermal necrolysis (TEN)**, **acute generalized exanthematous pustulosis (AGEP)**, and **drug-induced hypersensitivity syndrome**. Commonly implicated drugs include antiepileptics, antibiotics, antivirals, nonsteroidal antiinflammatories, and allopurinol. TEN should be suspected in patients with dusky erythema, bullae, a positive Nikolsky sign, or mucosal involvement. Evolution within hours to a diffuse pustular eruption is indicative of AGEP. While generalized erythema could also be due to a benign drug reaction, if a patient presents with a full-body erythema, it is best to withdraw the offending medication.

C. Generally, high fevers alone can cause whole-body redness. Therefore constant fever and generalized erythema in a patient could be the result of any infectious or inflammatory process. Nevertheless, toxic shock syndrome (TSS), scarlet fever, dengue, and staphylococcal scalded skin syndrome (SSSS) can present with distinct morphologies and vital sign alterations that can be clues to diagnosis.

TSS should be suspected in patients with hypotension, tachycardia, and a "sunburn-like" rash that starts on the chest or intertriginous sites before spreading to the rest of the body. Oropharyngeal, conjunctival, and vaginal mucosa may be hyperemic but rarely develop bullae or erosions. The erythema of TSS is caused by superantigenic toxins (commonly produced by *Staphylococcus aureus* or group A *Streptococcus*) and can result in multiorgan failure.

Discrete gritty papules with surrounding erythema (sandpaper-like rash) is found in **scarlet fever**. Other unique features of this rash are perioral sparing and distinct red lines located in skin creases, particularly the antecubital fossa ("Pastia lines"). Desquamation may occur as the rash begins to resolve. Since scarlet fever is due to group A *Streptococcus* exotoxin, patients will likely have either an accompanying pharyngitis or a soft tissue infection.

Dengue virus should be considered in travelers returning from Central/South America, sub-Saharan Africa, and Asia who develop a morbilliform rash 3 to 6 days after the onset of fever. This rash can become markedly confluent, resulting in generalized erythema with isolated patches of unaffected skin ("islands of white in a sea of red"). Other symptoms include headaches, retro-orbital eye pain, arthralgias, and myalgias.

SSSS typically begins with facial and/or flexural erythema that can generalize to the rest of the body. Other features of SSSS include positive Nikolsky sign, evolution to flaccid bullae in flexural areas, and superficial desquamation that occurs within days. SSSS occurs more commonly in children; when it is present in adults, patients typically have renal dysfunction or are immunosuppressed.

D. If the erythema coincides with recurrent febrile episodes, it is important to consider systemic autoinflammatory diseases such as **adult-onset Still disease (AOSD)**. AOSD is characterized by polyarticular arthritis, pharyngitis, and daily fever spikes accompanied by an evanescent salmon-pink erythema. Generalized lymphadenopathy, hepatosplenomegaly, abnormal liver function tests, myalgia, and serositis may also be observed. Other systemic autoinflammatory diseases, including familial Mediterranean fever, may also present with periodic and relapsing fevers.

E. **Sézary syndrome** should be suspected when older patients present with persistent redness, weight loss, and generalized lymphadenopathy. While more commonly presenting as an erythroderma (see Chapter 42), it can also present as a diffuse erythema without scale.

F. The differential for flushing should be considered in patients without fever and with episodic erythema most pronounced on the face, neck, and chest. Generalized flushing can occur due to pheochromocytomas, medullary thyroid cancer, and pancreatic neuroendocrine tumors. **Carcinoid syndrome**, occurring in approximately 10% of patients with carcinoid tumors, is characterized not only by flushing, but also by abdominal cramping, fatigue, and diarrhea.

See Appendix 1 for Further Reading and Image References.

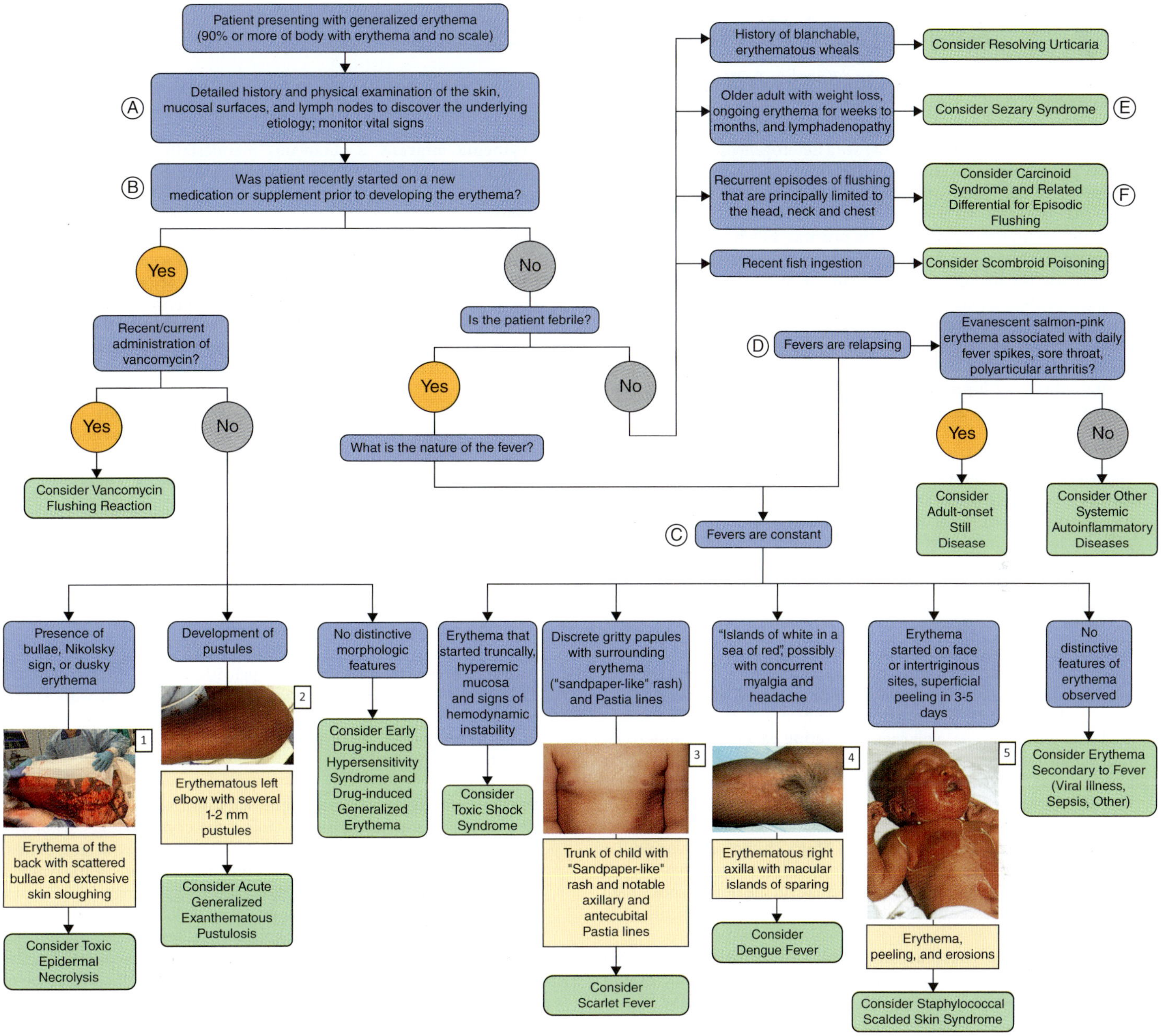
Patient presenting with generalized erythema (90% or more of body with erythema and no scale)
(A) Detailed history and physical examination of the skin, mucosal surfaces, and lymph nodes to discover the underlying etiology; monitor vital signs
(B) Was patient recently started on a new medication or supplement prior to developing the erythema?
Yes
Recent/current administration of vancomycin?
Yes
Consider Vancomycin Flushing Reaction
No
Presence of bullae, Nikolsky sign, or dusky erythema
1
Erythema of the back with scattered bullae and extensive skin sloughing
Consider Toxic Epidermal Necrolysis
Development of pustules
2
Erythematous left elbow with several 1-2 mm pustules
Consider Acute Generalized Exanthematous Pustulosis
No distinctive morphologic features
Consider Early Drug-induced Hypersensitivity Syndrome and Drug-induced Generalized Erythema
No
Is the patient febrile?
Yes
What is the nature of the fever?
No
History of blanchable, erythematous wheals
Consider Resolving Urticaria
Older adult with weight loss, ongoing erythema for weeks to months, and lymphadenopathy
Consider Sezary Syndrome (E)
Recurrent episodes of flushing that are principally limited to the head, neck and chest
Consider Carcinoid Syndrome and Related Differential for Episodic Flushing (F)
Recent fish ingestion
Consider Scombroid Poisoning
(D) Fevers are relapsing
Evanescent salmon-pink erythema associated with daily fever spikes, sore throat, polyarticular arthritis?
Yes
Consider Adult-onset Still Disease
No
Consider Other Systemic Autoinflammatory Diseases
(C) Fevers are constant
Erythema that started truncally, hyperemic mucosa and signs of hemodynamic instability
Consider Toxic Shock Syndrome
Discrete gritty papules with surrounding erythema ("sandpaper-like" rash) and Pastia lines
3
Trunk of child with "Sandpaper-like" rash and notable axillary and antecubital Pastia lines
Consider Scarlet Fever
"Islands of white in a sea of red," possibly with concurrent myalgia and headache
4
Erythematous right axilla with macular islands of sparing
Consider Dengue Fever
Erythema started on face or intertriginous sites, superficial peeling in 3-5 days
5
Erythema, peeling, and erosions
Consider Staphylococcal Scalded Skin Syndrome
No distinctive features of erythema observed
Consider Erythema Secondary to Fever (Viral Illness, Sepsis, Other)

7 Annular and Figurate Erythemas

Amber Y. Bo and Karolyn A. Wanat

Annular and figurate erythemas (FEs) are a heterogeneous group of skin eruptions presenting with annular, concentric, polycyclic, or arciform erythematous lesions that are associated with multiple dermatologic entities. The classic FE starts as small pink-red papules on the legs. They are typically asymptomatic but can be pruritic. FEs have equal occurrence among both sexes and all ages and have a fluctuating course over weeks to years. The diagnosis requires clinical and histopathologic correlation and is often a diagnosis of exclusion.

The characteristic changes, type of scale, and time course of lesions can help differentiate these entities.

If there is peripheral scale, **tinea** infections should be considered. **Subacute cutaneous lupus, annular erythema of Sjogren, psoriasis,** and **mycosis fungoides** also can present with annular lesions, with or without scale.

A. Superficial **erythema annulare centrifugum** presents with slowly growing patches/plaques with scale (annular/polycyclic red-pink patches/plaques on the trunk and extremities that spread centrifugally up to 6 cm in diameter over days to weeks). They have a pale central clearing and a "trailing scale," a white inner margin on the advancing edge. While typically asymptomatic, they can be pruritic and occasionally vesicles develop on the margin.

B. **Necrolytic migratory erythema (NME)** presents as erythematous, well-demarcated scaly plaques/patches with erosion of the advancing edge. Lesions are often present in intertriginous and periorificial areas and can be intensely pruritic or painful. It is classically associated with glucagonoma, a glucagon-secreting pancreatic tumor causing weight loss, new-onset diabetes mellitus, glossitis, and angular cheilitis. Rarely, NME appears with liver or gastrointestinal disease (pseudoglucagonomas).

C. **Purpura annularis telangiectodes of Majocchi** presents as annular plaques (up to 3 cm in diameter) with central clearing, punctuate telangiectasias, and cayenne pepper petechiae on the border most often on the legs of adolescent or young females. It is a type of capillaritis.

D. **Disseminated superficial actinic porokeratosis** presents as smaller papules (2–7 mm) that grow radially with a hyperkeratotic border and predilection for sun-exposed areas, most often on the legs of adult females.

E. **Erythema gyratum repens (EGR)** presents as rapidly migrating concentric rings of erythematous plaques with scaling edges that cover large areas of the trunk and extremities, while sparing the face, palms, and soles, in a "wood grain" pattern. EGR is intensely pruritic. This rare disorder affects adults and is associated with an underlying malignancy in 85% of cases, most commonly a neoplasm of the breast, lung, stomach, or esophagus.

F. **Erythema migrans**, a cutaneous manifestation of Lyme disease, presents 3 to 30 (median 7) days after a tick bite as an erythematous circular patch with a pale ring around a dark center ("bull's eye" appearance). The targetoid lesions expand over several weeks (growing up to a diameter of 70 cm) and most spontaneously resolve after 4 weeks. Lesions notably spare the palms and soles. Although some patients report tingling/burning, most lesions are asymptomatic and rarely pruritic or painful. Secondary erythema migrans lesions are smaller, without indurated centers, and spread from the initial tick bite. A similar lesion may appear in southern tick-associated rash illness, spread by *Amblyomma americanum*.

G. **Deep gyrate erythema** manifests as static or slowly expanding annular plaques with a cord-like border. The indurated and elevated presentation corresponds to the deeper dermis involvement on histopathology with a mononuclear infiltrate in the mid-lower dermis.

H. **Annular erythema of infancy (AEI)** is an uncommon disorder that typically presents as bilateral, symmetrical, annular erythema on the trunk in children. **Eosinophilic annular erythema** is an entirely different diagnosis and is found in adults, but like AEI, it tends to present with annular erythema without scale.

I. **Annular urticaria** are short-lived pruritic lesions resolving under 24 hours with a wheal-like appearance and associated with multiple morphologies. The rapidly migratory and short-lived nature of these, in addition to multiple morphologies, can help differentiate from other entities.

J. **Erythema marginatum** is a manifestation of acute rheumatic fever (RF) that presents as migratory polycyclic erythematous eruptions on the trunk and proximal extremities while sparing the face, palms, and soles. The lesions spread peripherally to form nonscaling patches and have a fluctuating course, fading and reappearing within hours. Hot showers often make the lesions more visible. Children younger than 5 years are more likely to manifest these lesions, although it can occur in adults. RF is a systemic autoimmune reaction to infection by group A β-hemolytic streptococci. Erythema marginatum resolves spontaneously and is unaltered by penicillin treatment of RF.

K. **Granuloma annulare, sarcoidosis, tuberculoid leprosy**, and other granulomatous disorders also are in the differential diagnosis for a patient with annular erythema. These typically are fixed, often more indurated. **Erythema multiforme** more often presents with targetoid, not annular, lesions.

See Appendix 1 for Further Reading and Image References.

Patient presenting with small, annular, erythematous spots
→ Detailed history and physical examination to rule out infectious, autoimmune, and malignant etiologies
→ Do the lesions have an associated scale?

Yes

- Rapidly growing and migratory
  - Concentric rings of erythematous plaques with scaling edges ("wood-grain" appearance) covering large areas of trunk and extremities

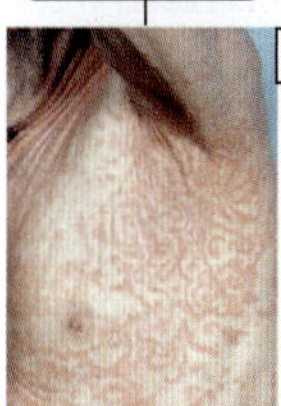

1

    - Multiple gyrate erythematous plaques, showing a wood-grain pattern.
    - Consider Erythema Gyratum Repens (EGR) (E)
    - Workup for underlying neoplasm (commonly lung, breast, stomach, and esophageal)
- Slowly growing over days to weeks
  - Trailing scale located on trunk and extremities
    - Nonindurated annular or polycyclic lesions enlarging centrifugally with a central clearing and a fine scale on the margin. Lesions can be pruritic and rarely, vesicular on the edges

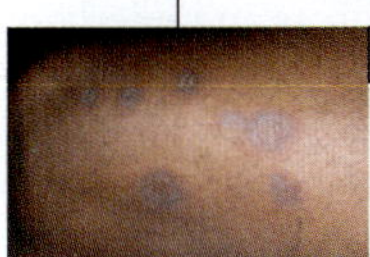

2

    - An annular plaque with delicate scaling on the inner margin of the advancing edge
    - Consider Superficial Erythema Annulare Centrifugum (EAC) (A)
  - Scaly patches in intertriginous areas
    - Intensely pruritic or painful. Associated with a glucagonoma; patient has weight loss, new-onset diabetes mellitus, glossitis, and angular cheilitis
    - Consider Necrolytic Migratory Erythema (NME) (B)
  - Lower extremities of adolescent or young females
    - Annular plaques (up to 3 cm in diameter) with central clearing, punctate telangiectasias, and a border of cayenne pepper petechiae
    - Consider Purpura Annularis Telangiectodes of Majocchi (C)
  - Lower extremities of adult females
    - Small papules (2–7 mm) with a hyperkeratotic border and predilection for sun-exposed areas
    - Consider Disseminated Superficial Actinic Porokeratosis (DSAP) (D)
  - Other differential diagnoses with an appearance of a peripheral or central scale and lesions are static or slow growing
    - KOH positive → Consider Tinea
    - KOH negative
      - Often in sun-exposed areas → Consider Subacute Cutaneous Lupus
      - Characteristic psoriasis lesions elsewhere → Consider Psoriasis
      - Consider Annular Erythema of Sjögren's
      - Sun-protected areas and distinct histopathology → Consider Mycosis Fungoides

No

- Slow, fixed lesions
  - Consider other differential diagnoses include granuloma annulare, sarcoidosis, Hansen disease (tuberculoid leprosy), and other granulomatous disorders which are fixed and often more indurated. Notably, erythema multiforme presents with targetoid, not annular lesions. (K)
  - "Bull's-eye" lesion that notably spares palms and soles. History of tick bite 3–30 days ago

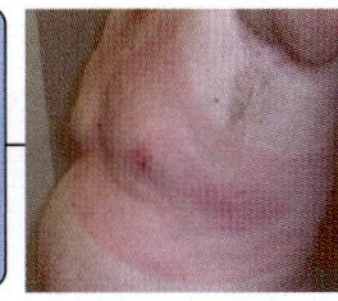

3

    - Annular erythema that spreads centrifugally. The peripheral erythematous border may or may not be sharply demarcated and is usually 1–2 cm in width
    - Consider Erythema Migrans (F)
  - Slowly expanding annular plaques with a "cord-like" border → Consider Deep Gyrate Erythema (G)
  - Bilateral, symmetric, annular erythema on the trunk

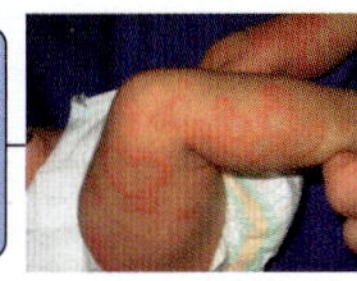

4

    - Expanding annular urticarial plaques in a 6-month-old boy.
    - Consider Annular Erythema of Infancy/ Eosinophilic Annular Erythema (H)
- Rapidly growing and migratory
  - Transient (<24 hours)
    - Lesions typically last <24 hours and are associated with multiple morphologies and a "wheal-like" appearance

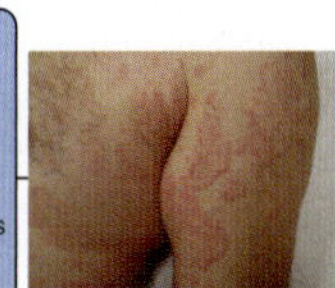

5

    - Lesions of urticaria are evanescent
    - Consider Annular Urticaria (I)
  - Migratory lesions
    - Migratory, polycyclic erythematous lesions, nonscaling, patches, fluctuating transient course within hours

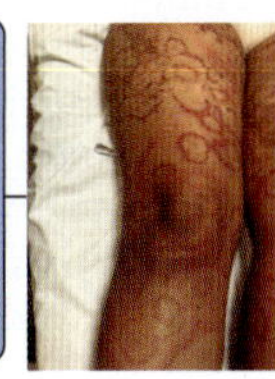

6

    - Faint evanescent annular and arciform erythema.
    - Consider Erythema Marginatum (J)

8 Flagellate Erythema

Ashley B. Crew and Natalia Vecerek

Flagellate erythema (FE) is a rare clinical finding, typically presenting as a truncal pruritic eruption of erythematous, violaceous, or hyperpigmented whiplike streaks. Diagnosing the underlying cause of FE commonly hinges on the history to examine for various exposures; in some instances, clinical findings can be helpful in ruling diagnoses in or out. Overall, this morphology is most commonly associated with ingestion of undercooked shiitake mushrooms, exposure to bleomycin, or underlying dermatomyositis, although other potential causes should not be overlooked.

A. When a patient presents with FE, a thorough history should be taken, particularly to evaluate for relevant exposures and ingestions, associated systemic symptoms, travel history, and pertinent medical history. Detailed examination of areas of FE can support certain diagnoses, while a comprehensive examination of the skin is needed to evaluate for underlying conditions.

B. Although there are limited data regarding **dermatomyositis (DM)**-induced FE, it is accepted as a common phenomenon and represents a sign of active disease. The pathophysiology of FE is unknown, but mechanical damage from pruritus may play a role. Clinically, the eruption presents on the trunk as red to violaceous streaks; typically the streaks are not hyperpigmented, reflecting ongoing inflammation in the skin. Additional physical examination findings of Gottron papules, heliotrope sign, poikilodermatous rash on sun-exposed skin, dilated nailfold capillaries, calcinosis cutis, and proximal muscle weakness can support a diagnosis of DM.

C. Patients with FE reporting a history of cyclical spiking fevers, joint pains, and sore throat should prompt a consideration of **adult-onset Still disease** (AOSD). While AOSD classically presents with asymptomatic, transient, evanescent, salmon-colored macular and papular rash, 15% to 65% of patients may exhibit chronic pruritic papules in a flagellate configuration. Some have noted that the classic evanescent eruption occurs early in the course of AOSD, while the linearly configured pruritic papules occur later in the disease course and may represent a more severe disease. Laboratory findings of leukocytosis, elevated ferritin, elevated inflammatory markers, and transaminitis can support the diagnosis of AOSD; infection, malignancy, and other autoimmune conditions must be excluded.

D. Testing for **dermatographism** can be a useful clinical tool, especially in patients presenting with edematous linear wheals. Positive testing can support the primary process of dermatographism or another pruritic dermatosis.

E. Streaky bullous dermatitis that fades into hyperpigmentation and is photodistributed should raise suspicion for **phytophotodermatitis**. Careful history is indicated to evaluate for photosensitizing exposures.

F. Approximately 1% to 2% of oncology patients who receive **antineoplastic agents** develop FE, which is generally truncal. While bleomycin is by far the most common cause, it has also been reported with docetaxel, trastuzumab, bendamustine, cisplatin, and doxorubicin. The pathophysiology is unclear; bleomycin may accumulate in the skin, which lacks the inactivating enzyme bleomycin hydrolase. The accumulation is enhanced by vasodilation from scratching. Bleomycin also reduces epidermal turnover, enhancing pigmentary incontinence and melanogenesis, which may explain why hyperpigmentation persists for months. Antineoplastic-related FE has been known to exhibit "heat recall," thus cooling of involved areas prevents recurrence during subsequent rounds of chemotherapy. It was previously thought that chemotherapy-related FE is dose dependent; however, there have been cases reported after low-dose injections of bleomycin given for plantar warts. Additionally, most patients develop FE after the first cycle of chemotherapy. The disease itself is self-limited, and cessation of chemotherapy is generally not recommended as this has been associated with increased mortality. Pruritus is typically treated with topical corticosteroids and oral antihistamines but occasionally requires oral steroids.

G. FE induced by **shiitake mushroom** (*Lentinus edodes*) is also predominantly truncal and occurs 1 to 2 days after ingestion of undercooked mushrooms. The pathogenesis is possibly due to increased interleukin secretion in response to the polysaccharide lentinan, which is denatured by cooking. FE secondary to shiitake mushroom ingestion generally resolves over the course of 1 to 3 weeks and, unlike bleomycin, does not typically cause persistent hyperpigmentation.

H. There have been two reported cases of flagellate plaques in **HIV** (human immunodeficiency virus) patients with hypereosinophilic syndrome. In the absence of other identifiable causes of FE, it is worth considering HIV infection as an underlying factor.

I. **Chikungunya fever** has been described to cause and worsen disorders of hyperpigmentation, including flagellate patterns. This likely represents a postinflammatory response after infection. The initial phase of FE related to chikungunya can be bullous. History to assess for travel to endemic areas and compatible systemic symptoms such as fevers, headaches, and joint pains is warranted.

J. Patients should be asked about their recent time spent in the ocean to evaluate for the possibility of **marine injury** causing flagellate dermatitis. Both jellyfish and Portuguese man-of-war tentacles have stinging nematocysts that produce bright red streaks and wheals in areas of skin contact.

See Appendix 1 for Further Reading and Image References.

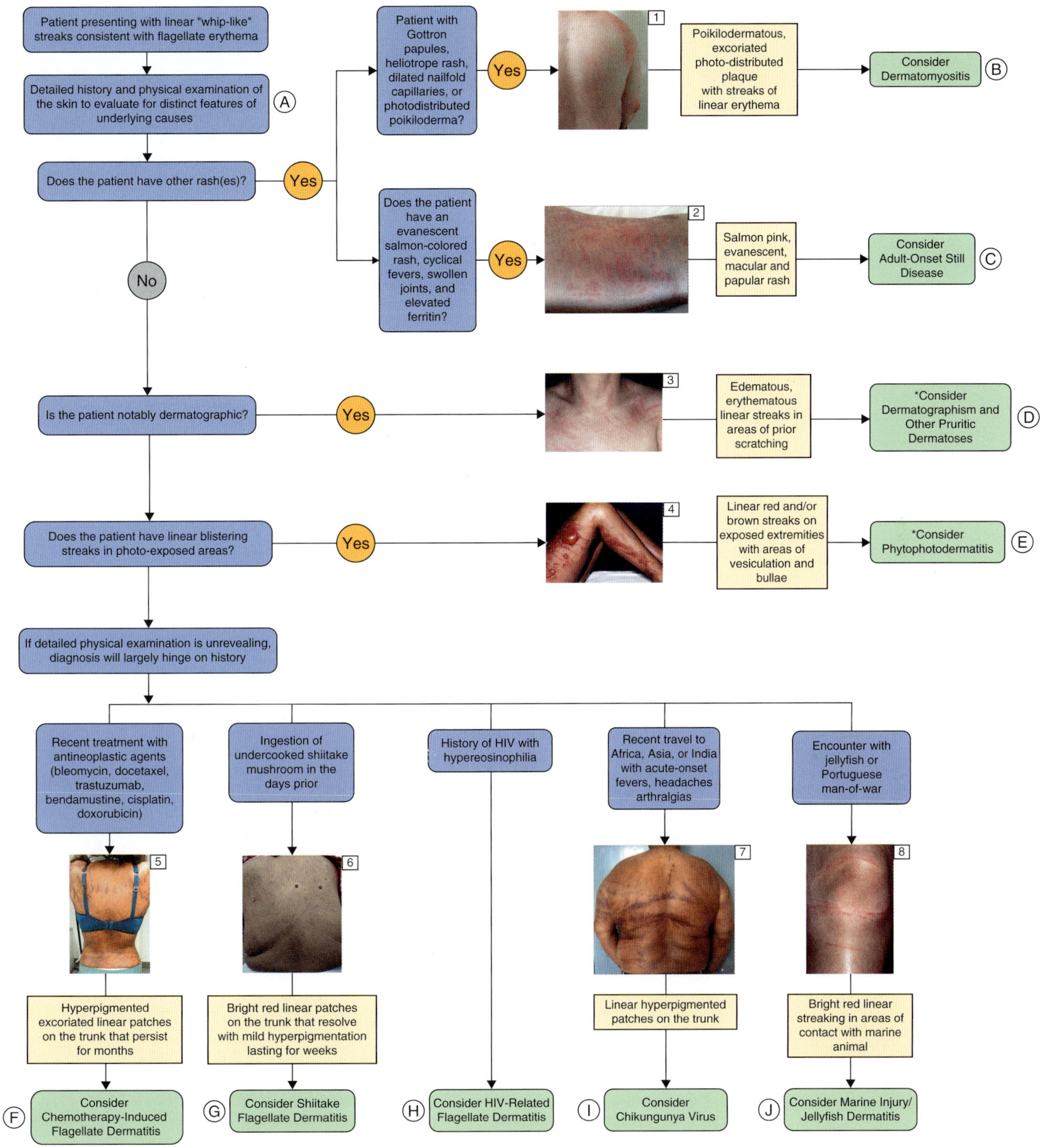

*Clinical Mimickers of Flagellate Erythema

PART II
Skin Hardening

9 Localized Skin Hardening

Neda Shahriari and Ruth Ann Vleugels

Localized skin hardening occurs most commonly due to inflammatory or genetic causes but can also be due to environmental factors or malignancy. The ability to accurately determine the cause of localized skin hardening is crucial to both treatment and ascertaining underlying systemic associations. Chapters 14 through 17 contain a more broad differential for skin nodules; in addition to the diagnoses discussed below, the diagnoses in Chapters 14 through 17 can also be considered in the differential for a patient with skin hardening.

A. The initial evaluation of a patient presenting with localized skin hardening should involve a thorough physical examination of the skin, nails, and mucosal surfaces to determine the geographic distribution of involvement. A detailed history, including a review of systems, can be helpful in determining the stage of onset and providing guidance in defining potential causes of hardening.

B. **En coup de sabre**, a form of linear morphea involving the frontoparietal scalp/forehead, appears as a hyperpigmented or hypopigmented linear streak (during the inflammatory stage, there may also be surrounding erythema). Although classically involving the forehead and scalp, it can also involve the eyebrows, nose, and lips. When extending into the scalp, a scarring alopecia can develop. As it progresses, the area of involvement develops an atrophic appearance. Given that en coup de sabre can involve underlying muscle, bone, and neurologic structures, including the eye, patients can develop headaches or seizures and should be closely monitored.

C. **Progressive hemifacial atrophy** (also known as Parry-Romberg syndrome) is often considered on a spectrum with en coup de sabre, and many patients have findings of both en coup de sabre and progressive hemifacial atrophy. The hallmark of progressive hemifacial atrophy is unilateral sclerosis and atrophy of the face due to involvement of underlying dermis, subcutaneous tissue, muscle, and bone yielding facial asymmetry. There can be alopecia involving the eyebrows and eyelashes. Patients with progressive hemifacial atrophy are at an increased risk for ophthalmic and neurologic pathology and should be closely followed by ophthalmology and neurology. A thorough regular dental evaluation is crucial as well to monitor for teeth alignment and jawbone changes. Given the degree of disfigurement, the disease can have a significant impact on quality of life.

D. **Alopecia porphyrinica** is a sclerodermiform manifestation of porphyria cutanea tarda (PCT). In PCT, patients can also develop sclerosis of the trunk, face, and neck, which can mimic morphea. Alopecia porphyrinica appears as white-yellow sclerotic plaques with surrounding hyperpigmentation and depressed scarring. Although not fully understood, an increase in uroporphyrin I is thought to increase collagen synthesis, yielding a sclerotic diathesis in some patients with PCT.

E. **Morphea** subtypes that do not involve the head and neck and present with localized skin hardening include the following major categories: plaque, guttate, and linear morphea of the extremities. Clinically, morphea can appear as erythematous to violaceous patches that evolve into ivory or hyperpigmented indurated plaques over time. In some instances, morphea can demonstrate the classic lilac-violaceous border indicative of continued inflammatory activity. Linear morphea that involves the extremities should be closely monitored as it may involve deeper structures—muscle, fascia, and bone—and if extending over joints, can cause joint deformity and mobility issues.

F. **Injection site sclerosis** can occur in the setting of injection with substances, including vitamin K (Texier's disease), interferon, bleomycin, silicone, or opioids. This can result in a localized sclerotic reaction at the site of injection.

G. **Chronic radiation dermatitis** occurs in the skin following irradiation to the area. In addition to skin induration, telangiectasias manifest, and the affected area can be prone to ulceration that may ultimately lead to necrosis. Development of chronic radiation dermatitis depends on several factors, including genetics, comorbidities, and radiation dose and method.

H. **Lipodermatosclerosis** occurs on the lower extremities in the setting of stasis dermatitis, which is due to incompetent valves leading to lower extremity edema. Due to this chronic edema and inflammation in the lower extremities, the skin and subcutaneous tissue become indurated and take on an "inverted wine bottle" appearance.

I. **Stiff skin syndrome (SSS)** is a genetic condition appearing at birth or in early childhood that involves a mutation in the fibrillin-1 gene (FBN1). The classic geographic distribution of SSS involves the buttocks and thighs, presenting with induration of the skin and subcutaneous tissues in these areas. There is classic sparing of the inguinal folds. Given the area of distribution, there is a restriction of joint mobility, yielding lumbar lordosis. Although most cases appear to bilaterally impact the shoulder and pelvic girdles, segmental SSS has recently gained attention as a subtype with delayed onset and segmental distribution, causing milder functional impairment.

J. **Carcinoma en cuirasse** presents as an induration of the chest wall and occurs due to the infiltration of malignant cells. This is most commonly seen in the setting of breast cancer.

See Appendix 1 for Further Reading and Image References.

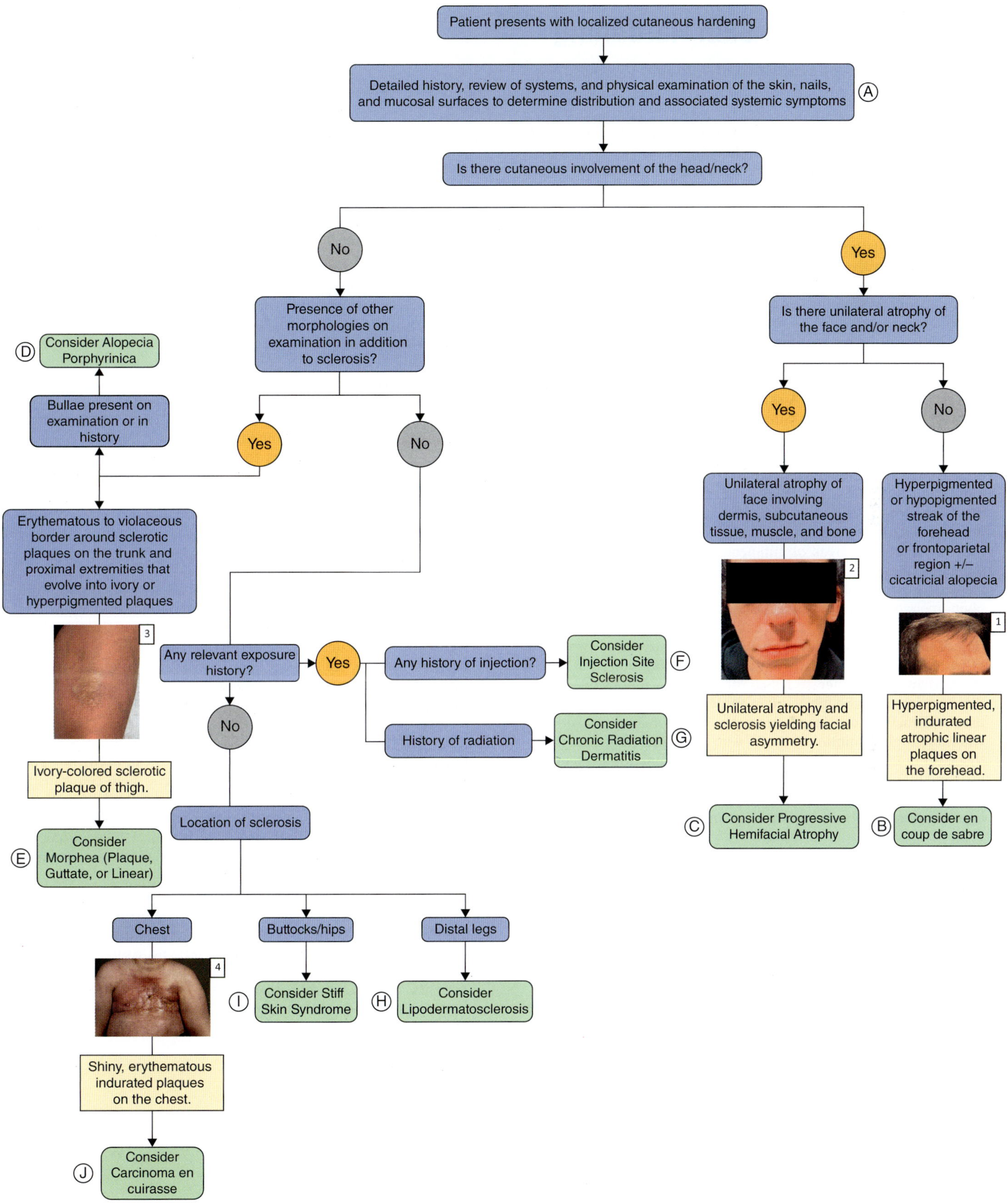
Patient presents with localized cutaneous hardening
Detailed history, review of systems, and physical examination of the skin, nails, and mucosal surfaces to determine distribution and associated systemic symptoms
A
Is there cutaneous involvement of the head/neck?
No
Presence of other morphologies on examination in addition to sclerosis?
Yes
Bullae present on examination or in history
Consider Alopecia Porphyrinica
D
Erythematous to violaceous border around sclerotic plaques on the trunk and proximal extremities that evolve into ivory or hyperpigmented plaques
3
Ivory-colored sclerotic plaque of thigh.
Consider Morphea (Plaque, Guttate, or Linear)
E
No
Any relevant exposure history?
Yes
Any history of injection?
Consider Injection Site Sclerosis
F
History of radiation
Consider Chronic Radiation Dermatitis
G
No
Location of sclerosis
Chest
4
Shiny, erythematous indurated plaques on the chest.
Consider Carcinoma en cuirasse
J
Buttocks/hips
Consider Stiff Skin Syndrome
I
Distal legs
Consider Lipodermatosclerosis
H
Yes
Is there unilateral atrophy of the face and/or neck?
Yes
Unilateral atrophy of face involving dermis, subcutaneous tissue, muscle, and bone
2
Unilateral atrophy and sclerosis yielding facial asymmetry.
Consider Progressive Hemifacial Atrophy
C
No
Hyperpigmented or hypopigmented streak of the forehead or frontoparietal region +/– cicatricial alopecia
1
Hyperpigmented, indurated atrophic linear plaques on the forehead.
Consider en coup de sabre
B

10 Diffuse Skin Hardening

Neda Shahriari and Ruth Ann Vleugels

Distinguishing the etiology of a patient presenting with diffuse skin hardening can be challenging. The underlying disease process is most predictive of the areas of involvement. Determining the cause is crucial for both establishing proper therapeutic management and investigating further systemic associations.

A. The initial evaluation of patients presenting with diffuse skin hardening should involve a detailed history. This includes understanding exposures, medical history, review of systems for any concurrent noncutaneous symptoms, prior infections, and nature and progress of cutaneous symptoms. It is crucial to do a thorough physical examination to better understand the distribution of skin hardening. Special attention should be paid to edema (puffy hand sign) or sclerosis (sclerodactyly) involving the fingers and the presence of Raynaud phenomenon. A skin biopsy and/or fascial biopsy may prove useful, depending on clinical suspicion.

B. The major variants of **systemic sclerosis (SSc)** include limited and diffuse, which are characterized by sclerodactyly. Preceding the induration and sclerosis of the fingers, patients may experience pitting edema of the digits and the puffy hand sign of SSc's edematous phase. Limited SSc involves the distal extremities and face. Diffuse SSc has additional areas of cutaneous involvement, typically also including the proximal extremities and trunk. Patients with SSc may also demonstrate other stigmata, including calcinosis, Raynaud phenomenon, matted telangiectasias, abnormal nailfold capillaroscopy, microstomia, bird facies, and salt-and-pepper dyspigmentation of the skin. Serologies are positive in approximately two-thirds of patients with SSc (usually anticentromere antibodies for limited SSc and antitopoisomerase I [Scl-70] and RNA polymerase III for diffuse SSc). A thorough workup must include evaluation of pulmonary function tests (e.g., spirometry, diffusion capacity, and lung volumes), high-resolution chest CT with interstitial lung disease protocol, echocardiogram, barium swallow, renal function tests, urinalysis, and blood pressure monitoring to assess for associated systemic processes, including interstitial lung disease, pulmonary arterial hypertension, esophageal dysmotility, and renal involvement.

C. Skin hardening can be observed in the setting of **eosinophilic fasciitis (EF)** typically presenting with woody induration involving the extremities. Patients typically note preceding pain and edema in affected areas with sparing of the face and digits. In a portion of patients, there is a notable history of strenuous physical activity preceding the onset of the disease process. More advanced sclerosis of the extremities results in the "groove sign," which is a linear depression at the site of veins within the indurated skin. A fascial biopsy can be obtained, typically showing fascial sclerosis in the context of a lymphocytic, histiocytic, and eosinophilic infiltrate. An alternative to a fascial biopsy is using magnetic resonance imaging to aid in the diagnosis of EF, which demonstrates fascial thickening and enhancement and can be utilized to follow a patient's response to treatment. Peripheral eosinophilia and concomitant plaque morphea are observed in some patients. Patients should also be screened for an associated monoclonal gammopathy.

D. **Scleredema** demonstrates woody induration of the affected skin, typically involving the upper back and neck. A tissue biopsy demonstrates widening of spaces between collagen bundles due to mucin deposition. There are three types of scleredema classified according to the association and/or precipitant. Type 1 typically follows an upper respiratory infection (most commonly strep pharyngitis), type 2 occurs in the context of IgGκ monoclonal gammopathy, and type 3 (i.e., scleredema diabeticorum) occurs in association with diabetes mellitus.

E. **Scleromyxedema** starts with linearly distributed waxy papules symmetrically progressing to diffuse induration most commonly involving the face (leading to leonine facies), ears, extremities, and upper trunk. A tissue biopsy helps to distinguish scleromyxedema from other entities in the differential, demonstrating increased fibroblasts in the dermis, collagen thickening, and increased mucin deposition. The most common extracutaneous manifestation is paraproteinemia (IgGλ most commonly), which can progress to multiple myeloma in approximately 10% of patients.

F. **Nephrogenic systemic fibrosis (NSF)** is a sclerosing disease mainly impacting the extremities. It occurs with gadolinium-based contrast exposure in the setting of renal disease or injury. Patients develop symmetric indurated and hyperpigmented plaques with irregular borders. Patients can also develop scleral plaques and fibrosis involving other organ systems, including the heart, lungs, and muscles. Histopathologically, NSF is similar to scleromyxedema; however, findings are deeper involving the subcutaneous fibrous septae.

G. **Sclerotic graft-versus-host disease (GVHD)** can occur in a patient who has received an allogeneic hematopoietic stem cell transplant. Sclerotic GVHD is characterized by indurated plaques that are patchy in comparison to systemic sclerosis. In addition, other characteristic cutaneous findings of SSc are absent. Histopathologically, deep dermal sclerosis, follicular plugging, and mild vacuolar changes at the basal layer can be observed.

H. Although quite rare, **diffuse sclerodermoid conditions due to exogenous substances** have occurred in toxic oil syndrome (i.e., ingestion of aniline-degraded rapeseed cooking oil) and eosinophilia-myalgia syndrome (i.e., ingestion of contaminated L-tryptophan), where patients are systemically ill preceding sclerosis. Other exposures leading to sclerodermatous skin changes include polyvinyl chloride, bleomycin, and taxanes.

See Appendix 1 for Further Reading.

Patient presents with sclerosis with significant body surface area involvement

↓

Detailed history, review of systems, and physical examination of the skin, nails, and mucosal surfaces to discover precipitators, exposures, additional systemic involvement, and precise area of skin involvement (A)

↓

Is there edema (puffy hand sign) or sclerosis (sclerodactyly) of the fingers and/or Raynaud phenomenon

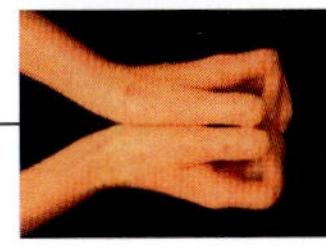
1

Sclerodactyly as evidenced by atrophic indurated skin of the fingers with joint contractures.

Yes → Evaluate for facial involvement (microstomia, bird facies), systemic associations, Raynaud phenomenon, and serologies.

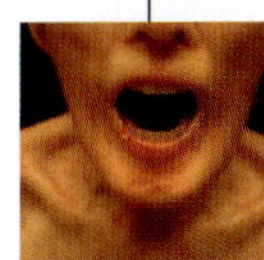
2

Microstomia as evidenced by decreased oral aperture.

→ Consider Systemic Sclerosis (B)

No → Is there history of exposure to drugs, chemicals, other exogenous substances, or transplant?

No →

- Rapid onset of woody induration of the extremities. "Groove sign" noted on examination. Peripheral eosinophilia sometimes present.

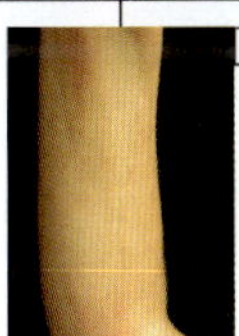
3

Indurated skin of the extremity with linear depression marking location of vein.

→ Consider Eosinophilic Fasciitis (C)

- Erythema and induration, typically most prominent over the upper back. Recent history of upper respiratory infection, diagnosis of monoclonal gammopathy, or diabetes mellitus.

→ Consider Scleredema (D)

- Widespread, monomorphic linearly distributed waxy papules. Progression leads to induration of the skin.

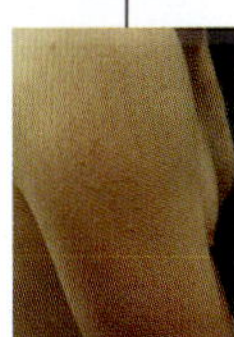
4

Numerous monomorphic pinpoint waxy papules on the upper arm.

→ Consider Scleromyxedema (E)

Yes →

- Gadolinium-based contrast exposure in the setting of kidney disease → Consider Nephrogenic Systemic Fibrosis (F)
- History of allogeneic hematopoietic stem cell transplant → Consider Sclerotic Graft-Versus-Host Disease (G)
- History of exogenous substance exposure → Consider Diffuse Sclerodermoid Conditions due to Exogenous Substances (H)

PART III
Sloughing Skin

11 Localized Skin Sloughing

Rebecca Sarac and Timmie R. Sharma

We define skin sloughing as an epidermis that is easily detached from underlying structures. This chapter on localized skin sloughing will address conditions in which the affected areas of skin sloughing are topographically isolated to a particular area of the body.

A. A number of conditions can present with isolated oral mucosal or gingival epidermal sloughing or erosions. These conditions may or may not have more generalized cutaneous involvement but are designated here because oral mucosal or gingival involvement may be the only sign at presentation.

B. Flaccid bullae in the oral cavity may be seen in several diseases. The **Pemphigus disorders** can present with oral erosions and ulcerations that are often described as "ragged."

Reactive infective mucocutaneous eruption (RIME) is a spectrum of diseases in which mucositis follows an infection. Patients tend to be young males presenting with polymorphous mucosal lesions affecting oral, ocular, and/or urogenital regions. Patients present with prodromal symptoms indicative of *Mycoplasma* infection (cough, fever, malaise) or another infection about 1 week prior to onset of mucositis. This can be difficult to distinguish from **Steven-Johnson syndrome (SJS)** and **erythema multiforme (EM)**. However, only a minority of patients with RIME have broader cutaneous involvement, and cutaneous lesions tend to lack the acral predominance seen in EM and tend to be less confluent than seen in SJS.

Hand-foot-and-mouth disease is an eruption caused by enteroviruses, presenting with erosive stomatitis and vesicles on the palms, soles, and genital area. Oral lesions are predominately located on the tongue, buccal mucosa, palate, uvula, and anterior tonsillar pillars.

Herpes simplex virus can be considered in a patient with grouped vesicles or ulcerations on an erythematous base. Coalescing lesions produce a larger ulceration with a characteristic "scalloped" border.

C. **Mucous membrane (cicatricial) pemphigoid** is characterized by "smooth" but irregular ulcers and erosions, desquamative gingivitis, and may or may not have intact vesicles or tense bullae. This is often contrasted with the "ragged" ulcerations noted in pemphigus.

D. Lacy-white plaques with ulceration and gingivitis can be seen in **oral lichen planus (LP)** and **chronic graft-versus-host disease (GVHD)**. Common associations with LP include middle age, coexistent hepatitis C viral (HCV) infection, and dental amalgam. Oral erosive LP is most commonly associated with HCV infection. In a patient with a history of stem cell transplant or exposure to nonirradiated blood products, chronic GVHD should be considered.

E. **EM major** presents not only with mucosal involvement, but also with typical (three-zone) targets, predominantly located on acrofacial sites.

F. **Oral candidiasis** presents with erythematous red plaques, which can be erosive, with satellite papules and pustules. Mucocutaneous candidiasis is often associated with a cottage cheese-like exudate. Intertriginous and genital areas may also be affected.

Patient presenting with localized skin or mucosal sloughing → Detailed history and physical examination of hair, skin, nails, and mucosa → Evidence of oral mucosal or gingival involvement on physical examination?

- No → *continued on next page*
- (A) Yes →
  - Smooth ulcers and erosions, with/without vesicles or tense bullae, desquamative gingivitis

    6

    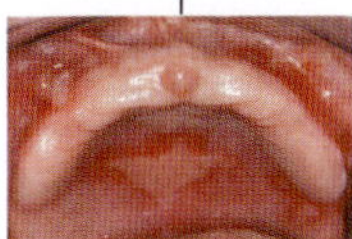

    → (C) Consider Mucous Membrane Pemphigoid
  - (D) Lacy-white plaques, ulceration, gingivitis
    - Middle-aged to elderly patient, history of HCV infection, history of dental amalgam

      7

      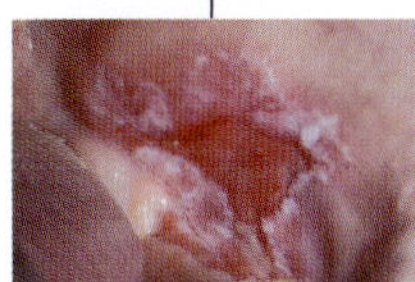

      → Consider Oral Lichen Planus
    - History of stem cell transplant or transfusion of nonirradiated blood products

      8

      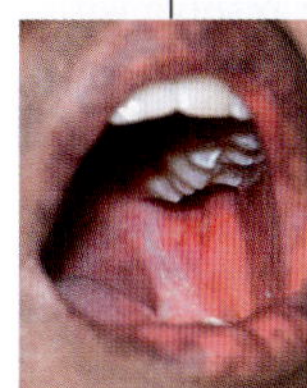

      → Consider Chronic Graft-Versus-Host Disease
  - (B) Flaccid vesicles/bullae
    - Ragged-appearing ulcers and erosions, desquamative gingivitis

      1

      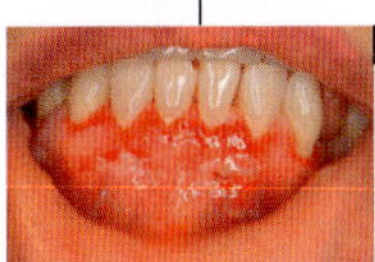

      → Consider Pemphigus Disorders
    - Prodromal symptoms, severe mucositis involving >2 sites, with/without cutaneous involvement

      2

      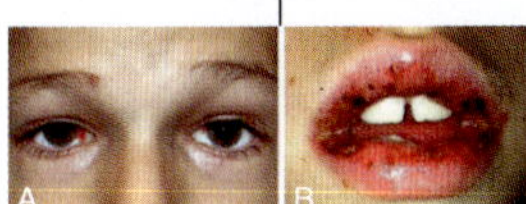

      → Consider Reactive Infective Mucocutaneous Eruption
    - Erythema, erosions, hemorrhagic crusts, with/without adjacent cutaneous involvement

      3

      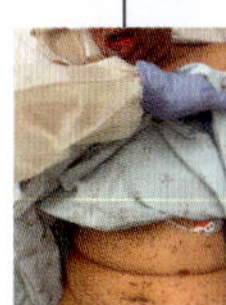

      → Consider Steven-Johnson Syndrome
    - Vesicles and macules on the hands, feet, oral mucosa, and genital area

      4

      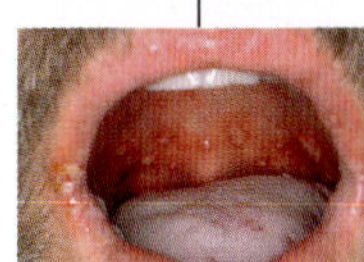

      → Consider Hand-foot-and-mouth Disease
    - Grouped vesicles or erosions on an erythematous base, scalloped border

      5

      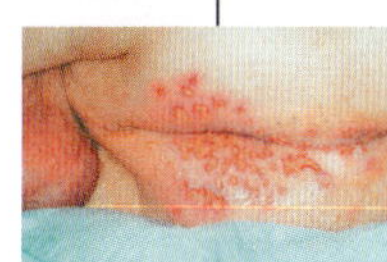

      → Consider Herpes Simplex Virus Infection
  - Three-zone target lesions

    9

    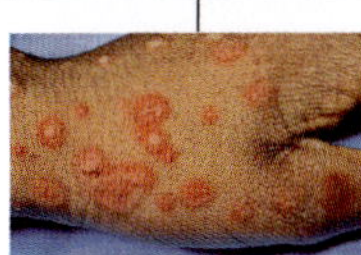

    → (E) Consider Erythema Multiforme
  - Deep red papules and pustules with satellite lesions

    10

    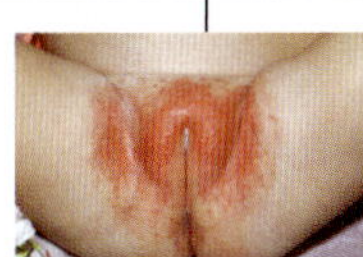

    → (F) Candidiasis

Continued

G. Sloughing that is localized to intertriginous areas is seen in benign familial pemphigus and toxic erythema of chemotherapy. **Benign familial pemphigus** presents with symmetric vesicles and characteristic "worm-eaten" erosions in the inframammary, axillary, and inguinal areas. **Toxic erythema of chemotherapy** is characterized by red to purple patches and plaques, which may slough; history will reveal a patient taking a chemotherapy drug.

H. Sloughing and blistering on the fingers can be seen with blistering dactylitis and herpetic whitlow. **Blistering dactylitis** is due to *Streptococcus* infection and presents with painful tense bullae on a background of erythema and edema. **Herpetic whitlow**, caused by herpes simplex virus, presents with painful grouped vesicles or erosions on a digit.

I. Localized skin sloughing may also be noted elsewhere but not necessarily in one of the specific locations noted above.

One or a few well-demarcated, round or oval, dusky patches, or atypical targets that resolve with hyperpigmentation are indicative of **fixed drug eruptions**. Re-exposure to the offending agent will cause recurrence of the lesion in the same location. Lesions resolve with residual hyperpigmentation.

Bullous impetigo is caused by *Staphylococcus aureus* and can be thought of as a localized form of staphylococcal scalded skin syndrome, as it is caused by the same exfoliative toxin. Lesions are painful erythematous patches with a typical collarette of scale.

Bullous cellulitis, most often caused by *Streptococcus pyogenes* and less often by *S. aureus*, presents with erythematous, edematous, and often hemorrhagic plaques with superimposed bullae.

J. Environmental injuries may present with localized skin sloughing at the site of injury. If there is erythema and sloughing noted in sun-exposed areas, consider **phototoxicity** from direct sun exposure. A medication history can also help elucidate whether the reaction could be drug-mediated. **Thermal** or **chemical burns** can also cause localized skin sloughing due to direct epidermal injury. Physical examination may reveal skin sloughing in a geometric or patterned distribution. Injury secondary to abuse should also be considered.

Sometimes localized skin sloughing occurs due to underlying acute inflammation due to other causes (see Chapters 2 to 6, 18, and 19 for potential other causes of skin sloughing not described in this chapter).

See Appendix 1 for Further Reading and Image References.

No → Involvement of intertriginous areas

(G) Yes

- Symmetric vesicles and "worm-eaten" erosions

11

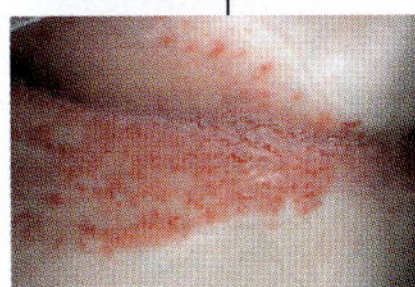

→ Consider Benign Familial Pemphigus

- Red-purple or dusky patches with central desquamation or blistering

12

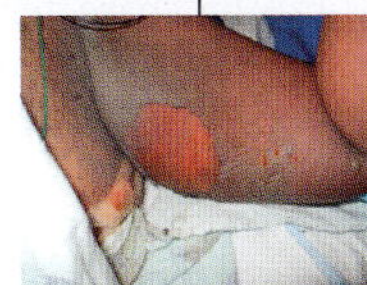

→ Consider Toxic Erythema of Chemotherapy

No

(H) Involvement of the fingers

- Painful tense bullae with erythema and edema on a digit

13

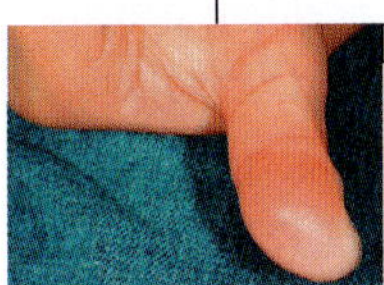

→ Consider Blistering Dactylitis

- Painful, grouped vesicles or erosions on a digit

14

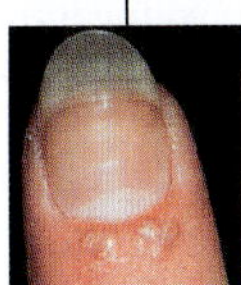

→ Consider Herpetic Whitlow

(I) Vesicles or bullae elsewhere on the body

- Atypical targets or dusky patches with postinflammatory hyperpigmentation upon resolution

15

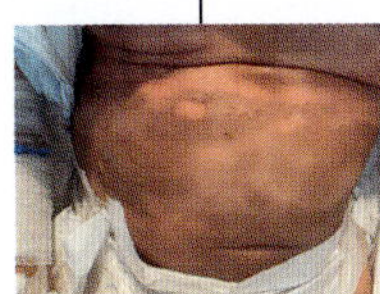

→ Consider Fixed Drug Eruption

- Round erosions or crusts with colarette of scale

16

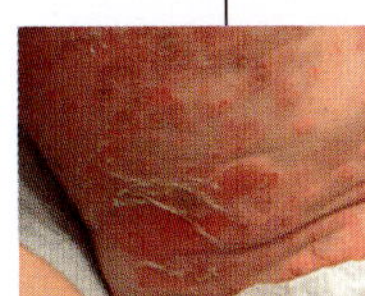

→ Consider Bullous Impetigo

- Bullae overlying edema, erythema, warmth, and tendernes

17

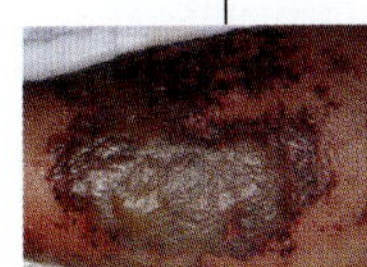

→ Consider Bullous Cellulitis

(J) Concern for environmental injury

- Sun-exposed distribution with history of sun exposure

18

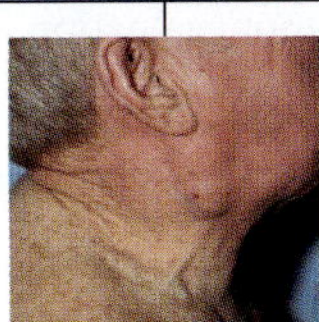

→ Consider Phototoxicity (Sunburn or Drug Induced)

- Exposure to hot water or objects

19

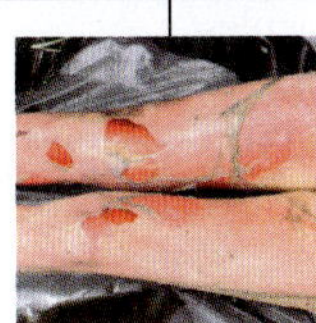

→ Consider Thermal Burn

- Exposure to caustic substance

20

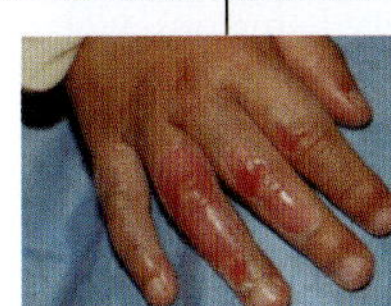

→ Consider Chemical Burn/ Severe Irritant Dermatitis

12 Generalized Sloughing Skin

Timmie R. Sharma and Rebecca Sarac

Epidermal sloughing is a clinical phenomenon which is defined as an epidermis that is easily detached from underlying structures. Pathologically, this can be characterized by an intraepidermal separation or full-thickness epidermal separation from the underlying dermis.

This chapter focuses on conditions which involve widespread skin sloughing. These conditions have varied etiologies and degrees of severity, ranging from severe cutaneous adverse reactions (SCAR) to nutritional deficiencies. As a result, accurate diagnosis is critical.

A. In **acute generalized exanthematous pustulosis (AGEP)** and **pustular psoriasis**, superficial coalescing pustules create "lakes of pus," which can cause superficial epidermal sloughing at the subcorneal layer.

In **AGEP**, patients develop numerous, tiny, sterile pustules on a base of edematous erythema that arises at the same time as fever. This usually occurs within 1 to 11 days of exposure to the causative medication.

There are four distinct clinical patterns of **pustular psoriasis**: von Zumbusch (abrupt onset of generalized painful erythema and pustulation), annular (pustules and scale at the advancing edge of an annular lesion), exanthematous (acute-onset eruption of tiny pustules and may overlap with AGEP), and localized (pustules arising within existing psoriatic plaques). Triggering factors include hypocalcemia, pregnancy, rapid taper of systemic corticosteroids, drugs, infections, and topical irritants.

B. Dusky macules and patches are the clinical presentation of epidermal necrosis. This is the hallmark clinical feature of the conditions listed below.

SJS/TEN is a life-threatening SCAR that presents as coalescing dusky macules and patches that may form atypical targets. Mucosal involvement is almost always present and typically involves more than two mucous membranes. Numerous medications are implicated. If there is concern for SJS/TEN, immediate withdrawal of the offending agent and consultation with urology/gynecology and ophthalmology are of critical importance.

Erythema multiforme (EM) tends to present with typical (three-zone) targets as opposed to the atypical (two-zone) targets noted in SJS/TEN or fixed drug reactions. Additional distinctions include that EM lesions tend to be papular and do not coalesce significantly. These lesions tend to be found on acral sites of the upper half of the body. EM major is characterized by severe mucosal involvement, which is absent in EM minor. The majority of cases are preceded by herpes simplex virus infection; however, other infectious agents have also been implicated.

Generalized bullous fixed drug reaction can present with round or oval sharply demarcated erythematous, violaceous, or dusky macules/patches, which may converge to form confluent large sheets of epidermal detachment and may resemble SJS/TEN. This reaction is typically noted asymmetrically, notably sparing various areas of the body. Lesions heal with postinflammatory hyperpigmentation. Reexposure to the offending drug will result in same-site recurrent lesions.

Toxic erythema of chemotherapy can present with red to purple patches and plaques in acral and intertriginous areas. There are case reports of associated skin sloughing as well. History will reveal a patient taking a chemotherapy drug. Although clinically the presentation is similar to SJS/TEN, the pathophysiology is proposed to be due to toxic effects of chemotherapy agents as opposed to a hypersensitivity reaction.

Widespread bullae and epidermal necrosis can also be seen in **acute graft-versus-host disease (aGVHD)**, which can resemble SJS/TEN. History will reveal a patient who has recently received a stem cell transplant or who has received nonirradiated blood products. Diarrhea, hyperbilirubinemia, and pancytopenia will also be seen in SJS/TEN-like aGVHD but are less likely to be seen in SJS/TEN.

C. If a patient presents with abrupt-onset confluent erythema, which may be localized periorally and in intertriginous areas, **staphylococcal scalded skin syndrome** should be considered. There is a lack of mucous membrane involvement, and the sloughing is more superficial than seen with the SJS/TEN spectrum. The epidermal sloughing is caused by a circulating staphylococcal exotoxin, which targets desmoglein 1 and causes widespread splitting of the epidermis at the granular layer distant from the site of primary infection. Patients affected typically include children younger than 5 years or elderly patients with an underlying medical condition, particularly renal disease.

D. Superficial epidermal sloughing due to acantholysis from autoantibodies directed toward desmogleins is seen in **pemphigus group disorders** (pemphigus vulgaris, foliaceous, and paraneoplastic). Patients with pemphigus vulgaris develop painful oral erosions and widespread flaccid blisters and erosions. They may form vegetative plaques overlying the erosions (pemphigus vegetans). In pemphigus foliaceous, mucosal involvement is not present, and lesions are characterized by superficial erosions, often seen on the trunk, with a distinct yellow scale-crust. Paraneoplastic pemphigus is characterized by severe stomatitis affecting all areas of the oropharynx and vermillion lips and is often treatment resistant. It is associated with hematologic malignancies, including most commonly non-Hodgkin lymphoma or chronic lymphocytic leukemia.

E. Nutritional deficiencies can cause epidermal sloughing due to reversible degeneration of the upper epidermis, which can lead to necrosis and thus sloughing of the epidermis. This is seen in **acrodermatitis enteropathica, pellagra, and protein-energy malnutrition**. Risk factors include alcoholism, HIV, anorexia, and restrictive diets, which should all prompt evaluation for nutritional deficiencies.

See Appendix 1 for Further Reading and Image References.

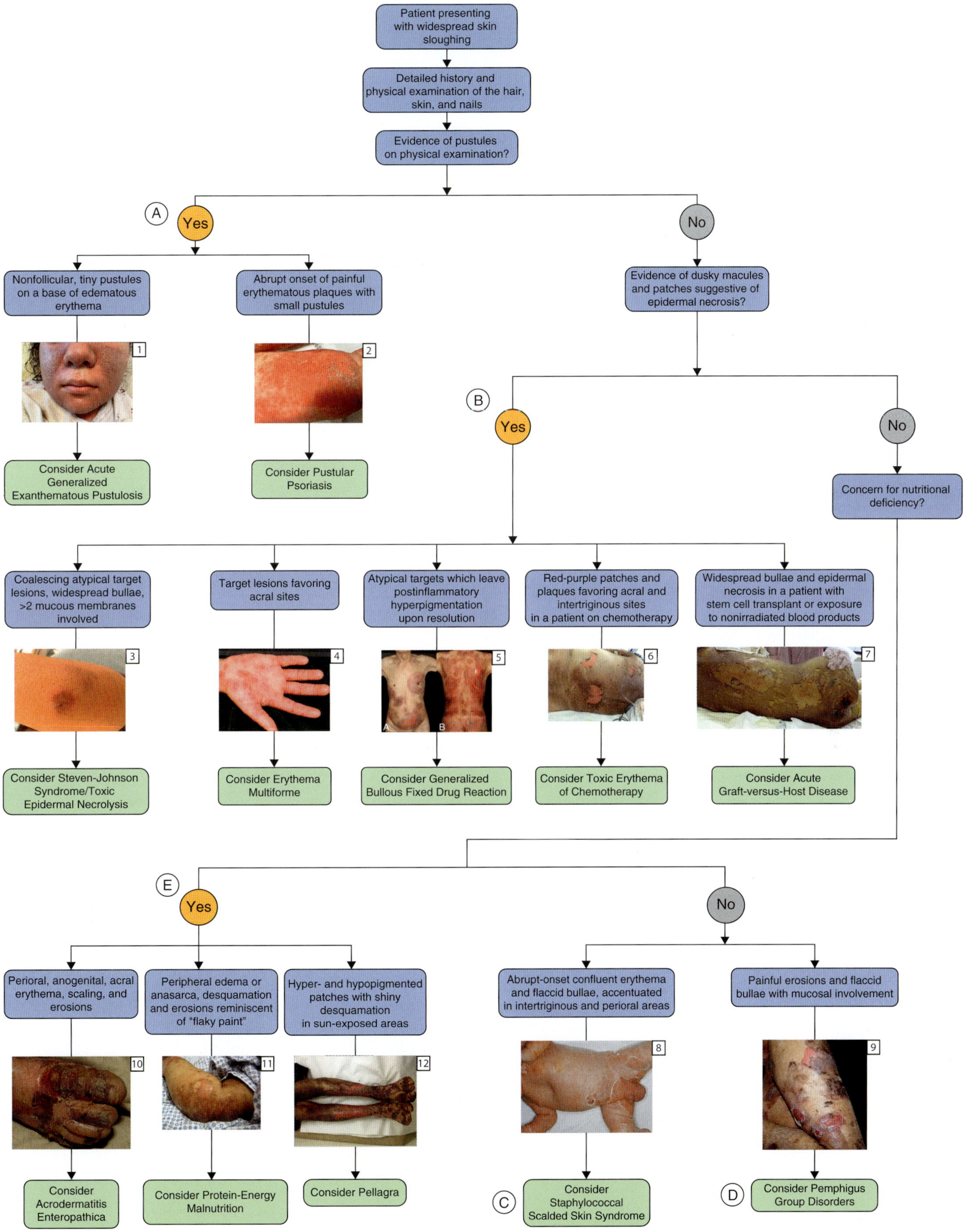
Patient presenting with widespread skin sloughing
Detailed history and physical examination of the hair, skin, and nails
Evidence of pustules on physical examination?
A
Yes
Nonfollicular, tiny pustules on a base of edematous erythema
1
Consider Acute Generalized Exanthematous Pustulosis
Abrupt onset of painful erythematous plaques with small pustules
2
Consider Pustular Psoriasis
No
Evidence of dusky macules and patches suggestive of epidermal necrosis?
B
Yes
Coalescing atypical target lesions, widespread bullae, >2 mucous membranes involved
3
Consider Steven-Johnson Syndrome/Toxic Epidermal Necrolysis
Target lesions favoring acral sites
4
Consider Erythema Multiforme
Atypical targets which leave postinflammatory hyperpigmentation upon resolution
5
A
B
Consider Generalized Bullous Fixed Drug Reaction
Red-purple patches and plaques favoring acral and intertriginous sites in a patient on chemotherapy
6
Consider Toxic Erythema of Chemotherapy
Widespread bullae and epidermal necrosis in a patient with stem cell transplant or exposure to nonirradiated blood products
7
Consider Acute Graft-versus-Host Disease
No
Concern for nutritional deficiency?
E
Yes
Perioral, anogenital, acral erythema, scaling, and erosions
10
Consider Acrodermatitis Enteropathica
Peripheral edema or anasarca, desquamation and erosions reminiscent of "flaky paint"
11
Consider Protein-Energy Malnutrition
Hyper- and hypopigmented patches with shiny desquamation in sun-exposed areas
12
Consider Pellagra
No
Abrupt-onset confluent erythema and flaccid bullae, accentuated in intertriginous and perioral areas
8
C
Consider Staphylococcal Scalded Skin Syndrome
Painful erosions and flaccid bullae with mucosal involvement
9
D
Consider Pemphigus Group Disorders

PART IV
Nodules

13 Purple Plums

Chen Yao and Lindy Fox

The "Purple plum" category encompasses a wide differential of various benign and malignant neoplasms or proliferations. Although many conditions may present as violaceous papules or plaques, only conditions presenting with violaceous or plum-like, soft to firm nodules are discussed in this chapter. Initial evaluation begins with history and physical examination, with attention to onset, distribution, lymph node involvement, and systemic symptoms. Basic laboratory studies, including complete blood count (CBC), blood urea nitrogen/creatinine, liver function tests, and lactate dehydrogenase, may be needed in patients with systemic symptoms. Ultimately skin biopsy is required, as a definitive diagnosis of "purple plum" nodules is made by histopathologic evaluation, and each of these entities can look quite similar morphologically.

If the patient presents with a single or few nodules on physical examination, particularly when present for longer than a few weeks, consider primary cutaneous neoplasms or early cutaneous metastases. These can be generally categorized into malignant, vascular, and benign neoplasms.

A. **Malignant tumors** include amelanotic melanoma, squamous cell carcinoma (SCC), Merkel cell carcinoma (MCC), sarcomas (e.g., Atypical Fibroxanthoma (AFX), Dermatofibrosarcoma Protuberans (DFSP), leiomyosarcoma), and cutaneous metastases. Cutaneous metastases of solid organ tumors can also present with many nodules depending on progression of the disease.

B. **Vascular neoplasms** with a single to a few purple plum nodules include those with a range of malignant potential. This category includes pyogenic granuloma, angiosarcoma, lymphangiosarcoma of Stewart-Treves syndrome, and tumors of Masson (intravascular papillary endothelial hyperplasia) and Dabska (endovascular papillary angioendothelioma). History of radiation therapy or lymph node dissection would be suggestive of angiosarcoma and lymphangiosarcoma, respectively.

C. **Benign neoplasms** that typically present with single to few purple plums include adnexal tumors (i.e., spiradenoma, cylindroma), tumors derived from collagen (keloids), elastin, muscle (leiomyoma), and nerves (schwannoma). These tumors are most often sporadic but may also present with many lesions in the setting of rare genetic syndromes. Certain adnexal tumors may be favored based on the location. Follicular and sebaceous neoplasms have a predilection for the face and scalp; eccrine neoplasms are most commonly found on the palms and soles; and apocrine tumors favor the eyelids, axilla, and anogenital region.

D. If the patient has a known history of HIV (particularly CD4 counts <500 cells/μL) or other immunocompromised condition and is presenting with several to many purple plums, always consider **Kaposi sarcoma** if chronic and **bacillary angiomatosis** if acute.

E. If CBC or peripheral smear demonstrates markedly elevated white blood cell counts or leukemic cells in the setting of several to many violaceous nodules on physical examination, **leukemia cutis** should be strongly considered. Leukemia cutis most commonly occurs in patients with acute myeloid leukemia, and its presence is associated with decreased overall survival. The specific subtype of leukemia can be further differentiated with immunohistochemistry, cytogenetics, or flow cytometry studies. Bone marrow biopsy is imperative for a definitive diagnosis of systemic leukemia.

F. If abnormal lymphocytes are detected on peripheral blood work or histopathology, **lymphoma cutis** should be suspected. Lymphoma cutis can be further categorized into primary cutaneous lymphoma or secondary cutaneous lymphoma, distinguished by the presence of simultaneous or preceding extracutaneous involvement such as lymphadenopathy. Cutaneous lymphomas include **T-cell lymphomas, B-cell lymphomas**, and **tumor-stage mycosis fungoides (MF)**. The presence of tumors and lymphadenopathy are key prognostic factors for MF. Lymphomatoid papulosis is considered on the spectrum and typically presents with papules or nodules that spontaneously resolve within 8 weeks. Very rarely, multiple myeloma can present in an aggressive form in which the monoclonal plasma cells infiltrate the skin to present as cutaneous **plasmacytoma. Blastic plasmacytoid dendritic cell neoplasm** is a rare, clinically aggressive, hematologic malignancy that can present with or without bone marrow involvement and leukemic dissemination.

G. If no malignant cells are seen under histopathology, inflammatory and infectious etiologies should be considered, including **cutaneous lymphoid hyperplasia, Sweet syndrome, exuberant granulation tissue**, and deep fungal or atypical **mycobacterial infection**. While most cases of cutaneous lymphoid hyperplasia lack clonality, monoclonality has occurred in both B-cell and T-cell cutaneous lymphoid hyperplasia and does not exclude this diagnosis. History can help identify the underlying etiology; cutaneous lymphoid hyperplasia can be induced by medications, infections, and foreign substances. Sweet syndrome is also associated with a wide range of disorders, including medications, infections, inflammatory bowel disease, pregnancy, and malignancy. Infections that can present as purple plums, including fungal and atypical mycobacteria, should not be overlooked as they can be life threatening and are not uncommon causes of this presentation.

See Appendix 1 for Further Reading and Image References.

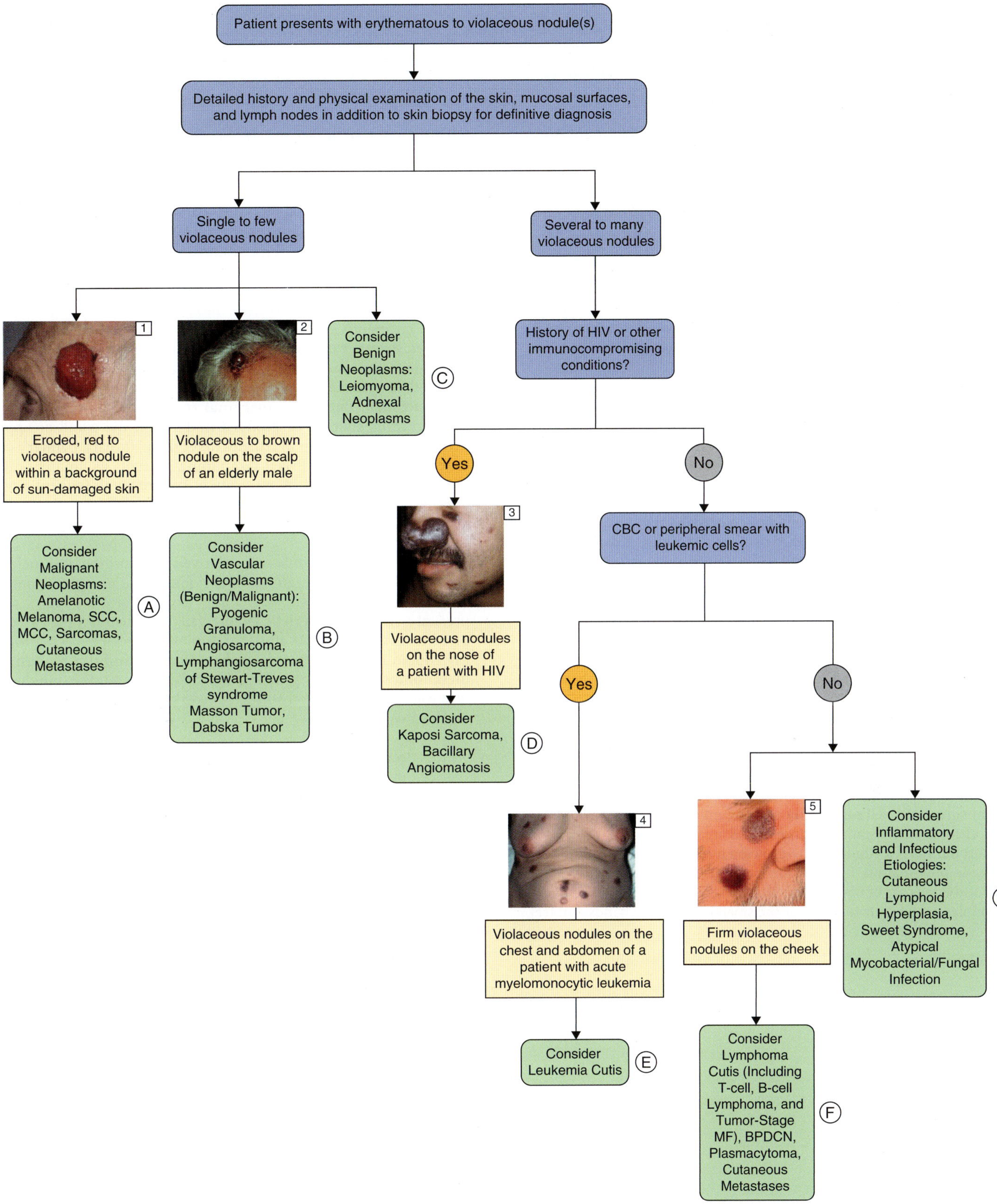
Patient presents with erythematous to violaceous nodule(s)
Detailed history and physical examination of the skin, mucosal surfaces, and lymph nodes in addition to skin biopsy for definitive diagnosis
Single to few violaceous nodules
Several to many violaceous nodules
1
Eroded, red to violaceous nodule within a background of sun-damaged skin
Consider Malignant Neoplasms: Amelanotic Melanoma, SCC, MCC, Sarcomas, Cutaneous Metastases
A
2
Violaceous to brown nodule on the scalp of an elderly male
Consider Vascular Neoplasms (Benign/Malignant): Pyogenic Granuloma, Angiosarcoma, Lymphangiosarcoma of Stewart-Treves syndrome Masson Tumor, Dabska Tumor
B
Consider Benign Neoplasms: Leiomyoma, Adnexal Neoplasms
C
History of HIV or other immunocompromising conditions?
Yes
No
3
Violaceous nodules on the nose of a patient with HIV
Consider Kaposi Sarcoma, Bacillary Angiomatosis
D
CBC or peripheral smear with leukemic cells?
Yes
No
4
Violaceous nodules on the chest and abdomen of a patient with acute myelomonocytic leukemia
Consider Leukemia Cutis
E
5
Firm violaceous nodules on the cheek
Consider Lymphoma Cutis (Including T-cell, B-cell Lymphoma, and Tumor-Stage MF), BPDCN, Plasmacytoma, Cutaneous Metastases
F
Consider Inflammatory and Infectious Etiologies: Cutaneous Lymphoid Hyperplasia, Sweet Syndrome, Atypical Mycobacterial/Fungal Infection
G

14 Hard Nodules

Katherine L. Wang and Olayemi Sokumbi

Multiple hard nodules may represent a variety of skin conditions, most notably metastases to the skin. Therefore, a thorough history needs to be elicited from any patient presenting with multiple hard nodules to rule out the possibility of dermal metastases. For patients presenting with a solitary hard nodule, refer to Chapter 15. Complete evaluation often includes biopsy with clinicopathologic correlation.

A. The initial evaluation of a patient presenting with multiple hard nodules involves a skin examination and a thorough history, including history of any malignancy. Note the clinical appearance, anatomical distribution, color, firmness, and whether the nodules are painful or pruritic. Constitutional symptoms, such as fatigue and weight loss, should be noted.

B. If the patient has a positive history of underlying malignancy, the nodules should be immediately biopsied and evaluated for the possibility of **cancer recurrence and/or metastasis**. Any malignancy can metastasize to the skin, but breast, lung, melanoma, lymphoma, and oropharyngeal cancers are most common.

C. The differential diagnosis for skin-colored hard nodules is broad and includes both benign and malignant entities. **Pilar cysts** are firm mobile nodules lacking a central punctum, classically found on the scalp. A minority of these cysts will develop into slow-growing benign tumors, and these are termed **proliferating pilar cysts**. **Hidradenomas** are slow-growing hyperpigmented nodules commonly found on the head and neck. A slowly growing nodule on the head or neck that is extremely painful is likely a **spiradenoma**. **Cylindromas** can present as coalescing nodules on the scalp with a striking turban tumor appearance.

While the aforementioned five tumors are commonly found on the head and neck, the remaining skin-colored nodules are usually found on the trunk or extremities. In **osteoma cutis**, bone grows within the skin. These lesions present as extremely hard nodules and may form secondary to inflammatory diseases, such as dermatomyositis. **Dermal squamous cell carcinoma** can present as growing scaly nodules, most commonly located in sun-exposed areas. **Dermatofibrosarcoma protuberans** is a painless slow-growing tumor that may be multinodular in presentation. It commonly occurs on the trunk. **Extraskeletal chondromas** are benign tumors that present as painless slow-growing nodules, commonly found near the small joints of the hands and feet. **Rheumatoid nodules** are firm nodules that appear near joints and are a classic symptom of rheumatoid arthritis.

D. Pink, red, or violaceous hard nodules include prurigo nodularis, Kaposi sarcoma, B-cell lymphomas, and leukemia cutis. **Prurigo nodularis** presents as highly pruritic symmetric lesions that grow in response to scratching/rubbing. **Kaposi sarcoma** should be considered in human immunodeficiency virus positive or organ transplant patients. It exhibits a wide range of cutaneous presentations, typically starting as a patch before evolving into plaques or reddish nodules.

The cutaneous B-cell lymphomas may range in color from pink to violet. **Primary cutaneous follicle center lymphoma** is the most common cutaneous B-cell lymphoma. It is present as solitary or grouped smooth nodules, typically arising on the head, neck, or trunk. **Primary cutaneous marginal zone lymphoma** may feature slow-growing, solitary, or grouped nodules on the trunk or upper extremities. Mostly seen in females older than 70 years, **primary cutaneous diffuse large B-cell lymphoma** presents as rapidly growing nodules on the legs. A minority of patients with **leukemia** will present with skin findings, potentially as asymptomatic widespread skin-colored to pink-plum nodules.

E. Hard blue or black nodules are relatively uncommon and include entities such as angiokeratomas and nodular malignant melanoma. **Angiokeratomas** are small, benign, hyperkeratotic papules that present with a characteristic "white veil" on dermoscopy. Patients presenting with multiple angiokeratomas and peripheral neuropathy should raise suspicion for **Fabry disease**. **Nodular malignant melanomas** are rapidly growing, bluish black to reddish-pink nodules found most often on sun-exposed skin. They frequently bleed and/or itch.

While this decision tree does not represent the exhaustive list of diagnoses that can present as hard nodules, it provides an approach to categorizing the diagnostic possibilities. Although morphologic classifications are beneficial, histopathologic examination remains the gold standard in diagnosing hard nodules with a degree of certainty.

See Appendix 1 for Further Reading.

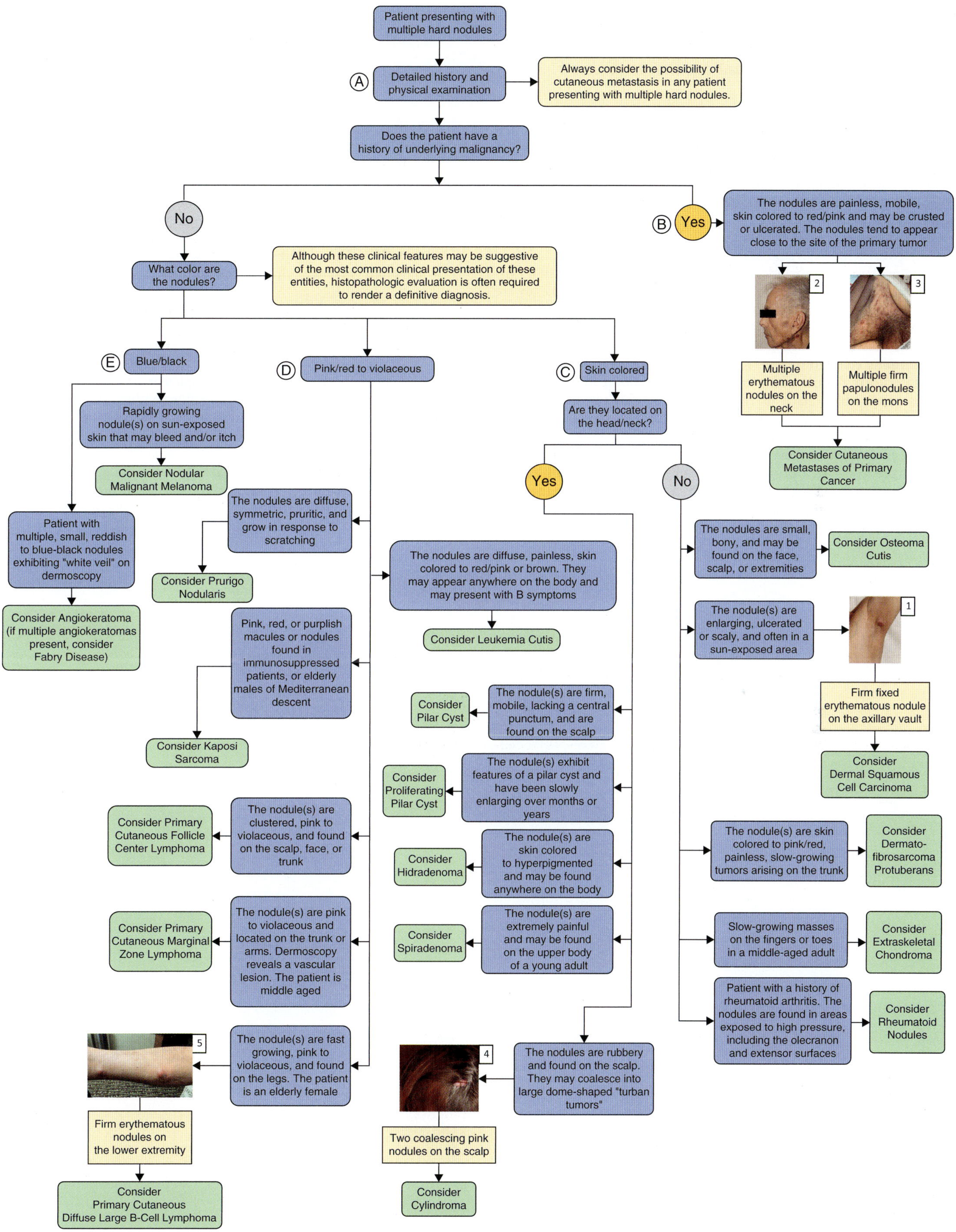
Patient presenting with multiple hard nodules
A
Detailed history and physical examination
Always consider the possibility of cutaneous metastasis in any patient presenting with multiple hard nodules.
Does the patient have a history of underlying malignancy?
No
What color are the nodules?
Although these clinical features may be suggestive of the most common clinical presentation of these entities, histopathologic evaluation is often required to render a definitive diagnosis.
B
Yes
The nodules are painless, mobile, skin colored to red/pink and may be crusted or ulcerated. The nodules tend to appear close to the site of the primary tumor
2
3
Multiple erythematous nodules on the neck
Multiple firm papulonodules on the mons
Consider Cutaneous Metastases of Primary Cancer
E
Blue/black
Rapidly growing nodule(s) on sun-exposed skin that may bleed and/or itch
Consider Nodular Malignant Melanoma
Patient with multiple, small, reddish to blue-black nodules exhibiting "white veil" on dermoscopy
Consider Angiokeratoma (if multiple angiokeratomas present, consider Fabry Disease)
D
Pink/red to violaceous
The nodules are diffuse, symmetric, pruritic, and grow in response to scratching
Consider Prurigo Nodularis
The nodules are diffuse, painless, skin colored to red/pink or brown. They may appear anywhere on the body and may present with B symptoms
Consider Leukemia Cutis
Pink, red, or purplish macules or nodules found in immunosuppressed patients, or elderly males of Mediterranean descent
Consider Kaposi Sarcoma
The nodule(s) are clustered, pink to violaceous, and found on the scalp, face, or trunk
Consider Primary Cutaneous Follicle Center Lymphoma
The nodule(s) are pink to violaceous and located on the trunk or arms. Dermoscopy reveals a vascular lesion. The patient is middle aged
Consider Primary Cutaneous Marginal Zone Lymphoma
The nodule(s) are fast growing, pink to violaceous, and found on the legs. The patient is an elderly female
5
Firm erythematous nodules on the lower extremity
Consider Primary Cutaneous Diffuse Large B-Cell Lymphoma
C
Skin colored
Are they located on the head/neck?
Yes
No
The nodule(s) are firm, mobile, lacking a central punctum, and are found on the scalp
Consider Pilar Cyst
The nodule(s) exhibit features of a pilar cyst and have been slowly enlarging over months or years
Consider Proliferating Pilar Cyst
The nodule(s) are skin colored to hyperpigmented and may be found anywhere on the body
Consider Hidradenoma
The nodule(s) are extremely painful and may be found on the upper body of a young adult
Consider Spiradenoma
The nodules are rubbery and found on the scalp. They may coalesce into large dome-shaped "turban tumors"
4
Two coalescing pink nodules on the scalp
Consider Cylindroma
The nodules are small, bony, and may be found on the face, scalp, or extremities
Consider Osteoma Cutis
The nodule(s) are enlarging, ulcerated or scaly, and often in a sun-exposed area
1
Firm fixed erythematous nodule on the axillary vault
Consider Dermal Squamous Cell Carcinoma
The nodule(s) are skin colored to pink/red, painless, slow-growing tumors arising on the trunk
Consider Dermato-fibrosarcoma Protuberans
Slow-growing masses on the fingers or toes in a middle-aged adult
Consider Extraskeletal Chondroma
Patient with a history of rheumatoid arthritis. The nodules are found in areas exposed to high pressure, including the olecranon and extensor surfaces
Consider Rheumatoid Nodules

15 Isolated Chronic Nodule

Ameije Ismaili and Olayemi Sokumbi

An isolated chronic nodule can present in a variety of forms. A thorough history is required to classify the chronicity of the nodule. Secondary characteristics of the nodule can help narrow the differential. Although distinct clinical features may help with sorting out the differential diagnosis, most isolated chronic nodules require histopathology for diagnostic confirmation.

A. Any patient may develop skin cancer, but risk factors that should heighten suspicion include a personal or family history of skin cancer, immunosuppression, or photodamage. Skin cancers typically are fast growing. A pearly nodule with telangiectasias is characteristic of **basal cell carcinoma**, while a dome-shaped nodule with a center that is ulcerated, scaly, verrucous, or eroded classically represents **squamous cell carcinoma. Keratoacanthoma** typically presents as a crateriform nodule with a keratotic core. **Nodular melanoma** may present as a blue-black or red-pink nodule that can be ulcerated, itchy, or bleed. Other nodules that may change rapidly over time include angiosarcoma, epithelioid sarcoma, and pyogenic granuloma. **Angiosarcoma** may present as a blue-black to red-pink nodule often preceded by a bruise-like appearance or edema. **Epithelioid sarcoma** is a firm skin-colored nodule typically seen in a young adult male with a nodule on the hands or wrist. **Pyogenic granuloma** is a red nodule and may be associated with pregnancy, medication, or preceding trauma. It is often associated with rapid growth and is typically surrounded by a collarette of scale. Violaceous to red rapidly changing nodules may represent lymphocytoma cutis, primary cutaneous marginal zone B-cell lymphoma (PCMZL), and primary cutaneous follicle center lymphoma (PCFCL). **Lymphocytoma cutis** may occur in the setting of irritant exposure, such as an insect bite. Histopathology reveals germinal centers with tingible body macrophages. **PCMZL** and **PCFCL** are indolent primary B-cell lymphomas, which often present as chronic red nodules.

B. The remaining nodules tend to be more slow-growing. **Angiolipoma** classically presents in young adults as a painful, skin-colored forearm nodule, while **lipomas** are typically painless.

C. Skin-colored nodules located in a periarticular area may be Dupuytren contracture or ganglion cyst. A transilluminating cyst on the dorsal aspect of the wrist favors a **ganglion cyst. Dupuytren contracture** characteristically shows pits or puckering over the palm.

D. Trichilemmal cysts present as soft, freely mobile, scalp nodules. **Epidermal inclusion cysts** are also soft and freely mobile and are the most common type of cyst.

Although these clinical features may be suggestive of the most common clinical presentation of these entities, histopathologic evaluation is often required to render a definitive diagnosis.

Patient presenting with an isolated chronic nodule

Detailed history and physical examination of the patient. Broadly assess the patient's underlying etiology and consider metastasis

Does the history reveal that the nodule has rapidly changed over time?

Yes

(A) Patient has risk factors for skin cancer such as a previous history of skin cancer (melanoma, SCC, BCC), old age, immunosuppression, and/or photodamage.

- Nodule is shiny, pearly with telangiectasias in a sun-exposed region → Consider BCC
- Non-tender, pink-red to violaceous, firm, dome-shaped nodule. It can be ulcerated and may be on the head/neck region → Consider Merkel Cell Carcinoma
- Red nodule in a Caucasian elderly patient with a dome-shaped nodule. It is most commonly located on the head and neck → Consider Atypical Fibroxanthoma
- Located in a sun-exposed area and has a core center that can be ulcerated, scaly, verrucous, or eroded. It may be painful → Consider SCC
- It has a crateriform architecture with a keratotic core → Consider Keratoacanthoma
- Blue, black, and/or pink nodule that is located in a sun-exposed region and portrays the ABCDEs →

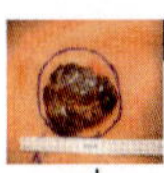

1

Brown-black multilobulated exophytic nodule on the abdomen → Consider Nodular Melanoma

- It may be located on the extremities such as the hands and wrist. It can be painful if there is nerve involvement. Positive for keratin, vimentin, and epithelial membrane antigen. Negative for S100, HMB45, CD31 → Consider Epithelioid Sarcoma
- Patient has a history of a bruise-like lesion prior to the nodule that may be located on the head or neck → Consider Angiosarcoma
- History reveals possible exposure to insect bites, metal implants, tattoos, vaccines; nodule is on the face or trunk → Consider Lymphocytoma Cutis
- Physical exam reveals nodule on the head/neck region → Consider Primary Cutaneous Follicle Center Lymphoma
- Physical exam reveals a smooth, tense, and shiny nodule that may be on the torso or upper extremities → Consider Primary Cutaneous Marginal Zone B-cell Lymphoma
- Dermoscopy reveals white linear rail lines and patient may be pregnant, have a medication adverse affect, or had recent injury to the site → Consider Pyogenic Granuloma

No

What color is the nodule? *continued on next page*

Yellow

The nodule is yellow and the patient has a history of paraproteinemia. The nodule may be ulcerated and located in the periorbital region → Consider Necrobiotic Xanthogranuloma

Skin-colored

Is it painful? (B)

Yes

- Younger adult patient with nodule on the forearms → Consider Angiolipoma
- Postmenopausal females with weakness and psychiatric symptoms → Consider Adiposis Dolorosa

No

- Soft, isolated, freely mobile nodule

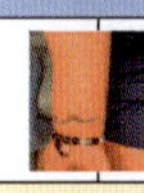

2

Skin-colored nodule on the volar forearm → Consider Lipoma

- Is it located in a periarticular area?

(C) **Yes**

- Physical exam findings show pits or puckering over the palm and the patient is unable to straighten fingers completely → Consider Dupuytren Contracture
- Physical exam shows transillumination of the nodule, and it is located on the dorsal aspect of the wrist → Consider Ganglion Cyst

No

Is it firm or soft? *continued on next page*

Soft (D)

- Physical examination shows a visible punctum on the nodule that may have a foul odor and cheesy consistency when ruptured → Consider Epidermal Inclusion Cyst
- It is located on the scalp and is freely mobile

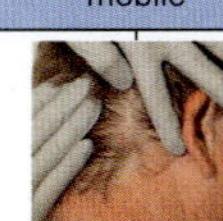

3

Skin-colored nodule on the scalp → Consider Trichilemmal Cyst

Continued

E. Giant cell tumor of tendon sheath, chondroid syringoma, epithelioid sarcoma, and **dermatofibrosarcoma protuberans (DFSP)** may present as firm skin-colored nodules. **Giant cell tumor of tendon sheath** is the most common benign tumor of the hand. **Chondroid syringomas** are often mistaken for cysts and are clinically indistinct. DFSP most commonly presents on the shoulder or pelvis region.

F. A skin-colored to red nodule may be **acanthoma fissuratum** if a glasses wearer has a nodule located on the postauricular sulcus or lateral nose with a groove or fissure. **Leiomyoma** should be considered in a patient with a movable nodule on the limbs that is sensitive after cold exposure. **Granular cell tumor** may present on the head or neck, and histology shows cells that are large, pale, and irregularly polygonal with periodic-acid Schiff (PAS)-positive granules.

G. In a middle-aged Caucasian adult with a yellow to red nodule that is located on the head or neck, consider **solitary reticulohistiocytoma**. Mucous membrane lesions may be present, and on histopathology, histiocytes demonstrate a "ground-glass" appearance.

H. Skin-colored to pink-white nodules may suggest a schwannoma or neurofibroma. A **schwannoma** may present as an asymptomatic nodule on the flexor part of an extremity, while a **neurofibroma** is a soft nodule with a clinical buttonhole sign.

I. Skin-colored to blue-black nodules may suggest a spiradenoma and trichoblastoma. **Spiradenomas** are common in young adults and often appear on the ventral upper half of the body. **Trichoblastoma** is a nodule associated with a hair follicle on the nose, face, or scalp.

J. Both hidradenoma and dermatofibroma may present as hyperpigmented nodules. **Hidradenomas** are clinically indistinctive but may be located on the head or neck. On histopathology, there are nests and nodules of large epithelial cells with abundant cytoplasm. **Dermatofibromas** frequently occur on the extremities and are easily recognized by central dimpling on lateral pressure.

K. Violaceous to red nodules may represent glomus tumor. A **glomus tumor** is usually painful and located on the subungual surface, hand, or palms.

L. A blue-black to red-pink nodule may be **intravascular papillary endothelial hyperplasia,** which is often painful and is commonly confused with angiosarcoma, but often presents around veins in the head, neck, or fingers. **Sinusoidal hemangioma** and **spindle cell hemangioma** may also present as blue-black to red-pink nodules.

See Appendix 1 for Further Reading and Image References.

- Is it firm or soft?
  - Firm (E)
    - It may be located on the hand or fingers in a middle-aged adult
      - Consider Giant Cell Tumor of Tendon Sheath
    - It may be located on the head or neck and does not have distinct clinical characteristics
      - Consider Chondroid Syringoma
    - It may be located on the trunk or proximal extremities in a young to middle-aged adult. It may turn into a violaceous to red-brown nodule

      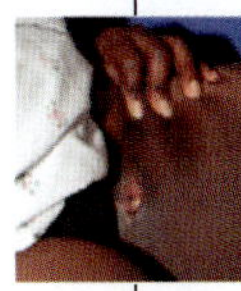

      4

      Red-brown nodule on the left medial thigh
      - Consider Dermatofibrosarcoma Protuberans

- What color is the nodule?
  - (F) Skin-colored to red
    - History reveals that the patient wears glasses and nodule is located on the postauricular surface or lateral nose

      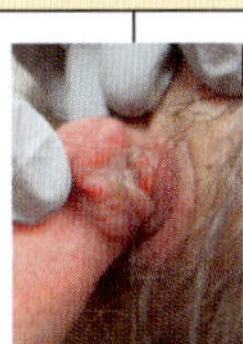

      5

      Ulcerated pink nodule with a central groove on the left postauricular sulcus
      - Consider Acanthoma Fissuratum
    - Patient has a movable nodule on the limbs with a history of pain on cold exposures
      - Consider Leiomyoma
    - Painless nodule on the head or neck
      - Consider Granular Cell Tumor
  - (G) Yellow to red
    - Most commonly in a middle-aged Caucasion adult and the nodule may be located on head or neck. Mucous membrane may have lesions
      - Consider Solitary Reticulohistiocytoma
  - (H) Skin-colored to pink to white
    - May be located on the flexor extremities
      - Consider Schwannoma
    - Soft nodule with the buttonhole sign
      - Consider Neurofibroma
  - (I) Skin-colored to blue-black
    - May be located on the ventral upper half of the body in a young adult and does not have distinct clinical characteristics
      - Consider Spiradenoma
    - Physical examination reveals association with a hair follicle and may be located on the nose or face/scalp
      - Consider Trichoblastoma
  - (J) Hyperpigmented
    - Where is it located?
      - Head and neck
        - Consider Hidradenoma
      - Lower Extremities
        - Physical exam reveals "dimple sign"
          - Consider Dermatofibroma
  - (K) Violaceous to red
    - May be located on the subungual surface, hand, or palms; can be painful
      - Consider Glomus Tumor
  - (L) Blue-black to red-pink
    - It may be located in the veins of the head, neck, or fingers and can be painful
      - Consider Intravascular Papillary Endothelial Hyperplasia
    - It may be located on the distal extremities and is firm
      - Consider Spindle Cell Hemangioma
    - It may be located on the breast or extremities

      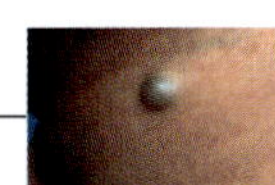

      6

      Bluish, compressible, well-demarcated nodule
      - Consider Sinusoidal Hemangioma

16 Acute or Recurrent Nodules

Milad Torabi and Maria Aleshin

A. The initial evaluation of a patient presenting with acute onset of nodules requires a detailed clinical history (including a history of recent infections, trauma), medication review, past medical history (to assess for associated conditions such as inflammatory bowel disease and malignancy), as well as a thorough physical examination to determine the morphology, secondary features (ulceration, drainage), and distribution of the lesions. There may be accompanying extracutaneous symptoms, such as abdominal pain, that may be more suggestive of a given etiology (e.g., pancreatic panniculitis). Often a biopsy for histopathology (with or without tissue culture) is needed alongside a thorough clinical history and physical examination to make the diagnosis.

B. **Infectious panniculitis** can occur secondary to direct inoculation or hematogenous spread of a microorganism. It is more commonly observed in immunocompromised patients with fever. When an infectious panniculitis is suspected, biopsies should be performed for both histopathology and tissue culture.

C. **Subcutaneous sweet syndrome** also often occurs in febrile immunocompromised patients and is associated with myelodysplastic syndrome, plasma cell dyscrasias, and leukemia. Consider this etiology in the appropriate clinical context once an infection has been ruled out.

D. Consider **medication-induced panniculitis** when lesions develop shortly after starting a new drug with improvement on cessation of the offending agent. Causative agents include oral contraceptive pills, antibiotics, leukotriene modifiers, small molecule inhibitors (BRAF inhibitors), and systemic steroids.

E. Patients presenting with tender nodules (occasionally ulcerative and draining oily brown liquid) on their lower extremities (although other areas may be affected) may have **pancreatic panniculitis** due to known or not yet diagnosed pancreatic disease, including cancer. **Alpha-1 antitrypsin deficiency panniculitis** can also present with ulcerative nodules draining oily material; however, distribution differs with a predilection for the lower trunk and thighs. It should be suspected in patients with a history of alpha-1 antitrypsin deficiency or in patients with emphysema and liver cirrhosis.

F. **Erythema induratum** is a rare form of panniculitis that occurs most commonly in adult females and presents with erythematous, tender, occasionally ulcerated nodules, classically occurring on the calves. It is often associated with tuberculosis; however, it can also be seen in the setting of other diseases, medications, or be idiopathic.

G. **Polyarteritis nodosa (PAN)** is a rare multisystem disorder characterized by small- and medium-vessel vasculitis. The cause of PAN is most often idiopathic but can be triggered by infections such as hepatitis B. Patients can present with fever, weight loss, malaise, and arthralgias with peripheral neuropathy and motor deficits. Cutaneous manifestations of PAN include palpable purpura (favoring the lower extremities) and erythematous nodules, which can ulcerate. Background livedo reticularis can also be seen.

H. **Primary cutaneous γ/δ T-cell lymphoma** is a rare type of lymphoma presenting in adults as rapidly progressive ulcerating and necrotic plaques that favor the extremities. Mucosal surfaces can be affected. Patients may present with fever, night sweats, and weight loss.

The remaining entities discussed on page 4 only rarely present with ulcerations or drainage, but please note that entities E to H do not always present with this morphology and can also present simply as nodules.

Patient presents with erythematous nodule(s) and/or plaque(s) (often painful)

(A) Detailed clinical history and physical examination +/– biopsy

Does patient have a history of immunosuppression or underlying malignancy and have fevers?

- Yes → Can infectious etiology be ruled out?
  - No → (B) Consider Infectious Panniculitis
  - Yes → (C) Consider Subcutaneous Sweet Syndrome
- No → Is there a causative relationship illustrated by previous drug intake and improvement on cessation?
  - Yes → (D) Consider Medication-Induced Panniculitis
  - No → Do the lesions favor the shins?
    - Yes → *continued on next page*
    - No → Does the lesion have ulceration +/– drainage?
      - Yes → Do the lesions have oily drainage?
        - Yes → Lesions occasionally ulcerated and draining oily brown liquid. Patient has a history of pancreatitis (acute or chronic) or pancreatic cancer. Can present with abdominal pain and/or joint pain

          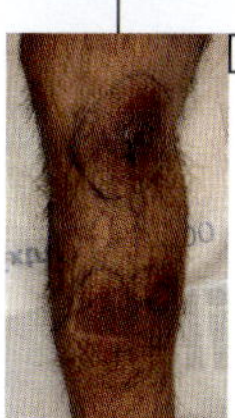

          Purpuric, tender, ulcerated nodules on the lower leg.

          → (E) Consider Pancreatic Panniculitis
        - Yes → Lesion on the trunk and proximal extremities (flanks, buttock, thighs). Occasionally ulcerated and draining oily material. History of liver cirrhosis and/or emphysema → (E) Consider Alpha-1 Antitrypsin Deficiency Panniculitis
        - No → Do the lesion favor the calves?
          - Yes → Lesion on the lower legs, particularly the calves. Occasionally ulcerated. Patient is often a women with a history of *Mycobacterium tuberculosis* infection

            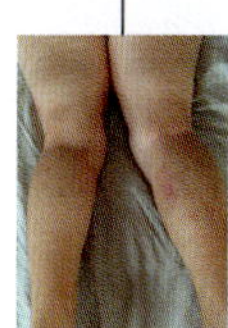

            Erythematous tender nodules on the bilateral calves.

            → (F) Consider Erythema Induratum
          - No → Are there livedo reticularis and palpable purpura?
            - Yes → Lesions include palpable purpura, nodules +/– ulceration, predominantly on the lower limbs frequently with livedo reticularis. Often accompanied by fevers, weight loss, arthralgias → (G) Consider Polyarteritis Nodosa
            - No → Lesions mostly on extremities. Can affect extranodal sites such as mucosa but spares the reticuloendothelial system → (H) Consider Primary Cutaneous γ/δ T-Cell Lymphoma

Continued

I. **Erythema nodosum** is one of the most common panniculitides. It presents as tender nonulcerated nodules on the bilateral shins, occasionally accompanied by joint pain. It is most often idiopathic but can be triggered by infections, medications, and chronic inflammatory diseases.

J. **Lipodermatosclerosis** is a panniculitis that develops secondary to chronic venous insufficiency. It classically presents as painful erythematous and indurated plaques with hyperpigmentation starting on the medial lower legs. There may be associated lower leg edema and varicosities. Consider these etiologies when patients have risk factors for venous insufficiency such as a history of smoking, prior DVTs, preexisting varicose veins, obesity, and a sedentary lifestyle.

K. Consider **lupus panniculitis** in patients, especially females, with a history of systemic lupus erythematosus and accompanying indurated erythematous nodules or plaques involving the face, trunk, proximal extremities, or buttocks (rarely the lower extremities). Once healed, these lesions can leave atrophic scars. Similarly, **subcutaneous panniculitis-like T-cell lymphoma (SPTCL)**, a rare cutaneous T-cell lymphoma, presents with indurated erythematous nodules or plaques that cause residual lipoatrophy on resolution. It is also associated with autoimmune conditions. However, SPTCL is less likely to develop lesions on the face, and patients present with constitutional symptoms, elevated erythrocyte sedimentation rate, and leukopenia.

L. Trauma to the skin can damage the subcutaneous fat and cause **traumatic panniculitis**. Cold panniculitis primarily occurs in young children exposed to cold climates and often presents with erythematous nodules and plaques in areas susceptible to decreased blood flow, such as the cheeks. Factitial panniculitis results from the injection of a foreign substance into the subcutaneous fat and should be considered when lesions occur in atypical locations.

See Appendix 1 for Further Reading and Image References.

Do the lesions favor the shins?

Yes

Bilateral lesions favoring shins in a young person. Triggered by infection, drugs, chronic inflammatory disease, or idiopathic

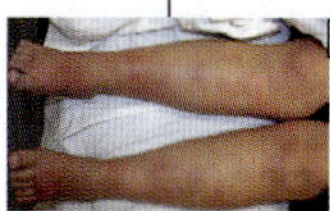

3

Erythematous, tender, nonulcerated nodules on the shins.

(I) Consider Erythema Nodosum

No → Do the lesions favor the face?

No

Lesions favor the lower leg above the medial malleolus. Associated with stasis changes (hemosiderin deposits; red-brown colored induration)

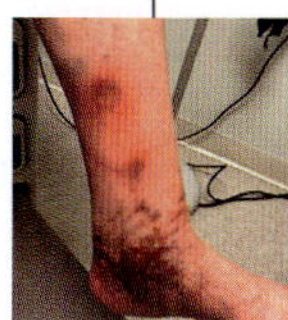

5

Tender erythematous nodules on the medial lower leg with background stasis changes and varicosities.

(J) Consider Lipodermatosclerosis

Deeply seated plaques involving the trunk and extremities that develop lipoatrophy after resolution. Constitutional symptoms may be observed

(K) Consider Subcutaneous Panniculitis-Like T-Cell Lymphoma

Lesion(s) preceded by a traumatic insult

(L) Consider Traumatic Panniculitis

Yes

Lesions favor proximal extremities and face and often precedes manifestation of SLE. Lesions heal with atrophic scarring. Female predominant

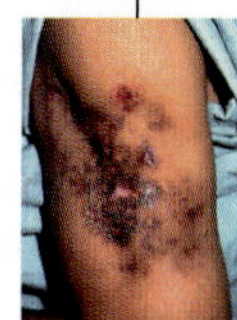

4

Hyperpigmented atrophic plaques on the proximal upper extremity.

(K) Consider Lupus Panniculitis

17 Diffuse Chronic Nodules

Henna Hundal and Maria Aleshin

For a patient presenting with diffuse chronic nodules, the recommended workup includes obtaining a detailed clinical history, including the frequency of scratching/rubbing, a past medical history, and a medication reconciliation. Close examination looking for blisters, burrows, and other clues can often provide the astute practitioner with the correct diagnosis. A skin biopsy should be considered if there is diagnostic uncertainty.

A. If the patient appears to present with both diffuse chronic nodules and blisters, **pemphigoid nodularis**, a rare nodular variant of bullous pemphigoid, may be considered. Pemphigoid nodularis typically presents with hyperkeratotic pruritic nodules resembling lesions seen in prurigo nodularis, while being accompanied by the blisters seen in classic bullous pemphigoid that are often distributed on the extremities and trunk. Blisters may not be apparent at all times.

B. *Sarcoptes scabiei* exposure can lead to the development of **nodular scabies**, a clinical variant of scabies that presents with strongly pruritic nodules with a predilection for the genitalia and scrotum. Other hallmark features of scabies infection, such as the presence of burrows or an eczematous morphology, can aid in the diagnosis. Patients should be evaluated for risk factors associated with scabies exposure, such as residence in a nursing home or other crowded living conditions.

C. **Reactive perforating collagenosis** is a rare autosomal dominant or autosomal recessive perforating dermatoses, which usually presents as pruritic variably sized papules and nodules with a central keratotic core, commonly present on the hands, elbows, and knees (although widespread involvement can occur). There is often a history of childhood lesions, and papules and nodules often develop after trauma or rubbing.

D. **Kyrle disease**, a subtype of an acquired perforating dermatosis, should be considered in patients with underlying kidney disease or diabetes mellitus. It is characterized by the transepidermal elimination of keratin. Patients present with strongly pruritic papulonodules with a central keratin plug, often distributed on the extensor surfaces of the lower extremities. However, lesions can be more widely distributed.

E. Multiple keratoacanthomas, which are often characterized by their umbilicated nature, can be seen due to various underlying disorders. **Ferguson-Smith syndrome** is an autosomal dominant disorder that typically presents in adolescence/early adulthood and is characterized by up to a hundred keratoacanthoma lesions (although some patients only develop one or two lesions). Lesions often occur on sun-exposed areas, although any site may be involved; they often spontaneously resolve and heal with deep scarring. **Generalized eruptive keratoacanthomas of Grzybowski** is a rare sporadic condition that presents in adulthood and is characterized by the sudden onset of numerous keratoacanthomas ranging from hundreds to thousands. Lesions are often small, pruritic, umbilicated, skin colored, contain a central keratotic core, and are distributed on the trunk and extremities, although mucosal (tongue, buccal mucosa, larynx) and intertriginous involvement may also occur.

F. If some or all lesions in a patient with diffuse nodules have a verrucous appearance, one should consider hypertrophic lichen planus and hypertrophic lupus erythematosus. **Hypertrophic lichen planus** presents with strongly pruritic, brown/violaceous, verrucous lesions typically on the lower extremities. **Hypertrophic lupus erythematosus**, a rare subset of lupus erythematosus, is characterized by chronic verrucous lesions, often presenting on the upper extremities and head.

G. Patients with a known history of malignancy or immunosuppression or those who present with concurrent fevers or other "B symptoms" and diffuse nodules should raise suspicion for an infectious etiology or cutaneous lymphoma of the skin. A biopsy for histopathology and tissue culture (bacteria, acid-fast bacilli, and fungal) is often required in these cases to distinguish between these two categories. **Cutaneous lymphomas** may be localized or may present with diffuse erythematous/violaceous papules, nodules, and tumors with occasional central ulceration and necrosis. **Infectious etiologies** should also be considered in patients presenting with diffuse nodules and underlying immunosuppression and/or fevers. Particular attention should be paid to the distribution of the lesions. If a sporotrichoid (lymphocutaneous) distribution to the lesions is observed, the differential for infectious causes includes sporotrichosis, pyogenic bacteria, tuberculosis, leishmaniasis, glanders, cat scratch disease, and anthrax, among others.

H. **Prurigo nodularis** presents with extremely pruritic papules that evolve into nodules over time, with lesions often distributed in easily accessible areas and sparing the upper-mid back. Prurigo nodularis can be seen in patients with underlying kidney disease or diabetes, but it has also been linked to other underlying conditions that can cause pruritus and/or a desire to scratch and rub the skin.

In many cases, patients with diffuse nodules require a biopsy and tissue culture for diagnosis. While the above represent some helpful clues to guide the differential, there are a myriad of other diagnostic possibilities not described here, including sarcoidosis, pseudolymphoma due to drugs, diffuse leiomyomas due to Reed syndrome, and nodular syphilis, to name a few.

See Appendix 1 for Further Reading and Image References.

Patient has broadly distributed nodules that have been present for several months

Does the patient have presence of other morphologies on examination?

Yes

- Burrows or eczematous morphology
  - Nodules and papules typically found on genitalia and scrotum. Strongly pruritic.

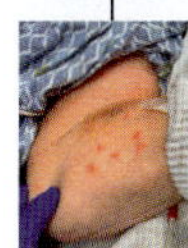

1

  - Pruritic erythematous nodules on the upper extremity
  - Consider Nodular Scabies (B)
- Blisters
  - Features of prurigo nodularis and bullous pemphigoid.
  - Consider Pemphigoid Nodularis (A)

No

Do the lesions have a central keratotic core or umbilication?

No

Are some or all lesions verrucous?

(F) **Yes** — Are some or all lesions purple and/or brown and mostly on the shins?

- **Yes**
  - Lesions are verrucous, brown, violaceous, lichenified, and on lower legs.

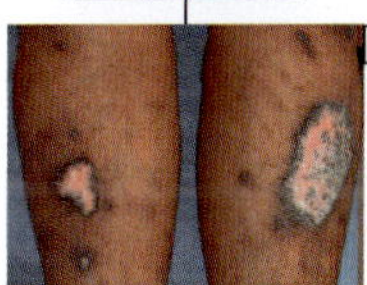

4

  - Verrucous hyperpigmented lichenified plaques on the shins
  - Consider Hypertrophic Lichen Planus
- **No**
  - Verrucous plaques typically found on the upper extremities and head.
  - Consider Hypertrophic Lupus Erythematosus

No — Does the patient have a history of immunosuppression or underlying malignancy and/or fevers?

- (G) **Yes**
  - Localized or diffuse pink-violaceous papules, nodules, tumors +/- central ulceration and necrosis.
    - Consider Lymphoma, Leukemia, and Other Metastasis
  - Can be sporotrichoid or more diffusely distributed.
    - Consider Infectious Etiology (Deep Fungal, Tuberculosis, Atypical Mycobacteria, etc.)
- (H) **No**
  - Often with secondary scale, crust, or ulceration. Spares the upper back. Strongly pruritic.

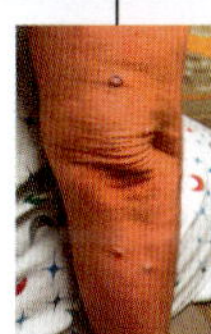

5

  - Diffusely scattered hyperpigmented keratotic papules and nodules
  - Consider Prurigo Nodularis

Yes

Keratotic — Developed in childhood?

- **Yes**
  - Pruritic papules and nodules with central keratotic core, arising after superficial trauma. Often on the upper extremities. Lesions present in childhood.

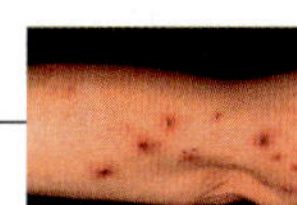

2

  - Scattered erythematous papules and nodules with central crust on the arm
  - Consider Reactive Perforating Collagenosis (C)
- **No**
  - Most common on the legs. Often with central keratotic core. Extensor surfaces favored. Often seen in patients with history of kidney disease or diabetes.

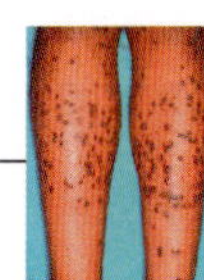

3

  - Pruritic papules and nodules with central keratotic core on the lower legs
  - Consider Acquired Perforating Disorder/ Kyrle Disease (D)

(E) **Umbilicated**

- Generalized
  - Generalized eruption (sometimes thousands) of dome-shaped papules and larger nodules in adulthood. Oral mucosa and larynx may be affected.
  - Consider Generalized Eruptive Keratoacanthomas of Grzybowski
- Limited
  - Oftentimes +family history. Few to hundred small red macules evolving into papules and nodules. Often on sites of trauma or sun-exposed areas. Heal spontaneously with scarring.
  - Consider Ferguson-Smith Syndrome

PART V
Vesicles/Bullae

18 Localized Vesicles/Bullae

Sophia Ly and Henry K. Wong

Localized vesiculobullous rashes may present in a variety of infectious, reactive, and autoimmune conditions. While several skin disorders may atypically manifest with blistering, this chapter focuses on common presentations of localized vesicles or bullae and common clinical clues that aid in diagnosis. Alongside diagnostic workup, management should broadly involve addressing the underlying etiology and symptomatic treatment (e.g., topical steroids).

A. Evaluation of a patient presenting with a localized vesiculobullous rash should begin with a detailed history, including comorbidities, drug intake, duration, and initial symptoms, and a thorough physical examination. The morphology, distribution, size, and evolution of lesions can help narrow the differential diagnoses. Some vesiculobullous rashes have preceding prodromes, including pruritis, burning pain, or systemic symptoms. Vesiculobullous presentations that are difficult to distinguish may require additional diagnostic testing, including skin biopsy, patch testing, or serological tests.

B. Patients with local bacterial skin infections may develop blistering lesions in rare or more severe cases. A visible break in the skin and systemic symptoms may be associated with these infections. **Bullous impetigo** should be suspected in children with flaccid bullae and minimal erythema, erosions with honey-colored crust, and collarette-like desquamation. An erythematous, edematous, tender unilateral plaque raises concern for **bullous erysipelas** or **cellulitis**, in which the latter lacks sharp margins and involves deeper tissues. **Bullous tinea** most commonly affects the feet and presents as an erythematous plaque with serous fluid-filled bullae.

C. A pruritic vesiculobullous eruption localized to the site of contact with an allergen or irritant is characteristic of **contact dermatitis**. Allergic contact dermatitis (ACD) causes a delayed vesicular rash after exposure to a sensitized allergen. In contrast, irritant contact dermatitis (ICD) manifests more immediately and is less likely to present with vesicles. ACD and ICD may sometimes be difficult to distinguish, in which case, patch testing may be necessary. Photocontact dermatitis is an allergic reaction to combined chemical and light exposure.

D. Chronic and relapsing eruptions of highly pruritic coin-shaped lesions are characteristic of **nummular eczema**. Acutely inflamed lesions develop vesicles and weeping. Nummular eczema usually occurs on the extremities of patients with diffusely dry skin or a history of atopic dermatitis.

E. In a patient with an acute, recurrent vesiculobullous rash localized to the hands or feet, consider a diagnosis of **dyshidrotic eczema**. Dyshidrotic eczema presents with sudden episodes of small, firm, and intensely pruritic vesicles, most commonly on the sides of the fingers and toes. Patients typically have a history of atopic or contact dermatitis.

F. **Insect bites** may present as vesiculobullous eruptions, typically on exposed skin. Characteristic lesion patterns, such as the "breakfast, lunch, and dinner" sign of three or more bites in a linear array or cluster after staying in a hotel or shelter, support the diagnosis of insect bites, particularly from fleas or bedbugs. Severe vesiculobullous reactions to insect bites may be associated with human immunodeficiency virus, Epstein-Barr virus, and hematologic malignancies.

G. **Localized bullous pemphigoid (LBP)** is an unusual form of bullous pemphigoid (BP). Like generalized BP, LBP commonly occurs in older adults and initially presents with intense pruritis followed by the development of tense fluid-filled bullae. LBP may occur at areas of trauma (surgical or accidental) and colostomy sites. Workup includes biopsy, direct immunofluorescence, and serological testing.

H. The following diagnoses should be considered in patients with bullae on normal-appearing skin localized to dependent sites. **Bullosis diabeticorum** is a complication of diabetes mellitus that manifests as sudden-onset, large tense bullae in the feet or hands. Blisters on pressure sites in comatose or chronically immobilized patients are likely **coma blisters**. During acute exacerbations of edema, patients with chronic venous insufficiency or cardiac insufficiency may develop **edema blisters** or tense bullae that respond with resolution of underlying edema.

I. In elderly or immunocompromised patients, a unilateral painful vesicular rash along a dermatome should raise concern for **herpes zoster**. Eruptions are preceded by burning or stabbing pain and progress to form grouped vesicles on a faint red base. Herpes zoster ophthalmicus is a form of herpes zoster that causes rash overlying the V1 dermatome and/or serious eye symptoms, such as keratitis, uveitis, or optic nerve palsies. Prompt evaluation and treatment can help reduce the severity of symptoms and risk of complications, which include postherpetic neuralgia, cranial neuropathies, polyneuritis, meningitis, and encephalitis.

J. Grouped vesicles on an erythematous base with prodromal pain and burning may also indicate **herpes simplex virus (HSV)**. HSV-1 infections typically affect the oral cavity and lips (e.g., herpes labialis), while HSV-2 localizes to anogenital areas. Lesions of HSV recur in the same sites as previous episodes. HSV may also manifest as erythema multiforme, characterized by "target" lesions with dark, occasionally bullous, centers.

K. **Fixed drug eruption** presents as singular or few round, well-demarcated violaceous macules, which may develop central blisters. Lesions characteristically recur in the same site on reexposure to the offending medication. Common culprits include antibiotics, nonsteroidal antiinflammatory drugs, and anticonvulsants. Lesions form within 48 hours of drug intake and resolve after discontinuation of the offending drug.

L. Bullous neutrophilic dermatoses, such as **bullous pyoderma gangrenosum (PG)** and **bullous Sweet syndrome (SS)**, should be considered in a febrile patient who presents with a rapidly developing tender erythematous rash. Bullous PG is a clinical variant of PG that manifests as painful superficial ulcers with blue-gray bullae and possible necrosis. The bullous variant of PG may localize to the face or upper extremities, particularly the dorsal hands. Bullous SS presents as tender papules or plaques with bullae, most commonly on the upper extremities, neck, or face. Bullous SS may cause ulcerations, similar to bullous PG. Bullous PG is variably considered a form of SS due to overlapping features. Pathergy is a sign of both PG and SS, in which lesions develop at sites of minor trauma. Bullous PG and bullous SS are usually associated with systemic disease or malignancy, warranting appropriate workup. The main treatments for bullous PG and bullous SS include corticosteroids and management of any underlying disorder or malignancy.

See Appendix 1 for Further Reading and Image References.

- Patient presenting with localized vesiculobullous rash
- (A) Detailed history and physical examination of skin, nails, lymph nodes, and mucosal surfaces to discover underlying etiology
  - → Management broadly involves addressing the underlying etiology and symptomatic treatment (e.g., topical steroids)
- Does the patient have signs of skin infection (e.g. erythema, edema, warmth, pain, pus, crust) +/– fever or other systemic symptoms?
  - **Yes** → Consider Bullous Skin Infections (e.g., Erysipelas, Impetigo, Tinea) (B) → Assess severity and treat appropriately (e.g., topical or systemic antibiotics)
  - **No** → Is the rash intensely pruritic?
    - **Yes**
      - Recent skin exposure to irritant or allergen causing acute rash confined to area of skin contact → 1 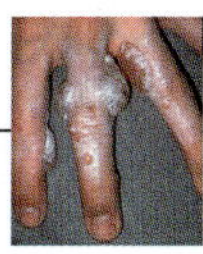 → Tense bullae with underlying erythema on the fingers → Consider Contact Dermatitis (C)
      - Chronic and relapsing coin-shaped plaques in a patient with diffusely dry skin → 2 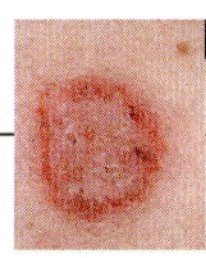 → Vesicles and papules coalescing into a coin-shaped plaque → Consider Nummular Eczema (D)
      - Episodes of intensely pruritic firm vesicles on the palms, fingers, or soles → 3 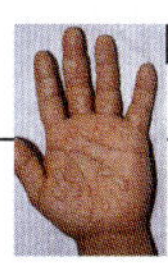 → Firm vesicles on palm and fingers → Consider Dyshidrotic Eczema (E)
      - Witnessed insect bite, high-risk exposures (wooded areas), or visible bite signs on the exposed skin → 4 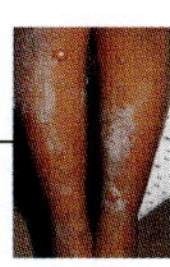 → Thick-walled vesicles and bullae on erythematous base on the lower legs → Consider Insect Bites (F)
      - Elderly patients with tense fluid-filled blisters with preceding intense pruritis on areas of trauma (surgical or accidental) or colostomy sites → Consider Localized Bullous Pemphigoid and Other Autoimmune Blistering Disorders (G)
    - **No** → Is the rash painful or burning?
      - **No** → Bullae on normal-appearing skin localized to dependent sites → Consider Bullosis Diabeticorum, Coma Blisters, or Edema Blisters (H)
      - **Yes**
        - Age >50 with fever, malaise, and vesicles along dermatome(s) that began as burning pain and/or erythematous papules → 5 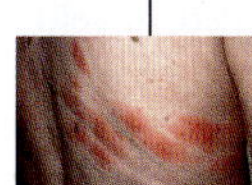 → Erythematous plaque with vesicles along dermatome → Consider Herpes Zoster (I)
        - Prodrome of fever, malaise, and grouped vesicles on an erythematous base; usually affects the oral, orbital, and genital areas → 6 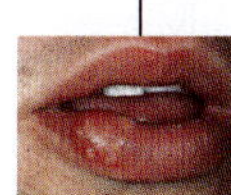 → Grouped vesicles on an erythematous base on the lips → Consider Herpes Simplex (J)
        - Round well-demarcated violaceous plaques with central blistering that recur at the same site upon re-exposure to the causative agent → 7 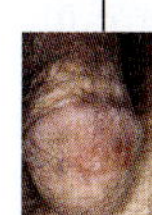 → Erythematous plaque with central blistering on the penis → Consider Fixed Drug Eruption (K)
        - Tender bullae and ulcers with necrotic borders +/- history of systemic disease or hematologic malignancy → 8 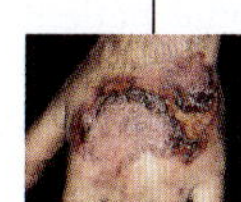 → Ulcer with necrosis and bulla, blue-gray margin on the dorsal hand → Consider Bullous Neutrophilic Dermatoses (L)

19 Generalized Vesicles and Bullae

Zachary D. Wendland and Noah Goldfarb

In this chapter, we provide a clinical approach to the diagnosis of conditions characterized by vesicles and bullae involving the skin and mucous membranes.

A. Evaluation of vesiculobullous eruptions begin with a detailed medical history and physical examination. Most immunobullous eruptions also require histopathology, direct and indirect immunofluorescence, and serology testing to confirm the diagnosis.

B. First, identify the primary lesion morphology: flaccid bullae, tense bullae, or vesicles.

C. For generalized vesiculobullous eruptions composed primarily of flaccid bullae, evaluate for prominent mucosal involvement.

D. Conditions typically lacking prominent mucosal involvement, including **multifocal bullous fixed drug eruption (FDE)**, **pemphigus foliaceus (PF)**, and **staphylococcal scalded skin syndrome (SSSS)**, can usually be differentiated clinically by their morphology and distribution.

Multifocal bullous FDE is a drug eruption recurring in the same area(s) on subsequent exposures. It presents as diffusely scattered, well-demarcated, circular or oval-shaped, targetoid patches that evolve into edematous plaques with an outer rim of erythema and a central dusky area forming bullae. Rarely mucosal lesions can occur.

PF presents with scattered crusted erosions in a seborrheic distribution (i.e., face, scalp, upper chest, and back). PF can progress to exfoliative erythroderma. Vesicles and bullae are rare, but when present, are flaccid and easily rupture (Nikolsky sign).

SSSS presents as painful, macular erythema in skin folds and perianal area that generalizes over 48 hours. Erythematous areas may become wrinkled in appearance and form flaccid bullae. Radial fissuring and crusting often develop around the eyes, nose, and mouth. Risk factors include immunosuppression and conditions associated with impaired renal clearance of toxin (e.g., infants less than 3 months of age, adults with kidney disease).

E. In patients with generalized flaccid bullae and prominent mucosal involvement, it is also important to evaluate for erosive cheilitis, with swelling, redness, erosions/ulcerations, as well as hemorrhagic and purulent exudate and crusting of the lips. While **pemphigus vulgaris (PV)** can involve the lips, severe erosive cheilitis is typically absent. PV presents with painful erosions involving the oral mucosa. While some patients only have mucosal involvement, most also develop painful cutaneous flaccid bullae (Nikolsky sign) and crusting developing on erythematous or normal-appearing skin, sparing the palms and soles. Rarely mucous membrane involvement is absent, making it difficult to distinguish PV from multifocal bullous FDE and, more rarely, PF.

The differential diagnosis of erosive cheilitis in patients with generalized flaccid bullae includes **bullous erythema multiforme (EM), reactive infectious mucocutaneous eruption (RIME), Stevens-Johnson syndrome/toxic epidermal necrolysis (SJS/TEN),** and **paraneoplastic pemphigus (PNP).**

F. **Bullous EM** presents with persistent or recurrent typical or atypical target lesions distributed symmetrically with a preponderance for the palms, soles, and extensor extremities. Typical target lesions are papules or plaques with three concentric zones of color; an outer ring of erythema surrounding an edematous region of pallor and a central dusky area forming bullae. The presence of typical target lesions is helpful in differentiating bullous EM from other flaccid bullous eruptions with erosive cheilitis.

G. History is important in differentiating between RIME (infection), SJS/TEN (new drug), and PNP (malignancy).

RIME is a mucocutaneous reaction to an infection, most commonly *Mycoplasma pneumoniae*. RIME has prominent mucosal involvement, typically with two or more mucosal sites involved. Oral involvement with erosive cheilitis is present in almost all patients. The second most common site involved is the eyes. Cutaneous findings are usually minimal or absent, but when present, a few vesiculobullous or targetoid lesions on the trunk and extremities may be noted, mimicking bullous EM, SJS/TEN, and PNP.

SJS/TEN is a severe adverse drug eruption representing the spectrum of epidermal necrolysis based on the extent of body surface area with epidermal detachment (<10% [SJS]; 10%–30% [SJS-TEN overlap]; >30% [TEN]). SJS/TEN typically occurs within 1 to 4 weeks after starting a new medication with erythematous macules and patches on the face and upper trunk. Macules and patches may develop into atypical targetoid lesions or coalesce into ill-defined diffuse erythematous patches that become painful, dusky, and/or purpuric and progress to epidermal detachment (Nikolsky sign). Prominent mucosal involvement occurs in almost all patients; 90% having oral involvement, typically with erosive cheilitis. In patients without recent initiation of a drug, consider conditions associated with TEN-like eruptions, including systemic lupus erythematosus (SLE), acute graft-versus-host disease, and PNP.

All patients with **PNP** present with prominent painful mucositis, most commonly with severe erosive cheilitis, stomatitis, and glossitis. Oral mucosal involvement is the initial presentation in over half of patients with PNP. In two-thirds of cases, malignancy precedes symptoms. The morphology of cutaneous findings associated with PNP is highly variable; most commonly flaccid bullae mimicking PV, targetoid lesions mimicking EM, or a lichenoid eruption mimicking lichen planus (LP); less commonly tense bullae, generalized morbilliform or lichenoid exanthems, or widespread flaccid bullae mimicking SJS/TEN.

H. For patients presenting with primarily tense bullae, mucous membrane involvement can again be helpful in differentiating these conditions. **Mucous membrane pemphigoid (MMP)** presents with prominent mucosal involvement, most notably the oral mucosa with buccal erosions and desquamative gingivitis, and scarring (e.g., conjunctival symblepharon). The majority of cases only involve the mucous membranes (75%), but in cases with cutaneous involvement, tense bullae most commonly present on the head, neck, and upper trunk. Other conditions that mimic MMP include mucous membrane epidermolysis bullosa acquisita (MM-EBA) and p200 bullous pemphigoid (BP), but both are rare.

I. Certain aspects of the medical history (e.g., history of LP, chronic lymphocytic leukemia [CLL], SLE, and pregnancy) can also be helpful in the diagnosis of eruptions composed of tense bullae.

Pemphigoid gestationis presents with new-onset tense bullae in the second or third trimester of pregnancy, most commonly starting in the periumbilical area. Bullae may spread to all body areas, including the palms and soles. It typically remits prior to delivery and worsens with subsequent pregnancies.

Continued

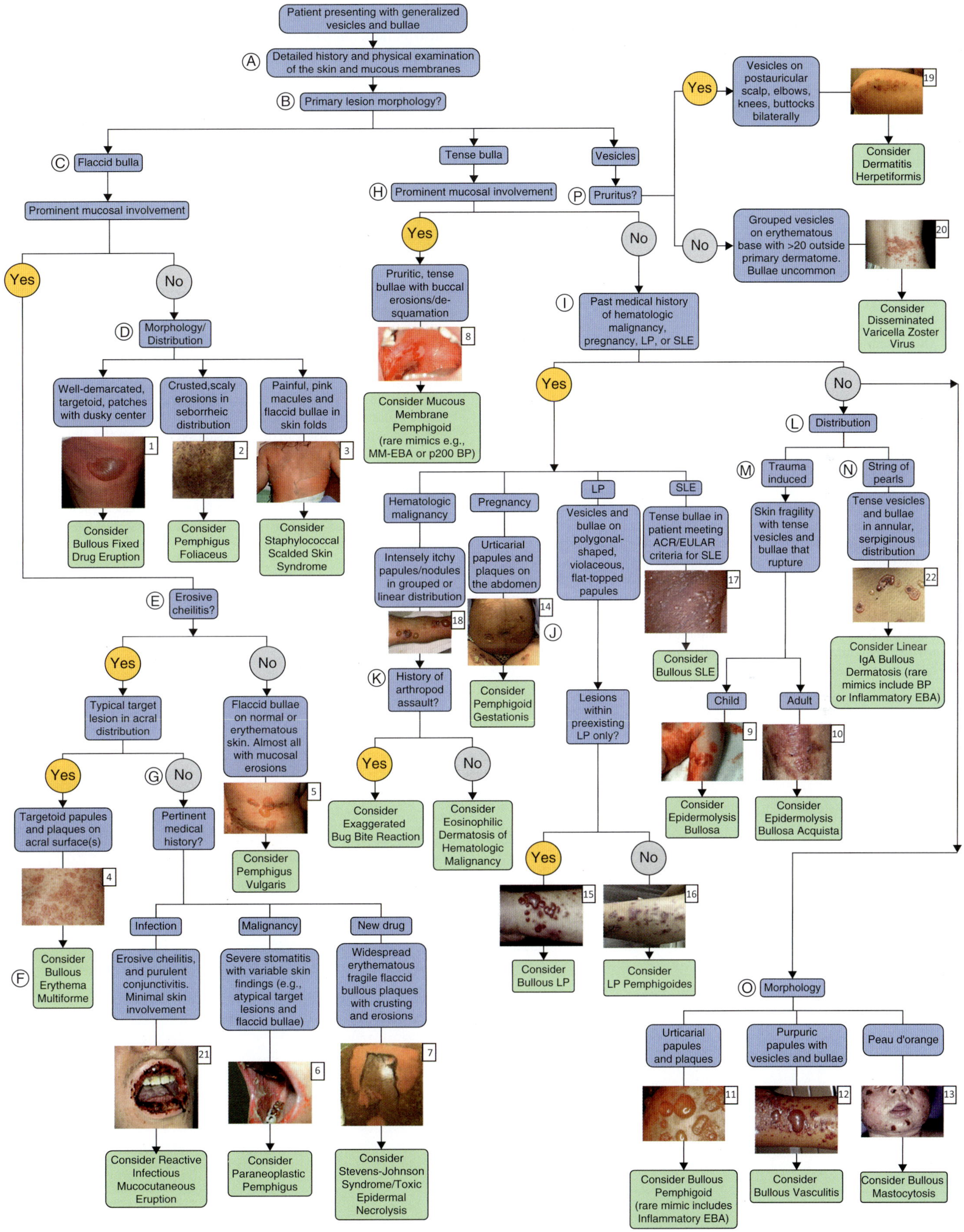
Patient presenting with generalized vesicles and bullae
A
Detailed history and physical examination of the skin and mucous membranes
B
Primary lesion morphology?
C
Flaccid bulla
Prominent mucosal involvement
Yes
No
D
Morphology/ Distribution
Well-demarcated, targetoid, patches with dusky center
1
Consider Bullous Fixed Drug Eruption
Crusted,scaly erosions in seborrheic distribution
2
Consider Pemphigus Foliaceus
Painful, pink macules and flaccid bullae in skin folds
3
Consider Staphylococcal Scalded Skin Syndrome
E
Erosive cheilitis?
Yes
Typical target lesion in acral distribution
Yes
Targetoid papules and plaques on acral surface(s)
4
F
Consider Bullous Erythema Multiforme
G
No
Pertinent medical history?
Infection
Erosive cheilitis, and purulent conjunctivitis. Minimal skin involvement
21
Consider Reactive Infectious Mucocutaneous Eruption
Malignancy
Severe stomatitis with variable skin findings (e.g., atypical target lesions and flaccid bullae)
6
Consider Paraneoplastic Pemphigus
New drug
Widespread erythematous fragile flaccid bullous plaques with crusting and erosions
7
Consider Stevens-Johnson Syndrome/Toxic Epidermal Necrolysis
No
Flaccid bullae on normal or erythematous skin. Almost all with mucosal erosions
5
Consider Pemphigus Vulgaris
Tense bulla
H
Prominent mucosal involvement
Yes
Pruritic, tense bullae with buccal erosions/de-squamation
8
Consider Mucous Membrane Pemphigoid (rare mimics e.g., MM-EBA or p200 BP)
No
I
Past medical history of hematologic malignancy, pregnancy, LP, or SLE
Yes
Hematologic malignancy
Intensely itchy papules/nodules in grouped or linear distribution
18
K
History of arthropod assault?
Yes
Consider Exaggerated Bug Bite Reaction
No
Consider Eosinophilic Dermatosis of Hematologic Malignancy
Pregnancy
Urticarial papules and plaques on the abdomen
14
J
Consider Pemphigoid Gestationis
LP
Vesicles and bullae on polygonal-shaped, violaceous, flat-topped papules
Lesions within preexisting LP only?
Yes
15
Consider Bullous LP
No
16
Consider LP Pemphigoides
SLE
Tense bullae in patient meeting ACR/EULAR criteria for SLE
17
Consider Bullous SLE
No
L
Distribution
M
Trauma induced
Skin fragility with tense vesicles and bullae that rupture
Child
9
Consider Epidermolysis Bullosa
Adult
10
Consider Epidermolysis Bullosa Acquista
N
String of pearls
Tense vesicles and bullae in annular, serpiginous distribution
22
Consider Linear IgA Bullous Dermatosis (rare mimics include BP or Inflammatory EBA)
O
Morphology
Urticarial papules and plaques
11
Consider Bullous Pemphigoid (rare mimic includes Inflammatory EBA)
Purpuric papules with vesicles and bullae
12
Consider Bullous Vasculitis
Peau d'orange
13
Consider Bullous Mastocytosis
Vesicles
P
Pruritus?
Yes
Vesicles on postauricular scalp, elbows, knees, buttocks bilaterally
19
Consider Dermatitis Herpetiformis
No
Grouped vesicles on erythematous base with >20 outside primary dermatome. Bullae uncommon
20
Consider Disseminated Varicella Zoster Virus

J. Patients with tense bullae and concomitant LP may have **bullous LP** or **lichen planus pemphigoides (LPP)**. Both have bullae develop within preexisting LP lesions. In LPP, bullae also develop outside LP lesions.

K. Bullous eruptions due to **exaggerated bug bite reactions** have been documented in patients with hematologic malignancies, most commonly CLL. Similar bullous eruptions mimicking bug bites (**eosinophilic dermatosis of hematologic malignancy**) have also been documented in patients with hematologic malignancies without a history of arthropod attack.

In patients with tense cutaneous bullae that meet the 2019 ACR/EULAR classification criteria for SLE, **bullous SLE** is the most likely diagnosis. Tense bullae may present on normal-appearing or inflamed skin, most commonly in photoexposed areas. Mucous membranes involvement may be present. Bullous SLE has a dramatic response to dapsone.

L. The distribution of bullous lesions can also help distinguish between tense bullous eruptions.

M. Tense bullae presenting in areas of trauma, most commonly on the scalp, elbows, knees, dorsal hands, and feet, include **epidermolysis bullosa (EB)** and **epidermolysis bullosa acquisita (EBA)**. EB is a heterogeneous group of genetic disorders, typically presenting soon after birth. An in-depth discussion on EB and its subtypes are outside the scope of this chapter. EBA, however, is an autoimmune disease that can occur at any age, but typically presents in older adults. EBA typically presents with bullae on normal-appearing or mildly erythematous skin in trauma-prone areas, healing with atrophic scarring and milia (classic EBA). Twenty percent of patients have scalp involvement resulting in scarring alopecia. Rarely, EBA can present with pruritic, inflammatory, urticarial plaques generalized throughout the body (inflammatory EBA), such as BP or linear IgA bullous dermatosis (LABD). Rarely, a mucosal-predominant EBA can occur that mimics MMP (MM-EBA). In MM-EBA, bullae are typically intact on presentation, compared with the fragile bullae of MMP.

N. Tense vesicles and bullae that line up in a serpiginous and annular distribution, referred to as "string of pearls", suggest **LABD**. In children, LABD presents most commonly as a self-limited autoimmune disease. LABD in adults is more commonly associated with drugs (e.g., vancomycin), malignancy (e.g., non-Hodgkins lymphoma, CLL), ulcerative colitis, and SLE. BP and inflammatory EBA may clinically mimic LABD. Prominent mucosal involvement is rare.

O. The morphology of lesions associated with tense bullae can also be an important clue. The presence of urticarial papules and plaques is suggestive of **BP**. BP is the most common autoimmune subepidermal blistering disease that predominantly affects older adults. BP typically presents with pruritus and urticarial papules and plaques (nonbullous phase). Later vesicles and bullae develop on normal or erythematous skin (bullous phase).

Other morphological findings that can help with the diagnosis of generalized vesicles and bullae are the presence of purpuric papules suggesting **bullous vasculitis** or diffuse edematous, dimpling (peau d' orange) appearance of the skin in patients with **bullous mastocytosis**.

P. In eruptions composed primarily of vesicles, the presence of pruritus versus pain is an important distinction. **Dermatitis herpetiformis** presents with intensely pruritic vesicles located on the elbows, knees, lower back, buttocks, and postauricular scalp. Intact vesicles are usually not appreciated due to scratching. **Disseminated varicella zoster virus**, however, is typically painful and presents with monomorphic grouped vesicles on an erythematous base with greater than 20 lesions outside the primary dermatome. Generalized vesicular eruptions and bullae are uncommon.

See Appendix 1 for Further Reading and Image References.

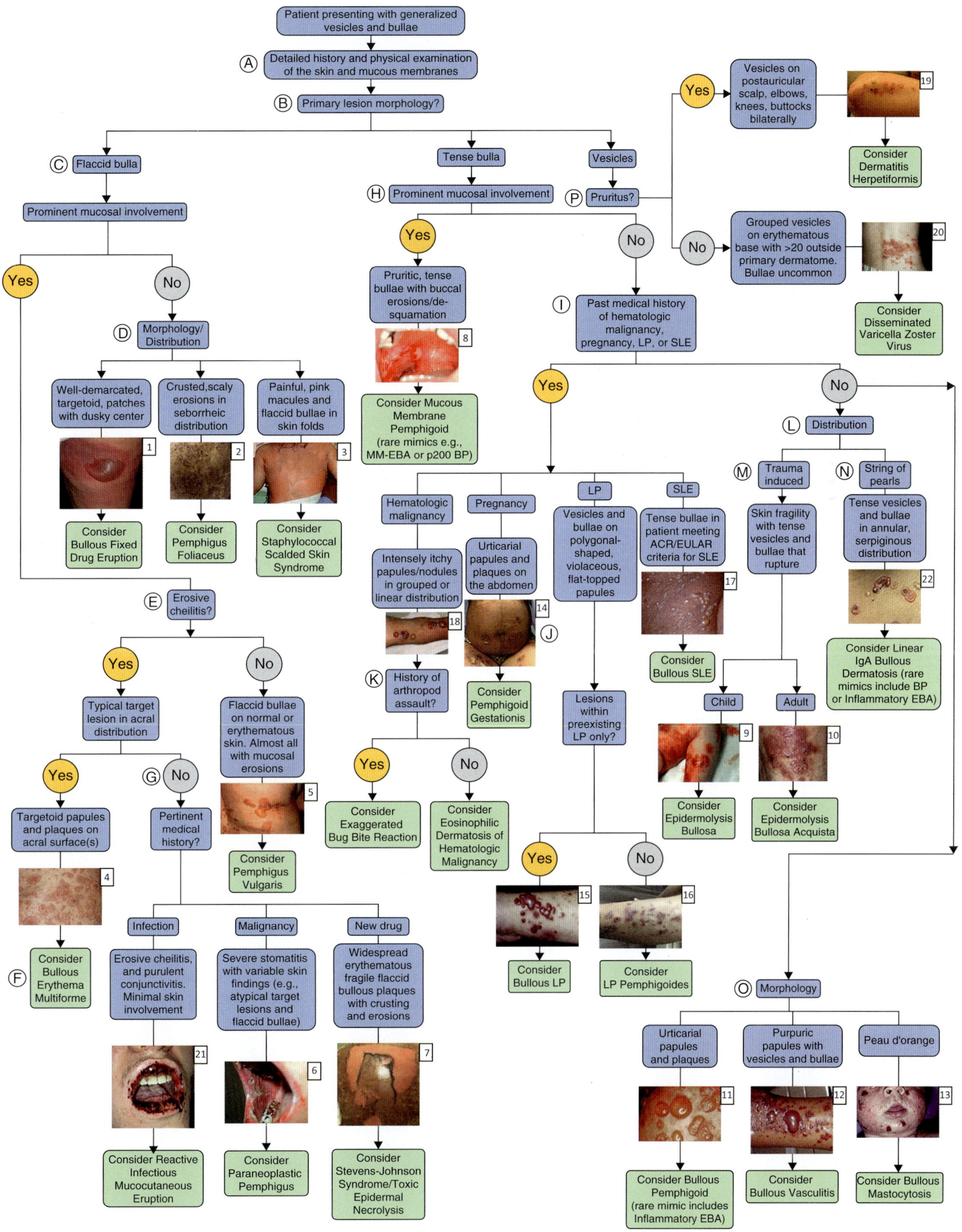
Patient presenting with generalized vesicles and bullae
A
Detailed history and physical examination of the skin and mucous membranes
B
Primary lesion morphology?
C
Flaccid bulla
Prominent mucosal involvement
Yes
No
D
Morphology/ Distribution
Well-demarcated, targetoid, patches with dusky center
1
Consider Bullous Fixed Drug Eruption
Crusted, scaly erosions in seborrheic distribution
2
Consider Pemphigus Foliaceus
Painful, pink macules and flaccid bullae in skin folds
3
Consider Staphylococcal Scalded Skin Syndrome
E
Erosive cheilitis?
Yes
Typical target lesion in acral distribution
Yes
Targetoid papules and plaques on acral surface(s)
4
F
Consider Bullous Erythema Multiforme
G
No
Pertinent medical history?
Infection
Erosive cheilitis, and purulent conjunctivitis. Minimal skin involvement
21
Consider Reactive Infectious Mucocutaneous Eruption
Malignancy
Severe stomatitis with variable skin findings (e.g., atypical target lesions and flaccid bullae)
6
Consider Paraneoplastic Pemphigus
New drug
Widespread erythematous fragile flaccid bullous plaques with crusting and erosions
7
Consider Stevens-Johnson Syndrome/Toxic Epidermal Necrolysis
No
Flaccid bullae on normal or erythematous skin. Almost all with mucosal erosions
5
Consider Pemphigus Vulgaris
Tense bulla
H
Prominent mucosal involvement
Yes
Pruritic, tense bullae with buccal erosions/de-squamation
8
Consider Mucous Membrane Pemphigoid (rare mimics e.g., MM-EBA or p200 BP)
No
I
Past medical history of hematologic malignancy, pregnancy, LP, or SLE
Yes
Hematologic malignancy
Intensely itchy papules/nodules in grouped or linear distribution
18
K
History of arthropod assault?
Yes
Consider Exaggerated Bug Bite Reaction
No
Consider Eosinophilic Dermatosis of Hematologic Malignancy
Pregnancy
Urticarial papules and plaques on the abdomen
14
J
Consider Pemphigoid Gestationis
LP
Vesicles and bullae on polygonal-shaped, violaceous, flat-topped papules
Lesions within preexisting LP only?
Yes
15
Consider Bullous LP
No
16
Consider LP Pemphigoides
SLE
Tense bullae in patient meeting ACR/EULAR criteria for SLE
17
Consider Bullous SLE
No
L
Distribution
M
Trauma induced
Skin fragility with tense vesicles and bullae that rupture
Child
9
Consider Epidermolysis Bullosa
Adult
10
Consider Epidermolysis Bullosa Acquista
N
String of pearls
Tense vesicles and bullae in annular, serpiginous distribution
22
Consider Linear IgA Bullous Dermatosis (rare mimics include BP or Inflammatory EBA)
O
Morphology
Urticarial papules and plaques
11
Consider Bullous Pemphigoid (rare mimic includes Inflammatory EBA)
Purpuric papules with vesicles and bullae
12
Consider Bullous Vasculitis
Peau d'orange
13
Consider Bullous Mastocytosis
Vesicles
P
Pruritus?
Yes
Vesicles on postauricular scalp, elbows, knees, buttocks bilaterally
19
Consider Dermatitis Herpetiformis
No
Grouped vesicles on erythematous base with >20 outside primary dermatome. Bullae uncommon
20
Consider Disseminated Varicella Zoster Virus

PART VI

Ulcers/Erosions

20 Oral Ulcers

Kathyana Paola Santiago Mangual and Jan M. Smogorzewski

The initial evaluation of patients presenting with oral lesions should include a thorough history and examination. In addition to considering the characteristics of the existing lesion, such as the location, time course, presence of pain, pruritus, and associated symptoms, it is also important to consider the prior history of erosive and ulcerative lesions. If oral ulcers are chronic and persist despite infectious and inflammatory workup and treatment, a biopsy to rule out malignancy should be an essential part of the diagnostic process.

Oral ulcers may involve the perioral region, lip, buccal mucosa, gingiva, palate, and/or tongue. The location, duration, progression, history of recurrence, and characteristics such as color are all important historical components the clinician should obtain, and there can be significant overlap in the location and morphology of the etiology of oral ulcers.

A. If the history reveals that the patient recently initiated a new medication or supplement, a drug-induced ulceration may be considered. **Stevens-Johnson syndrome (SJS)/toxic epidermal necrolysis (TEN)** may present with mucosal involvement prior to a skin eruption. On the oral mucosa, it will appear as a hemorrhagic erosion covered with a grayish-white membrane. Medications that are known to trigger SJS/TEN include allopurinol, sulfonamide antibiotics, and antiepileptics. Exposure to other new drugs, vaccines, and supplements should also be considered as potential triggers. Certain medications, including nonsteroidal anti-inflammatory medications and sulfonamide antibiotics, may cause a **bullous fixed drug eruption**, characterized by circular dusky patches that reoccur in the same locations on drug rechallenge and typically involve other cutaneous sites as well. If no drug culprit is evident, **reactive infectious mucocutaneous eruption** can be considered.

B. A single lesion in the oral mucosa may have a broad differential, including infectious, neoplastic, or inflammatory causes. An individual lesion to the lip or tongue may represent a **syphilitic chancre** and will have indurated margins and a clean base and will be painless. With an appropriate travel history or in endemic areas, **leishmaniasis** can also result in a single ulcerative lesion on the lip. **Aphthous ulcers** are painful, round, shallow, and oval-shaped with a yellow central exudate. If these are recurring, **recurrent aphthous stomatitis** may be the diagnosis. However, if they are recurrent and extensive, **Behçet syndrome (BS)** should be considered, particularly if the patient also has genital ulcers in addition to a positive pathergy test, other skin lesions (e.g., erythema nodosum-like lesions or folliculitis), and/or a history of uveitis. If the criteria for diagnosis of BS are not met, but there is evidence of recurrent oral aphthous ulcers, **complex aphthosis** may be considered. Any nonhealing oral ulcer that persists despite infectious and inflammatory workup or has accompanying concerning symptoms or history, such as weight loss, lymphadenopathy, and history of tobacco or alcohol use, should be biopsied to rule out malignancy, in particular **squamous cell carcinoma**.

Oral erosion/ulceration

A thorough history of the onset, progression, and duration of the lesion should be obtained. A thorough medication history, medical history, and previous drug reactions may also elicit essential information to arrive at the proper diagnosis.

(A) Suspicious drug history (e.g., antimicrobial, anticonvulsant, or NSAID started within the past 4–6 weeks), + Nikolsky sign?

- Yes → Ulceration preceded by circular discrete dusky patches that recur in the same place on drug rechallenge
  - Yes → 2

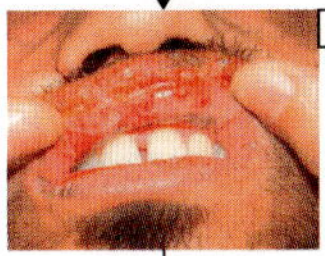

    Consider Bullous/Ulcerative Fixed Drug Eruption
  - No → 1

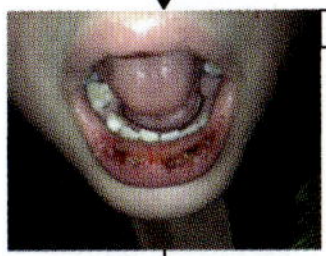

    Consider Stevens-Johnson Syndrome/Toxic Epidermal Necrolysis
- No → Recent history of viral/bacterial infection; sparse, polymorphic eruption; hemorrhagic crusting, – Nikolsky sign?
  - Yes → 3

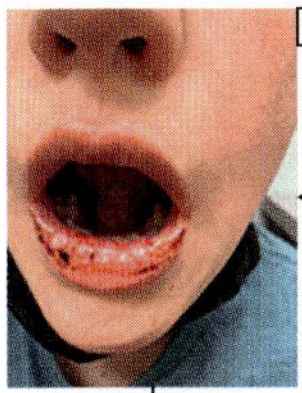

    Consider Reactive Infectious Mucocutaneous Eruption
  - No → Single lesion?
    - No → Multiple lesions *continued on next page*
    - (B) Yes →
      - Painful, shallow, oval shaped; yellow central exudate; located on superior or inferior mucosal lip; progresses to gray-white color; past episodes of similar ulceration
        - Yes → Past episodes of similar ulceration in genitals
          - Yes → Presence of other cutaneous lesions; +pathergy test; history of uveitis
            - Yes → Consider Behçet Syndrome
            - No → Consider Complex Aphthosis
          - No → Consider Recurrent Aphthous Stomatitis
        - No → 5

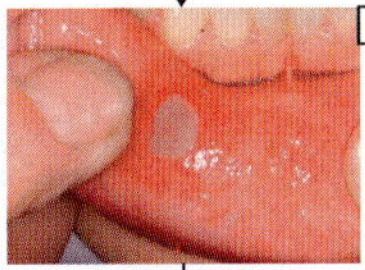

          Consider Aphthous Ulcer
      - Clean base, indurated margins, painless → 4

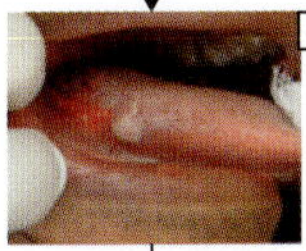

        Consider Syphilitic Chancre
      - Ulceration causing disfigurement; prior history of cutaneous leishmaniasis and/or history of recent travel to South America, East Africa, and/or India → 6

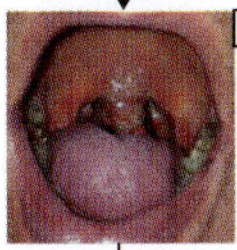

        Consider Leishmaniasis
      - Firm mass or thick plaque with keratosis and/or erythema and ulceration; history of chronic tobacco/alcohol use → 7

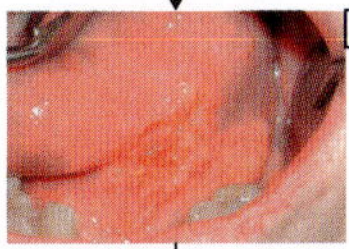

        Consider Malignancy, especially Squamous Cell Carcinoma (SCC)

Continued

C. Lesions of discoid lupus begin with a violaceous hue and inflammatory borders and can be seen on the mucosal and cutaneous lip. In the appropriate clinical context, palatal ulcers can be a diagnostic clue for **systemic lupus erythematosus**.

D. Mucosal ulcerations with concomitant vesicles on the palms and soles and a viral prodrome may lead to a diagnosis of **hand-foot-and-mouth disease**.

E. Patients may present with grouped vesicles that rapidly rupture to form erosions and ulcers with a scalloped border. If these are recurring and appear with prodromal signs such as tingling, **herpes simplex virus** may be considered. If these occur in a dermatomal pattern along the palate or mucosa, **herpes zoster** may be considered.

F. Painful erosions and ulcerations can also be seen in **erosive oral lichen planus (OLP)**. This can affect one or multiple areas of the mouth, including the lips, mucosa, palate, and tongue. It often presents with striated white lesions. In the gums, it can lead to desquamative gingivitis. Patients with OLP may also have cutaneous lesions that are typically pruritic, violaceous, and flat-topped papules with Wickham striae. Histopathologic assessment with direct immunofluorescence may reveal cystoid bodies or a linear pattern of fibrin and shaggy fibrinogen deposits at the epithelial basement membrane. OLP may coexist with cutaneous lichen planus.

G. **Mucous membrane pemphigoid (MMP)** and **pemphigus vulgaris (PV)** are immune-mediated diseases that manifest with blisters and ulcerations in mucous membranes and gingiva. The blisters/ulcerations may be recurrent and may be visibly distinguished from OLP lesions by the absence of mucocutaneous reticular lesions and the presence of Nikolsky sign. MMP can also cause desquamative gingivitis in the gums. Diagnosis of MMP and PV is confirmed by histopathology and direct immunofluorescence.

See Appendix 1 for Further Reading and Image References.

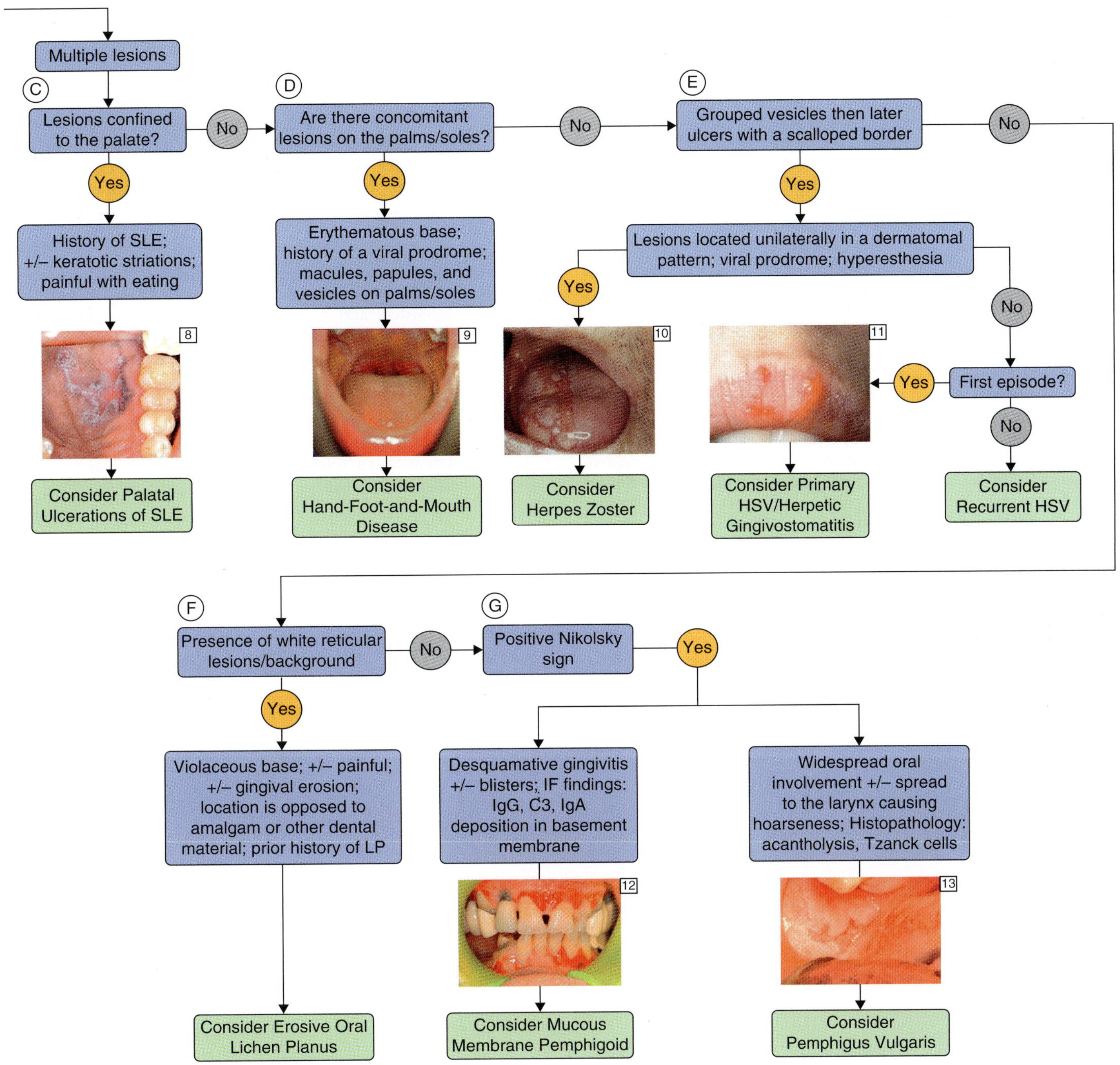
Multiple lesions
C
Lesions confined to the palate?
No
Yes
History of SLE; +/– keratotic striations; painful with eating
8
Consider Palatal Ulcerations of SLE
D
Are there concomitant lesions on the palms/soles?
No
Yes
Erythematous base; history of a viral prodrome; macules, papules, and vesicles on palms/soles
9
Consider Hand-Foot-and-Mouth Disease
E
Grouped vesicles then later ulcers with a scalloped border
No
Yes
Lesions located unilaterally in a dermatomal pattern; viral prodrome; hyperesthesia
Yes
10
Consider Herpes Zoster
No
First episode?
Yes
11
Consider Primary HSV/Herpetic Gingivostomatitis
No
Consider Recurrent HSV
F
Presence of white reticular lesions/background
No
Yes
Violaceous base; +/– painful; +/– gingival erosion; location is opposed to amalgam or other dental material; prior history of LP
Consider Erosive Oral Lichen Planus
G
Positive Nikolsky sign
Yes
Desquamative gingivitis +/– blisters; IF findings: IgG, C3, IgA deposition in basement membrane
12
Consider Mucous Membrane Pemphigoid
Widespread oral involvement +/– spread to the larynx causing hoarseness; Histopathology: acantholysis, Tzanck cells
13
Consider Pemphigus Vulgaris

21 Anogenital Ulcers

Kathyana Paola Santiago Mangual and Jan M. Smogorzewski

The majority of anogenital ulcers have an infectious etiology and are sexually transmitted. It is therefore important to elicit a thorough sexual history and perform a physical examination that includes the evaluation of other mucosal regions, such as the oral mucosa, as well as the assessment of the lymphatics surrounding the genital region.

A. Anogenital ulcerations primarily affecting mucosal sites have a broad differential. In the uncircumcised male with bright red ulceration of the glans penis, **Zoon balanitis** should be considered. **Pemphigus vulgaris** will typically present as painful erosions with the involvement of other mucosal sites. **Erosive lichen planus** is characterized by the presence of violaceous or erythematous plaques with a white reticulate border. **Lichen sclerosus et atrophicus** presents with pruritus and significant pain with scarring and the potential for ablation of physiologic anatomy. Oval-shaped, shallow yellow ulcerations that progress to gray-white may be caused by **aphthous ulcers**. If the erosive or ulcerative lesion is recurrent, **complex aphthosis** and **Behçet syndrome** may be considered. The presence of other cutaneous lesions, positive pathergy test, and history of uveitis are suggestive of Behçet syndrome.

B. If there is a suspicious medication history, including nonsteroidal anti-inflammatory drugs or sulfonamide antibiotics, along with cutaneous lesions that are circular, well-defined and appear on medication rechallenge in the same locations, a **fixed drug eruption** should be considered.

C. Painless ulcers may present with and without inguinal lymphadenopathy (LAD). In the presence of painful LAD and an ulcer with indurated borders and a clean base, **syphilitic chancre** may be considered. The presence of buboes in the inguinal region, or the presence of anal pain, discharge, bleeding, tenesmus, or constipation, may be indicative of **lymphogranuloma venereum**, which can be confirmed with nucleic acid amplification testing. In the absence of inguinal LAD, **granuloma inguinale/donovanosis** may be considered, particularly in endemic regions. **Malignancy** must be considered in the differential of a nonhealing ulcer in the anogenital area.

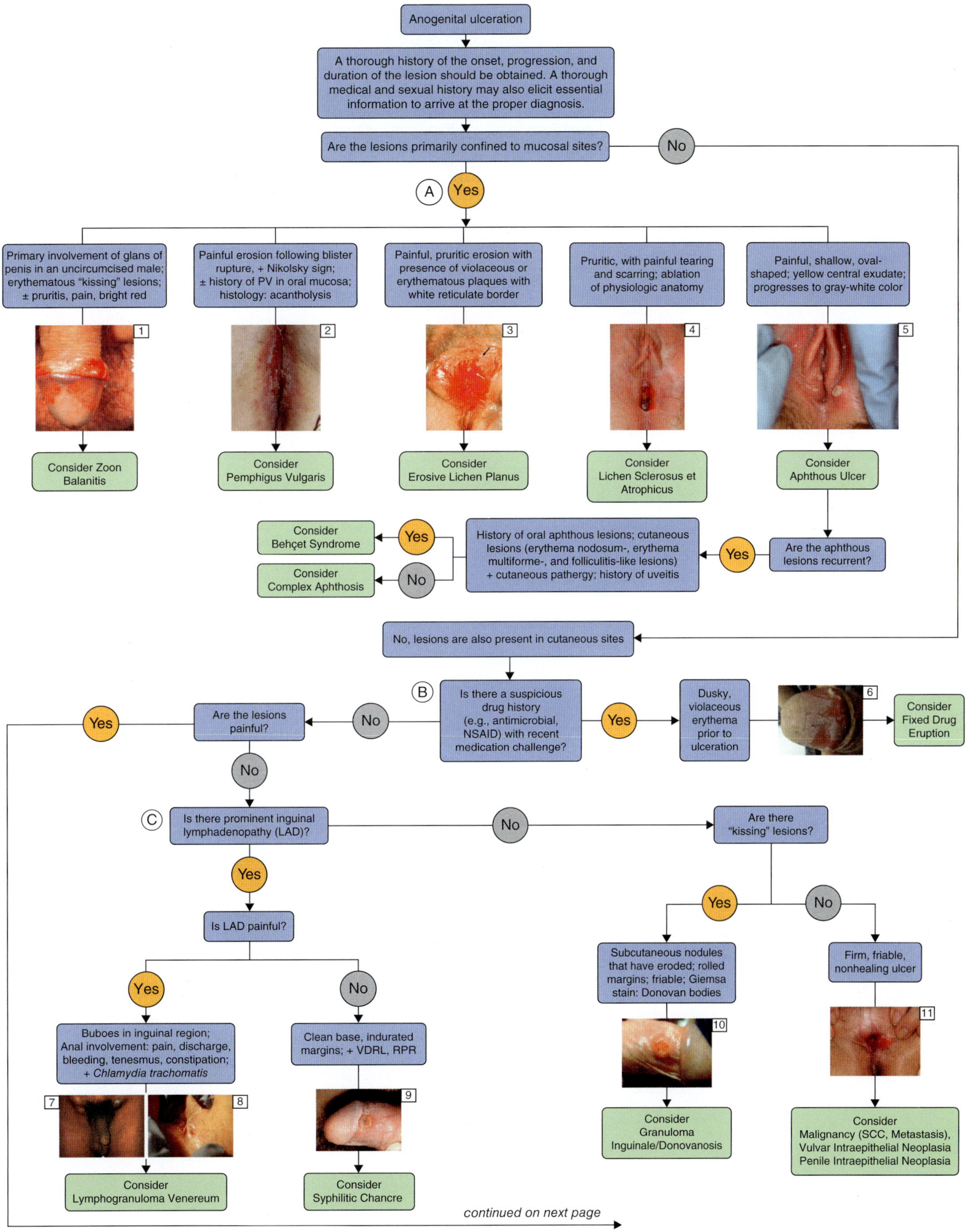
Anogenital ulceration
A thorough history of the onset, progression, and duration of the lesion should be obtained. A thorough medical and sexual history may also elicit essential information to arrive at the proper diagnosis.
Are the lesions primarily confined to mucosal sites?
No
A
Yes
Primary involvement of glans of penis in an uncircumcised male; erythematous "kissing" lesions; ± pruritis, pain, bright red
1
Consider Zoon Balanitis
Painful erosion following blister rupture, + Nikolsky sign; ± history of PV in oral mucosa; histology: acantholysis
2
Consider Pemphigus Vulgaris
Painful, pruritic erosion with presence of violaceous or erythematous plaques with white reticulate border
3
Consider Erosive Lichen Planus
Pruritic, with painful tearing and scarring; ablation of physiologic anatomy
4
Consider Lichen Sclerosus et Atrophicus
Painful, shallow, oval-shaped; yellow central exudate; progresses to gray-white color
5
Consider Aphthous Ulcer
Are the aphthous lesions recurrent?
Yes
History of oral aphthous lesions; cutaneous lesions (erythema nodosum-, erythema multiforme-, and folliculitis-like lesions) + cutaneous pathergy; history of uveitis
Yes
Consider Behçet Syndrome
No
Consider Complex Aphthosis
No, lesions are also present in cutaneous sites
B
Is there a suspicious drug history (e.g., antimicrobial, NSAID) with recent medication challenge?
Yes
Dusky, violaceous erythema prior to ulceration
6
Consider Fixed Drug Eruption
No
Are the lesions painful?
Yes
No
C
Is there prominent inguinal lymphadenopathy (LAD)?
No
Are there "kissing" lesions?
Yes
Subcutaneous nodules that have eroded; rolled margins; friable; Giemsa stain: Donovan bodies
10
Consider Granuloma Inguinale/Donovanosis
No
Firm, friable, nonhealing ulcer
11
Consider Malignancy (SCC, Metastasis), Vulvar Intraepithelial Neoplasia Penile Intraepithelial Neoplasia
Yes
Is LAD painful?
Yes
Buboes in inguinal region; Anal involvement: pain, discharge, bleeding, tenesmus, constipation; + *Chlamydia trachomatis*
7
8
Consider Lymphogranuloma Venereum
No
Clean base, indurated margins; + VDRL, RPR
9
Consider Syphilitic Chancre
continued on next page

Continued

D. An extremely painful ulcer that has a friable base with yellow-gray exudate and a violaceous ragged border, in addition to inguinal LAD, may be **chancroid** caused by *Haemophilus ducreyi*. It is common for patients to have more than one ulcer. The involved lymph nodes may present as painful fluctuant buboes. **Herpes simplex virus (HSV)** presents as recurrent grouped vesicles that rupture to form erosions and ulcerations. In a young female patient with viral prodrome in whom HSV has been ruled out, an **acute genital ulcer** may be considered. This has been associated with Epstein-Barr virus, cytomegalovirus, influenza, mycoplasma, or COVID-19 infection. Recurrent nodules and abscesses, and presence of sinus tracts in the anogenital region are indicative of **hidradenitis suppurativa**, and other intertriginous areas of the body should be examined.

Patients who present with a painful purulent ulcer that progressed from an erythematous papule and have a history of inflammatory bowel disease may have **cutaneous Crohn's disease (CD)**. Biopsy of the ulcer will reveal discrete, noncaseating, sarcoidal granulomas with Langhans-type multinucleated giant cells. Although genital involvement in CD is rare, cutaneous disease may be the primary manifestation.

Pyoderma gangrenosum presents as pustules that erode into necrotic ulcers and exhibit pathergy and heal with cribriform scarring. Workup for possible underlying systemic disease is indicated.

See Appendix 1 for Further Reading and Image References.

Yes

D

Friable ulcer with yellow-gray exudate with LAD

12
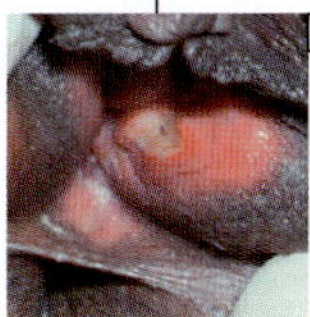

Consider Chancroid

Grouped vesicles on erythematous base and/or ulcers with scalloped borders

13
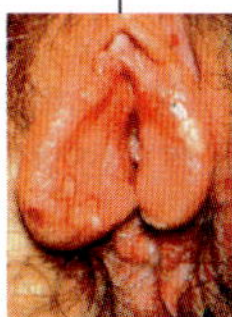

Consider Herpes Simplex Virus

Negative sexual history; ± young female; recent viral or bacterial infection

14
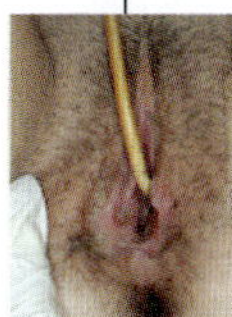

Consider Acute Genital Ulcer

Firm nodules, deep abscesses and cysts, and purulent sinus tracts; ± presence of similar lesions in other intertriginous regions

15
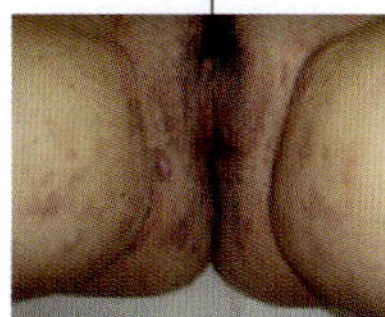

Consider Hidradenitis Suppurativa

Knife-cut fissures, granulomatous infiltration of the skin; ± GI manifestations; histopathology noncaseating granulomas

16
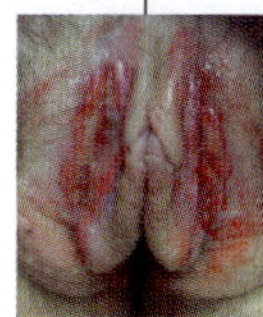

Consider Cutaneous Crohn's Disease

Pustules erode into necrotic ulcers; dusky violaceous hue; undermined margins; purulent coating in center; +pathergy; cribriform scarring; neutrophilic infiltrate on histopathology

17
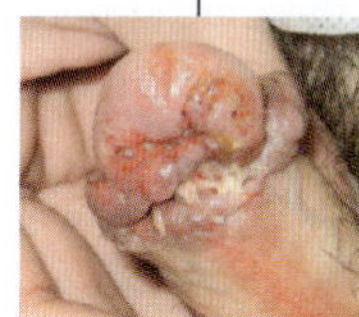

Consider Pyoderma Gangrenosum

22 Cutaneous Ulcer(s)

Smriti Prasad and Alex G. Ortega-Loayza

Cutaneous ulcers are full-thickness open wounds that are associated with both epidermal and dermal tissue loss. They are a major cause of patient morbidity and sometimes mortality, a significant financial burden on the healthcare system, and can represent a therapeutic challenge for dermatologists. Ulcers appear most commonly on the lower legs due to venous or arterial insufficiency, pressure ulcers, or neuropathy; however, there are also less common causes for ulcers. A thorough history and physical examination are required to help identify and address the underlying cause of the chronic ulcer.

The initial step when seeing a patient with cutaneous ulcers is to perform a thorough history and examination to help determine the underlying cause. Important points to consider include patient age, sex, duration of ulcer, and medical history, such as comorbidities (e.g., diabetes, heart disease, kidney disease), history of cancer, autoimmune or psychiatric conditions, and any recent procedures. Consider other factors that could be contributing, such as nutritional status, genetic factors, and medications. For chronic ulcers that do not respond to standard wound care, skin biopsies are useful in ruling out malignancy and deep infections.

Key features of the ulcer to examine and subsequent next steps to consider include:

- Take note of anatomical region (for example, malleoli, pressure sites, or distal parts of the leg)
- Evaluate perfusion: check pulses and temperature of feet; consider calculating an ankle brachial index (ABI) or performing venous reflux studies or venous Doppler scans
- Evaluate for edema, stasis dermatitis changes, and varicosities: if present, consider compression
- Evaluate for signs of infection/inflammation: if present, consider cultures, imaging studies, and antibiotics
- Evaluate for drainage: if abundant, consider hyperabsorbable dressings
- Examine for biofilm: if present, consider sharp/surgical debridement

A. The most frequent chronic ulcer in an ambulatory setting is a **venous ulcer**, commonly located over the medial malleolus. Physical examination will often show other signs of venous insufficiency (varicose veins, pitting edema), brown discoloration, and telangiectasias. Duplex ultrasonography can be useful to diagnose venous reflux.

B. **Neuropathic ulcers** are commonly located over pressure points. Diabetes is a common cause of neuropathic ulcers. On examination, they are often malodorous with exudate, and the surrounding skin notably has impaired sensation.

C. **Peripheral artery disease** can also lead to cutaneous ulcers and is a common manifestation of atherosclerosis. Unlike many other ulcers, arterial ulcers are usually painless, although patients often have concurrent claudication. There is a notable lack of hair on the legs. Physical examination reveals a sharply demarcated ulcer on the distal extremities that rarely bleeds. Pedal pulses are often diminished or absent. ABI is often reduced (<0.91).

D. **Hidradenitis suppurativa (HS)** and **cutaneous Crohn's disease** may present with chronic deep nodules and painful ulcers, often in intertriginous areas. Evaluating for other clinical signs of HS such as double-headed comedones, abscesses, sinus tracts, and other cutaneous comorbidities of HS such as dissecting cellulitis of the scalp and pilonidal cyst is helpful. In a patient with suspected cutaneous Crohn's disease, a gastrointestinal work-up and a skin biopsy may be useful.

E. **Pyoderma gangrenosum** commonly presents in middle-aged adults as a painful ulcer on the lower extremities with violaceous borders. History of trauma may be present in up to one-third of patients, and the ulcer usually worsens with debridement. Concurrent rheumatoid arthritis, inflammatory bowel disease, or monoclonal gammopathy may be noted in the history, and a full review of systems is needed to evaluate for potential underlying conditions.

F. There are various types of **panniculitis** that can cause ulcers, but the most common one is lipodermatosclerosis. Most panniculitides also have indurated skin surrounding the ulcer, which can be a helpful clue. However, a deep (telescoping) biopsy is needed to confirm diagnosis.

G. In terms of **vasculitis**, understanding the size of the involved vessels is key, as small vessel involvement clinically manifests as palpable purpura, whereas medium or mixed vessel involvement presents with livedo recularis or retiform purpura. Biopsies, including the ulcer edge, should be performed and sent for hematoxylin and eosin and direct immunofluorescence, preferably on early lesions within 24 to 48 hours of appearance.

H. Various microbes can cause **infectious ulcers**, such as *Pseudomonas* (e.g., ecthyma), *Mycobacterium*, fungi, and parasites (e.g., leishmaniasis). Detailed travel and social histories are needed. Tissue cultures can help identify the causal organism.

I. Ulcers may also be caused by **cutaneous malignancies**. Squamous cell carcinomas may present as keratotic or ulcerated nodules, most commonly on sun-exposed areas. They can also develop in the setting of previously traumatized or chronically inflamed skin (e.g., Marjolin ulcers). Basal cell carcinomas are also often present on sun-exposed areas and commonly have central ulceration. They may bleed spontaneously or with minimal trauma.

J. Ulcers can also form due to **mechanical trauma**, such as pressure, friction, or skin picking. These ulcers can be treated after removing the inciting cause. Pressure ulcers occur over bony prominences and are improved with position changes and support surfaces along with general wound care. Skin picking causes angulated ulcers most commonly on the face and extremities and requires comprehensive history taking to elicit the cause and best treatment course.

K. There are various **iatrogenic** causes of ulcers. For instance, medications such as kinase inhibitors and hydroxyurea may be culprits. Exposure to radiation may lead to nonhealing ulcers. Ulcers can also be seen at injection sites of certain medications, such as heparin.

L. Rarely, **genetic** causes such as beta-thalassemia, sickle cell, and spherocytosis may also lead to ulcers. There are few clinical clues that are specific for these conditions; therefore, a careful personal medical and family history should be conducted.

See Appendix 1 for Further Reading.

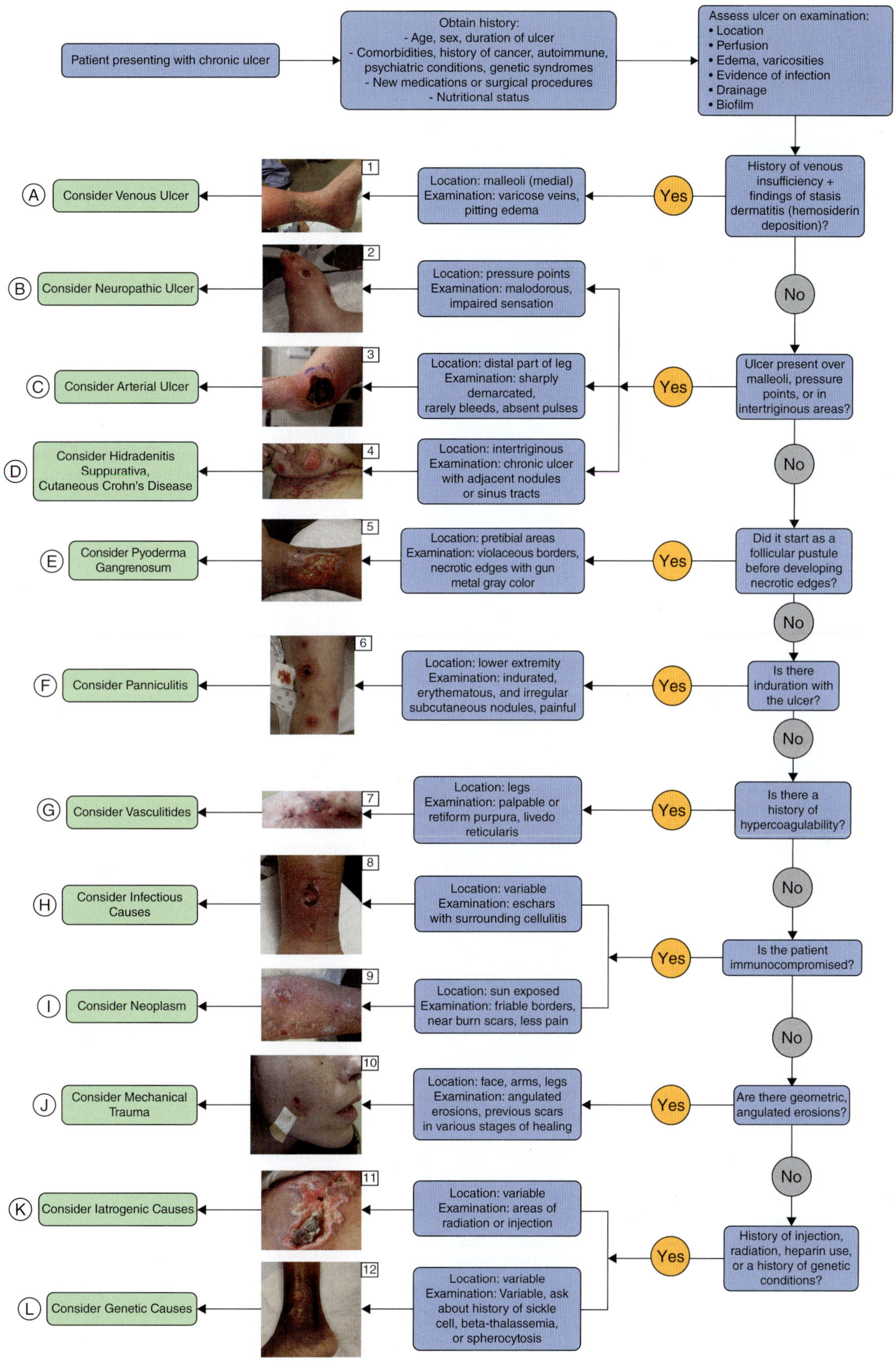
Patient presenting with chronic ulcer
Obtain history:
- Age, sex, duration of ulcer
- Comorbidities, history of cancer, autoimmune, psychiatric conditions, genetic syndromes
- New medications or surgical procedures
- Nutritional status
Assess ulcer on examination:
• Location
• Perfusion
• Edema, varicosities
• Evidence of infection
• Drainage
• Biofilm
History of venous insufficiency + findings of stasis dermatitis (hemosiderin deposition)?
Yes
Location: malleoli (medial) Examination: varicose veins, pitting edema
1
A
Consider Venous Ulcer
No
Ulcer present over malleoli, pressure points, or in intertriginous areas?
Yes
Location: pressure points Examination: malodorous, impaired sensation
2
B
Consider Neuropathic Ulcer
Location: distal part of leg Examination: sharply demarcated, rarely bleeds, absent pulses
3
C
Consider Arterial Ulcer
Location: intertriginous Examination: chronic ulcer with adjacent nodules or sinus tracts
4
D
Consider Hidradenitis Suppurativa, Cutaneous Crohn's Disease
No
Did it start as a follicular pustule before developing necrotic edges?
Yes
Location: pretibial areas Examination: violaceous borders, necrotic edges with gun metal gray color
5
E
Consider Pyoderma Gangrenosum
No
Is there induration with the ulcer?
Yes
Location: lower extremity Examination: indurated, erythematous, and irregular subcutaneous nodules, painful
6
F
Consider Panniculitis
No
Is there a history of hypercoagulability?
Yes
Location: legs Examination: palpable or retiform purpura, livedo reticularis
7
G
Consider Vasculitides
No
Is the patient immunocompromised?
Yes
Location: variable Examination: eschars with surrounding cellulitis
8
H
Consider Infectious Causes
Location: sun exposed Examination: friable borders, near burn scars, less pain
9
I
Consider Neoplasm
No
Are there geometric, angulated erosions?
Yes
Location: face, arms, legs Examination: angulated erosions, previous scars in various stages of healing
10
J
Consider Mechanical Trauma
No
History of injection, radiation, heparin use, or a history of genetic conditions?
Yes
Location: variable Examination: areas of radiation or injection
11
K
Consider Iatrogenic Causes
Location: variable Examination: Variable, ask about history of sickle cell, beta-thalassemia, or spherocytosis
12
L
Consider Genetic Causes

23 Acral Ulcers

Raveena Ghanshani and Ashley B. Crew

Acral ulcers will be defined, for the purposes of this chapter, as ulcers affecting the skin of the hands and/or feet. Acral ulcers, an uncommon presentation in dermatology, have an extensive differential diagnosis that includes diagnoses in the inflammatory, infectious, mechanical, and malignant categories. Evaluation of a patient with acral ulcers requires a thorough patient history and careful evaluation of the characteristics of the ulcer(s). Certain morphological features can help guide differential diagnosis and subsequent workup. Management of acral ulcers begins with treating pertinent underlying conditions, wound care, and utilization of appropriate topical and, in some cases, systemic therapies.

A. Initial assessment involves eliciting a detailed history with a focus on the history of chronic illness, such as diabetes, peripheral arterial disease (PAD), or autoimmune diseases. Occupational and travel history are also important components of the diagnosis. The practitioner should assess the characteristics of the ulcer(s) (unilateral or bilateral, single or multiple, painful or painless, eschar present or absent) as well as any other cutaneous findings, such as changes to the skin surrounding the ulcer or other findings on a complete skin examination.

B. Initial physical examination should assess whether the patient has cutaneous sensation that is grossly intact in the areas of the ulcer(s). If sensation is not intact, the diagnoses of **diabetic ulcers** or **lepromatous leprosy** should be considered. Further physical examination can be helpful in distinguishing between these etiologies in a patient with symmetric sensory loss. In addition to "glove and stocking" sensation loss in the extremities, patients with leprosy may exhibit leonine facies, hypopigmented macules, and madarosis. History of living in or traveling to areas that are endemic for *Mycobacterium leprae* can also support this diagnosis. Patients with long-standing diabetes may present with painless ulcers on weight-bearing bony regions of the body (i.e., the plantar metatarsal head). The patient may also demonstrate other findings of long-standing diabetes, such as acral fissuring and xerosis, hammer toes, and cheiroarthropathy. Further history may reveal other diagnoses associated with long-standing poorly controlled diabetes, such as chronic kidney disease and diabetic retinopathy.

C. In patients with grossly intact peripheral sensation, check whether the ulcers are singular and/or unilateral or multiple and/or bilateral. In the category of single or unilateral ulcers, infectious and malignant etiologies should be considered initially. For patients with a single, abruptly arising ulcer, orf, brown recluse spider bite, and **pyoderma gangrenosum (PG)** should be considered. **Orf** presents as an erythematous nodule that appears 3 to 7 days after exposure to sheep, goats, or reindeer. The erythematous papule evolves over several weeks into a crusted and ulcerated nodule, typically healing 4 to 8 weeks after onset. A **brown recluse spider bite** presents with pain in the initial hours and then advances from an erythematous papule to a dusky necrotic ulcer. PG characteristically presents as a rapidly expanding ulcer with pain out of proportion to the lesion. PG typically has an irregular, undermined, violaceous border and heals with a cribriform scar. Patients with suspected PG should be assessed for inflammatory bowel disease, arthritis, and hematologic conditions or malignancies. While PG frequently presents asymmetrically or as a single lesion, it can present diffusely with multiple lesions.

For singular lesions that progress slowly, over months to years, cutaneous malignancies should be considered. Squamous cell carcinomas arising within a scar or wound, also known as **Marjolin ulcers**, are most often seen in elderly patients and should be considered in chronic ulcers (>3 months) that are unresponsive to treatment. If an ulcer arises on the sole of the foot, or less frequently on the palmar surface of the hand, in the context of an irregularly bordered, often multicolored (brown, black, blue-gray) plaque, a diagnosis of **acral lentiginous melanoma** should be considered.

D. If a patient presents with multiple and/or bilateral acral ulcers, they should be assessed for additional signs and symptoms of connective tissue disease (CTD). If the ulcers are on the palmar or distal fingers and accompanied by background findings of sclerodactyly, proximal nailfold changes (e.g., erythema, cuticular fraying, capillary dilation, and dropout), or telangiectasias, a diagnosis of **systemic sclerosis** should be considered. If patients have palmar and/or extensor ulcerations, they should be assessed for other signs of **dermatomyositis (DM)**, including heliotrope sign, Gottron papules/sign, or poikiloderma of the scalp, shoulders (shawl sign), lateral thighs (holster sign), and general photosensitivity. These patients should also be assessed for painful palmar papules, and when extensor ulcerations or painful palmar papules are noted in the context of suspected DM, the **MDA5** subtype should be considered. In these cases, the clinician should have a high level of concern for associated rapidly progressive interstitial lung disease and should expediently refer to rheumatology and pulmonology colleagues.

E. If patients lack signs or symptoms of CTD, a thorough social history can help to determine the risk of possible **frostbite** from cold exposure or the risk of **cholesterol embolism** that is often associated with preceding invasive arterial procedures, prolonged anticoagulation, or acute thrombolytic therapy. Frostbite may present with bullae and neuropathy with deeper injuries. Cholesterol embolism may present with other systemic findings associated with embolism, such as renal compromise, gastrointestinal ulcers, altered mental status, or eosinophilia, in addition to other cutaneous manifestations such as retiform purpura and livedo reticularis.

Clinical features, including location over pressure points and overlying eschar, and associated symptoms, such as pain with ambulation (claudication) and elevation, can help to support a diagnosis of **peripheral arterial disease (PAD)**. Retiform appearance, associated proximal ulcerations, and history of chronic dialysis support a diagnosis of **calciphylaxis**. Involvement of the distal phalanges with dry gangrenous change and history of smoking in a patient younger than 50 years can help to support the diagnosis of **Buerger disease**. Punched-out ulcers, palpable purpura, and subcutaneous nodules can tip the clinician off to the diagnostic category of **vasculitis**.

See Appendix 1 for Further Reading and Image References.

Patient presents with full-thickness focal loss of skin on acral* surfaces

→ Perform a detailed history and physical examination with special focus on ulcer characteristics, other acral regions, and other cutaneous findings. Evaluate the distribution, size, shape, and color of ulcer. (A)

→ Management typically involves treating underlying disorder, wound care, and biopsy and subsequent excision if necessary

→ Is cutaneous sensation intact in the ulcerated extremities? (B)

Yes → Is the ulcer single/unilateral or multiple/bilateral?

(C) Single/unilateral

- Most common on the lower extremities, older patients with burns/scars, history of skin cancer; chronic ulcer >3 months, unresponsive to/recurrence after treatment; increasing size, bleeding, induration, and everted edges; lymphadenopathy

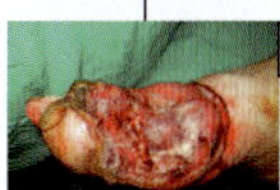
4

→ Consider Marjolin Ulcer (SCC in Scar/Wound)

- Often on the sole of foot; can present as bleeding, irregularly bordered, multicolored (brown, black, blue-gray, red, etc.) plaque with central ulceration; can be amelanotic; lymphadenopathy

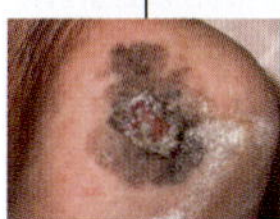
5

→ Consider Acral Lentiginous Melanoma

- Contact exposure to sheep, goats, reindeer (i.e., farmers, veterinarians); weeping erythematous ulcerated nodule often on the dorsal hand, no scar +/– erythema multiforme eruption after 1.5–2 weeks

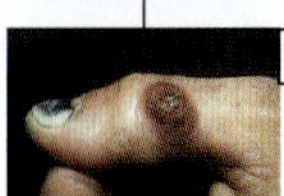
1

→ Consider Orf (Parapoxvirus)

- Pain begins few hours after bite; can advance from erythematous papule (within hours) to large dusky necrotic ulcer; can rarely progress to systemic shock/DIC

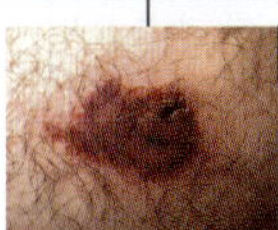
2

→ Consider Brown Recluse Spider Bite

- Necrotic, rapidly expanding; ulcer border is irregular, undermined, violet-gray, pain out of proportion to size, cribiform scarring, history of IBD, arthritis, hematologic condition/malignancy

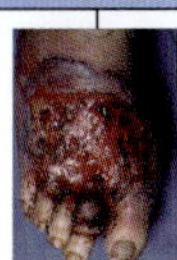
3

→ Consider PG

Multiple/bilateral → Are there signs of CTD?

(D) **Yes**

- Ulceration at tips and interphalangeal joints of hands; Females > Males; Sclerodactyly, Raynaud, calcinosis cutis, fingertip pitting, telangectasias, pruritus; antibodies (anticentromere, anti-Scl-70, anti-RNA pol III)

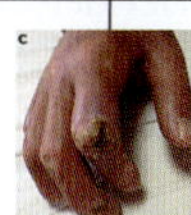
14

→ Consider Scleroderma/ Systemic Sclerosis

- Ulcers found on knuckles, elbows, hands; Gottron papules and mechanic's hands; association with interstitial lung disease, high CK, muscle weakness, and anti-MDA5 antibody (confirms diagnosis)

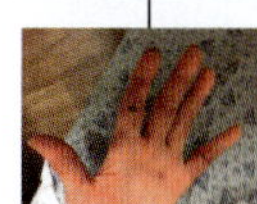
15

→ Consider MDA5 Dermatomyositis

(E) **No**

- Skin temperature below −2°C (28°F) from cold exposure/arsine gas; ulceration, hemorrhage, and edema of extremities; bullae and neuropathy with deeper injury

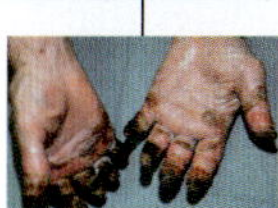
8

→ Consider Frostbite

- Sudden onset of altered mental status, fever, hypertension; cyanotic blue toes, livedo reticularis, multiple irregularly bordered ulcers encircled by retiform purpura; eschar present

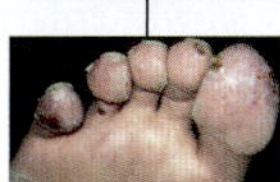
9

→ Consider Cholesterol Embolism

- History of atherosclerosis, smoking; weak/absent peripheral pulses; round punched out ulcers surrounded by shiny skin; sharply demarcated with no bleeding

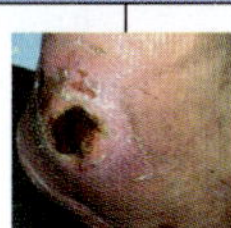
10

→ Consider PAD

- History of chronic kidney disease; severely painful, large violaceous plaques with irregular border, accompanied by retiform purpura; leather-like eschars can be present

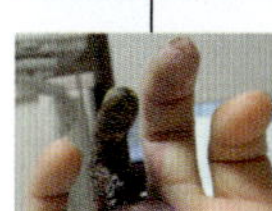
11

→ Consider Calciphylaxis

- Onset at under 50 years old, history of smoking/tobacco use, claudication; digital gangrene and painful ulcerations from ischemia, ulcers on both the upper and lower extremities

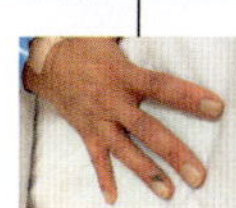
12

→ Consider Buerger Disease

- Erythematous punched out ulcer, may see palpable purpura, subcutaneous nodules; in PAN: livedo racemosa, retiform purpura, ulcers, and subcutaneous nodules

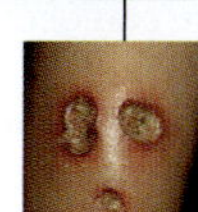
13

→ Consider Vasculitis

No

- Painless ulcer, glove and stocking sensory neuropathy; travel history to endemic areas; other features: Leonine facies, hypopigmented macules, claw hand, madarosis

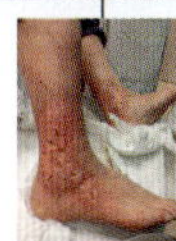
6

→ Consider Leprosy

- Painless ulcer, common on surface of heel or big toe (weight-bearing regions over bony prominence), callus formation; long-standing history of diabetes; peripheral neuropathy; other features: dryness, fissures, hammer toe

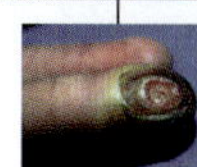
7

→ Consider Diabetic Ulcer

*Defined for these purposes as hands/feet.

24 Punched-Out Erosions

McKayla J. Poppens and Marcia Hogeling

Punched-out erosions (POEs) are secondary lesions that develop within hours to days as a sequela of inflammatory and infectious disorders, particularly following vesicular eruptions. The severity and distribution of cutaneous to mucocutaneous POEs vary widely. Many presentations may be the consequence of viral or superficial bacterial infections, but POEs may also present as the cutaneous manifestation of serious systemic disease.

A. Initial evaluation should include a complete history, including any underlying dermatosis, chronic conditions, medications, recent illnesses, and travel. Details about primary lesions will aid in diagnosis. Inquiring about systemic and prodromal symptoms such as fever, pruritus, arthralgia, myalgia, neuralgia, and lymphadenopathy is important. Examine the erosions of concern but also mucosal surfaces and lymph nodes, while making note of signs indicating systemic disease. When building a differential diagnosis, consider the lesion distribution in context of prior lesion morphology, medical history, and systemic signs. Clinical diagnosis is often possible, but serology, polymerase chain reaction (PCR) assays, and skin biopsy can support the diagnosis.

B. The presence of active or inactive dermatosis (often atopic dermatitis or Darier disease) or recent skin injury are clues to secondary infections, such as Kaposi varicelliform eruption, impetigo, or ecthyma.

Kaposi varicelliform eruptions are caused most frequently by herpes simplex virus (HSV) type-1 (**eczema herpeticum**) but also by HSV-2, coxsackievirus A16 (**eczema coxsackium**), vaccinia virus, varicella zoster virus (VZV), smallpox virus, or monkeypox virus that infects a preexisting dermatosis and can disseminate. Systemic symptoms such as malaise, fever, and lymphadenopathy may be present. Diagnosis is clinical, but PCR or Tzanck smear of lesional fluid is confirmatory.

Impetigo is a superficial staphylococcal or streptococcal infection. Risk factors include crowded living conditions, poor hygiene, underlying scabies, and skin barrier defects. Impetigo first presents as a bullous or nonbullous eruption. Diagnosis can be made clinically to initiate empiric antibiotic coverage. Gram stain and bacterial culture of the exudate help guide antibiotic treatment. **Ecthyma** is an ulcerative and deeper form of impetigo. Early lesions appear as POEs that progress to deep ulcerations with adherent yellow crusting and raised violaceous margins.

C. For older, nonimmunized, or immunocompromised patients presenting with acute neuritis and POE in a dermatomal distribution, **herpes zoster** should be considered. Diagnosis can be made clinically and confirmed by VZV PCR.

D. **Hydroa vacciniforme**, a rare chronic photodermatitis associated with Epstein-Barr virus (EBV) infection, typically presents in childhood, although late-onset cases have been described. Blisters on sun-exposed skin are reproduced by repetitive ultraviolet A exposure. Facial swelling, fever, mosquito bite hypersensitivity, and liver damage can occur.

E. For erosions confined to mucous membranes, early aphthous stomatitis can present as POE. **Recurrent aphthous stomatitis** affects up to 20% of the population, often immunocompromised patients or those with anemia, neutropenia, or enteropathies (malabsorption, gluten sensitivity, ulcerative colitis, Crohn's disease). Oral aphthae are painful and persistent for 7 to 14 days. **Major aphthous stomatitis (Sutton disease)** is a rare form of aphthous stomatitis that frequently presents in patients with HIV with remitting or persistent (2–12 weeks) painful oral, esophageal, anal, or genital lesions. **Oculo-oral-genital syndrome (Behçet syndrome)** is a rare vasculitis syndrome more common in patients with eastern Asian or Mediterranean descent that presents as recurrent oral and genital erosions. As HLA-B51 remains the most important genetic factor associated with Behçet syndrome, HLA typing is helpful in diagnosis.

F. With an estimated prevalence of 90%, **HSV** infections are common causes of POEs. HSV may present as orolabial herpes, herpetic sycosis, herpetic whitlow, ocular HSV, or Kaposi varicelliform eruption. Pruritis and pain may precede vesicular eruptions. Fever and regional lymphadenopathy may also occur. Oral and genital erosions can also be from **EBV** (often unifocal) or, more rarely, **cytomegalovirus** (unifocal or dispersed) in patients with chronic immunosuppression. PCR assays confirm etiology.

Erythema multiforme is a type IV hypersensitivity reaction triggered mostly by infection (especially HSV, but also histoplasmosis, EBV, mycoplasma) that presents with three-ringed targets and variable mucosal involvement (POE with hemorrhagic sloughing). Severe presentation may require hospitalization.

Reactive infectious mucosal eruption is a postinfectious (respiratory viruses, mycoplasma, or *Chlamydophila pneumoniae*) vesiculobullous or erosive mucosal-predominant eruption. Evidence of a preceding infection is necessary for diagnosis, so clinical workup should begin with chest radiography and laboratory tests for acute infection.

Consider **disseminated histoplasmosis** in immunocompromised or elderly patients who reside near or have traveled to the Ohio or Mississippi River Valleys. Urinary ELISA (enzyme-linked immunosorbent assay) or PCR assays confer diagnosis.

G. In patients with celiac disease, pruritic excoriated POEs on the scalp, buttocks, or extensor surfaces are pathognomonic for **dermatitis herpetiformis**. Diagnosis is made based on clinical signs and immunofluorescence microscopy showing dermal IgA deposition.

H. Aside from **pitted keratolysis** (associated with hyperhidrosis), POEs on the lower extremities are commonly associated with diabetes (**early neuropathic ulcerations**), metabolic disease and smoking (**early arterial insufficiency**), or systemic disease (**polyarteritis nodosa, tertiary syphilis**).

Numbness is a clue to early neuropathic ulcers. Consider early arterial insufficiency in patients with skin fragility, hair loss, dependent edema, and intermittent claudication. The ankle-brachial index test is a sensitive screening tool for arterial insufficiency. Polyarteritis nodosa presents with systemic symptoms and cutaneous manifestations: subcutaneous nodules, palpable purpura, livedo reticularis, and POE or ulceration. Diagnosis of polyarteritis nodosa is confirmed by biopsy. In high-risk groups with slowly enlarging nodules that become POEs or ulcers in different stages of healing on the lower legs, tertiary cutaneous syphilis should be considered. Serological testing confirms the diagnosis.

See Appendix 1 for Further Reading and Image References.

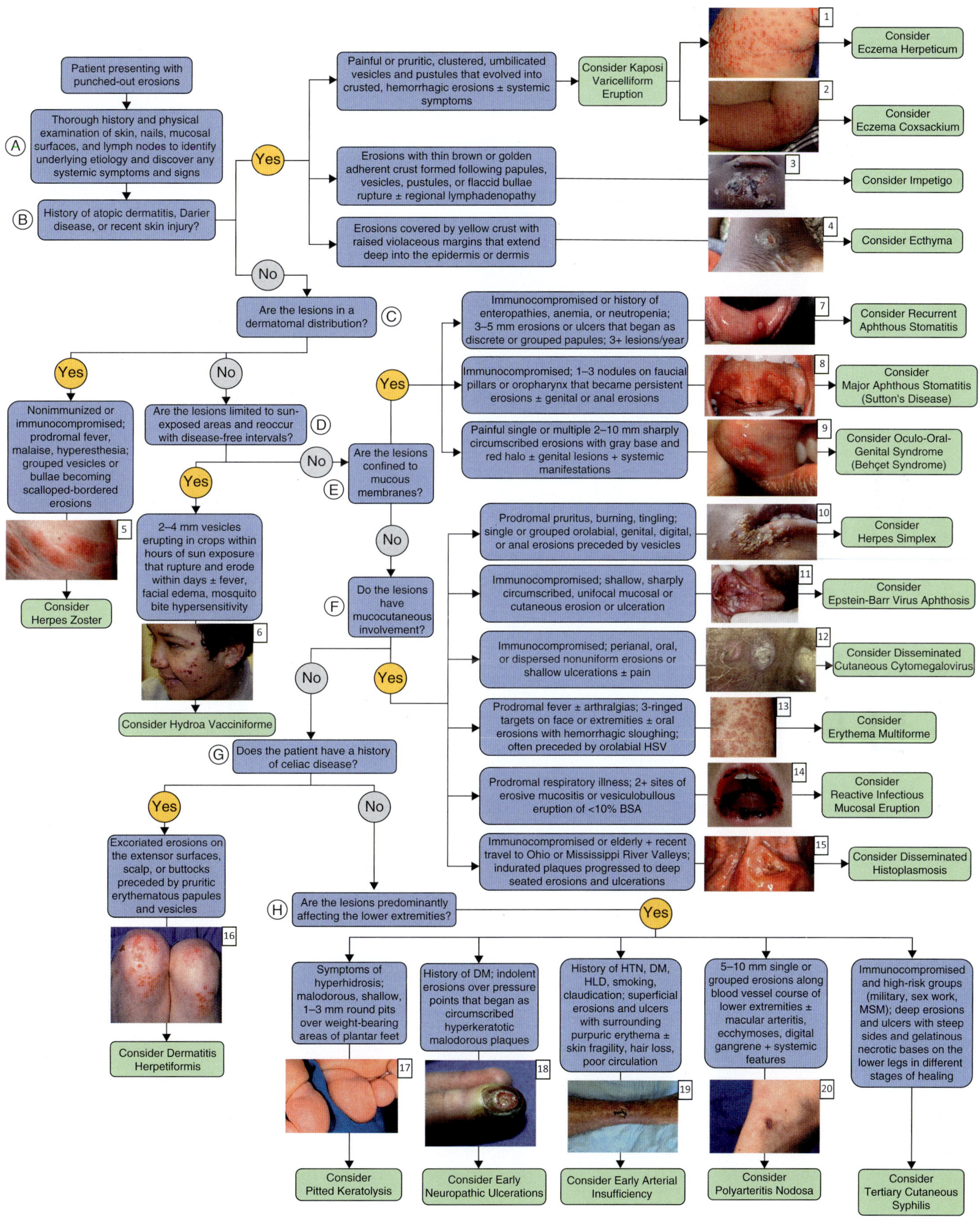
Patient presenting with punched-out erosions
A
Thorough history and physical examination of skin, nails, mucosal surfaces, and lymph nodes to identify underlying etiology and discover any systemic symptoms and signs
B
History of atopic dermatitis, Darier disease, or recent skin injury?
Yes
Painful or pruritic, clustered, umbilicated vesicles and pustules that evolved into crusted, hemorrhagic erosions ± systemic symptoms
Consider Kaposi Varicelliform Eruption
1
Consider Eczema Herpeticum
2
Consider Eczema Coxsackium
Erosions with thin brown or golden adherent crust formed following papules, vesicles, pustules, or flaccid bullae rupture ± regional lymphadenopathy
3
Consider Impetigo
Erosions covered by yellow crust with raised violaceous margins that extend deep into the epidermis or dermis
4
Consider Ecthyma
No
Are the lesions in a dermatomal distribution?
C
Yes
Nonimmunized or immunocompromised; prodromal fever, malaise, hyperesthesia; grouped vesicles or bullae becoming scalloped-bordered erosions
5
Consider Herpes Zoster
No
Are the lesions limited to sun-exposed areas and reoccur with disease-free intervals?
D
Yes
2–4 mm vesicles erupting in crops within hours of sun exposure that rupture and erode within days ± fever, facial edema, mosquito bite hypersensitivity
6
Consider Hydroa Vacciniforme
No
Are the lesions confined to mucous membranes?
E
Yes
Immunocompromised or history of enteropathies, anemia, or neutropenia; 3–5 mm erosions or ulcers that began as discrete or grouped papules; 3+ lesions/year
7
Consider Recurrent Aphthous Stomatitis
Immunocompromised; 1–3 nodules on faucial pillars or oropharynx that became persistent erosions ± genital or anal erosions
8
Consider Major Aphthous Stomatitis (Sutton's Disease)
Painful single or multiple 2–10 mm sharply circumscribed erosions with gray base and red halo ± genital lesions + systemic manifestations
9
Consider Oculo-Oral-Genital Syndrome (Behçet Syndrome)
No
Do the lesions have mucocutaneous involvement?
F
Yes
Prodromal pruritus, burning, tingling; single or grouped orolabial, genital, digital, or anal erosions preceded by vesicles
10
Consider Herpes Simplex
Immunocompromised; shallow, sharply circumscribed, unifocal mucosal or cutaneous erosion or ulceration
11
Consider Epstein-Barr Virus Aphthosis
Immunocompromised; perianal, oral, or dispersed nonuniform erosions or shallow ulcerations ± pain
12
Consider Disseminated Cutaneous Cytomegalovirus
Prodromal fever ± arthralgias; 3-ringed targets on face or extremities ± oral erosions with hemorrhagic sloughing; often preceded by orolabial HSV
13
Consider Erythema Multiforme
Prodromal respiratory illness; 2+ sites of erosive mucositis or vesiculobullous eruption of <10% BSA
14
Consider Reactive Infectious Mucosal Eruption
Immunocompromised or elderly + recent travel to Ohio or Mississippi River Valleys; indurated plaques progressed to deep seated erosions and ulcerations
15
Consider Disseminated Histoplasmosis
No
G
Does the patient have a history of celiac disease?
Yes
Excoriated erosions on the extensor surfaces, scalp, or buttocks preceded by pruritic erythematous papules and vesicles
16
Consider Dermatitis Herpetiformis
No
H
Are the lesions predominantly affecting the lower extremities?
Yes
Symptoms of hyperhidrosis; malodorous, shallow, 1–3 mm round pits over weight-bearing areas of plantar feet
17
Consider Pitted Keratolysis
History of DM; indolent erosions over pressure points that began as circumscribed hyperkeratotic malodorous plaques
18
Consider Early Neuropathic Ulcerations
History of HTN, DM, HLD, smoking, claudication; superficial erosions and ulcers with surrounding purpuric erythema ± skin fragility, hair loss, poor circulation
19
Consider Early Arterial Insufficiency
5–10 mm single or grouped erosions along blood vessel course of lower extremities ± macular arteritis, ecchymoses, digital gangrene + systemic features
20
Consider Polyarteritis Nodosa
Immunocompromised and high-risk groups (military, sex work, MSM); deep erosions and ulcers with steep sides and gelatinous necrotic bases on the lower legs in different stages of healing
Consider Tertiary Cutaneous Syphilis

PART VII
Papules and Plaques

25 Verrucous Papules and Plaques

Kirk Williams and Steven Daveluy

The term verrucous means "wartlike" and describes skin lesions with a hyperkeratotic surface. A variety of diseases can present with verrucous papules and plaques.

A. **Verruca** presents as hyperkeratotic papules with thrombosed capillaries, seen as small red/black dots that can often be better appreciated when lesions are pared down. Verruca is common in children and the immunocompromised. Recalcitrant lesions should raise suspicion for **squamous cell carcinoma (SCC)** or **verrucous carcinoma**.

B. Rough wartlike papules in a linear or whorled configuration, present since birth or childhood, are typical of **epidermal nevi**, which are benign hamartomas that often follow the lines of Blaschko. Changes in texture or color over time can occur.

C. **Angiokeratomas** are vascular red-purple papules with either a smooth or verrucous surface. They have a predilection for the scrotum and vulva but can present anywhere.

D. **Seborrheic keratoses** can have a variety of appearances, including stuck-on-appearing papules/plaques with a verrucous surface. They increase in number with age and present anywhere except the palms and soles.

E. **SCC** can present as a verrucous papule that enlarges and may ulcerate. It can present anywhere but is most common in areas of chronic sun damage. Biopsy is required for diagnosis. **Keratoacanthoma** is a subtype of SCC with a distinct history and morphology. It presents as a dome-shaped papulonodule with a central depression with rapid growth.

F. **Actinic keratoses** can present as hyperkeratotic papules or plaques in areas of sun damage. Patients often have several actinic keratoses in the same anatomic area.

G. Skin tags, otherwise known as **acrochordons**, present as skin-colored or hyperpigmented pedunculated papules that typically have a smooth surface but may present with a verrucous or hyperkeratotic surface.

H. **Dermatosis papulosa nigra** typically presents as monomorphic, small round papules on the cheeks of individuals of African or Asian descent.

I. The entities that cause verrucous papules on the palms and soles can be distinguished by their distinct morphology. **Punctate palmoplantar keratoderma** presents with hyperkeratotic papules on the palms and soles. **Spiny keratoderma** is a variant that presents with spine-like projections.

Patient presenting with a verrucous papule or plaque

↓

Detailed history and physical examination of the skin, nails, lymph nodes, and mucosal surfaces to discover classification of lesion

↓

Is the lesion a papule?

No → *continued on next page*

Yes ↓

(A) Thrombosed capillaries; Hyperkeratotic papule, red/black dots

1

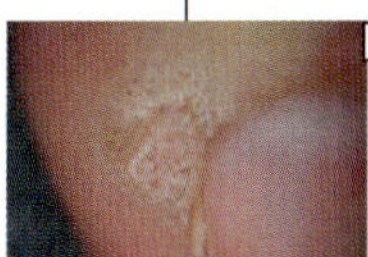

→ Consider Verruca, SCC, or Verrucous Carcinoma

(B) Linear or whorled configuration

2

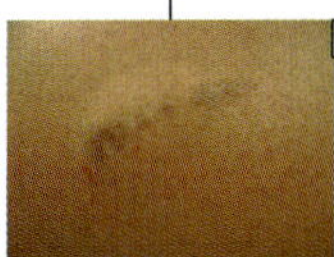

→ Consider Epidermal Nevus

(C) Purple/red in color, often located on the scrotum or vulva

3

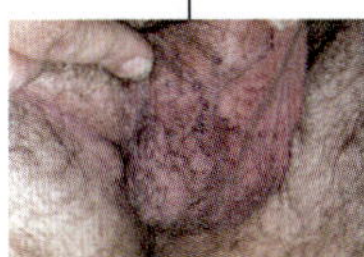

→ Consider Angiokeratoma

(D) Waxy, stuck-on appearance; anywhere except the palms/soles

4

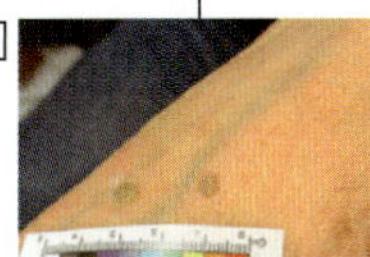

→ Consider Seborrheic Keratosis

(E) Papules or plaques, variegated in color, +/– ulceration; Erythematous, hyperkeratotic; Background of chronic sun damage

5

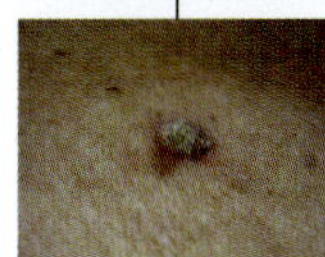

→ Consider Squamous Cell Carcinoma, Verrucous Carcinoma, Keratoacanthoma

(F) Photodistributed hyperkeratotic macules and papules, fair skin and sun damage

6

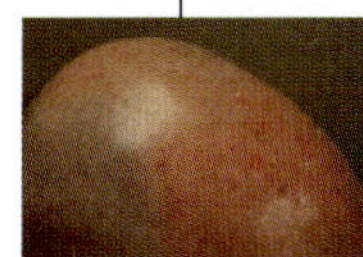

→ Consider Actinic Keratosis

(G) Pedunculated papule with hyperkeratosis on tip, often surrounded by soft pedunculated papules

7

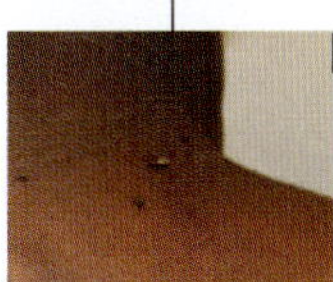

→ Consider Acrochordon

(H) 1-3 mm brown papules on the face

8

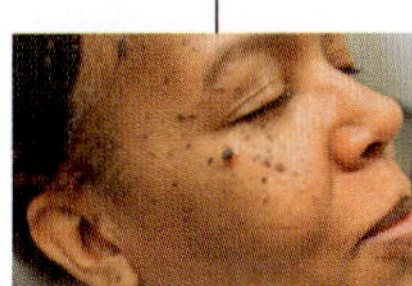

→ Consider Dermatosis Papulosa Nigra

(I) 1-2 mm palmoplantar spine-like keratotic papules resembling a music box

9

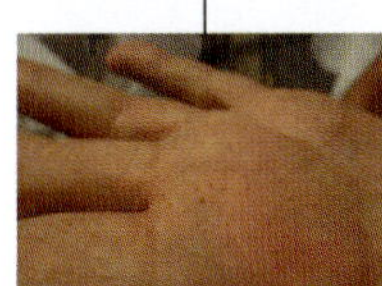

→ Consider Spiny Keratoderma

(I) Keratotic papules on the palms and soles; Confined to the creases of the palms and heel

10

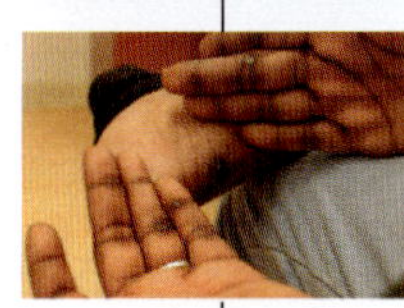

→ Consider Punctate Palmoplantar Keratoderma

Continued

J. In a patient with prior exposure to *Mycobacterium tuberculosis*, repeat exposure via inoculation of the skin can lead to **tuberculosis verrucosa cutis**, which presents as a verrucous plaque, often on the hands.

K. Lesions with a predilection for the lower legs include **hypertrophic lichen planus** and verrucous **Kaposi sarcoma (KS)**. Intensely pruritic plaques with a surface resembling an igneous rock are seen in hypertrophic lichen planus. This condition typically presents on the shins and can also involve the ankles, arms, or trunk. Verrucous KS is a rare variant of KS that can present in patients with the HIV-associated form.

L. Vegetating **pyodermatitis vegetans** is often associated with inflammatory bowel disease and presents with erosive vegetating plaques, often in intertriginous areas. Flaccid bullae and pustules may also be present.

M. **Bromoderma**, resulting from systemic exposure to bromides, often presents as erythematous, edematous plaques, which may evolve into vegetating or ulcerated plaques. Early lesions resemble an acneiform eruption.

N. Multiple **infectious diseases** of the skin can present with verrucous plaques, either owing to direct inoculation or hematogenous spread. A thorough history regarding travel to endemic areas and assessing for systemic symptoms, such as fever and cough, can help narrow the differential. Biopsy with tissue culture is needed for diagnosis.

O. There are rare reports of **mycosis fungoides** presenting with verrucous plaques, either de novo or in the presence of a known disease. Cutaneous **sarcoidosis** can present as verrucous papules and plaques and can be misdiagnosed as SCC or verruca. The rare perforating variant of granuloma annulare presents with erythematous papules and plaques with central hyperkeratosis, as opposed to the smooth-topped annular plaques seen in classic granuloma annulare. Histology is needed for the diagnosis of these conditions.

See Appendix 1 for Further Reading and Image References.

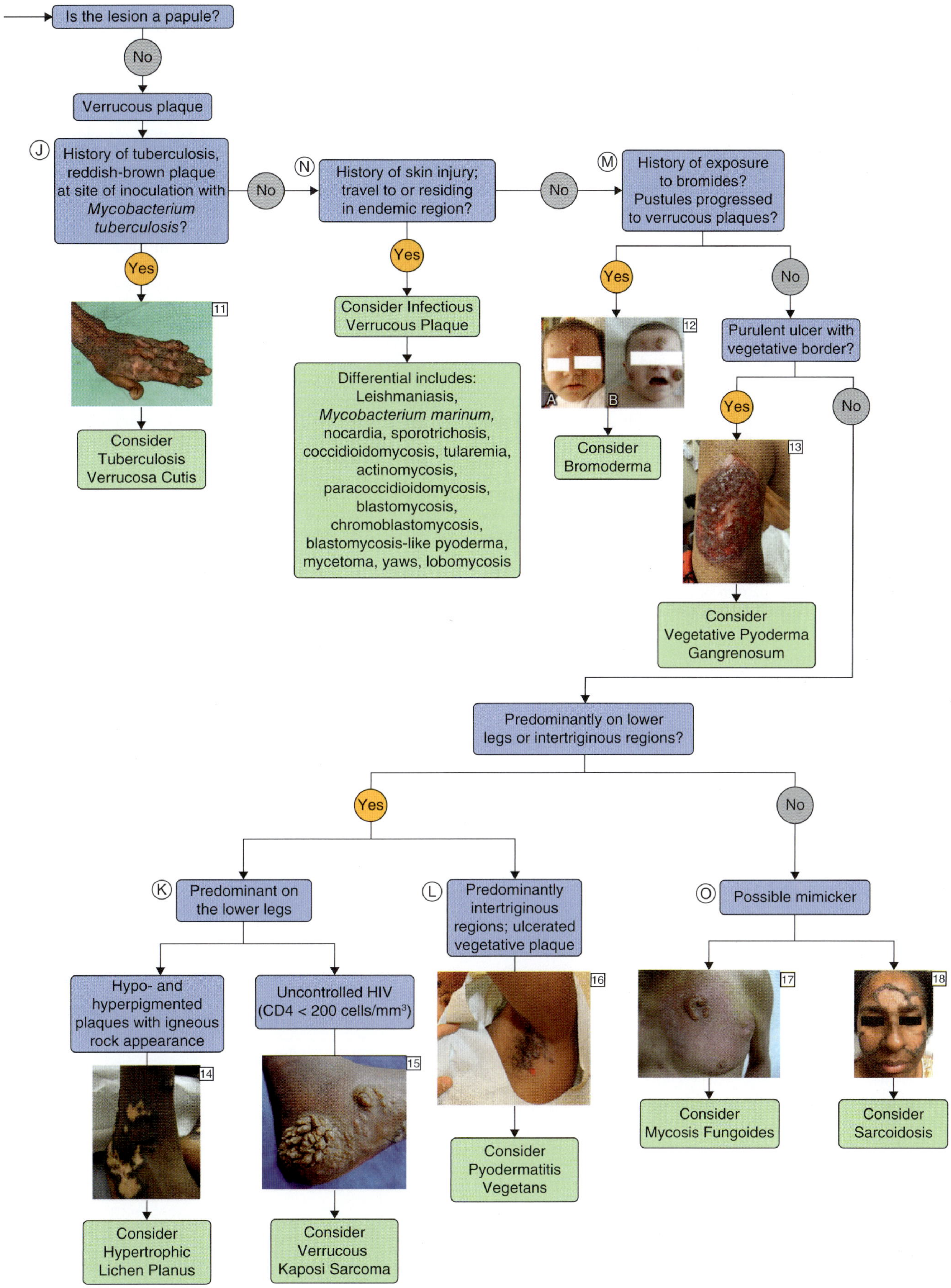
Is the lesion a papule?
No
Verrucous plaque
J
History of tuberculosis, reddish-brown plaque at site of inoculation with *Mycobacterium tuberculosis*?
Yes
11
Consider Tuberculosis Verrucosa Cutis
No
N
History of skin injury; travel to or residing in endemic region?
Yes
Consider Infectious Verrucous Plaque
Differential includes: Leishmaniasis, *Mycobacterium marinum,* nocardia, sporotrichosis, coccidioidomycosis, tularemia, actinomycosis, paracoccidioidomycosis, blastomycosis, chromoblastomycosis, blastomycosis-like pyoderma, mycetoma, yaws, lobomycosis
No
M
History of exposure to bromides? Pustules progressed to verrucous plaques?
Yes
12
A
B
Consider Bromoderma
No
Purulent ulcer with vegetative border?
Yes
13
Consider Vegetative Pyoderma Gangrenosum
No
Predominantly on lower legs or intertriginous regions?
Yes
K
Predominant on the lower legs
Hypo- and hyperpigmented plaques with igneous rock appearance
14
Consider Hypertrophic Lichen Planus
Uncontrolled HIV (CD4 < 200 cells/mm³)
15
Consider Verrucous Kaposi Sarcoma
L
Predominantly intertriginous regions; ulcerated vegetative plaque
16
Consider Pyodermatitis Vegetans
No
O
Possible mimicker
17
Consider Mycosis Fungoides
18
Consider Sarcoidosis

26 Spiny Papules

Rahul Masson and Jennifer L. Hsiao

Spiny papules are primary lesions that may be seen in a variety of different cutaneous conditions. They may be associated with systemic conditions, such as vitamin deficiency, diabetes, or renal disease. Drugs and infections may also trigger eruptions with spiny papules. A key clinical feature to consider is whether the distribution of spiny papules is follicular or not.

A. During the initial evaluation of a patient presenting with spiny papules, a comprehensive history should be elicited, including any underlying medical conditions, current and past medications, and social history. Conduct a complete review of systems to identify any systemic signs or symptoms. Perform a thorough physical examination of the face, trunk, extremities, and palmoplantar regions. Evaluate for alopecia.

B. Spiny papules may present in patients with a history of atopy. **Keratosis pilaris (KP)** usually presents with erythematous minute follicular keratotic papules on the extensor surfaces of the arms and thighs. Older patients who present with dome-shaped pruritic nodules on the trunk and extremities may have **prurigo nodularis**. Prurigo nodularis tends to spare the upper mid-back resulting in a characteristic "butterfly sign," and irritants such as heat or sweat can worsen the pruritis. Of note, patients with prurigo nodularis may also present without history of atopy. If a patient has atopic dermatitis with a predominant pattern of pruritic follicular accentuation, consider a diagnosis of **follicular eczema**.

C. **Arsenical keratosis** presents as keratotic papules on the pressure points of the palms and soles. A thorough social and occupational history should be obtained to elicit potential exposure to arsenic through medication, water, or other sources of contamination.

D. Targeted immunotherapies can trigger the onset of spiny papules in KP-like or pityriasis rubra pilaris (PRP)-like distributions. **KP-like drug eruptions** present with diffuse minute follicular papules that spare the palms and soles. In contrast, **PRP-like drug reactions** present with pink- or salmon-colored follicular papules coalescing into large plaques with islands of sparing, typically on the trunk and extremities.

E. If a patient presents with discrete, nonfollicular, keratotic papules confined to sites of previous irradiation, the patient may have **postirradiation digitate keratosis**. This condition has mainly been reported in older female patients who have received radiation treatment for breast cancer.

F. **KP atrophicans** is a group of disorders that include KP atrophicans faciei (also called ulerythema ophryogenes), atrophoderma vermiculatum, and keratosis follicularis spinulosa decalvans. These conditions are characterized by inflammatory hyperkeratotic papules followed by scarring and possibly alopecia.

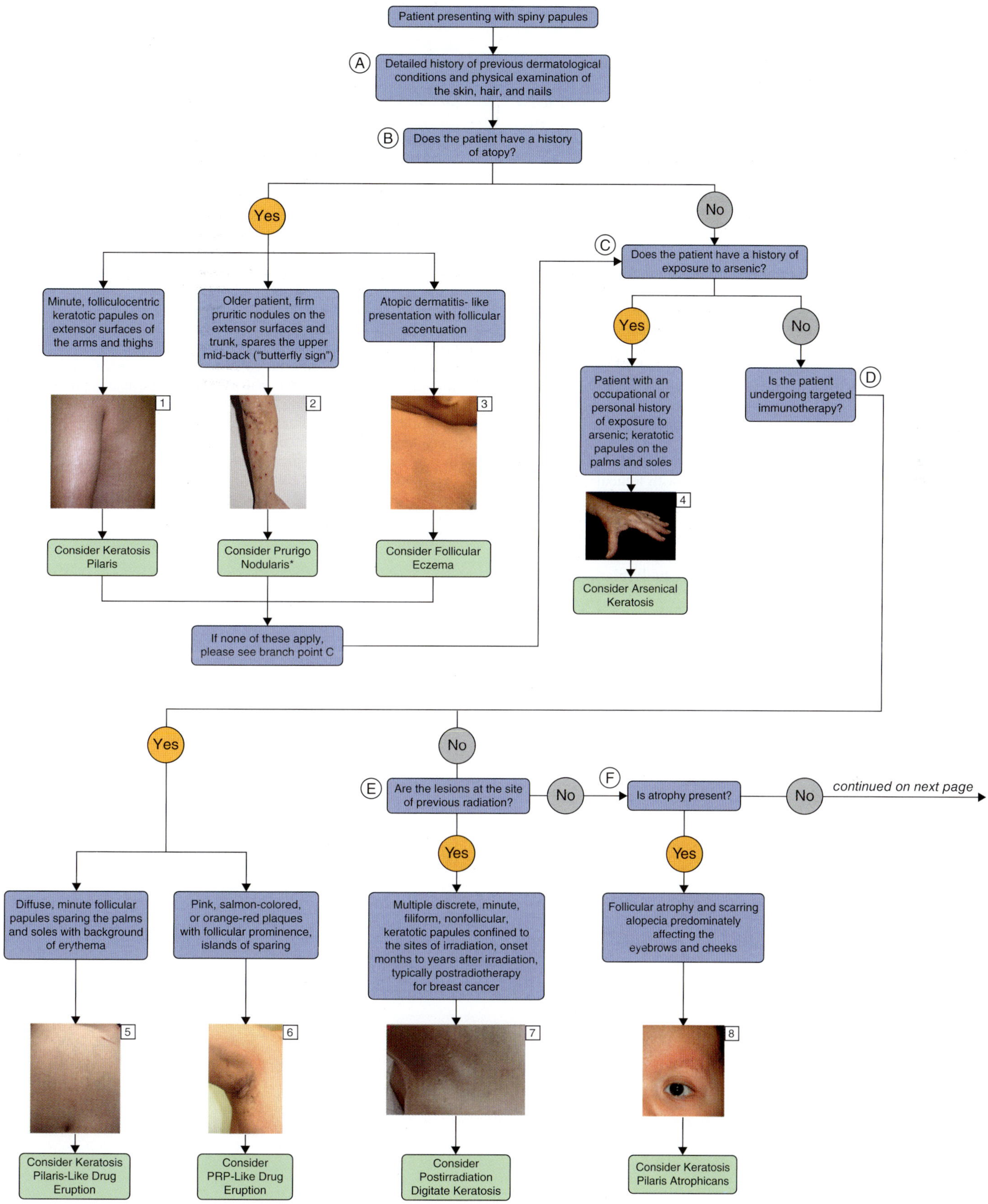

*May also occur in individuals without a history of atopy

Continued

G. **Lichen spinulosus** presents with skin-colored follicular papules that can coalesce into larger plaques on the trunk and extremities. If generalized, it may occur as part of type VI, human immunodeficiency virus (HIV)–associated PRP.

Phrynoderma presents with generalized follicular keratotic papules and can present with a characteristic "toad skin" appearance. It is caused by nutritional deficiencies, most often vitamin A deficiency. Other clinical features of vitamin A deficiency may be present, such as night blindness or xerophthalmia.

PRP has a bimodal distribution with most patients presenting in the first or fifth/sixth decade of life. Key features include reddish-orange follicular papules coalescing into plaques with "islands of sparing." There is typically craniocaudal spread, and some patients will progress to erythroderma. Waxy reddish-orange or yellow palmoplantar keratoderma may be present.

Disseminate and recurrent infundibulofolliculitis is characterized by 1 to 2 mm pruritic, monomorphic, skin-colored, folliculocentric papules, resembling "goosebumps," on the neck, trunk, and extremities. This condition predominantly occurs in young adult males of African descent.

Erythromelanosis follicularis presents as reddish-brown patches on the face (particularly the lateral cheeks) and neck, with minute follicular papules within the patches. There may be associated alopecia in the patches. Most cases were originally reported among people of Asian descent.

Folliculotropic mycosis fungoides may present with pruritic patches and plaques on the head and neck with follicular accentuation and associated alopecia.

For older patients reporting a history of multiple myeloma or paraproteinemia and presenting with follicular spicules on the face, a diagnosis of **hyperkeratotic spicules** should be considered. The spiny, skin- to pink-colored papules of **trichodysplasia spinulosa** also localize to the head (especially the central face) and neck regions, and concomitant alopecia of the eyebrows and eyelashes may be seen. Trichodysplasia spinulosa is caused by a polyomavirus infection, and immunocompromised patients are most affected.

H. A central hyperkeratotic plug is a key clinical characteristic of acquired perforating dermatoses, which include Kyrle disease, **reactive perforating collagenosis (RPC)**, perforating folliculitis, and **elastosis perforans serpiginosa (EPS)**. These dermatoses are generally associated with underlying medical conditions, such as diabetes mellitus or chronic kidney disease. Both **Kyrle disease** and **RPC** present with hyperkeratotic papules, typically on the lower extremities and are most common in those with long-standing diabetes or renal disease. RPC has an inherited form that has onset in childhood. The Koebner phenomenon may occur in RPC. **Perforating folliculitis** presents with keratotic follicular papules, typically on the extremities and buttocks. Finally, consider **EPS** in younger male patients with nonpruritic, skin-colored, or slightly erythematous keratotic papules, some with an overlying central crust, in an annular or serpiginous pattern. EPS may be associated with genetic disorders, such as Down syndrome, Ehlers-Danlos syndrome, Marfan syndrome, or drug induced.

I. **Multiple filiform verrucae** typically present as skin-colored filiform papules on the face. A history of HIV or other underlying immunodeficiency may be considered if the verrucae are extensive. **Spiny keratoderma** is a subtype of punctate palmoplantar keratoderma, which may be inherited or acquired. It presents with pinpoint keratotic projections on the palms and/or soles. Finally, consider a diagnosis of **multiple minute digitate hyperkeratosis** in patients with spiny projections on the trunk and/or extremities in a nonfollicular distribution.

See Appendix 1 for Further Reading and Image References.

Does the patient have lesions in a follicular distribution?

(G) Yes

- Skin-colored follicular papules coalescing into larger plaques, symmetric involvement of the trunk and extremities

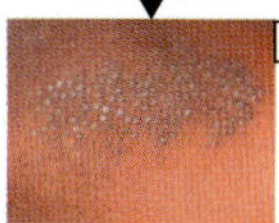

9

  → Consider Lichen Spinulosus

- Deficiency in vitamin A or general malnutrition, may have night blindness and xerophthalmia, generalized involvement

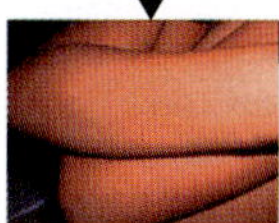

10

  → Consider Phrynoderma

- Follicular red-orange or salmon papules coalescing into plaques, +/- palmoplantar keratoderma, +/- erythroderma, and islands of sparing

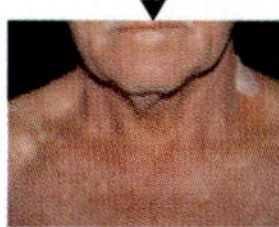

11

  → Consider Pityriasis Rubra Pilaris

- Patient of African descent with solitary and confluent skin-colored papules in a follicular distribution on the neck, trunk, and extremities

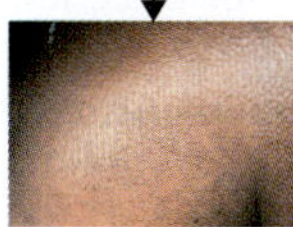

12

  → Consider Disseminate and Recurrent Infundibulofolliculitis

- Bilateral erythematous patches with follicular papules on lateral cheeks, associated with hyperpigmentation and alopecia

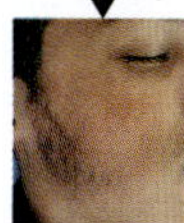

13

  → Consider Erythromelanosis Follicularis Faciei

- Patches and plaques mainly on the head and neck with follicular accentuation; alopecia may be present +pruritic

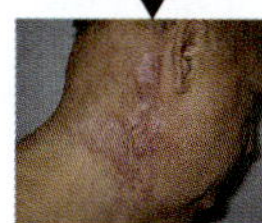

14

  → Consider Folliculotropic Mycosis Fungoides

- Older patient with a history of multiple myeloma, paraproteinemia, or cryoglobulinemia; presents with follicular spicules

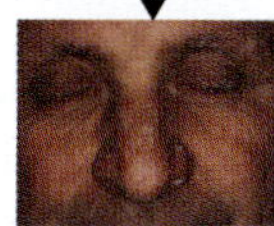

15

  → Consider Hyperkeratotic Spicules

- Immuno-compromised patient with skin-colored papules and follicular spines on the central face, +/- alopecia of the eyebrows and eyelashes

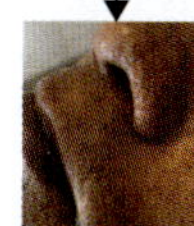

16

  → Consider Trichodysplasia Spinulosa

No →

(H) Is a central hyperkeratotic plug present?

Yes

- Skin-colored, erythematous, or hyperpigmented umbilicated papules with tightly adherent central crust or plug; grouped in linear, arcuate, or serpiginous patterns; most common on neck and arms; associated with Down syndrome, D-penicillamine use, and other genetic disorders

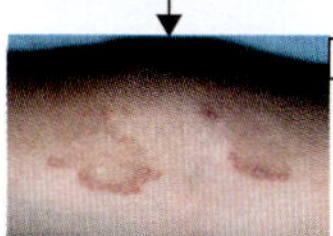

17

  → Consider Elastosis Perforans Serpiginosa

- Erythematous or brown follicular papules with central keratotic plug on the extremities and buttocks; has also been described in the setting of psoriasis and HIV infection

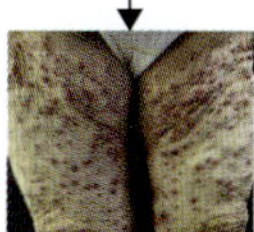

18

  → Consider Perforating Folliculitis

- Skin-colored or hyperpigmented papules with central keratotic plug, + koebnerization, history of chronic kidney disease, diabetes, or rarely malignancy or medication induced; typically on the legs or generalized

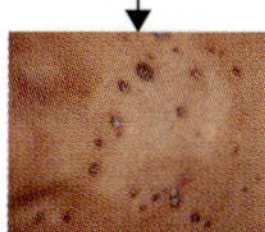

19

  → Consider Reactive Perforating Collagenosis

- History of long-standing diabetes or chronic renal disease, large hyperkeratotic papules on the lower extremities

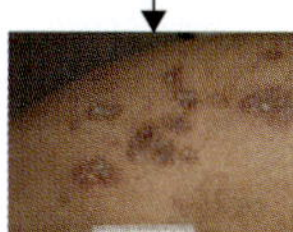

20

  → Consider Kyrle Disease

No → **(I)**

- Lesions predominately on the face and/or neck
  - Multiple filiform verrucous papules, mainly on the face and neck; potential history of HIV if extensive

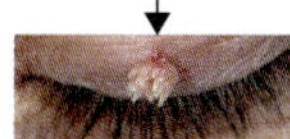

21

  → Consider Multiple Filiform Verrucae (Warts)

- Lesions predominately on the palmoplantar regions
  - Discrete pinpoint keratotic projections on the palms, soles, or both; +/- positive family history; if acquired, +/- associated malignancy

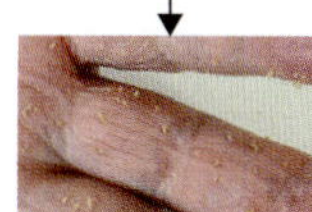

22

  → Consider Spiny Keratoderma (Palmoplantar Keratoderma)

- Lesions predominately on the trunk and/or extremities
  - White, yellow, or brown spicules in a nonfollicular distribution on the trunk and limbs

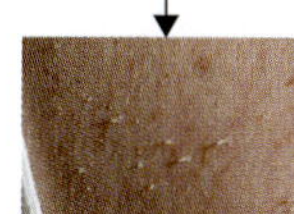

23

  → Consider Multiple Minute Digitate Hyperkeratosis

27 Targetoid Papules

Jesse J. Keller

Targetoid papules are a distinct cutaneous finding that can represent a variety of skin conditions depending on the nature, location, distribution, and context of the targets. They may be seen in the setting of uncomplicated urticaria to life-threatening conditions, such as Stevens-Johnson syndrome.

A. The first step is to confirm whether the target fits the description of a "typical target." A typical target features three complete zones—a central dusky red dot surrounded by a circumferential edematous zone of pallor, which is surrounded further by a final erythematous rim. Atypical targets, which can display incomplete rings and may not feature all three complete zones, are often seen in **Stevens-Johnson syndrome/toxic epidermal necrolysis (SJS/TEN)**. Atypical targets of SJS/TEN may be macular and progress to the development of bullae and epidermal desquamation. Common medication culprits include allopurinol, antibiotics, anticonvulsants, and nonsteroidal antiinflammatory drugs (NSAIDs). Skin biopsy is important to promptly confirm this diagnosis, as patients are likely to require specialized care in a burn unit setting.

B. **Urticaria** is a common condition that may occasionally present in targetoid form. Reassuring findings include pruritus and a migratory nature, with individual lesions clearing completely in less than 24 hours.

C. Targetoid lesions that are fixed, painful, and leave behind hyperpigmentation may be suggestive of **urticarial vasculitis**. Workup for urticarial vasculitis includes a thorough review of systems that may reveal fatigue, malaise, and joint pain. Additionally, serum and urine testing may demonstrate reduced complement and/or proteinuria. Histology classically shows a neutrophilic infiltrate, leukocytoclasis, and fibrinoid necrosis.

D. The prototypical targetoid rash is **erythema multiforme (EM)**. EM is most commonly a sequela of orolabial or genital herpes simplex virus reactivation and classically presents with typical targets on the palms and soles. Less commonly, EM may be precipitated by other viral infections, vaccinations, antibiotics, systemic inflammatory conditions, or malignancy. Skin biopsy often demonstrates lymphocytic infiltrate and interface change.

E. **Bites from *Cimex lectularius* (bedbugs)** can result in targetoid papules, typically presenting with a mostly acral distribution. Grouping of three lesions together may serve as a clue. A biopsy showing a superficial and deep eosinophilic infiltrate supports a diagnosis of arthropod bite, and home inspection may be necessary to identify the infestation.

F. Intermittent same-site targetoid papules may be seen in the case of a **fixed drug eruption (FDE)**, which is a reaction to an intermittently ingested medication. Common culprits include antimicrobials and NSAIDs. FDE may present with blistering and typically heals with hyperpigmentation. Common areas of involvement include mucosal sites (e.g., oral mucosa, genitals) as well as interdigital spaces. Skin biopsy showing interface change, pigment incontinence, and melanophages may be confirmatory. A thorough review of over-the-counter and intermittently ingested medications that the patient may not immediately recall is helpful to identify and eliminate the causative agent.

See Appendix 1 for Further Reading and Image References.

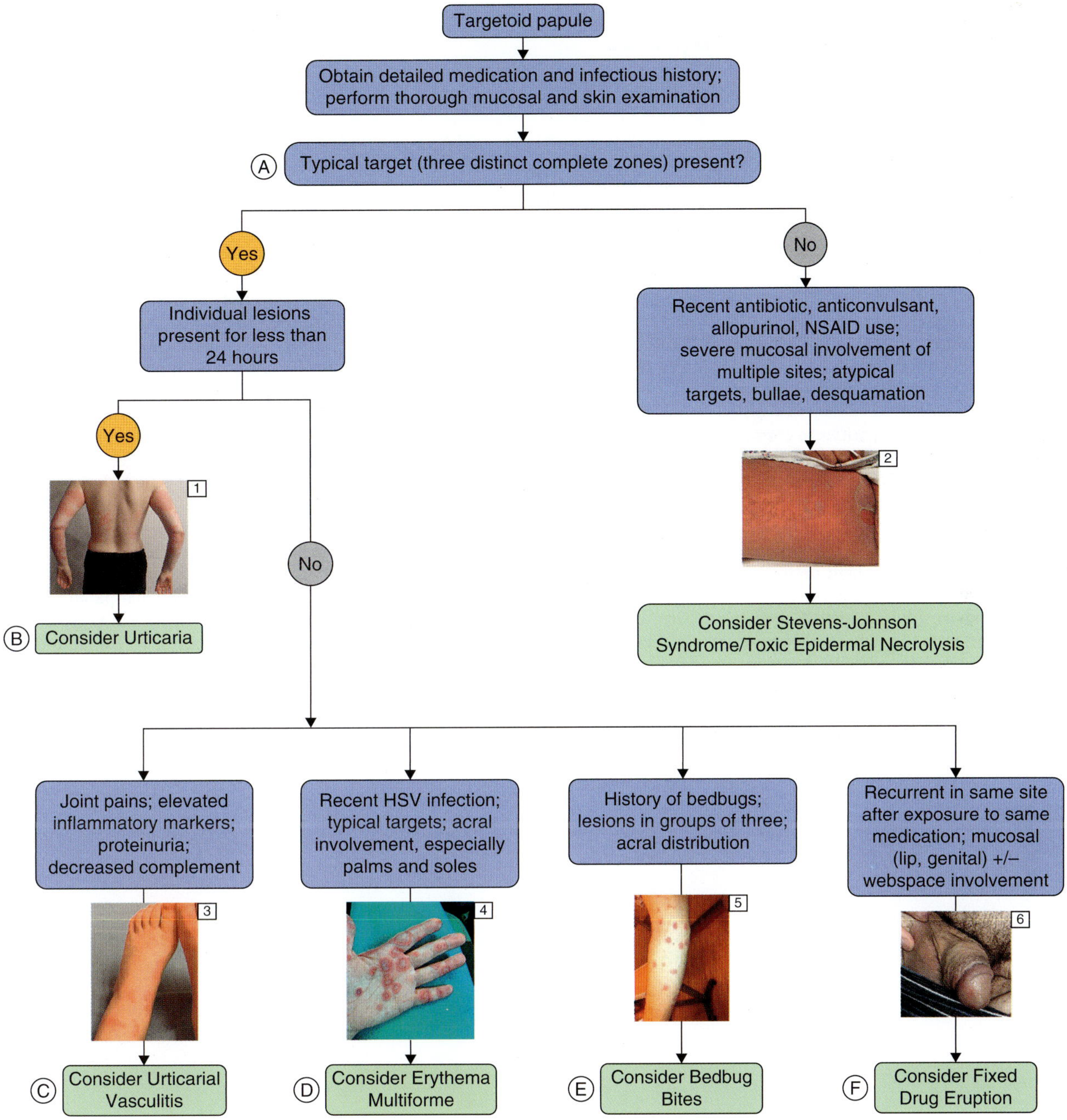
Targetoid papule
Obtain detailed medication and infectious history; perform thorough mucosal and skin examination
(A) Typical target (three distinct complete zones) present?
Yes
Individual lesions present for less than 24 hours
Yes
1
(B) Consider Urticaria
No
No
Recent antibiotic, anticonvulsant, allopurinol, NSAID use; severe mucosal involvement of multiple sites; atypical targets, bullae, desquamation
2
Consider Stevens-Johnson Syndrome/Toxic Epidermal Necrolysis
Joint pains; elevated inflammatory markers; proteinuria; decreased complement
3
(C) Consider Urticarial Vasculitis
Recent HSV infection; typical targets; acral involvement, especially palms and soles
4
(D) Consider Erythema Multiforme
History of bedbugs; lesions in groups of three; acral distribution
5
(E) Consider Bedbug Bites
Recurrent in same site after exposure to same medication; mucosal (lip, genital) +/– webspace involvement
6
(F) Consider Fixed Drug Eruption

28 Monomorphic Papules

Linnea Westerkam and Christopher Sayed

Monomorphic papule(s) are defined as raised solid lesions ≤10 mm in diameter with little variation in appearance. There is a broad differential for a patient presenting with monomorphic papules, so further medical history, examination, and diagnostic testing are often needed to elucidate the correct diagnosis and management strategies.

A. A detailed history (particularly onset, symptoms, and prior similar lesions) and thorough examination should be included in the initial evaluation. Skin biopsy may also be useful but is not necessary for most diagnoses. Eliciting progression, chronicity, and distribution will likely lead down specific diagnostic pathways.

B. If a viral cause is suspected, entities to consider include **molluscum contagiosum (MC)**, **flat wart**, and **common wart**. MC is a skin infection caused by the DNA poxvirus and is typically self-limited in healthy individuals. Infection is most commonly seen in children; however, in adults, anogenital-predominant lesions may be transmitted via sexual contact or MC may indicate an underlying immunodeficiency. MC lesions are firm umbilicated papules and can be found anywhere on the body. Flat and common warts, caused by the human papillomavirus, have a predilection for the hands and feet, although they can occur anywhere and be widespread. Flat warts are typically smooth, whereas common warts are hyperkeratotic with a rough surface.

C. Asymptomatic monomorphic papules that tend to appear in grouped distributions include **keratosis pilaris** and **lichen nitidus**. Keratosis pilaris presents as minute skin-colored to erythematous follicular papules, typically occurring symmetrically on the posterior upper arms and thighs. Lesions may also appear on the cheeks and buttocks and often improve with age. Lichen nitidus lesions are 1- to 2 mm papules with a potentially more widespread asymmetric distribution, usually in a clustered or linear configuration.

D. Differential diagnosis for diffuse asymptomatic monomorphic papules includes **perforating disorders**, **hyperkeratosis lenticularis perstans**, **disseminated superficial actinic porokeratosis**, and **vitamin deficiencies**. Perforating disorders present as larger spinier papules, often associated with underlying syndromes or chronic disease (i.e., end-stage renal disease). The lesions of hyperkeratosis lenticularis perstans, also known as Flegel disease, are commonly seen on the distal lower extremities. Disseminated superficial actinic porokeratosis is typically multiple, erythematous, flat papules on the extremities with a double-edged ring of scale at the border. Vitamin deficiencies causing hyperkeratotic follicular papules on the extremities include both scurvy (vitamin C), which is typically associated with impaired wound healing, gingival bleeding, and coiled hairs, and phrynoderma (vitamin A), which typically has associated eye findings.

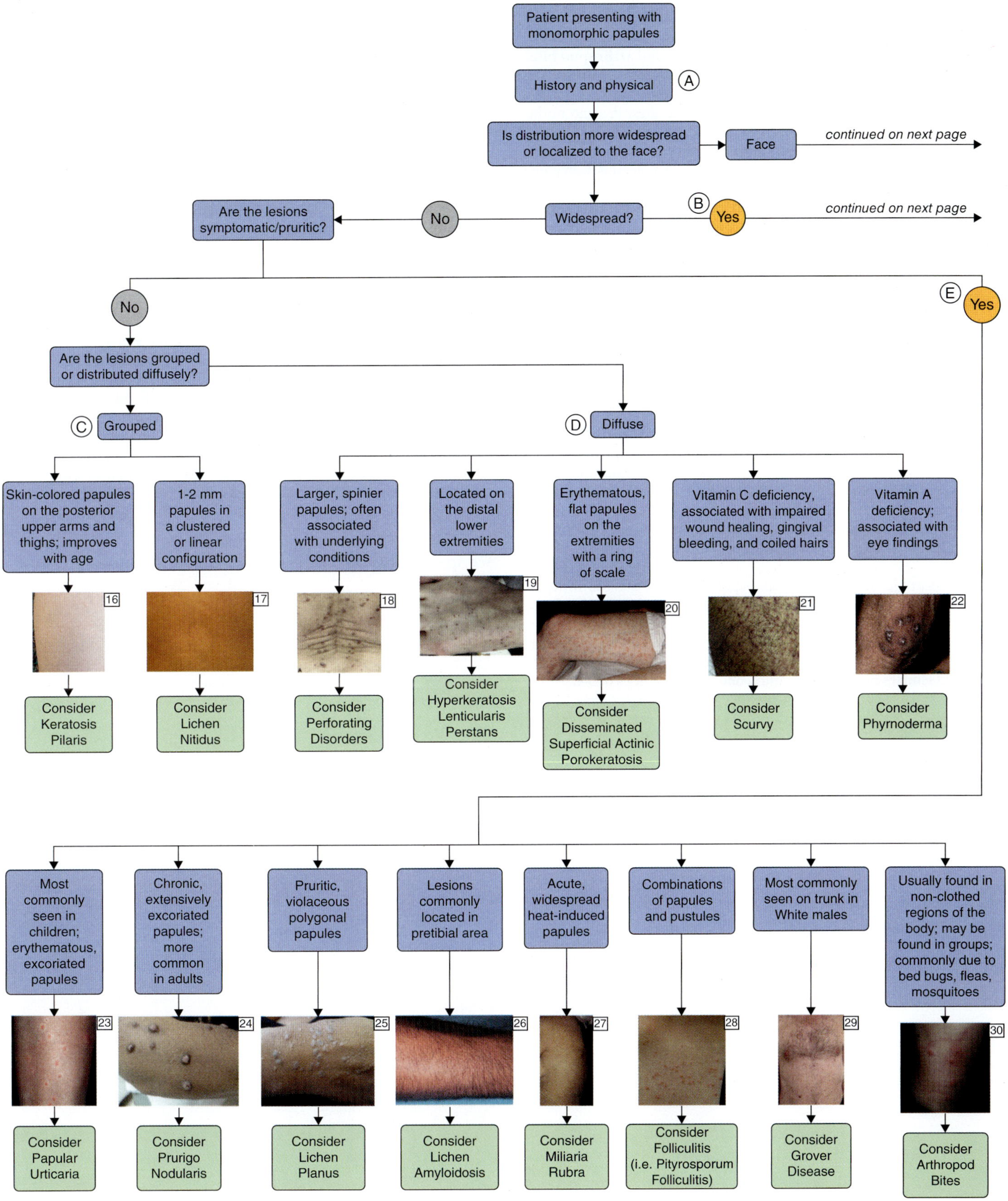
Patient presenting with monomorphic papules
History and physical
A
Is distribution more widespread or localized to the face?
Face
continued on next page
Widespread?
B
Yes
continued on next page
No
Are the lesions symptomatic/pruritic?
No
E
Yes
Are the lesions grouped or distributed diffusely?
C
Grouped
D
Diffuse
Skin-colored papules on the posterior upper arms and thighs; improves with age
16
Consider Keratosis Pilaris
1-2 mm papules in a clustered or linear configuration
17
Consider Lichen Nitidus
Larger, spinier papules; often associated with underlying conditions
18
Consider Perforating Disorders
Located on the distal lower extremities
19
Consider Hyperkeratosis Lenticularis Perstans
Erythematous, flat papules on the extremities with a ring of scale
20
Consider Disseminated Superficial Actinic Porokeratosis
Vitamin C deficiency, associated with impaired wound healing, gingival bleeding, and coiled hairs
21
Consider Scurvy
Vitamin A deficiency; associated with eye findings
22
Consider Phyrnoderma
Most commonly seen in children; erythematous, excoriated papules
23
Consider Papular Urticaria
Chronic, extensively excoriated papules; more common in adults
24
Consider Prurigo Nodularis
Pruritic, violaceous polygonal papules
25
Consider Lichen Planus
Lesions commonly located in pretibial area
26
Consider Lichen Amyloidosis
Acute, widespread heat-induced papules
27
Consider Miliaria Rubra
Combinations of papules and pustules
28
Consider Folliculitis (i.e. Pityrosporum Folliculitis)
Most commonly seen on trunk in White males
29
Consider Grover Disease
Usually found in non-clothed regions of the body; may be found in groups; commonly due to bed bugs, fleas, mosquitoes
30
Consider Arthropod Bites

Continued

E. For patients presenting with pruritic monomorphic papules, **papular urticaria**, **prurigo nodularis**, **lichen planus**, **lichen amyloidosis**, **miliaria rubra**, **folliculitis**, **Grover disease**, and **arthropod bites** should be considered. Papular urticaria is most commonly seen in patients aged 2 to 10 years as erythematous papules and most likely represents a hypersensitivity reaction to insect bites. Prurigo nodularis appears as chronic, extensively excoriated lesions and is more common in adults and patients with a history of atopic dermatitis. If a patient presents with intensely pruritic, violaceous polygonal papules, lichen planus should be considered. The pretibial area is most commonly affected by lichen amyloidosis, which presents with hyperpigmented papules that coalesce into rippled plaques. Miliaria rubra presents as acute heat-induced papules common in warm, humid climates or on the back of hospitalized patients who are mostly immobile in beds. Folliculitis, specifically pityrosporum folliculitis, usually consists of a mix of follicular papules and pustules on the upper trunk. Papules of Grover disease, also called transient acantholytic dermatosis, are most commonly seen on the trunk and are most prevalent in White males. Arthropod bites (e.g., bed bug, flea, mosquito) are usually located in unclothed areas of the body and may be grouped, particularly with bed bugs.

F. For patients presenting with facial monomorphic papules, the color of the lesions is an important distinguishing feature. The differential diagnosis for whitish yellow papules on the face includes **osteoma cutis** and **milium**. Osteoma cutis presents as shiny erythematous to yellowish to skin-colored papules that may coalesce into plaques, often associated with trauma or prior inflammation. Milium are described as 1- to 2-mm smooth white papules.

G. Monomorphic acneiform facial papules include **steroid-induced acne** and **periorificial dermatitis**. Steroid-induced acne should be considered in adults using corticosteroids; lesions may also be widespread on the chest and back. Periorificial dermatitis typically presents as erythematous papules around the nose and mouth and is most common in females in the second, third, and fourth decades of life.

H. **Dermatosis papulosa nigra (DPN)** should be considered for hyperpigmented facial papules. DPN is most frequently seen on the cheeks in Black people, and lesions are typically 1 to 3 mm. Reddish brown firm papules on the face may reflect **lupus miliaris disseminatus faciei**.

I. The differential diagnosis for skin-colored facial papules includes **sebaceous hyperplasia**, **angiofibroma**, **trichoepithelioma** and **trichilemmoma**, **fibrofolliculoma** and **trichodiscoma**, **syringomas**, **eccrine hidrocystoma**, and **apocrine hidrocystoma**. If lesions are umbilicated, sebaceous hyperplasia should be considered. Lesions are most commonly located on the face and are skin colored or yellowish, usually 1 to 4 mm in size, and typically found in older adults. Angiofibromas usually present as one or a few papules on the nose of adults or multiple on the face of patients with tuberous sclerosis. Trichoepithelioma can present as solitary or multiple smooth, skin-colored papules. If lesions are found in a periorbital distribution, syringoma, eccrine hidrocystoma, and apocrine hidrocystoma should be considered. The presence of many widespread, skin-colored papules on the face that grow in number from childhood or young adulthood through later adulthood should prompt consideration of evaluation and biopsy to rule out underlying syndromic causes. Multiple trichilemmomas could indicate Cowden syndrome; multiple angiofibromas may suggest tuberous sclerosis; and fibrofolliculomas/trichodiscomas may be a sign of Birt-Hogg-Dube syndrome. Each of these syndromes requires further workup for associated malignancy and other serious health risks.

See Appendix 1 for Further Reading and Image References.

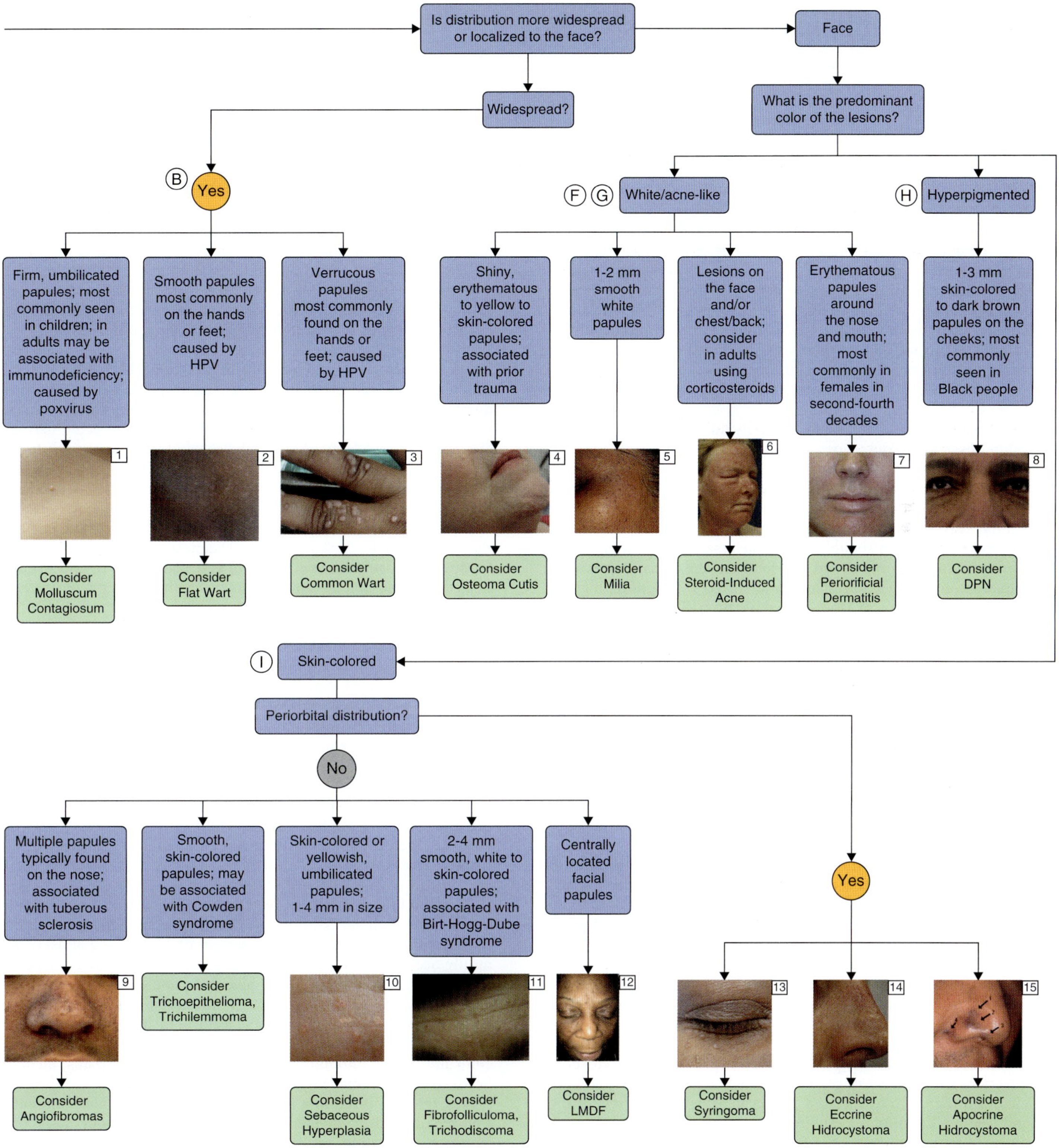
Is distribution more widespread or localized to the face?
Face
Widespread?
What is the predominant color of the lesions?
B
Yes
F G
White/acne-like
H
Hyperpigmented
Firm, umbilicated papules; most commonly seen in children; in adults may be associated with immunodeficiency; caused by poxvirus
Smooth papules most commonly on the hands or feet; caused by HPV
Verrucous papules most commonly found on the hands or feet; caused by HPV
Shiny, erythematous to yellow to skin-colored papules; associated with prior trauma
1-2 mm smooth white papules
Lesions on the face and/or chest/back; consider in adults using corticosteroids
Erythematous papules around the nose and mouth; most commonly in females in second-fourth decades
1-3 mm skin-colored to dark brown papules on the cheeks; most commonly seen in Black people
1
2
3
4
5
6
7
8
Consider Molluscum Contagiosum
Consider Flat Wart
Consider Common Wart
Consider Osteoma Cutis
Consider Milia
Consider Steroid-Induced Acne
Consider Periorificial Dermatitis
Consider DPN
I
Skin-colored
Periorbital distribution?
No
Multiple papules typically found on the nose; associated with tuberous sclerosis
Smooth, skin-colored papules; may be associated with Cowden syndrome
Skin-colored or yellowish, umbilicated papules; 1-4 mm in size
2-4 mm smooth, white to skin-colored papules; associated with Birt-Hogg-Dube syndrome
Centrally located facial papules
Yes
9
Consider Trichoepithelioma, Trichilemmoma
10
11
12
13
14
15
Consider Angiofibromas
Consider Sebaceous Hyperplasia
Consider Fibrofolliculoma, Trichodiscoma
Consider LMDF
Consider Syringoma
Consider Eccrine Hidrocystoma
Consider Apocrine Hidrocystoma

29 Umbilicated Lesions

Erika T. McCormick and Adam J. Friedman

Umbilicated lesions, characterized by a central depression, occur in infectious, inflammatory, benign, and malignant dermatologic conditions. Viral infections that commonly cause umbilicated lesions include members of the *Poxviridae* family (molluscum contagiosium, monkeypox, cowpox, orf, and paravaccinia) and members of the *herpesvirus* family (varicella zoster virus [VZV], herpes simplex virus [HSV]). Benign epidermal tumors or proliferations such as sebaceous gland hyperplasia (SGH), sebaceous adenoma (SA), warty dyskeratoma (WD), and desmoplastic trichoepithelioma (DT) present as umbilicated lesions. Basal cell carcinoma (BCC) can present with umbilication. Differential diagnosis of umbilicated lesions in the immunocompromised patient can include cutaneous or disseminated infections with dimorphic fungi (cryptococcosis, histoplasmosis, or talaromycosis). Diagnostic and treatment approaches vary by diagnosis.

A. Initial evaluation of umbilicated lesions includes a detailed history of lesion onset, time course, progression, local symptoms, and assessment for constitutional symptoms. Full medical and medication history should be obtained with emphasis on identifying immunocompromised states. Other considerations may include age, sexual history, travel, exposures, country of residence, and occupation. Physical examination should include the assessment of lesion location, appearance, number, and distribution, vital signs, lymph node palpation, and inspection of mucosal surfaces. Diagnosis may be aided by dermoscopy or laboratory evaluation. Skin biopsy may be indicated to confirm diagnosis or rule out malignancy.

B. **Molluscum contagiosum (MC)** is the most common infectious cause of umbilicated papules. Risk factors for MC include conditions that alter skin barrier (e.g., atopic dermatitis, Darier disease) or immune function. Although typically seen in children, adults may develop MC due to sexual transmission or immunocompromised status. Lesions are pink to skin-colored, pearly, umbilicated, firm, rounded papules or nodules with a caseous plug. MC develops anywhere on the body, commonly in the anogenital region in adults, and is asymptomatic or mildly pruritic. Dermoscopy reveals polylobular white-yellow amorphous structures or peripheral crown vessels. Diagnosis is clinical but can be confirmed with potassium hydroxide test or biopsy demonstrating intracytoplasmic viral inclusion bodies ("molluscum bodies"). MC is often self-limiting; lesions should resolve after 6 to 9 months. In immunocompromised patients, MC may be greater than 1 cm ("giant MC") and unresponsive to conventional treatments. Decision to treat depends on numerous patient and clinical factors. Treatment options include mechanical, chemical, immune-modulating, and antiviral therapies.

C. Cutaneous lesions of cowpox and mpox (previously monkeypox) infections (*Orthopoxvirus* genus) begin as painful macules and papules that progress to vesicles and umbilicated pustules before crusting and healing. **Cowpox** is a rare infection found primarily in Europe, typically found on the hands from contact with infected animals (rodents). Fever, flu-like symptoms, or lymphadenopathy may be present. **Mpox** is endemic to Africa; endemic infections are acquired from animals (e.g., rodents, monkeys). During the 2022 global outbreak, human-to-human transmission via contact with lesions, body fluids, respiratory droplets, and possibly fomites has been well documented. Men who engage in sexual activity with men are currently a high-risk population. Mpox may be considered in patients with epidemiological risk factors that present with prodromal symptoms (e.g., respiratory symptoms, fever, malaise) followed by a vesiculopustular, painful rash lasting 14 to 21 days. Lymphadenopathy and mucosal lesions may occur. Endemic cases classically spread centrifugally, while cases from the 2022 outbreak often spread from the anogenital area. Diagnoses can be confirmed by orthopoxvirus or viral-specific polymerase chain reaction (PCR) assays. Mild mpox infections are self-limited and managed supportively; however, severe disease can occur in children and immunocompromised individuals. Antiviral drugs developed to treat smallpox, another orthopoxvirus, are used to treat severe mpox infections. Vaccines are available for mpox prevention and postexposure prophylaxis.

D. **Herpes zoster (HZ)** and **eczema herpeticum (EH)** present with vesicular eruptions that may be umbilicated. HZ, a neurocutaneous disorder resulting from VZV reactivation, typically occurs in immunocompromised or elderly individuals. HZ causes an acute dermatomal eruption of herpetiform umbilicated vesicles along with fever, malaise, dysesthesia, allodynia, and pain. EH, most commonly caused by HSV, is a disseminated infection affecting patients with preexisting dermatoses. Clinical features include widespread painful clusters of umbilicated vesicles and pustules that evolve into crusted, hemorrhagic, "punched out" skin erosions. Diagnosis of these infections can be clinical or confirmed with PCR of vesicular fluid. HZ and EH are treated with antiviral therapy; EH can be life threatening if untreated.

E. **Orf** ("ecthyma contagiosum") and **paravaccinia virus** ("milker's nodule") cause localized cutaneous infection. At-risk occupations include farm workers caring for goats/sheep (Orf) or cattle (paravaccinia virus), butchers, and veterinary surgeons. In these infections, one to few firm red/violaceous papules appear at the site of contact with infected animals, typically on the hands. Orf lesions enlarge to form a hemorrhagic pustule or bulla with central umbilication. Paravaccinia virus causes milker's nodule, a tender nodule with a depressed umbilicated center and overlying crust. Lymphangitis, regional lymphadenopathy, fever, or malaise may be present. Diagnosis can be clinical or confirmed with parapoxvirus or viral-specific PCR assays. Infections typically resolve spontaneously within 6 weeks.

F. Solitary umbilicated lesions on the head, neck, and upper trunk may represent epidermal tumors or proliferations. **Sebaceous gland hyperplasia (SGH)**, benign enlargement of sebaceous glands, commonly occurs on the central or upper face of adults. SGH presents as one or multiple painless, umbilicated papules with yellow hue; umbilication represents a follicular infundibular ostium. Papules may be telangiectatic. Dermoscopic features include yellow globules, indicative of sebaceous glands, and crown vessels. SGH is diagnosed clinically. Other umbilicated benign adnexal neoplasms include **Sebaceous Adenoma (SA)**, **Warty Dyskeratoma (WD)**, and **desmoplastic trichoepithelioma (DT)**. SA appears as a painless, smooth, well-circumscribed papule or nodule with a yellow hue, polypoid appearance, crusting, or central umbilication. WD is a solitary, verrucous, often crusted, skin-colored to red-brown papule or nodule with a central keratotic plug. DT presents as a solitary, firm, skin-colored to erythematous annular plaque with central depression/umbilication. DT requires close monitoring due to potential for malignant transformation to BCC. Diagnosis of SA requires biopsy; complete excision may be indicated to rule out BCC with sebaceous differentiation or sebaceous carcinoma. WD and DT can be diagnosed clinically, but biopsy can rule out BCC or other adnexal carcinoma.

Continued

Patient presenting with umbilicated lesion(s)

(A) Detailed history and thorough physical examination with attention to lesion location, appearance, evolution (including photos if provided), number and distribution of lesions, characterization of the composition of the umbilicated center, vital signs, lymph node palpation, inspection of mucosal surfaces

→ Management will be based on the underlying etiology of the lesions

Does the history reveal that the patient is immunosuppressed or immunocompromised?

- **Yes** → *continued on next page*
- **No** → Are there multiple lesions?
  - **No** → *continued on next page*
    - (E) Consider cutaneous viral infections if:
      - History of occupational exposure (workers who deal with dairy cattle, sheep, or goats); Examination shows isolated lesions (commonly) on hands
        - Hemorrhagic pustule or bullae with umbilicated center and overlying crust +/– Fever, malaise, LAD, lymphangitis → Consider Orf
        - Tender nodule with umbilicated center and overlying crust +/– LAD, lymphangitis → Consider Milker's Nodule
  - **Yes** → Suspect cutaneous viral infections
    - Painful lesions/rash
      - (C) Painful papules which evolve to form a vesicle, then umbilicated pustule +/– Fever, LAD
        - Lesions at the site of contact with infected animal host (rodents) in endemic area (Europe) → Consider Cowpox
        - History of exposure to infected animal in endemic area (Africa) or part of high-risk group (i.e., MSM for 2022 outbreak) Prodromal flu-like symptoms followed by rash development
          - 2 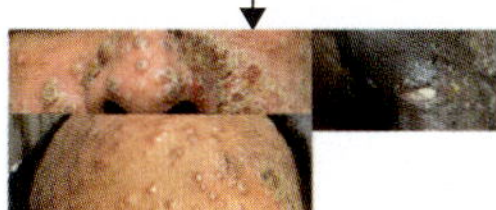
          - Umbilicated lesions on the nose/cheeks, base of ventral side of penis, and forehead → Consider Mpox (previously Monkeypox)
      - (D) Dermatomal eruption of herpetiform, umbilicated vesicles, local dysesthesia/allodynia/pain +/– Fever, malaise
        - Risk factors include old age, immunocompromised (autoimmune diseases, cancer, HIV/AIDS, treatment with biologics/immunosuppressants)
        - 3 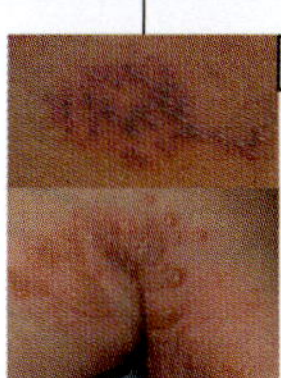
        - Umbilicated vesicular and bullous eruptions → Consider HZ
      - (D) Clusters of painful umbilicated vesicles and pustules that evolve into crusted, hemorrhagic, "punched out" skin erosions +fever → History of atopic dermatitis or other dermatosis that disrupts skin barrier → Consider Eczema Herpeticum
    - Asymptomatic to mildly pruritic lesions
      - Common in children, may be associated with sexual transmission in adults
      - 1 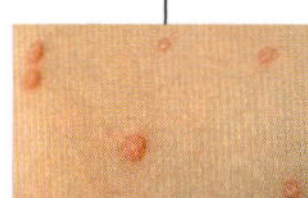
      - Discrete, dome-shaped, shiny papules with central umbilication → (B) Consider Molluscum Contagiosum

Continued

G. **BCC**, the most common malignant cutaneous neoplasm, arises from sun-damaged skin and typically occurs in older adults or immunocompromised individuals. Nodular BCC, the most common subtype, presents as a pearly papule or nodule with smooth surface, central umbilication, and arborizing telangiectasias. Biopsy should be performed if BCC is suspected. Most BCCs are managed with standard surgical excision, although certain cases require Mohs micrographic surgery.

H. Differential diagnosis of umbilicated lesions in the immunocompromised patient should include opportunistic infections, particularly disseminated fungal infections (e.g., **cryptococcosis, histoplasmosis, or talaromycosis**). These infections occur in susceptible individuals through inhalation of fungus in endemic regions. *Cryptococcus* is found globally, *Histoplasma* is endemic to central/south central United States, and *Talaromyces* is endemic to Southeast/South Asia. Infections begin with fever, weight loss, hepatosplenomegaly, lymphadenopathy, and respiratory and gastrointestinal symptoms. On examination, cutaneous lesions of histoplasmosis and cryptococcosis are polymorphic papules, plaques, pustules, nodules, ulcers, and erosions, some of which can be umbilicated. Histoplasmosis may cause oral ulcers. In talaromycosis, characteristic lesions are papules with central necrosis and umbilication on the face, trunk, and extremities. Diagnosis of dimorphic fungal infections can be established by tissue biopsy, imaging, and culture of involved tissue, sputum, and serum. Treatment relies on systemic antifungal therapy; these infections can be fatal if untreated.

See Appendix 1 for References and Image References.

Does the history reveal that the patient is immunosuppressed or immunocompromised?

Yes

(H) Consider all applicable differential diagnoses for immunocompetent patients and additionally consider opportunistic infections

- Sick patient with various skin lesions including papules or nodules with umbilication +Fever, LAD +/–HSM, symptoms from other organ involvement
  - Association with oral ulcers; risk factors include travel or residence in endemic area (central/south central United States), CD4 count <150 cells/mm³
    - Consider Disseminated Histoplasmosis
  - May be associated with CNS symptoms, and risk factors include CD4 count <100 cells/mm³
    - Consider Disseminated Cryptococcus
- Papules with central necrosis and umbilication +Fever, LAD, HSM +/– symptoms from other organ involvement; travel or residence in endemic region (South and Southeast Asia), CD4 count <100 cells/mm³
  - Consider Talaromycosis (previously Penicilliosis)

Are there multiple lesions?

No

(F) Consider benign epidermal tumors and proliferations and rule out BCC

- One or multiple yellowish papules with central umbilication on the central/upper face; Relatively common in middle-aged to older adults

  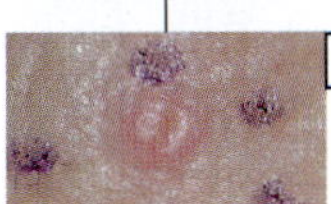

  4

  Solitary SH on the nose

  - Consider Sebaceous Hyperplasia
- History of sun/UV exposure, past skin cancers, often older adults; Smooth, pearly papule/nodule with central umbilication, telangiectasias

  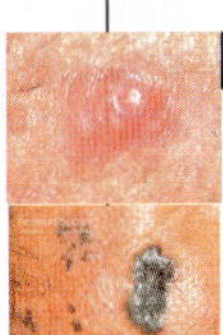

  5

  Nodular (top) and pigmented (bottom) BCC

  - (G) Consider BCC
- Smooth, well-circumscribed papule or nodule with yellowish hue +/– polypoid appearance, crust, central umbilication; On the head/neck/upper trunk; middle-aged to older adults, uncommon
  - Consider Sebaceous Adenoma
- Solitary, skin-colored to red-brown verrucous papule or nodule with crust and a central, keratotic umbilicated pore on the head/neck; middle-aged to older adults, uncommon
  - Consider Warty Dyskeratoma
- Solitary, firm skin-colored to erythematous, annular, indurated papule/plaque with a central depression/umbilication; middle-aged female, uncommon

  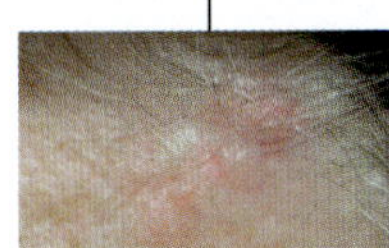

  6

  DT on forehead

  - Consider DT

30 Acneiform Papules

Sapana Desai and Adam J. Friedman

Acneiform papules are follicular eruptions clustered within a group of versatile dermatoses, characterized by papules that gradually transcend into pustules and cystic nodules resembling acne vulgaris. A variety of etiologies, including infections, hormonal and/or metabolic abnormalities, genetic syndromes, and drug eruptions may present as acneiform papules. The key distinguishing factor of acneiform diagnoses (with a few exceptions) compared to true acne is the absence of comedones. Patient evaluation is predominantly clinical, with an emphasis on a history of new medications and/or exposures to chemical irritants, but may also entail performing biopsies or cultures in rare/challenging circumstances. Management and therapeutic approaches are specific to the individual diagnosis and contributing cause.

There are several acneiform eruptions that are characterized as chronic inflammatory in nature.

A. **Acne conglobata** is a severe variant of acne vulgaris predominantly seen in males. Physical examination may unveil groups of multiple inflammatory, dusky-colored papules that transform into pustules and nodules involving the trunk, limbs, and buttocks. Interconnecting abscesses and draining sinuses may become secondarily infected, causing pain and malodor. Healing is slow and results in both depressed and hypertrophic scars. Isotretinoin is the first-line therapy.

B. **Hidradenitis suppurativa (HS)**, part of the follicular occlusion tetrad, is a multifactorial disease characterized by occlusion of hair follicles and presents with a chronic cycle of inflammation, healing, and scarring. While it occurs in both genders, there is an increased incidence in females in the United States. HS presents as recurrent, exquisitely tender, erythematous papulonodules typically affecting the intertriginous and anogenital regions, which can then progress to draining abscesses with subsequent bridge scarring and tunnel formation. HS is often progressive, with marked morbidity from factors such as chronic pain, restricted mobility, and depression. Diagnosis is based on clinical signs and symptoms as well as disease chronicity and family history. Treatment includes antiseptic washes, topical and systemic antibiotics, hormonal and metabolic modulators, biologics, and procedural interventions such as intralesional steroid injections, deroofings, and surgical excisions.

C. **Periorificial dermatitis** is characterized by discrete, irregularly grouped, symmetric clusters of 1- to 2-mm erythematous papulopustules on the face. Lesions increase in number with central confluence and satellite pattern that predictably exhibit perioral distribution with sparing of the vermillion border but may also present in a periorbital or perinasal distribution. Confluent plaques appear eczematous with tiny scales, and associated pruritus and burning. Diagnosis is based on clinical examination, and KOH preparation from a pustule may yield an increased density of *Demodex* mites. Although self-limiting, cessation of occlusive facial cosmetics is encouraged. Treatment is determined by disease severity and may include nonsteroidal antiinflammatory agents, including calcineurin inhibitors, as well as topical and systemic antibiotics and/or antiparasitic agents such as ivermectin.

D. **Rosacea** is a recurrent episodic inflammatory disorder resulting from barrier dysfunction, heightened innate immune response, and inappropriate neurovascular reactivity. Cutaneous presentation includes centrofacial erythema with telangiectasias, acneiform papules, and phymatous changes. Papulopustules measuring 2 to 3 mm can evolve into dusky-red edematous papules and nodules with symmetric facial localization. Phymatous changes comprising rhinophyma, metophyma, and blepharophyma may follow from marked sebaceous hyperplasia. Diagnosis is determined by cutaneous manifestations; increased density of *Demodex* mites on KOH preparation is common but not diagnostic. Although therapy is noncurative, treatment modalities concentrate on diminishing facial redness and inflammatory lesions using topical creams (i.e., ivermectin, azelaic acid, oxymetazoline), systemic antibiotics, isotretinoin, and cosmetic lasers.

E. **Eosinophilic folliculitis (EF)** is an idiopathic recurrent dermatosis with an unknown etiology and is most prevalent among individuals with HIV but may also occur in HIV-negative patients, regarded as **Ofuji disease**. Characterized by very pruritic, erythematous dome-shaped papulopustules and less commonly urticarial patches localized to face and upper truncal body, the diagnosis is confirmed with skin biopsy that unveils lymphocytic and eosinophilic inflammation around hair follicles. Treatment in a patient with HIV requires the initiation of highly active antiretroviral therapy to help reconstitute immune systems. Other treament modalities focus on antiinflammatory effects via a multitude of topical creams, antihistamines, antifungals, antibiotics, and isotretinoin.

F. **Pseudofolliculitis barbae (PFB)** is a chronic inflammatory disease of hair-bearing areas most commonly involving the beard line with increased predilection among African-American males and females. Following hair removal, regrowing hairs penetrate the skin through extrafollicular and transfollicular mechanisms and evoke a foreign body reaction. PFB is characterized by painful, pruritic, erythematous 2- to 5-mm papules and pustules. Although treatment is tricky, patients inclined to shave are advised to use a multiblade razor that maintains hair lengths of 1 to 3 mm (five o'clock shadow), with an alternative being to allow the facial hair to grow out.

G. **Acne keloidalis nuchae** is a chronic inflammatory dermatosis affecting the nuchal region characterized by firm follicular-based papulopustules with associated hypertrophic scarring, scarring alopecia, and postinflammatory hyperpigmentation. It is most commonly seen in African-American males. Management includes topicals, intralesional corticosteroids, systemic antibiotics, lasers, and surgical excisions.

Besides chronic inflammatory eruptions, there are also several forms of acute acneiform papular eruptions.

H. **Gram-negative folliculitis** is often the consequence of long-term treatment of acne vulgaris with antibiotics, with *Escherichia coli, Pseudomonas aeruginosa, Serratia marcescens, Klebsiella*, and *Proteus* species serving as the chief causative microbes. Patients present with eruptive papulopustules localized to the cheeks, chin, and nasal ala. Definitive diagnosis is accomplished via microscopy and bacterial cultures, and the treatment of choice is isotretinoin.

I. **Pityrosporum folliculitis** is an infection of the pilosebaceous unit caused by overgrowth of *Mallasezia furfur*, a lipophilic yeast inhabitant of the normal skin flora. The disease manifests in adolescents and young adult males with increased risk factors attributed to humidity, excessive sebum production, occlusion from emollients, antibiotic usage, or preexisting seborrheic dermatitis. Lesions are classified as uniform, pruritic erythematous papules and papulopustules exhibiting a perifollicular pattern and involve the upper truncal region as well as the forehead and neck. While diagnosis is determined by clinical examination, positive KOH scrapings are confirmatory, revealing budding yeasts, which is followed by treatment with oral antifungals.

Patient presenting with acneiform eruption

→ Detailed history and thorough physical examination with attention to lesion location and distribution, characteristic appearance, and evolution

→ Management and therapeutic approaches are specific to the diagnosis and contributing cause

continued on next page

Chronic in nature

- Recalcitrant nodulocystic acne; groups of multiple dusky-colored papulopustules and nodules leading to interconnecting abscesses and draining sinuses; Distribution: trunk/limbs/buttocks (-) systemic manifestations

  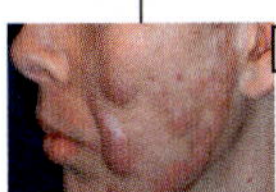
  1

  → Consider Acne Conglobata (A)

- Exquisitely tender, deep-seated erythematous papulonodules that can progress to draining abscesses with subsequent bridge scarring and tunnel formation; Distribution: intertriginous and anogenital regions

  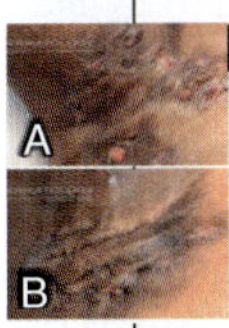

  2

  → Consider HS (B)

- Discrete, irregularly grouped, symmetric clusters of 1–2 mm erythematous papulopustules, (+) central confluence and satelliting; Distribution: perioral/periorbital/perinasal

  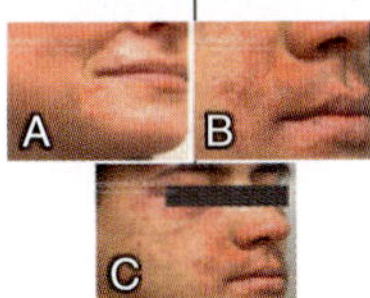

  3

  → Consider Periorificial Dermatitis (C)

- Episodic centrofacial erythema, 2–3 mm papulopustules, and phymatous changes; (+) KOH with Demodex mites >5/cm^2

  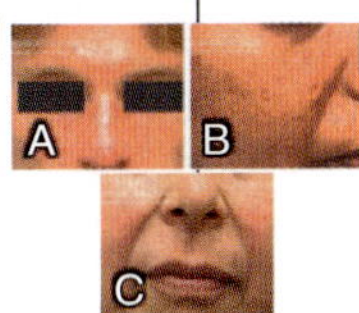

  4

  → Consider Rosacea (D)

- Noninfectious, pruritic, erythematous dome-shaped papulopustules with possible urticarial patches; Distribution: face and truncal region (+/–) HIV

  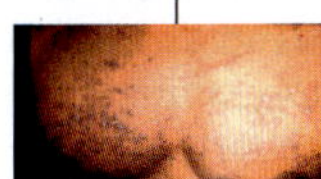
  5

  → Consider Eosinophilic Folliculitis (E)

- Painful, pruritic, erythematous papules and pustules following hair removal; Distribution: beard line

  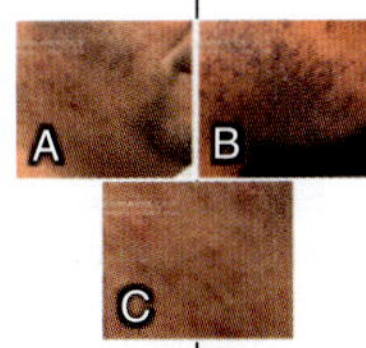

  6

  → Consider PFB (F)

- Firm papulopustules with associated hypertrophic scarring, scarring alopecia, and PIH; Distribution: posterior neck and scalp

  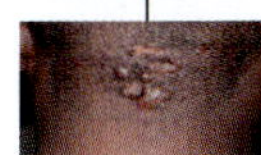
  7

  → Consider AKN (G)

Acute in nature

- Infectious, superficial eruptive papulopustules; Distribution: cheeks/chin/nasal ala; (+) History of long-term treatment of acne with antibiotics

  → Consider Gram-Negative Folliculitis (H)

- Infectious, uniform, pruritic, erythematous papules and papulopustules with perifollicular pattern; Distribution: upper trunk/forehead/and neck, (+) KOH

  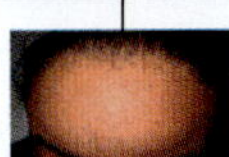
  8

  → Consider Pityrosporum Folliculitis (I)

- Infectious, monomorphic, pruritic, erythematous papules and pustules with follicular scaling; Distribution: forehead/cheeks/eyelashes/nasal ala; (+) KOH with Demodex mites >5/cm^2

  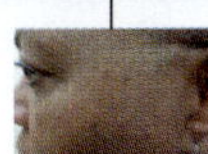
  9

  → Consider Demodex Dermatitis (J)

Continued

J. Overlapping components of rosacea often coexist with adult patients diagnosed with ***Demodex* dermatitis**. *Demodex* spp., a genus of human mites in the family of Demodecidae that live within the infundibulum of hair follicles and sebaceous glands, are often found on facial skin, with primary involvement of the forehead, cheeks, nasal region, and eyelashes. Patients exhibit nonspecific clinical features including small monomorphic papules and pustules, follicular scaling, erythema, and associated pruritus. Diagnosis is confirmed via performing KOH scrapings yielding a high density of *Demodex* mites (>5/cm^2) and is treated with acaricides including permethrin and ivermectin.

Some inflammatory acneiform eruptions are secondary to iatrogenic causes.

K. Drug-induced acneiform eruptions are nonallergic reactions that develop in association with recent initiation of a culprit medication such as topical corticosteroids, glucocorticoids, antiepileptics (i.e., carbamazepine, phenytoin), lithium, isoniazid, cyclosporine, anabolic steroids, JAK inhibitors, and cyanocobalamin. Clinical presentation includes monomorphic erythematous papules or papulopustules with truncal and upper extremity distribution. Treatment rarely necessitates disruption of the culprit drug.

L. HER1/epidermal growth factor receptor (EGFR) and **HER2 inhibitor-induced papulopustular eruptions** are cutaneous adverse effects of epidermal growth factor receptor inhibitors (EGFRis) affecting 65% to 90% of patients treated with targeted therapies for various malignancies. EGFR belongs to a family of tyrosine kinase receptors, which regulate tumor cell differentiation, survival, and proliferation and are inhibited by monoclonal antibodies and tyrosine kinase inhibitors. EGFRis evoke dose-dependent papulopustular reactions within the first 2 weeks of drug administration, affecting sebaceous-rich regions including the head, neck, and upper body. Photoprotection, topical antibiotics, retinoids, steroids, and oral tetracyclines are first-line for management and potential prevention. Isotretinoin can be advantageous in more severe cases.

M. Chloracne eruptions are rare dermatoses that manifest due to occupational and/or accidental environmental exposure to certain halogenated aromatic compounds, including chlorinated dioxins and dibenzofurans, and develop within a few months after swallowing, inhaling, or touching the responsible agent. Inflammatory processes lead to the formation of keratinous plugs within pores, resulting in yellow papulopustules and cysts that localize to the face, as well as the axillae and groin in advanced cases. Diagnosis is primarily clinical, and biopsies may exhibit decreased sebaceous gland density and development of hamartomas. Principal treatment mandates removal from the source of contamination followed by oral antibiotics or isotretinoin, and symptomatic management.

N. Acne cosmetica is a mild but persistent form of acne triggered via the usage of comedogenic cosmetics that elicit chemically induced plugging of pilosebaceous orifices. Acneiform comedones, micropapules, and low-grade folliculitis ensue on the face, neck, and hairline. Diagnosis requires identifying the culprit product, and treatment necessitates the use of noncomedogenic products, and benzoyl peroxide or salicyclic acid, as both have comedolytic properties.

O. Acne aestivalis is a seasonal ultraviolet A radiation-induced polymorphous light eruption (PMLE) occurring in spring and summer that leads to idiopathic monomorphic eruptions consisting of multiple, uniform, keratotic, erythematous papules and papulovesicles localized to the lateral aspects of the upper arms, shoulder girdle, back and chest, with facial sparing. PMLE is a delayed-type hypersensitivity from solar exposure or artificial sources and equally affects both genders. Diagnosis is by visual examination, history of sun exposure, and sometimes biopsy, and treatment entails topical retinoids and/or benzoyl peroxide.

P. Miliaria results from blockage of eccrine sweat glands and is characterized by pruritic, erythematous, 2- to 4-mm nonfollicular papules and papulovesicles involving the trunk and skin folds. Regarded as a common ailment in humid climates, the disease affects individuals of all ages and is especially common among children and infants due to their underdeveloped glands. Diagnosis is clinical, and treatment includes avoiding sweat-provoking activities and occlusive clothing, taking cool showers, and application of keratolytics and topical antibacterials.

Acneiform eruptions may also occur secondary to acneiform syndromes.

Q. Acne fulminans is a rare subtype of severe inflammatory acne primarily affecting adolescent males and presents clinically with an abrupt eruption of painful, hemorrhagic papulopustules and ulceronecrotic nodules associated with systemic symptoms. Patients are febrile and present with leukocytosis, polyarthralgia, hepatosplenomegaly, and anemia, with radiological examinations often demonstrating osteolytic lesions of the clavicle and sternum. While disease pathogenesis is well described, it is presumed to be associated with increased androgen levels, explosive hypersensitivity reaction to surface bacteria *Cutbacterium acnes*, genetic predisposition, as well as complex diseases including **SAPHO, PAPA, PASH**, and **PAPASH** syndromes, respectively. Management is arduous, requiring immediate attention with a combination of oral corticosteroids and isotretinoin.

R. SAPHO syndrome is a rare polygenic disease that encompasses a variety of autoinflammatory bone disorders and may present with **S**ynovitis, **A**cne, **P**ustulosis, **H**yperostosis, and **O**steitis. Acneiform eruptions include acne conglobata and/or acne fulminans, with other skin conditions such as HS and dissecting cellulitis of the scalp. Diagnosis is clinical, though often accompanied by radiological imaging, and should be suspected in the setting of pustular disease in association with rheumatic pain. Osteoarticular manifestations are managed via various antiinflammatory agents and bisphosphonates, while cutaneous features are treated with isotretinoin and acitretin.

S. PAPA syndrome is a rare, autosomal dominant, autoinflammatory disorder characterized by **P**yogenic **A**rthritis, **P**yoderma gangrenosum, and **A**cne. Acneiform eruptions are prominent from puberty and are classically of the severe nodulocystic type. Clinical features along with familial tendency are adequate to make a conclusive syndrome diagnosis, and treatment options include tumor necrosis factor (TNF) inhibitors and interleukin-1 antagonists, and oral tetracycline or isotretinoin.

T. PASH syndrome is a rare, autoinflammatory disorder characterized by **P**yoderma gangrenosum, **A**cne conglobata, and **S**uppurative **H**idradenitis (HS), with links to mutations in the PSTPIP1 gene. While no standard treatment has been determined, current management modalities utilize systemic antibiotics, immunosuppressants, and/or biologics.

U. PAPASH syndrome is an uncommon autoinflammatory condition characterized by **P**yogenic **A**rthritis, **P**yoderma gangrenosum, **A**cne vulgaris, and **S**uppurative **H**idradenitis. Presumed to result due to a mutation in the PSTPIP1 gene that affects the innate immune system, there exists a common mechanism of interleukin-1-driven episodes of neutrophil-predominated sterile inflammation. Effective treatment is similar to that of PASH syndrome and includes more frequently TNF inhibitors and interleukin-1 antagonists.

See Appendix 1 for Further Reading and Image References.

Patient presenting with acneiform eruption

→ Detailed history and thorough physical examination with attention to lesion location and distribution, characteristic appearance, and evolution

→ Management and therapeutic approaches are specific to the diagnosis and contributing cause

History reveals iatrogenic origin

- Monomorphic erythematous papules and papulopustules with recent initiation of culprit medication; Distribution: truncal and upper extremity

  10 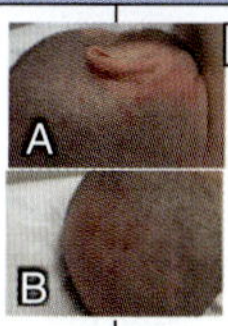

  → Consider Drug-Induced Acneiform Eruption (K)

- Dose-dependent papulopustular eruptions within the first 2 weeks of EGFR Inhibitor initiation; Distribution: sebaceous-rich regions (e.g., head/neck/upper body)

  11 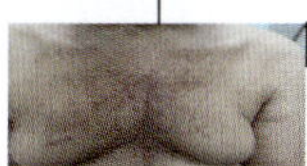

  → Consider HER1/EGFR and HER2 Inhibitor-Induced Eruption (L)

- Yellow papulopustules and cysts that manifest due to exposure to certain halogenated aromatic compounds; Distribution: face/axillae/groin

  12 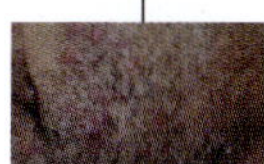

  → Consider Chloracne (M)

- Acneiform comedones, micropapules, and low-grade folliculitis triggered by comedogenic cosmetics, Distribution: pilosebaceous orifices

  13 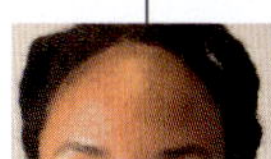

  → Consider Acne Cosmetica (N)

- Idiopathic, monomorphic, keratotic, erythematous papules and papulovesicles from seasonal UVA radiation-induced PMLE; Distribution: lateral aspects of upper arms/shoulder girdle/back/chest

  → Consider Acne Aestivalis (O)

- Pruritic, erythematous, 2–4 mm nonfollicular papules and papulovesicles due to blockage of eccrine sweat glands; Distribution: trunk and skin folds

  14 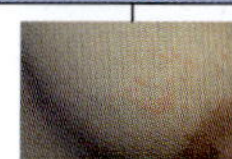

  → Consider Miliaria (P)

History reveals an associated syndrome

- Variant of severe nodulocystic acne; painful hemorrhagic papulopustules and ulcerated nodules and (+) systemic manifestations

  → Consider Acne Fulminans (Q)

- Synovitis, acne, pustulosis, hyperostosis, and osteitis; (+) acne conglobata or acne fulminans

  15 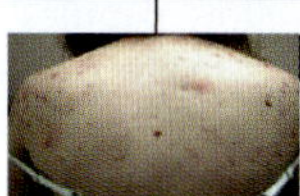

  → Consider SAPHO Syndrome (R)

- Pyogenic arthritis, pyoderma gangrenosum, and acne; (+) AD inheritance

  → Consider PAPA Syndrome (S)

- Pyoderma gangrenosum, acne conglobata, and hidradenitis suppurativa

  → Consider PASH Syndrome (T)

- Pyogenic arthritis with PASH syndrome

  → Consider PAPASH Syndrome (U)

31 Perforating Papules

Megana Rao and Edita M. Newton

A. A diverse group of diseases can present as crusted papules and nodules, including perforating disorders, infection, autoimmune disease, and malignancy. Clinicians should consider the timing of onset, distribution of lesions, morphology, and associated symptoms to determine the diagnosis.

Perforating papules are a group of papulonodular skin disorders characterized by transepidermal elimination of dermal components, presenting as keratotic papules often associated with pruritus. Perforating diseases are classically differentiated based on the type of eliminated fibers identified histologically, as well as differentiating inherited versus acquired onset. Historically, there are four classic forms of perforating papules: **Elastosis perforans serpiginosa (EPS), reactive perforating collagenosis (RPC), Kyrle disease, and perforating folliculitis**. However, more recently, both Kyrle disease and perforating folliculitis are recognized as forms of **acquired perforating dermatosis**. Further, acquired RPC and rarely acquired EPS also fall into the diagnosis of acquired perforating dermatosis despite histopathologic similarity to the inherited forms.

B. Inherited or primary perforating disorders include EPS and RPC. **EPS** is characterized by 2- to 5-mm keratotic papules arranged in an annular or serpiginous pattern, most commonly on the lateral neck, face, and flexural areas in male patients. Individual papules may be asymptomatic or have mild pruritus, and spontaneous resolution may take multiple years. Histologically, elastin is identified as the perforating substance. While primary EPS often presents in childhood or early adulthood, drug-induced EPS as well as presentation with associated syndromes are more variable in timing of onset and can occur later in life. **Drug-induced EPS** is most commonly associated with penicillamine in the treatment of Wilson disease, cystinuria, and rheumatoid arthritis. The underlying mechanism is suspected to be drug-mediated disruption of cross-linking of elastin fibers leading to transepidermal elimination. Genetic syndromes associated with EPS include Ehlers-Danlos syndrome, Down syndrome, Marfan syndrome, osteogenesis imperfecta, pseudoxanthoma elasticum, Rothmund-Thomson syndrome, cutis laxa, acrogeria, and Moyamoya disease.

Inherited **RPC** typically presents with 5- to 8-mm papules with central keratotic plug following superficial trauma on the arms and hands with childhood onset. The keratotic papules of RPC may develop in linear array, demonstrating the Koebner phenomenon in response to trauma. Inciting trauma can include scratching, insect bites, or even resolving herpes zoster infection. Associated pruritus is typically severe. There is often spontaneous resolution within weeks or months. Histologically, collagen is identified as the perforating substance. While acquired RPC arising in adulthood can be identical histologically to the inherited form, it is best classified as acquired perforating dermatosis.

C. **Acquired perforating dermatosis** includes acquired EPS, acquired RPC, perforating folliculitis, and Kyrle disease. For simplicity, acquired perforating dermatosis is used as a unifying term due to the similar clinical presentation and associated risk factors despite underlying histopathologic variations or overlap. Clinically, patients present with firm papules and nodules with a central keratotic core, most commonly on the lower legs, although they can also be generalized. There are often prurigo nodules, and pruritus can be severe. Acquired perforating dermatosis in adulthood typically arises in patients with advanced chronic kidney disease receiving maintenance hemodialysis or diabetes mellitus with associated nephropathy. Unlike inherited perforating disorders, acquired perforating dermatosis is common, affecting upward of 10% of patients receiving maintenance hemodialysis. Other systemic disorders, such as liver dysfunction, hypothyroidism, and HIV infection, have also been reported in association with acquired perforating dermatosis. There are several associated medications, including sirolimus, antivirals such as indinavir, monoclonal antibodies, kinase inhibitors such as erlotinib, tumor necrosis factor inhibitors, and epidermal growth factor receptor inhibitors.

D. **Perforating calcific elastosis** is a rare, distinct perforating disorder that typically presents as a plaque on the periumbilical skin of multiparious females. The plaque can have peripheral keratotic papules or verrucous surface. While involvement of the abdomen is most common, perforating calcific elastosis of the breasts has been described. Histological findings are unique with transepidermal elimination of calcified elastin fibers, similar to those found in the lesion skin of pseudoxanthoma elasticum.

E. Other dermatologic disorders can present with clinical features of keratotic papules concerning for perforating disorders. If a lesion is localized, one can consider **squamous cell carcinoma**, which can present as a new-onset keratotic papule in the background of actinic damage. If the patient has a history of an underlying dermatologic condition, there are a variety of conditions one may consider. In patients with a history of pruritus and eroded or crusted dome-shaped papules or nodules, consider **prurigo nodularis**. Patients with **sarcoidosis** may present with asymptomatic red-brown papules and plaques. Well-defined, annular, pink plaques on the face/scalp/neck may indicate **discoid lupus erythematosus**. Patients with skin-colored or yellow papules on flexural areas may have **pseudoxanthoma elasticum**. In patients who have plaques with trailing scale and associated papules and pustules, consider **dermatophytosis**. Patients who present with annular plaques without scale may have **granuloma annulare**. Further, there may be features of transepidermal elimination within distinct dermatoses histopathologically, such as perforating granuloma annulare and chondrodermatitis nodularis helicis. Ultimately, histological evaluation aids in diagnostic confirmation.

See Appendix 1 for Further Reading and Image References.

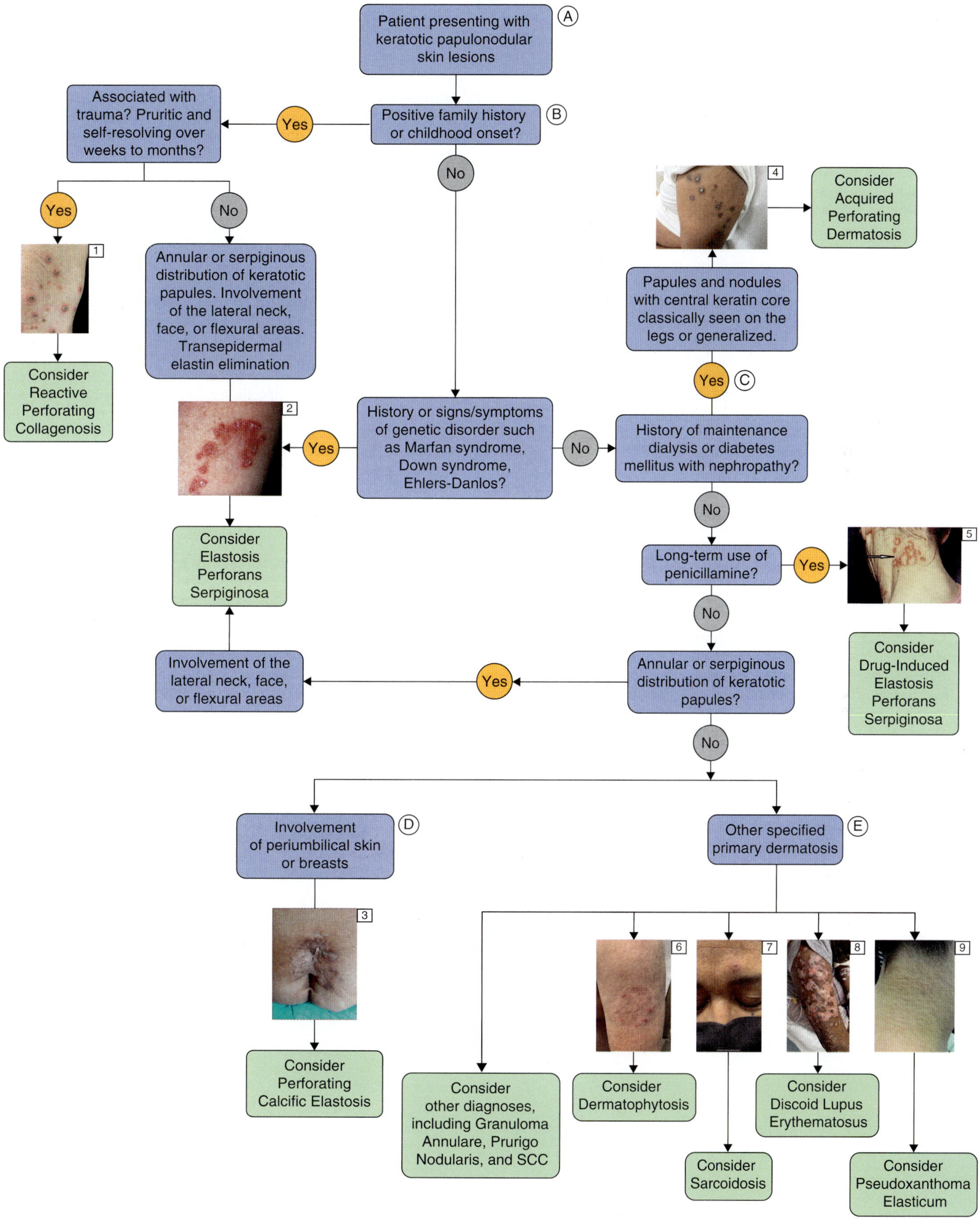
Patient presenting with keratotic papulonodular skin lesions
A
Positive family history or childhood onset?
B
Yes
Associated with trauma? Pruritic and self-resolving over weeks to months?
Yes
1
Consider Reactive Perforating Collagenosis
No
Annular or serpiginous distribution of keratotic papules. Involvement of the lateral neck, face, or flexural areas. Transepidermal elastin elimination
2
Consider Elastosis Perforans Serpiginosa
No
History or signs/symptoms of genetic disorder such as Marfan syndrome, Down syndrome, Ehlers-Danlos?
Yes
No
History of maintenance dialysis or diabetes mellitus with nephropathy?
Yes
C
Papules and nodules with central keratin core classically seen on the legs or generalized.
4
Consider Acquired Perforating Dermatosis
No
Long-term use of penicillamine?
Yes
5
Consider Drug-Induced Elastosis Perforans Serpiginosa
No
Annular or serpiginous distribution of keratotic papules?
Yes
Involvement of the lateral neck, face, or flexural areas
No
Involvement of periumbilical skin or breasts
D
3
Consider Perforating Calcific Elastosis
Other specified primary dermatosis
E
Consider other diagnoses, including Granuloma Annulare, Prurigo Nodularis, and SCC
6
Consider Dermatophytosis
7
Consider Sarcoidosis
8
Consider Discoid Lupus Erythematosus
9
Consider Pseudoxanthoma Elasticum

32 Edematous, "Juicy" Papules

Shae Margulies and Kiran Motaparthi

A. The evaluation of a patient with edematous lesions initially involves eliciting the duration of the rash, the presence or absence of systemic symptoms, and a thorough drug history. A physical examination should be performed of the skin, mucosal surfaces, and nails. It is helpful to first determine if there are additional superficial (epidermal) changes, such as scale or crust, or strictly deep (dermal) processes with no visible epidermal changes.

B. A patient with mucous membrane edematous lesions, specifically in the genital region, should raise suspicion for **genital herpes simplex virus (HSV) infection**. Some patients experience painful genital ulcers and local lymphadenopathy, while other patients are asymptomatic. Skin lesions are characterized by 2- to 4 mm vesicles on an erythematous base, which often progress to erosions and ulcerations with scalloped borders. Diagnosis can be supported with polymerase chain reaction. In a patient who presents with a diffuse painful rash, oral mucosal involvement, and lesions in the same stage of development, **monkeypox** should be considered. Monkeypox is preceded by fever, malaise, and lymphadenopathy, followed by the progression of papules, vesicles, pustules, and eventually eschars.

C. Grouped painful lesions on an acral surface are characteristic of **herpetic whitlow**, which occurs following inoculation of HSV through a skin defect. A solitary, painful erythematous nodule on the hand in a patient exposed to sheep or goats is classic for **orf**. Painful vesicular lesions that follow a dermatomal distribution are pathognomonic for **herpes zoster**, which is more common in older or immunosuppressed patients.

D. Clinical findings associated with **varicella** are preceded by fever and malaise. The associated pruritic rash first appears as macules that progress to papules and then vesicles, which often become crusted. Characteristically, lesions are in different stages of development and diffusely present on the face, extremities, and trunk. **Allergic contact dermatitis** is common and often presents with erythematous crusted or weeping plaques localized to an area in contact with an allergen.

E. **Arthropod bite reaction** presents with localized papules with or without a central vesicle; treatment is often symptomatic. A symmetric distribution of multiple pruritic, monomorphous, pink or red-brown papules in a child between the ages of 2 and 6 years is characteristic of **Gianotti-Crosti syndrome (GCS)**. The trunk, palms, and soles are typically spared, and lesions may last for many weeks. GCS is typically associated with Epstein-Barr virus or hepatitis B virus.

F. Multiple circumscribed, dermal, erythematous, and highly pruritic plaques located anywhere on the body are indicative of urticaria or a dermal hypersensitivity reaction. **Urticaria** is transient, with individual plaques described as migratory and lasting for less than 24 hours. Acute urticaria occurs for less than 6 weeks, and a precipitating factor is found in less than 50% of cases. Alternatively, chronic urticaria lasts for more than 6 weeks. By comparison, nonmigratory plaques lasting longer than 24 hours are characteristic of **dermal hypersensitivity reaction**, which can recur over months to years.

G. Nonpruritic dermal edematous lesions may be painful or tender. **Cellulitis** is a poorly demarcated area of skin erythema, edema, and warmth. Caused by bacteria that gain access to the dermis through a breach in the skin barrier, cellulitis is often treated empirically to cover beta-hemolytic streptococci and methicillin-susceptible *Staphylococcus aureus*. In contrast, **erysipelas** is a more superficial, sharply demarcated form of cellulitis. The abrupt appearance of tender erythematous plaques and nodules on the upper trunk, proximal extremities, and neck in association with fever is classic for **Sweet syndrome**. Patients require evaluation for associated inflammatory and hematologic conditions.

H. Dermal edematous lesions that are nontender may be associated with dysesthesia. Patients with **urticarial vasculitis (UV)** have systemic symptoms, including arthralgias, hematuria, and abdominal pain. Laboratory findings commonly include decreased complement levels and serological findings of systemic lupus erythematosus. In a patient with a history of Still disease, cryopyrin-associated period syndrome, or Schnitzler syndrome, **neutrophilic urticarial dermatosis (NUD)** should be considered. In contrast to urticaria, UV and NUD are nonmigratory, last for more than 24 hours, are not responsive to antihistamines, and are associated with purpura and postinflammatory hyperpigmentation. In contrast, dermal edematous lesions may be asymptomatic. Isolated recurrent swelling confined to the lips is characteristic of **granulomatous cheilitis**. Initially, the swelling may resolve within days; over time, the swelling becomes persistent. While there is no definitive treatment, corticosteroids have been used to prevent recurrence.

See Appendix 1 for References.

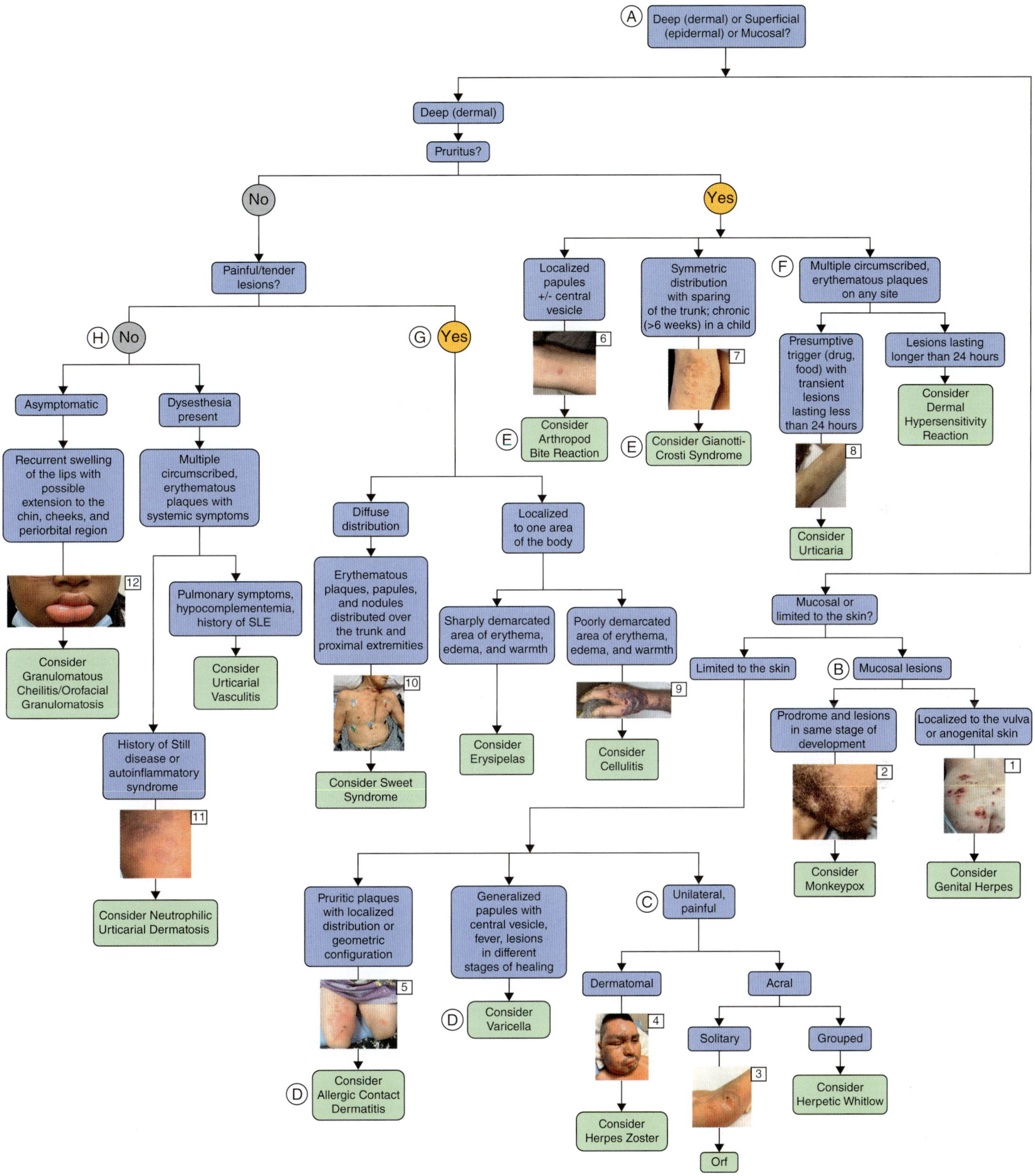
A
Deep (dermal) or Superficial (epidermal) or Mucosal?
Deep (dermal)
Pruritus?
No
Painful/tender lesions?
H
No
Asymptomatic
Recurrent swelling of the lips with possible extension to the chin, cheeks, and periorbital region
12
Consider Granulomatous Cheilitis/Orofacial Granulomatosis
Dysesthesia present
Multiple circumscribed, erythematous plaques with systemic symptoms
Pulmonary symptoms, hypocomplementemia, history of SLE
Consider Urticarial Vasculitis
History of Still disease or autoinflammatory syndrome
11
Consider Neutrophilic Urticarial Dermatosis
G
Yes
Diffuse distribution
Erythematous plaques, papules, and nodules distributed over the trunk and proximal extremities
10
Consider Sweet Syndrome
Localized to one area of the body
Sharply demarcated area of erythema, edema, and warmth
Consider Erysipelas
Poorly demarcated area of erythema, edema, and warmth
9
Consider Cellulitis
Yes
Localized papules +/- central vesicle
6
E
Consider Arthropod Bite Reaction
Symmetric distribution with sparing of the trunk; chronic (>6 weeks) in a child
7
E
Consider Gianotti-Crosti Syndrome
F
Multiple circumscribed, erythematous plaques on any site
Presumptive trigger (drug, food) with transient lesions lasting less than 24 hours
8
Consider Urticaria
Lesions lasting longer than 24 hours
Consider Dermal Hypersensitivity Reaction
Mucosal or limited to the skin?
Limited to the skin
Pruritic plaques with localized distribution or geometric configuration
5
D
Consider Allergic Contact Dermatitis
Generalized papules with central vesicle, fever, lesions in different stages of healing
D
Consider Varicella
C
Unilateral, painful
Dermatomal
4
Consider Herpes Zoster
Acral
Solitary
3
Orf
Grouped
Consider Herpetic Whitlow
B
Mucosal lesions
Prodrome and lesions in same stage of development
2
Consider Monkeypox
Localized to the vulva or anogenital skin
1
Consider Genital Herpes

33 Annular Papules and Plaques

Margaret A. O'Brien and Sylvia Hsu

A. Annular lesions are common in dermatology and have a broad differential diagnosis. The term "annular" refers to a ring-shaped lesion. Dermatophyte infections (colloquially known as "ringworm") are one of the most common presentations of annular lesions. However, other inflammatory processes and conditions can manifest as annular lesions. It is important to accurately diagnose these annular lesions to mitigate a prolonged time to diagnosis and prevent incorrect treatment strategies.

B. Patients with **dermatophytosis** present with a gradually enlarging, erythematous papule or plaque that has raised borders with scale. These fungal infections thrive in warm, moist environments and are spread by direct contact. Viewing a scraping of the scaly edge of a lesion with potassium hydroxide under a microscope is an easy in-office method to confirm the diagnosis. A dermatophyte infection should prompt evaluation for onychomycosis. Treatment involves topical or oral antifungals.

C. **Pityriasis rosea (PR)** presents in young patients with an enlarging, erythematous, oval-shaped lesion with fine or "powdery" scale and a border of scale inside an erythematous border, known as trailing "collarette" of scale. This collective pattern of scale is referred to as "pityriasiform." This initial lesion is called the "herald patch." A more widespread eruption of similar but smaller lesions can occur hours to weeks after the herald patch. These additional lesions erupt along Langer lines, which is why it is referred to as a "Christmas tree" distribution. A quarter of patients will have significant pruritus. PR usually self-resolves in 6 to 8 weeks, and treatment involves supportive care.

D. Patients with **Superficial erythema annulare centrifugum (EAC)** are typically adults with nonindurated annular lesions with trailing scale inside erythematous borders that can coalesce into polycyclic patches. These lesions are commonly present on the trunk, buttocks, thighs, and legs, sparing the hands, feet, and face. While the pathogenesis is unknown, EAC is most commonly associated with a cutaneous fungal infection. Malignancy as the cause of EAC is extremely rare, so exhaustive workup for occult malignancy is not recommended or warranted. EAC can last weeks to decades and can recur.

E. Clinicians should suspect **plaque psoriasis** in patients with well-demarcated erythematous plaques with silvery scale on the scalp, elbows, or knees. Psoriasis can have an annular appearance when the center of the lesion heals before the active edges. It can also present with a papular morphology, as in guttate psoriasis. Although not a diagnostic test, the Auspitz sign is pathognomonic for psoriasis and is defined as pinpoint bleeding after removal of scale. A combination of topical, oral, and injectable medications can be used, depending on the severity and recalcitrance of a patient's psoriasis.

F. **Subacute cutaneous lupus erythematosus (SCLE)** should be considered in patients with annular plaques that have raised, scaly borders, and central clearing on sun-exposed areas. These lesions are most commonly found on the face, lower neck, upper trunk, and extensor surfaces of the arms. Approximately half of these patients will also meet the American Rheumatology Association criteria for systemic lupus erythematosus (SLE) and should be further evaluated for systemic disease.

G. **Granuloma annulare (GA)** typically presents in young children and adults before age 40. The lesions begin as smooth, indurated, skin-colored to dull-red papules that progress into plaques with central clearing. The lesions are mostly found on the upper or lower extremities, rarely affecting the palms and soles. GA usually self-resolves within 2 years.

H. **Sarcoidosis** has a wide range of clinical presentations, from localized to widespread disease. It typically presents in young adults with a higher incidence in Black patients. The lesions are red-brown to violaceous papules that can coalesce to form annular plaques, affecting mainly the face, neck, upper trunk, and upper extremities. A skin biopsy showing the presence of noncaseating granulomas is a major diagnostic criterion. Cutaneous findings are among the first signs of systemic disease; however, some patients have skin-limited disease. For most patients, symptoms are not disabling. Oral corticosteroids are the first-line treatment for those with disfiguring or disabling cutaneous sarcoidosis. Patients should also be evaluated for pulmonary involvement and uveitis.

I. **Erythema migrans** should be considered for patients with one or several expanding erythematous annular lesions after being exposed to a tick bite or traveling to wooded regions where the deer tick (*Ixodes scapularis* or *Ixodes pacificus*) is native. Erythema migrans is the characteristic rash of Lyme disease due to the spirochete *Borrelia burgdorferi*. The onset of the rash after the tick bite is anywhere from 3 to 30 days. While the rash is asymptomatic, some patients may report having an influenza-like prodrome preceding the rash. Prompt treatment with antibiotics is essential to avoid progression of the disease.

J. One should suspect **Erythema multiforme (EM)** in patients with mucocutaneous ulcers or a known history of herpes simplex virus (HSV) infection who present with many target lesions on the palms, soles, elbows, and knees. While HSV is the most common etiology of EM, other infections, such as mycoplasma, have been associated with EM as well. Typically, the lesion will have three zones: a raised outer border, an erythematous middle zone, and a dusky or necrotic center. However, some lesions can appear annular rather than targetoid. The lesions will usually resolve in 3 to 5 weeks without any treatment.

K. A clinician should consider **tumid lupus erythematosus** in a patient presenting with burning to asymptomatic, erythematous, annular papules or plaques without scale in a photosensitive distribution. Lesions can last for days to weeks but can spontaneously regress without scarring. Besides photoprotection, hydroxychloroquine is the first-line treatment. For localized disease, topical corticosteroids and intralesional steroids are additional options.

L. **Nummular dermatitis** is common in patients with dry skin, especially with xerosis on the lower extremities. Nummular dermatitis presents with coin-shaped patches, with or without vesicles, that can have central clearing. While nummular dermatitis is typically circular or round, it can also appear annular. Treatment involves education on proper dry skin care, topical corticosteroids for flares, and biologics or JAK inhibitors for patients with debilitating disease.

Continued

(A) Patient presenting with annular papule(s) or plaque(s)

→ Presence of scale?

- **Yes**
  - Leading scale with raised borders → Gradually enlarging annular plaques or papules with raised borders
    - 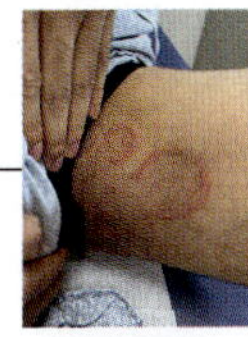 1 → Consider Dermatophytosis (B)
  - Trailing scale
    - Trailing scale is in "collarette" distribution within oval-shaped lesion, on the trunk and proximal limbs
      - 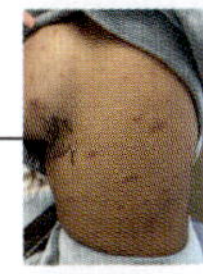 2 → Consider Pityriasis Rosea (C)
    - Trailing scale is inside erythematous borders of annular plaque(s); commonly associated with a cutaneous fungal infection
      - 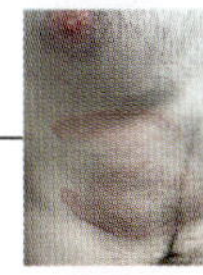 3 → Consider Superficial EAC (D)
  - Silvery scale → Silvery scale on erythematous, well-demarcated plaques commonly on the scalp, elbows, and/or knees
    - 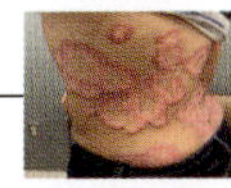 4 → Consider Plaque Psoriasis (E)
  - Fine scale → Fine scale on raised borders of annular papulosquamous plaques on photosensitive areas
    - 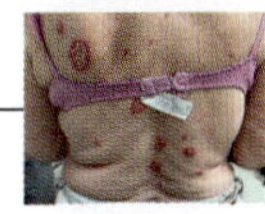 5 → Consider Subacute Cutaneous Lupus Erythematosus (F)
- **No**
  - Dull red-brown and indurated
    - Smooth, indurated, annular lesions on the upper or lower extremities sparing the palms and soles
      - 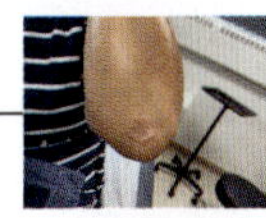 6 → Consider Granuloma Annulare (G)
    - Central clearing with disease progression, frequently located on the face, extensor surfaces, or within tattoos
      - 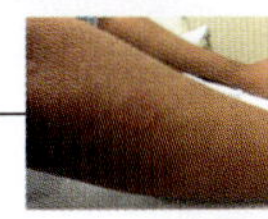 7 → Consider Sarcoidosis (H)
  - Erythematous
    - Asymptomatic
      - Expanding lesion(s) with or without center zone erythema, in patient with recent travel to the NE United States
        - 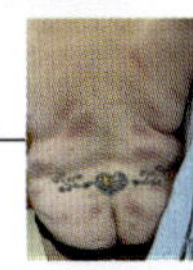 8 → Consider Erythema Migrans (I)
      - Target lesion with necrotic or dusky center in patient with oral ulcers or known prior HSV infection
        - 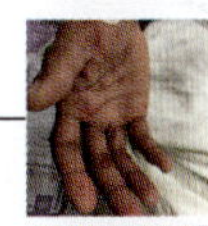 9 → Consider Erythema Multiforme (J)
    - Symptomatic
      - Burning, annular to arcuate configuration, in a photosensitive distribution
        - 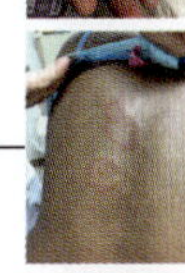 10 → Consider Tumid Lupus (K)
      - Pruritic, coin-shaped lesion(s) on dry skin with or without vesicles that favor the lower extremities
        - 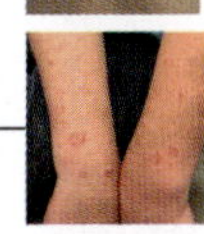 11 → Consider Nummular Dermatitis (L)
      - Transient, pruritic lesions with raised borders lasting <24 hours
        - 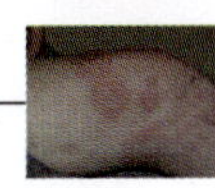 12 → Consider Urticaria (M)
  - Violaceous → Pruritic, purple to red, annular lesions with raised borders and atrophic centers, commonly located on male genitalia and intertriginous regions
    - 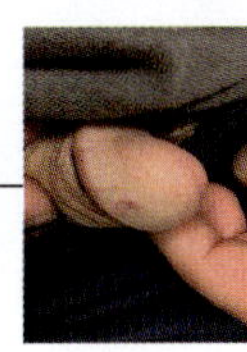 13 → Consider Annular Lichen Planus (N)

M. **Urticaria** should be considered in patients with transient pruritic, blanchable, well-circumscribed, erythematous plaques with raised borders. Individual lesions last less than 24 hours. Urticaria is classified as spontaneous or inducible. Spontaneous urticaria is the most common and is often idiopathic or less commonly precipitated by upper respiratory tract infections, medications, or food. Physical examination should incorporate screening for angioedema and referral to emergency care if concern for airway swelling or anaphylaxis arises. Further evaluation and workup are warranted if lesions last longer than 24 hours. Urticarial vasculitis (UV) can mimic urticaria, but UV plaques last longer than 24 hours. UV may be associated with an underlying disease such as SLE; further diagnostic workup should be considered.

N. One should consider **annular lichen planus (LP)** in patients with purple, pruritic annular plaques with purple-to-white raised borders and central clearing on the axilla, groin, or penis. Distal aspects of the extremities and trunk may also be involved. Treatment involves symptomatic control of pruritus and targeting inflammation with corticosteroids.

See Appendix 1 for References and Image References.

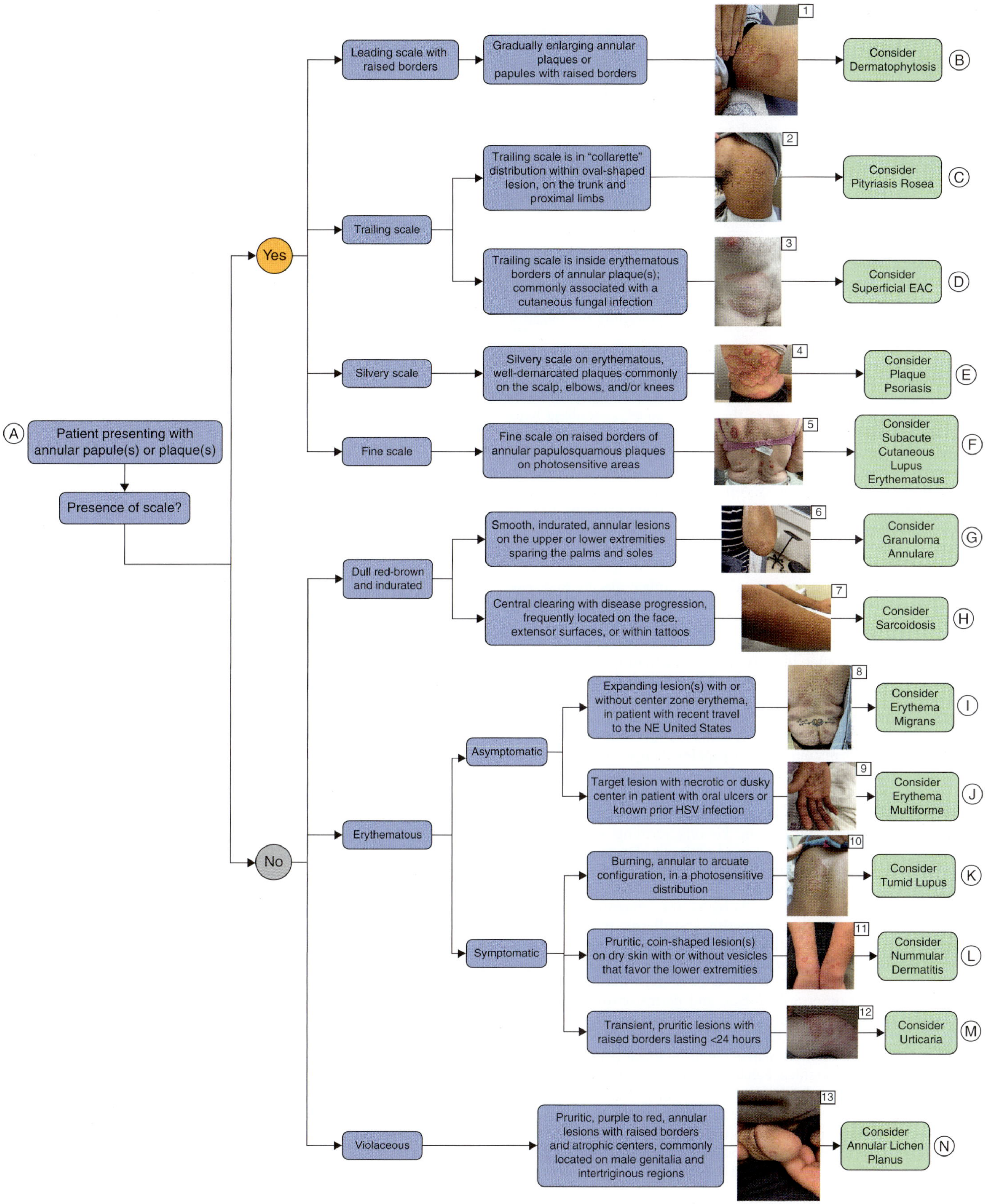
(A) Patient presenting with annular papule(s) or plaque(s)
Presence of scale?
Yes
Leading scale with raised borders
Gradually enlarging annular plaques or papules with raised borders
1
Consider Dermatophytosis (B)
Trailing scale
Trailing scale is in "collarette" distribution within oval-shaped lesion, on the trunk and proximal limbs
2
Consider Pityriasis Rosea (C)
Trailing scale is inside erythematous borders of annular plaque(s); commonly associated with a cutaneous fungal infection
3
Consider Superficial EAC (D)
Silvery scale
Silvery scale on erythematous, well-demarcated plaques commonly on the scalp, elbows, and/or knees
4
Consider Plaque Psoriasis (E)
Fine scale
Fine scale on raised borders of annular papulosquamous plaques on photosensitive areas
5
Consider Subacute Cutaneous Lupus Erythematosus (F)
No
Dull red-brown and indurated
Smooth, indurated, annular lesions on the upper or lower extremities sparing the palms and soles
6
Consider Granuloma Annulare (G)
Central clearing with disease progression, frequently located on the face, extensor surfaces, or within tattoos
7
Consider Sarcoidosis (H)
Erythematous
Asymptomatic
Expanding lesion(s) with or without center zone erythema, in patient with recent travel to the NE United States
8
Consider Erythema Migrans (I)
Target lesion with necrotic or dusky center in patient with oral ulcers or known prior HSV infection
9
Consider Erythema Multiforme (J)
Symptomatic
Burning, annular to arcuate configuration, in a photosensitive distribution
10
Consider Tumid Lupus (K)
Pruritic, coin-shaped lesion(s) on dry skin with or without vesicles that favor the lower extremities
11
Consider Nummular Dermatitis (L)
Transient, pruritic lesions with raised borders lasting <24 hours
12
Consider Urticaria (M)
Violaceous
Pruritic, purple to red, annular lesions with raised borders and atrophic centers, commonly located on male genitalia and intertriginous regions
13
Consider Annular Lichen Planus (N)

34 Linear Papules and Plaques

Samuel A. Stetkevich and Jason E. Hawkes

Papules and plaques arranged in a linear configuration are a common clinical presentation and highly suggestive of an external cause, although several inherent inflammatory conditions may also form a linear pattern in response to skin trauma. In this chapter, we discuss a stepwise approach to linear papules and plaques that teaches providers key dermatological findings essential for establishing a diagnosis.

A. Initial evaluation of linear papules or plaques begins with an inquiry into any known or suspected acute environmental exposures. This includes recent outdoor activities, travel, animal contacts, changes in lifestyle or diet, and any new exposures preceding the onset of symptoms.

B. Suspicion of an environmental exposure should prompt evaluation for a sporotrichoid spreading pattern in the skin. This pattern is a linear ascending extension of the papules or plaques along lymphatic chains. **Sporotrichosis**, ***Mycobacterium marinum***, and ***Mycobacterium chelonae*** **infections** spread in a sporotrichoid pattern. A recent rose or thorn prick with subsequent painless lesions suggests sporotrichosis. A recent water exposure with tender lesions suggests *M. marinum* infection. A recent exposure to cosmetic instrumentation (tattoo or piercings) with tender lesions suggests *M. chelonae* infection.

C. In the absence of a sporotrichoid pattern, other specific high-risk environmental exposures should be assessed. A history of sleeping in a hotel or infested environment followed by diffuse pruritus and/or linearly grouped papules may suggest a diagnosis of **bed bugs**. Consider **scabies** after identifying poor sanitation or communal living with concomitant generalized pruritus and papules worse at night and involving the interdigital web spaces, genitals, or skin folds. Dermoscopy or a skin scraping can assist in visualizing mites, eggs, or scybala (brown feces). A history of outdoor exposure and erythematous, edematous, pruritic papules often arranged in a linear pattern supports **arthropod assault**.

D. If obvious environmental exposures are ruled out, determine the duration of individual lesions. Lesions forming and resolving within <24 hours are indicative of **urticaria**. **Dermatographism**, or pressure-induced urticaria, is the most common form of physical urticaria and is reproduced by rubbing or scratching the skin. If individual lesions persist for >24 hours, the remaining differential includes **keloids, flagellate dermatitis**, and **allergic/irritant contact dermatitis**. Keloids are smooth fibrous plaques forming at areas of known trauma and may be linear. Flagellate dermatitis will resemble "whip" marks and can appear after shiitake mushroom ingestion, with adult-onset Still disease and dermatomyositis, or after exposure to medications (e.g., bleomycin, doxorubicin, cisplatin, or docetaxel). Allergic/irritant contact dermatitis should be considered for any remaining environmentally induced linear papule or plaque that is not already classified. Patch testing may be required to identify a chemical or irritant that is present in specific products.

E. If environmental exposures are not suspected, the provider should assess whether the papules and plaques follow the normal lines of embryonic cellular migration and development, also known as the Blaschko lines.

F. The presence of a Blaschkonian distribution prompts the provider to evaluate whether the lesions appeared in early childhood. Consider **incontinentia pigmenti** in a young female at any of the four distinct stages. Stage 1 involves linear vesicles within erythematous plaques, stage 2 presents as verrucous linear plaques, stage 3 transitions to linear hyperpigmentation, and stage 4 includes linear hypopigmentation and atrophic plaques. **Linear porokeratosis** can also be considered in a young child with unilateral hyperkeratotic papules or plaques surrounded by a peripheral, thick, ridge-like scale. **Inflammatory linear verrucous epidermal nevus** may be diagnosed in early childhood as well and classically appears as hyperkeratotic erythematous plaques, often on the lower extremities and left side of the body. An **epidermal nevus** presents as well-circumscribed, smooth, velvety, or verrucous papules and plaques along Blaschko lines. The diagnoses uncommon in childhood include **linear lichen planus, lichen striatus**, and **linear morphea**. Linear lichen planus occurs along Blaschko lines as purple, pruritic, flat-topped plaques and papules. Lichen striatus presents as red, pink, or flesh-colored, pinpoint, flat-topped papules with a slight scale. Linear morphea characteristically presents as a band-like, firm, erythematous or violaceous plaque.

G. Koebnerization (or an isomorphic response) is the appearance of new skin lesions on previously unaffected skin in response to trauma and is an important diagnostic clue. **Hypertrophic lichen planus** koebnerizes and presents as thickened verrucous plaques that favor the extremities. Consider **lichen nitidus** when asymptomatic, pinhead-sized, shiny papules koebnerize. **Flat warts** and **molluscum contagiosum** may present very similarly and koebnerize, but flat warts will be distinctly flat topped, whereas molluscum contagiousum will have a distinct central umbilication or white core. **Plaque psoriasis** is also associated with Koebner phenomenon and should be considered in patients with a known history of sharply demarcated, erythematous, silver-scaled plaques, as well as involvement of the scalp, umbilicus, trunk, gluteal fold, acral skin, or extensor surfaces. **Guttate psoriasis** will also koebnerize, but the patient will often have an antecedent streptococcal infection followed by eruptive, small, oval-shaped papules with fine scale. **Darier disease** is one final condition that koebnerizes and should be considered when gritty, yellow-brown papules are present in a "seborrheic distribution," with a history of nail chipping, cobblestoning of the hard palate, and family members with similar lesions.

H. Lesions involving the genitals are another important diagnostic clue. Small, dome-shaped, flesh-colored, asymptomatic papules, usually on the corona of the glans penis suggest **pearly penile papules**. Small, shiny papules easily separated at the base on the labia minora or vestibule suggest **vestibular papillomatosis**. In the absence of genital involvement, consider **linear focal elastosis, striae distensae**, or **papular mucinosis**. Linear focal elastosis will present as asymptomatic linear plaques, often on the trunk with a yellowish hue and may develop in preexisting striae. Striae distensae (or stretch marks) present as depressed, atrophic, wrinkled plaques parallel to lines of skin relaxation. Papular mucinosis presents as erythematous or flesh-colored, dome-shaped, or flat-topped papules associated with leonine faces, doughnut proximal interphalangeal joint sign, or paraproteinemia (most often IgGλ).

See Appendix 1 for Further Reading and Image References.

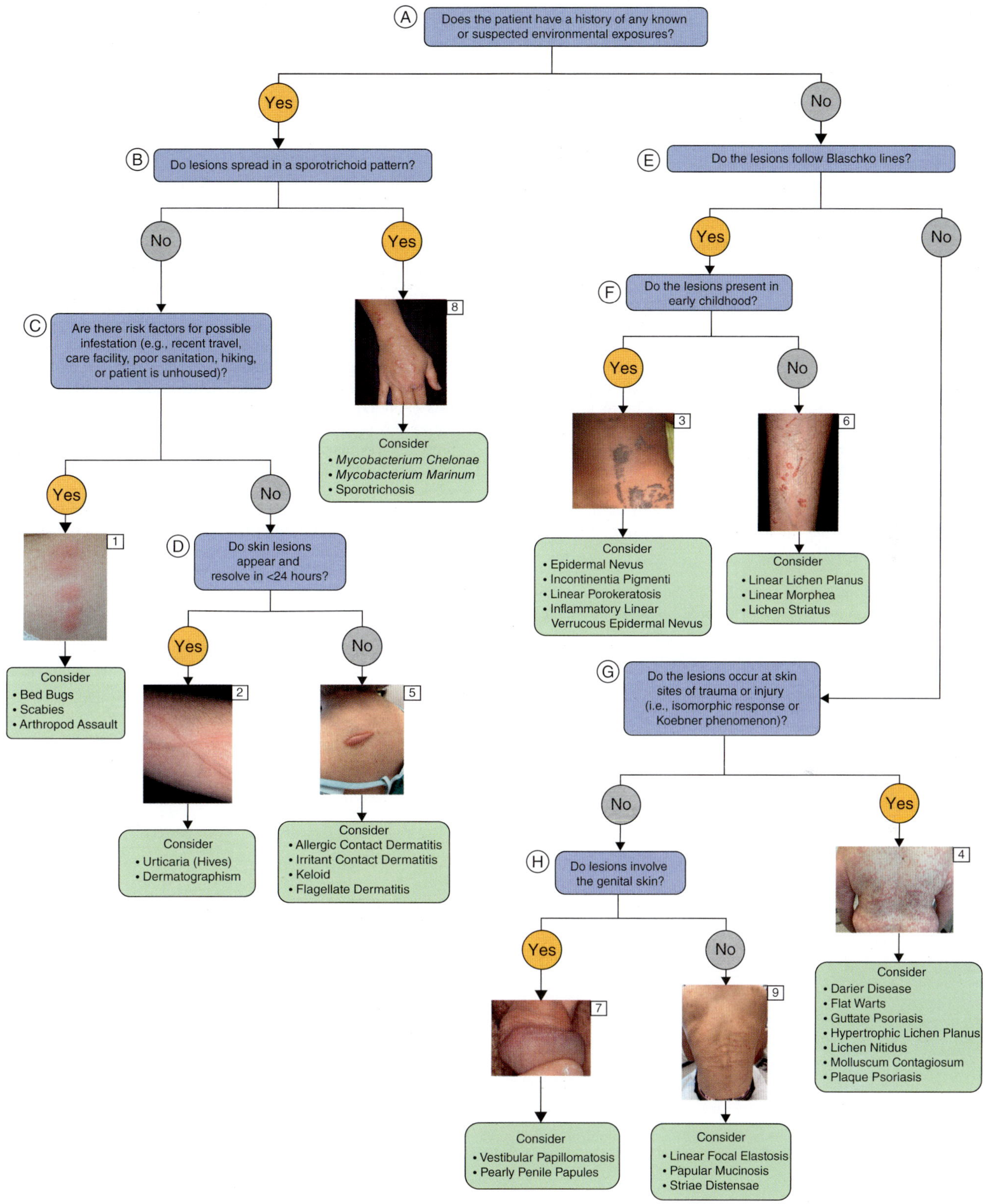
A
Does the patient have a history of any known or suspected environmental exposures?
Yes
B
Do lesions spread in a sporotrichoid pattern?
No
C
Are there risk factors for possible infestation (e.g., recent travel, care facility, poor sanitation, hiking, or patient is unhoused)?
Yes
1
Consider
• Bed Bugs
• Scabies
• Arthropod Assault
No
D
Do skin lesions appear and resolve in <24 hours?
Yes
2
Consider
• Urticaria (Hives)
• Dermatographism
No
5
Consider
• Allergic Contact Dermatitis
• Irritant Contact Dermatitis
• Keloid
• Flagellate Dermatitis
Yes
8
Consider
• Mycobacterium Chelonae
• Mycobacterium Marinum
• Sporotrichosis
No
E
Do the lesions follow Blaschko lines?
Yes
F
Do the lesions present in early childhood?
Yes
3
Consider
• Epidermal Nevus
• Incontinentia Pigmenti
• Linear Porokeratosis
• Inflammatory Linear Verrucous Epidermal Nevus
No
6
Consider
• Linear Lichen Planus
• Linear Morphea
• Lichen Striatus
No
G
Do the lesions occur at skin sites of trauma or injury (i.e., isomorphic response or Koebner phenomenon)?
No
H
Do lesions involve the genital skin?
Yes
7
Consider
• Vestibular Papillomatosis
• Pearly Penile Papules
No
9
Consider
• Linear Focal Elastosis
• Papular Mucinosis
• Striae Distensae
Yes
4
Consider
• Darier Disease
• Flat Warts
• Guttate Psoriasis
• Hypertrophic Lichen Planus
• Lichen Nitidus
• Molluscum Contagiosum
• Plaque Psoriasis

35 Dermal Papules and Plaques

Amina Ziad and Alexandra Philippa Charrow

The initial evaluation of patients with dermal papules should include a detailed history and thorough examination, including timing of onset, evolution, and associated symptomatology. The differential for dermal papules is broad, and as such, the color (taking into account the patient's baseline skin tone), morphology, and distribution of lesions are critical in determining a diagnosis. Histological evaluation is often needed for definitive diagnosis.

A. **Variable presentation and great imitators**: Both **syphilis** and **sarcoidosis** have variable presentations and should remain on the differential for widespread dermal rashes. Similarly, **mycosis fungoides** can be mistaken for several other skin conditions and should be considered in patients with pruritic, erythematous patches and plaques with overlying fine scale and a predilection for the buttocks/trunk.

B. **Skin colored**: **Lipoid proteinosis** is a rare, autosomal recessive deposition disorder in which skin-colored papules and nodules appear on the face and axilla within the first 2 years of life. **Leiomyomas** and **angioleiomyomas** are benign smooth muscle tumors that present as firm, solitary nodules on the lower extremities and are generally diagnosed via histology.

C. **Red-brown (granulomatous):** Granulomatous lesions appear red-brown on examination and apple jelly colored on diascopy. While, on occasion, history and risk factors can differentiate these conditions, biopsy and infectious workup are generally needed for definitive diagnosis. **Sarcoidosis** has variable cutaneous manifestations and should be included in any red-brown papule differential. **Secondary syphilis** has a granulomatous variant that presents with red-brown papules and minimal scale. **Granuloma annulare** presents with red-brown dermal papules that form annular plaques, preferentially on the extremities. **Necrobiosis lipoidica diabeticorum** most commonly presents in middle-aged females as yellow-brown telangiectatic plaques with elevated brown-violaceous borders, usually in the pretibial area, sometimes ulcerating. **Multicentric reticulohistiocytosis** presents as firm red-brown papules and nodules on acral surfaces and is associated with erosive arthritis. **Palisaded neutrophilic granulomatous dermatitis (PNGD)** and **interstitial granulomatous dermatitis (IGD)** are commonly seen in association with rheumatologic conditions. PNGD presents symmetrically with tender erythematous to violaceous papules and plaques on extensor surfaces, especially elbows and fingers, while IGD presents as plaques in annular patterns or linear cords ("rope sign"), favoring the lateral trunk, axillae, buttocks, and medial thighs. **Interstitial granulomatous drug reaction** which presents with annular plaques and indurated borders is usually found in intertriginous regions and is associated with antihypertensive medications and tumor necrosis factor-alpha inhibitors.

Patient presenting with dermal papule(s)

Initial evaluation with complete history, chronic medical conditions and medications, and thorough physical examination to identify potential underlying etiology.

(A) Is the lesion a possible imitator?

Yes → What is the distribution of the lesion(s)?

- Red-brown lesions that favor the face and nose. Patient likely to have systemic symptoms.

  1
  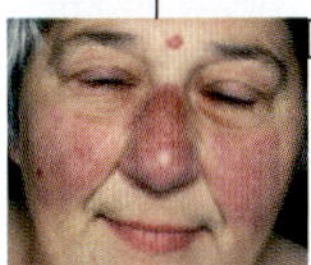

  → Consider Sarcoidosis

- Red-brown papules with little overlying scale that favor the palms, soles, and shins. Patients may also have moth-eaten alopecia.

  2
  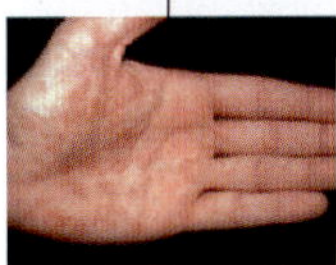

  → Consider Syphilis

- Favors the trunk and buttocks and presents with pruritic, erythematous patches and plaques with overlying fine scale.

  3
  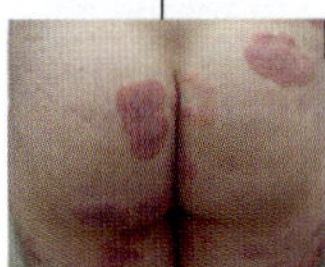

  → Consider Mycosis Fungoides

No → What is the primary color?

continued on next page

Red-brown (C)

Does the patient have a history of any rheumatologic condition?

Yes

- Patient with symmetrical tender erythematous to violaceous papules and plaques on extensor surfaces, especially the elbows and fingers.

  4
  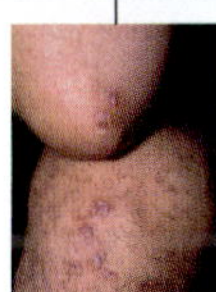

  → Consider Palisaded Neutrophilic Granulomatous Dermatitis (PNGD)

- Patient presenting with plaques in annular patterns or linear cords ("rope sign"), favoring the lateral trunk, axillae, buttocks, and medial thighs.

  5
  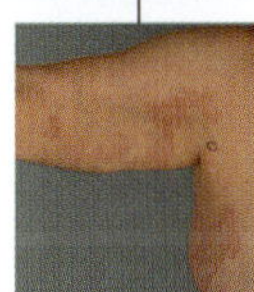

  → Consider Interstitial Granulomatous Dermatitis (IGD)

No → Is the patient taking antihypertensives or TNF-α-inhibitors?

- **Yes** → Patient with annular plaques and indurated borders favoring intertriginous regions.

  6
  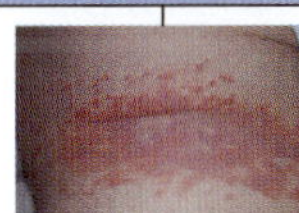

  → Consider Interstitial Granulomatous Drug Reaction (IGDR)

- **No** → Do the lesions favor the extremities?

  Yes

  - Patient with red-brown dermal papules that form annular plaques, preferentially on the extremities.

    7
    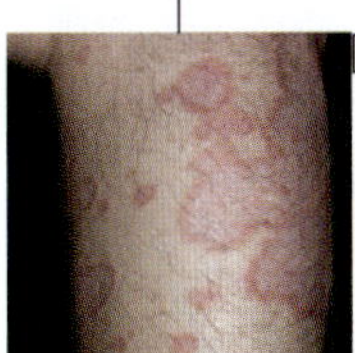

    → Consider Granuloma Annulare (GA)

  - Patient is most commonly a middle-aged female presenting with yellow-brown telangiectatic plaques with elevated brown-violaceous borders, usually in the pretibial area, that may ulcerate.

    8
    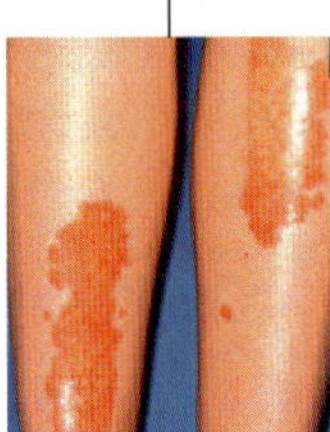

    → Consider Necrobiosis Lipoidica Diabeticorum (NLD)

  - Patient presenting with firm, red-brown papules and nodules on acral surfaces that are associated with erosive arthritis.

    9
    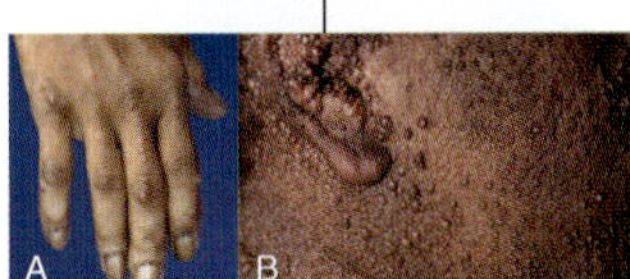

    → Consider Multicentric Reticulohistiocytosis (MRH)

Skin colored (B)

Do the lesions affect the face?

- **No** → Firm solitary nodules favoring the lower extremities.

  10
  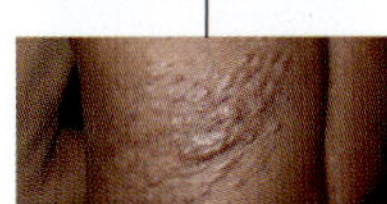

  → Consider Leiomyoma or Angioleiomyoma

- **Yes** → Papules and nodules appear within the first two years of life and there may be a family history

  11
  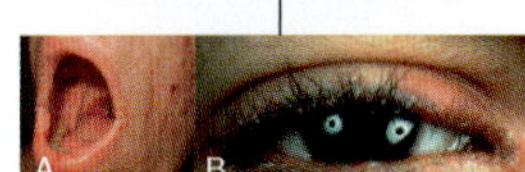

  → Consider Lipoid Proteinosis

Continued

D. **Yellow**: Papules that appear yellow tend to be related to sebaceous glands or are xanthomatous. **Xanthomas** are a broad category of lipid deposits in the tissue and include eruptive, tuberous, tendinous, palmar, and planum subtypes. **Eruptive xanthomas** are red-yellow papules on the extensor surfaces of the extremities, buttocks, and hands and can be seen in the setting of primary or secondary hypertriglyceridemia. **Tuberous xanthomas** present as pink-yellow papules usually on the elbows and knees, while **tendinous xanthomas** are clinically similar but occur on the Achilles tendon and extensor tendons of the hands, knees, and elbows. Both are associated with familial conditions of high cholesterol. **Palmar xanthomas** present as yellowish plaques involving the palms and are associated with familial lipid disorders, multiple myeloma, and primary biliary cirrhosis. **Plane xanthomas** are yellow-orange macules, papules, patches, and plaques most commonly affecting intertriginous areas of the body, seen in patients with both normal and elevated lipid levels. **Necrobiotic xanthogranuloma** presents as yellow-red-brown papules around the eyes in those with hypergammaglobulinemia. **Juvenile xanthogranuloma** are solitary yellow-brown papules preferentially presenting on the head and neck of children, but adult-onset cases do occur.

E. **Brown**: **Urticaria pigmentosa** presents with monomorphic tan-brown papules and plaques of varying sizes. A firm stroke of the lesions will induce an urticarial wheal and flare known as Darier sign.

F. **Violaceous or erythematous: Erythema elevatum diutinum** is an uncommon vasculitis that presents with arthralgias and symmetric plaques favoring extensor surfaces and periarticular sites. **Leukemia cutis** presents in those with leukemia with red firm papules, plaques, and sometimes hemorrhagic ulcers. **Cutaneous B-cell lymphoma** presents as asymptomatic solitary or clustered pink to purple papules and arcuate plaques and is generally diagnosed histologically. **Cutaneous metastases** can present as skin-colored, pink to red-purple papules, plaques, or nodules and may be eroded or with overlying alopecia. **Wells syndrome** presents with acute onset, pruritic, erythematous plaques and can mimic cellulitis. It may persist for weeks and typically recurs. Erythematous lesions on the chest or arms may represent **tumid lupus**, a rare skin condition presenting with edematous, firm, erythematous, and annular plaques. No scaling or follicular plugging is present. **Reticulate erythematous mucinosis** is a similar appearing clinical entity, presenting with papules and plaques coalescing into a reticular or net-like configuration, typically on the midchest and back. **Lymphomatoid papulosis** also commonly affects the extremities appearing as red papules, which become more vesicular or pustular and eventually necrotic over days to weeks. It can be associated with an underlying lymphoma.

G. **White**: **Dystrophic calcinosis cutis** usually occurs in a preexisting lesion or skin region affected by an inflammatory process and presents as deposits of chalky granular material on the fingers, elbows, and areas of trauma.

See Appendix 1 for Further Reading and Image References.

What is the primary color?

(E) Brown
- Appearance of urticarial wheal and flare lesion after stroking skin lesion (Darier sign).

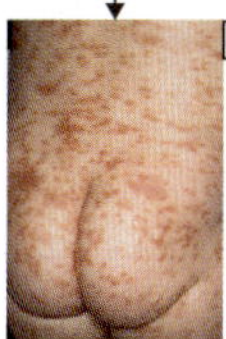

12

- Consider Urticaria Pigmentosa

(F) White
- Chalky, granular deposits in areas of prior inflammation or trauma.

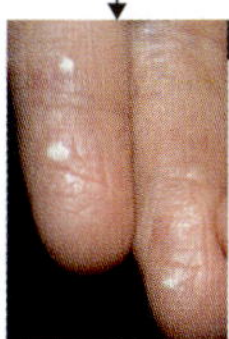

13

- Consider Dystrophic Calcinosis Cutis

(G) Erythematous/violaceous
- Does the patient have symmetric plaques on extensors and periarticular areas with arthralgias?
  - Yes

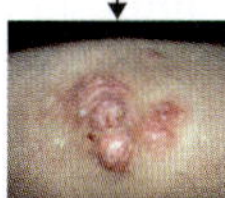

14

- Consider Erythema Elevatum Diutinum (EED)
  - No → Are the lesions pruritic?
    - Yes → Acute onset of erythematous plaques that may mimic cellulitis but tend to last for several weeks and may recur.

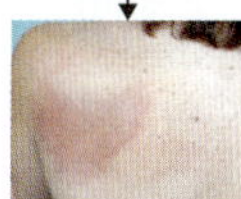

15

- Consider Wells Syndrome
    - No → Do the lesions become more pustular or ulcerate?
      - Yes → Favors the extremities and presents with red papules that progressively ulcerate.

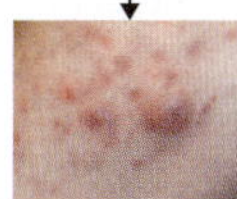

16

- Consider Lymphomatoid Papulosis
      - No → Is it a solitary lesion or is there a history of leukemia or lymphoma?
        - Yes → Asymptomatic solitary pink to purple papules and arcuate plaques.

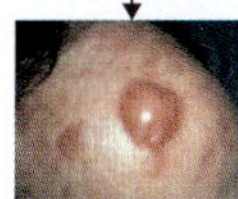

17

- Consider Cutaneous B-Cell Lymphoma
        - Yes → Pink to red-purple papules, plaques, and/or nodules in patient with history of cancer.

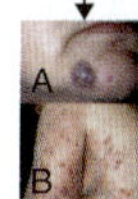

18

- Consider Cutaneous Metastases
        - Yes → Red, firm papules and plaques; hemorrhagic ulcers may or may not be present.

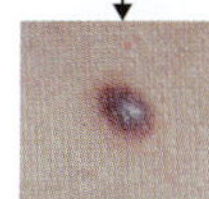

19

- Consider Leukemia Cutis
        - No → Are the lesions primarily distributed on the chest and back?
          - Yes → Papules and plaques coalescing into a reticular configuration favoring the mid chest and back.

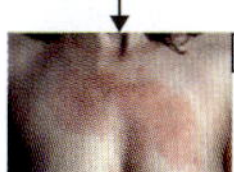

20

- Consider Reticulate Erythematous Mucinosis
          - Yes → Red, edematous, annular plaques favoring the chest and arms without scaling or follicular plugging.

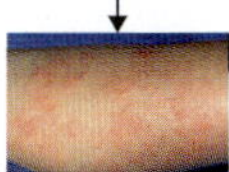

21

- Consider Tumid Lupus

(D) Yellow
- Are the lesions primarily distributed on the head and neck?
  - Yes → Adult patient with yellow-red papules typically around the eyes and hypergammaglobulinemia.

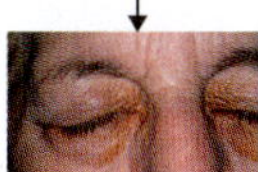

22

- Consider Necrobiotic Xanthogranuloma (NXG)
  - Yes → Child or adult with single or multiple yellow-brown papules typically on the head and neck.

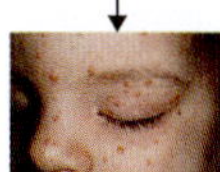

23

- Consider Juvenile Xanthogranuloma (JXG)
  - No → Patient with red-yellow papules on extensor surfaces of the extremities and elevated triglycerides.

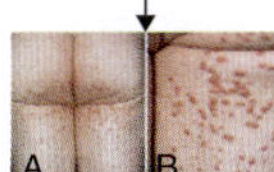

24

- Consider Eruptive Xanthomas
  - No → Patient with pink-yellow papules on the Achilles tendon and extensor tendons of the hands, knees, and the elbows. May also be associated with elevated cholesterol.

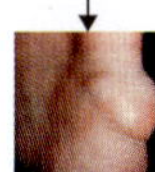

25

- Consider Tendinous Xanthomas
  - No → Patient with pink-yellow papules typically favoring the knees and the elbows.

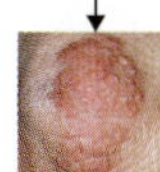

26

- Consider Tuberous Xanthomas
  - No → Patient presenting with yellowish plaques involving the palms. Associated with familial lipid disorders, multiple myeloma, and primary biliary cirrhosis.

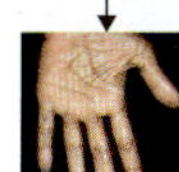

27

- Consider Palmar Xanthomas
  - No → Patient with yellow-orange macules, papules, patches, and plaques that favor intertriginous areas. Seen in patients with both normal and elevated lipid levels.

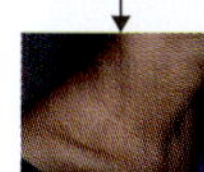

28

- Consider Plane Xanthomas

36 Perifollicular Papules

Kirk Williams and Steven Daveluy

Perifollicular papules can be seen in a variety of skin conditions caused by inflammation or occlusion of the hair follicle. The anatomic distribution allows accurate diagnosis of some entities, while others, such as folliculitis, can have a widely variable distribution.

A. The presence of comedones is a clue to consider acne and hidradenitis suppurativa (HS). **Acne vulgaris** is a common cause of perifollicular papules and pustules on the face and upper trunk. Follicular papules and double-headed comedones can be seen in **HS**, particularly the "follicular" subtype of HS. The typical lesions (e.g., nodules, abscesses, sinus tracts) seen in typical anatomic locations (intertriginous regions) and history of chronicity and recurrence help point to a diagnosis of HS.

B. Erythematous perifollicular papules and/or pustules on the face can be caused by **rosacea** or **demodex folliculitis**, which may represent a spectrum of the same disease. Persistent erythema and facial flushing are hallmarks of rosacea. Perifollicular scaling may be a clue to the presence of demodex mites.

C. Tiny flat-topped perifollicular papules can be seen in **papular eczema**. It is more common in patients of African or Asian descent. Classic atopic dermatitis is often also present on examination.

D. **Pityriasis rubra pilaris** presents with progressive, well-demarcated, reddish-orange scaly papules and plaques that spread in a craniocaudal pattern, often with distinct "islands of sparing." The papulosquamous eruption often has a follicular accentuation. Palmoplantar keratoderma and nail dystrophy may be present. The clinical course is highly variable with occasional pruritus.

E. **Folliculotropic mycosis fungoides** is a distinct variant of mycosis fungoides that occurs most commonly in adult male patients. It presents as erythematous plaques with follicular accentuation and acneiform or keratosis pilaris-like follicular papules, sometimes associated with alopecia.

F. **Majocchi granuloma** presents with papules and nodules caused by dermatophyte infection of the hair follicle, often in patients with tinea corporis.

G. The hallmark of **eosinophilic folliculitis** is intense pruritus. Physical findings appear similar to acne, with erythematous papules and pustules most commonly occurring on the head, neck, and upper trunk. It may be associated with advanced HIV.

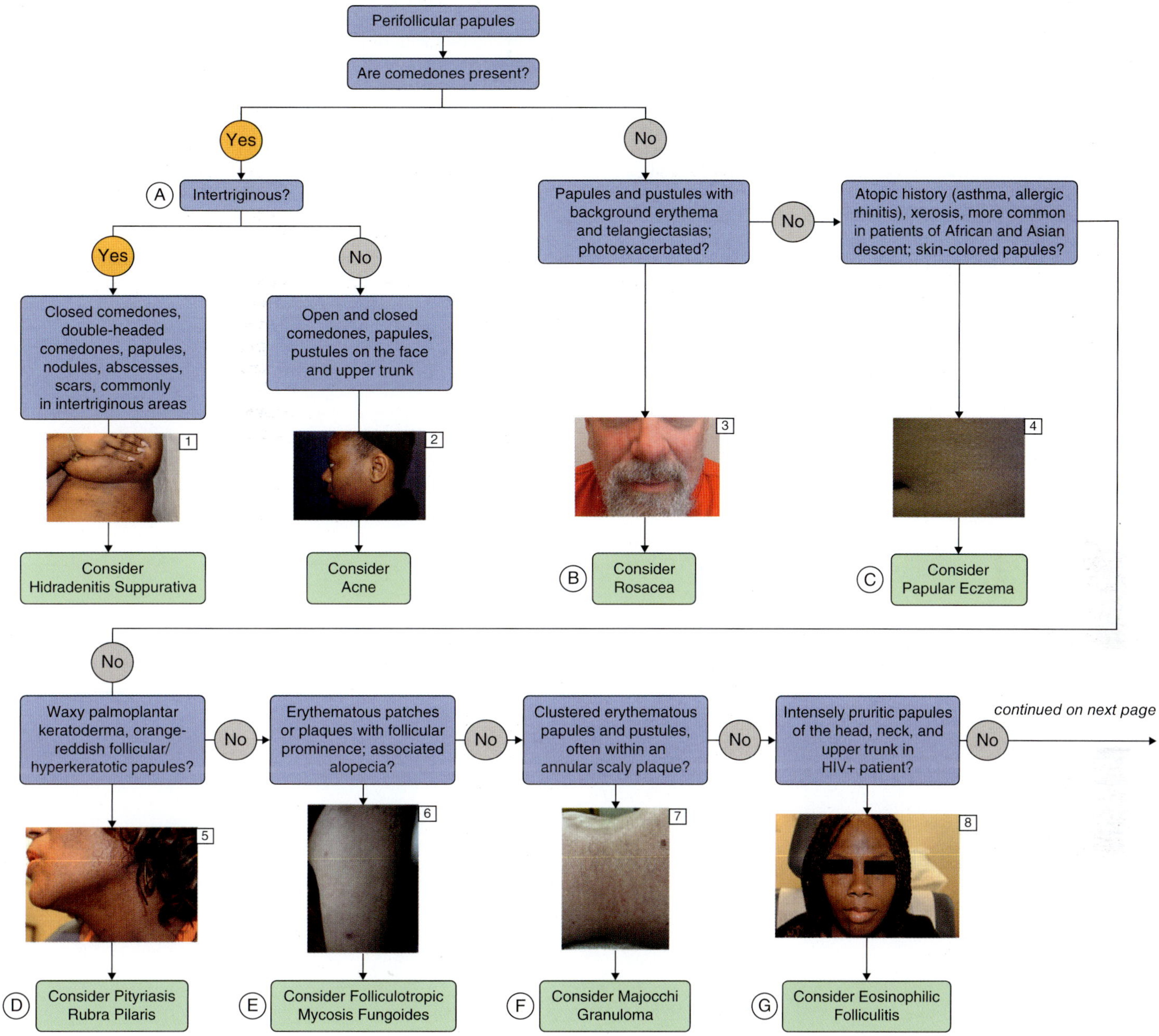
Perifollicular papules
Are comedones present?
Yes
A Intertriginous?
Yes
Closed comedones, double-headed comedones, papules, nodules, abscesses, scars, commonly in intertriginous areas
1
Consider Hidradenitis Suppurativa
No
Open and closed comedones, papules, pustules on the face and upper trunk
2
Consider Acne
No
Papules and pustules with background erythema and telangiectasias; photoexacerbated?
3
B Consider Rosacea
No
Atopic history (asthma, allergic rhinitis), xerosis, more common in patients of African and Asian descent; skin-colored papules?
4
C Consider Papular Eczema
No
Waxy palmoplantar keratoderma, orange-reddish follicular/hyperkeratotic papules?
5
D Consider Pityriasis Rubra Pilaris
No
Erythematous patches or plaques with follicular prominence; associated alopecia?
6
E Consider Folliculotropic Mycosis Fungoides
No
Clustered erythematous papules and pustules, often within an annular scaly plaque?
7
F Consider Majocchi Granuloma
No
Intensely pruritic papules of the head, neck, and upper trunk in HIV+ patient?
8
G Consider Eosinophilic Folliculitis
No
continued on next page

Continued

H. The differential for monomorphic follicular papules includes steroid acne, disseminate and recurrent infundibulofolliculitis, and pityrosporum folliculitis. The acute onset of monomorphic acneiform papules or pustules 2 to 5 weeks after starting corticosteroid therapy is typical of **steroid acne**. Skin-colored monomorphic 1- to 2 mm papules resembling "goose bumps" are seen in **disseminate and recurrent infundibulofolliculitis**, most common in young males of African descent on the neck, trunk, buttocks, and proximal extremities. Intense pruritus and acute onset of monomorphic follicular papules and/or pustules on the face and upper trunk should lead to consideration of **pityrosporum folliculitis**, particularly in the context of recent antibiotic use.

I. **Phrynoderma** is caused by vitamin A deficiency and presents with spiny papules on the extensor extremities that may spread to the trunk and spare the hands/feet.

J. Several diseases have sites of anatomic predilection. In **keratosis pilaris**, rough pinpoint papules are most commonly seen on the upper arms and thighs. **Erythromelanosis follicularis faciei et colli** presents on the lateral cheeks and neck with erythema and/or hyperpigmentation with tiny follicular papules within. **Pseudofolliculitis barbae** presents with skin-colored, erythematous, or hyperpigmented follicular papules in areas that are shaved, typically the beard region. **Folliculitis decalvans** presents with erythematous papules and pustules on the scalp that progress to scarring alopecia with tufted hairs. Early disease can be indistinguishable from folliculitis. **Acne keloidalis nuchae** presents with perifollicular erythematous papules and keloid-like papules on the occipital scalp and posterior neck, most commonly in young men of African descent.

K. Finally, **folliculitis** due to a variety of causes, including irritants, bacteria, fungi, viral, drug-induced, should stay on the differential of any skin condition with follicular papules.

See Appendix 1 for Further Reading and Image References.

No

(H) Monomorphic papules?

Yes

Acute onset of acneiform papules with recent exposure to steroids

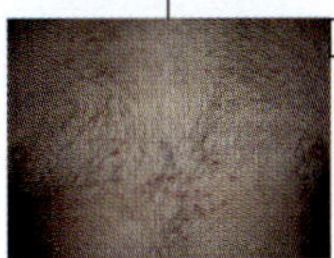
9

Consider Steroid Acne

Skin-colored papules on the neck, trunk, buttocks, and proximal extremities

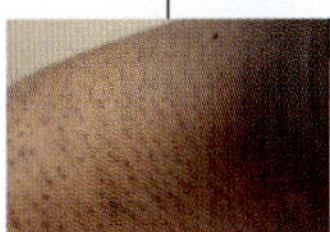
10

Consider Disseminate and Recurrent Infundibulofolliculitis

Intensely pruritic pink papules; history of immunosuppression or recent antibiotic use

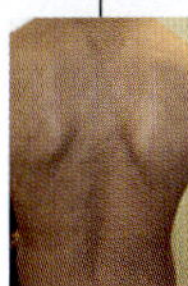
11

Consider Pityrosporum Folliculitis

No

Poor vitamin A intake; spiny papules primarily on extensor surfaces that can spread to the trunk?

Yes

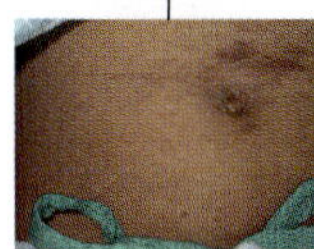
12

(I) Consider Phrynoderma

No

History of iodine administration; acneiform eruption most commonly in sebaceous areas?

Yes

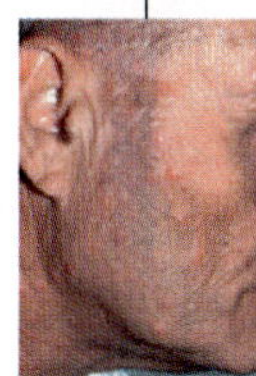
13

Consider Iododerma

No

(J) Localized to a specific anatomic region?

No → Nonspecific papules and pustules → Consider folliculitis and rule out underlying etiologies (bacterial, fungal, candida, herpes, irritant, drug induced, etc.) (K)

Yes

Pinpoint keratotic papules on the upper outer arms and anterior thighs?

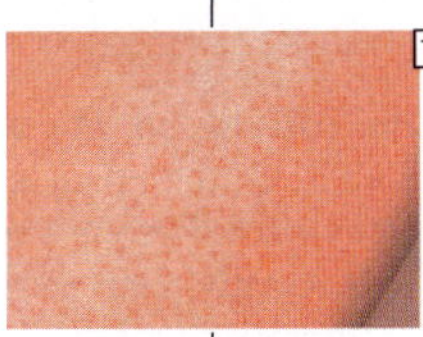
14

Consider Keratosis Pilaris

No

Erythematous or hyperpigmented papules on the beard and neck region, triggered by shaving?

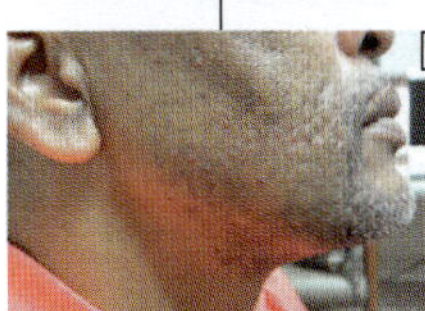
15

Consider Pseudofolliculitis Barbae

No

Papules, pustules, and keloid-like scars on the occipital scalp/ neck; exacerbated by shaving hair?

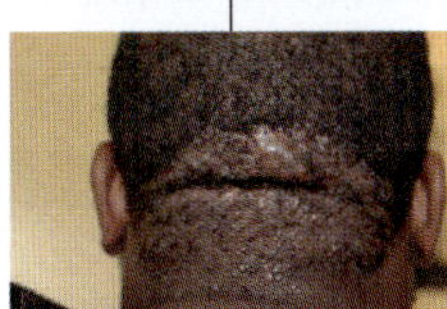
16

Consider Acne Keloidalis Nuchae

No

Papules, pustules, scars, alopecia, and tufted hairs on the scalp?

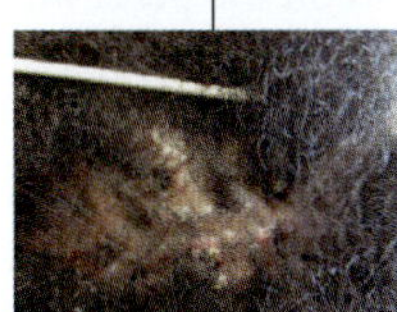
17

Consider Folliculitis Decalvans

No

Lateral cheeks/neck with pinpoint follicular/keratotic papules on background of red-brown skin

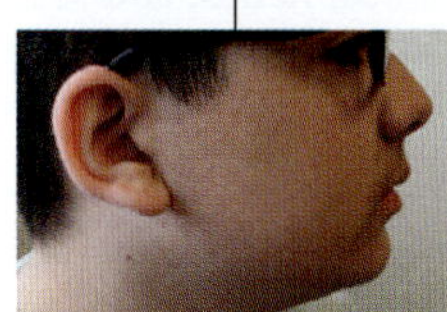
18

Consider Erythromelanosis Follicularis Faciei Et Colli

37 Pityriasiform Papules and Plaques

Hana Ahmed and Tiffany Mayo

The description of pityriasiform can be thought of as pityriasis rosea (PR)-like. The general clinical appearance is pink papules or plaques with associated fine scale. A thorough history and examination of the palms, soles, nails, and mucosa will help guide the clinician to a more specific diagnosis.

A. In the clinical setting of pink scaly papules with a central collarette of trailing scale following Langer lines, the two primary diagnoses to consider are **PR** and **PR-like drug eruptions**. The former often has a herald patch, which is a larger scaly plaque that precedes the general eruption by about a week. **PR** also frequently has a prodrome, can follow an upper respiratory infection, and is thought to be due to the reactivation of human herpesvirus 7 and 8. Of note, it is more commonly seen on the trunk, but an inverse variant exists and involves the axilla and groin.

B. In comparison, **PR-like drug eruptions** must be distinguished from an occurrence of PR in the setting of a new drug. Making this distinction is important as medication cessation is recommended if the rash is thought to be drug-related. In general, PR-like drug eruptions may be more likely to involve the face and mucosa, have severe pruritus, and peripheral eosinophilia compared to PR, while less likely to have a herald patch.

Biopsy can be helpful as PR will have mounds of non-adherent parakeratosis, spongiosis, perivascular lymphohistiocytic infiltrate, and erythrocyte extravasation. PR-like drug eruptions have been reported to have an interface dermatitis and eosinophils.

C. In the setting of pityriasiform lesions with palmar and plantar involvement, additional entities to consider are **secondary syphilis** and **reactive arthritis** (formerly Reiter syndrome). **Secondary syphilis** is a chronic systemic infection that progresses through active and latent stages and is acquired through inoculation at mucosae and abraded skin. Secondary syphilis can mimic guttate psoriasis and occurs about 3 to 10 weeks after the initial chancre. Red-brown papules and plaques with collarettes of scale may be present on the palms and soles. There can be other signs, including alopecia, mucosal involvement, and condyloma lata. Serum testing and/or biopsy can further aid in diagnosis.

D. **Reactive arthritis** classically presents with urethritis, arthritis, ocular findings, oral ulcers, and psoriasiform skin lesions. It is often triggered by *Chlamydia trachomatis* but is also seen in response to other infections, including shigellosis.

Patients may present with psoriatic plaques on the extensor legs, dorsal hands, and scalp, as well as on the penis, which is known as balanitis circinata. Keratoderma blennorrhagicum, initially appearing as pustules and then later as hyperkeratotic pink plaques, may be seen on the palms and soles.

E. **Tinea versicolor** is a common superficial mycosis caused by *Malassezia globosa* and *Malassezia furfur*. Patients present with asymptomatic macules and patches or thin papules and plaques. The lesions may be brown, tan, or pink and have overlying thin scale. In darker skin types, lesions may be hypopigmented. The chest, back, and upper arms are most commonly involved. A KOH preparation of the scale will demonstrate hyphae and spores. Wood's lamp may show fluorescence due to the fluorochrome present (pityrialactone).

F. **Mycosis fungoides (MF)** is a type of cutaneous T-cell lymphoma (CTCL), which typically affects patients in the sixth to seventh decade; however, it can also be seen in younger patients. MF may present as patches, plaques, and tumors, and in some cases, a stepwise progression through these stages is observed. We will focus on patch-stage MF for this pityriasiform chapter. MF may present with erythematous patches and plaques with fine scale. The buttocks and sun-protected areas of the trunk and extremities are favored anatomical sites. Clinicians should have a low threshold to biopsy, and in this setting, a tangential biopsy is preferred. Histology classically depicts a lichenoid infiltrate with atypical lymphocytes within vacuoles in the epidermis. The degree of lymphocytic involvement becomes more pronounced in plaque- and tumor-stage lesions.

G. The term pityriasis lichenoides refers to a group of disorders that includes pityriasis lichenoides et varioliformis acuta (PLEVA), febrile ulceronecrotic Mucha-Habermann disease (subtype of PLEVA), and **pityriasis lichenoides chronica (PLC)**. These all fall within the realm of clonal T-cell disorders that can rarely be associated with MF.

PLC presents as recurrent crops of erythematous or reddish brown papules with a central scale. The papules spontaneously flatten and regress, leaving behind postinflammatory pigment alteration, which can last for weeks. The course of disease can last for several years. Unlike PLEVA, the eruption is often asymptomatic.

Histopathology is often necessary for diagnostic purposes. Importantly, this entity is CD30 negative, helping differentiate from lymphomatoid papulosis.

H. Small and large plaque parapsoriasis are chronic idiopathic dermatoses that overlap with cutaneous lymphomas and pityriasis lichenoides. Both conditions can be widespread or more focal and favor sun-protected sites. **Small plaque parapsoriasis** presents with 1- to 5 cm well-demarcated, ovoid, pink, or hyperpigmented patches, sometimes with a yellow hue. There is a variant known as digitate dermatosis, in which elongated finger-like plaques are seen on the trunk and flanks oriented along the skin cleavage lines. There is a lower risk of progressing to CTCL when compared with large plaque parapsoriasis.

I. **Large plaque parapsoriasis** presents as erythematous, round scaly patches or plaques that are larger than 5 cm in size. Poikiloderma may be present. These patients require long-term follow-up as there is a risk of developing overt CTCL, usually MF.

J. **Pityriasis rotunda** presents as asymptomatic, large, well-demarcated circular to polycyclic hyperpigmented or hypopigmented patches or thin plaques, measuring 10 cm to even 30 cm in diameter. There is an overlying fine scale, and the trunk and extremities are favored. It has been reported in association with malnutrition, mycobacterial infection, and malignancy.

K. If nail changes are present, psoriasis should be considered. We will focus on **guttate psoriasis**, which often mimics PR. Guttate psoriasis presents as well-demarcated pink or red papules with adherent white to silvery scale with a diffuse distribution. It is mostly seen in the setting of recent infection, often streptococcal pharyngitis; however, a host of other infectious etiologies have been cited. Additionally, medications may exacerbate or induce psoriasis.

L. **Pityriasis rubra pilaris (PRP)** presents with follicularly based reddish-orange papules coalescing into plaques with "islands of sparing." There may be a reddish-orange waxy keratoderma of the palms and soles. PRP frequently demonstrates cephalic to caudal spread.

See Appendix 1 for Further Reading and Image References.

Adult patient presenting with papules and plaques with fine scale

↓

Detailed history with pertinent positives, negatives, and thorough physical examination of the skin, hair, nails, and mucosal surfaces

↓

Pink scaling papules with central trailing scale following Langer lines (Christmas tree pattern)?

Yes

- Preceded by larger herald/mother patch
  Trunk involvement
  +/– Prodromal symptoms
  +/– Pruritus (mild)
  +/– Previous URI

  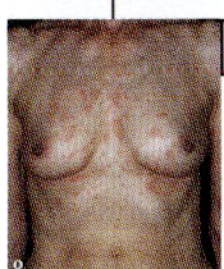

  1

  → Consider Pityriasis Rosea (A)

- Recent exposure to drug/vaccine
  Dusky-red scaly macules, papules, or plaques
  +/– Facial involvement
  +/– Mucosal involvement
  +/– Pruritus
  No prodrome

  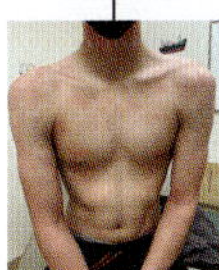

  2

  → Consider Pityriasis Rosea-like Drug Eruption (B)

No

Does the patient have palmar/plantar or nail involvement?

Yes

- Preceded by chancre by 3–4 weeks;
  Prodrome of fever, LAD, arthralgias;
  Red-brown papules and plaques with collarettes of scale on the palms and soles
  +/– Alopecia
  +/– Mucosal involvement
  +/– Condyloma lata

  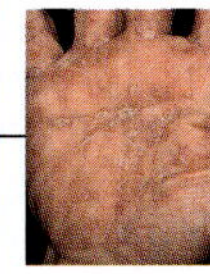

  3

  → Consider Secondary Syphilis (C)

- Keratoderma blennorrhagicum: initially pustules on the palms and soles, later scaly pink plaques
  Preceded by *Chlamydia, Shigella,* or other infection
  +/– Urethritis
  +/– Arthritis
  +/– Balanitis circinata

  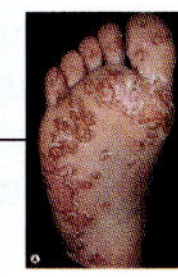

  4

  → Consider Reactive Arthritis (D)

No

Yes

- Drop-like pink papules with micaceous scale on the scalp, face, neck, trunk, and extremities
  +/– Koebner phenomenon
  +/– Nail changes: onycholysis, pitting, subungual hyperkeratosis, oil spots
  +/– Arthritis
  +/– Auspitz sign
  +/– Annulus migrans

  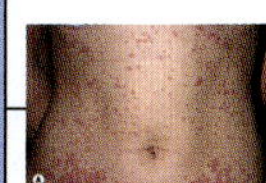

  10

  → Consider Guttate Psoriasis (K)

- Follicular-based papules
  Islands of sparing
  Cranio-caudal spread
  +/– Waxy keratoderma
  +/– Thickened nails
  (no nail pitting)

  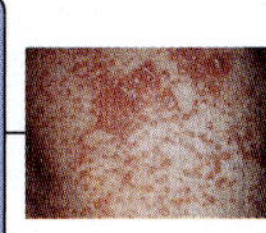

  11

  → Consider Pityriasis Rubra Pilaris (L)

No

- Oval to round macules/patches or thin papules/plaques which coalesce
  Color can vary between brown, tan, pink, or hypopigmented
  Fine scale
  Seborrheic region of the upper trunk and shoulders

  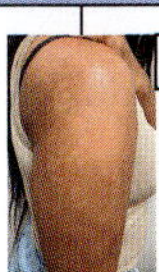

  5

  → Consider Tinea Versicolor (E)

- Patients in sixth to seventh decade with irregular erythematous scaly patches, often in bathing suit distribution
  Can progress to plaques
  +/– Atrophy
  +/– Poikiloderma
  +/– Pruritus

  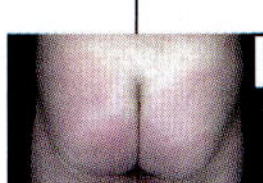

  6

  → Consider Mycosis Fungoides (F)

- Recurrent crops of red-brown papules with micaceous scale
  Postinflammatory pigment alteration
  Regresses over weeks to months
  Often chronic or relapsing
  Distribution can vary from diffuse to peripheral

  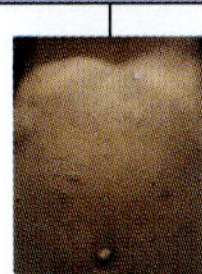

  7

  → Consider Pityriasis Lichenoides Chronica (G)

- 1–5 cm well-demarcated pink or hyperpigmented scaly patches, some with yellow hue, predominantly on the trunk and flanks

  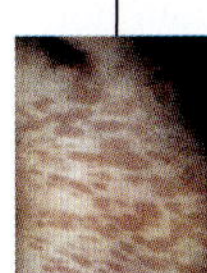

  8

  → Consider Small Plaque Parapsoriasis (H)

- >5 cm erythematous scaly patches or plaques on sun-protected sites
  +/– Poikiloderma
  +/– risk of developing into CTCL

  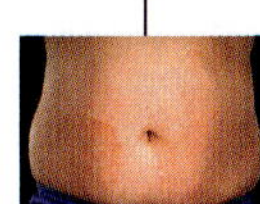

  9

  → Consider Large Plaque Parapsoriasis (I)

- Asymptomatic and large (10–30 cm) round scaly patches or thin plaques
  +/– Malnutrition
  +/– Mycobacterial infection
  +/– Malignancy
  More common in Far East, Mediterranean basin, or patients of African descent

  → Consider Pityriasis Rotunda (J)

38 Lichenoid Papules and Plaques

Corey L. Snyder and Martina Porter

Lichenoid rashes are typically described as purplish, flat-topped, and somewhat scaly. Classically, lichenoid rashes often share features on biopsy, including a band-like lymphocytic infiltrate in the papillary dermis that obscures the dermal-epidermal junction. However, other conditions may look similar clinically despite not having a lichenoid pattern on histopathology.

A. Initial evaluation of patients with a lichenoid rash should include a comprehensive history and physical examination. Important components of a patient's history that should be considered include comorbidities, other systemic symptoms, sexual history, list of medications, and previous laboratory studies. A detailed physical examination should inspect the genital/perianal region and oral mucosa.

B. The defining feature of **lichen simplex chronicus (LSC)** is the intense pruritus that is typically triggered by the itch-scratch cycle. LSC most commonly occurs in areas of the body that are easily accessible to scratching, which leads to excoriations and lichenified plaques.

C. Lesions limited to the oral mucosa should prompt a detailed history of dental fillings and medications. **Lichenoid amalgam reaction** is a type IV hypersensitivity reaction to amalgam/mercury-containing dental fillings. It is clinically and histologically similar to oral lichenoid drug reactions. Definitive diagnosis can be confirmed when removal of fillings leads to resolution of symptoms.

Oral lichenoid drug reactions appear clinically similar to oral lichen planus (LP), especially the erosive and reticular forms of LP. Histology resembles lichenoid drug eruption and is distinguished from LP by damage to the basal epidermal keratinocytes with multiple apoptotic cells, focal parakeratosis, focal interruption of the granular layer, cytoid bodies in the cornified and granular layers, and the presence of eosinophils. Medications commonly associated with drug-induced LP include angiotensin-converting enzyme inhibitors, nonsteroidal anti-inflammatory drugs, antimalarials, beta-blockers, gold salts, penicillamines, and thiazides.

Oral LP is a variant of LP that predominantly occurs on the buccal mucosa and lateral tongue, with characteristic Wickham striae. Clinical subtypes include reticular oral LP with Wickham striae, erythematous oral LP, and erosive oral LP. Oral LP can be distinguished on histology with parakeratosis of the epithelium, sawtooth rete ridges, and Civatte bodies in the basal layer.

D. **Plaque psoriasis** is characterized by well-demarcated plaques with overlying silvery scale predominantly affecting the extensor surfaces. The Koebner phenomenon and Auspitz sign are common features of psoriasis. Pruritus is typical of psoriasis, which can trigger the itch-scratch cycle that leads to a concurrent LSC.

Prurigo nodularis is characterized by firm pruritic nodules typically on the extensor surfaces but sometimes occuring on the trunk or elsewhere on the body. It is often associated with atopic dermatitis.

Lichen amyloidosis predominantly affects the shins and other extensor surfaces and is characterized by pruritic, scaly, dome-shaped papules that can form plaques with a rippled appearance. Histology demonstrates amyloid deposition in the superficial dermis, especially in the dermal papillae between epidermal rete ridges.

E. **Lichen sclerosus** can affect many regions of the body but predominates in the genital and perianal regions. Female patients who are peri- or postmenopausal are most commonly affected. Lichen sclerosus presents with white flat plaques with a purple border and then progresses to become atrophic and crinkled before becoming shiny with scar formation.

F. If lesions are not concentrated in a specific anatomical location, the color of the papule/plaque should be carefully examined. If violaceous lesions are present, a history of immunodeficiency should be queried.

G. A history of acquired immunodeficiency syndrome (AIDS) or other immunodeficiency puts patients at increased risk for **Kaposi sarcoma**, a vascular tumor often associated with human herpesvirus 8 infection. Lesions are often asymptomatic with reddish-purple papules that can occur on the lower extremities, nose, oral mucosa, and genitals.

H. **Lichenoid drug eruption** should be considered in patients with a positive medication history (common offending medications are discussed in section C above). Clinically, **lichenoid drug eruptions** resemble LP, with differences on histology including focal parakeratosis and presence of eosinophils.

If there is no recent medication change, and the patient presents with flat-topped, violaceous, polygonal, pruritic papules with Wickham striae, LP should be considered. There are several subtypes of LP, including annular, actinic, hypertrophic, bullous, inverse, atrophic, nail, oral, and genital as well as LP pigmentosus and lichen planopilaris. When nails are involved, thinning is common and can manifest as ridges, grooves, or splitting. LP predominantly affects the ventral wrists, lower back, and ankles. Mucosal involvement is common and can distinguish LP from clinically similar conditions, such as psoriasis and lichen sclerosus.

Keratosis lichenoides chronica (KLC) has a chronic progressive course and presents with brownish-purple, thick, scaly papules that can be distinguished from LP by an absence of pruritus, lack of response to corticosteroids, and focal parakeratosis on histology. KLC often occurs on the trunk and limbs and can be associated with seborrheic dermatitis on the face.

I. If the patient's lesions are not violaceous, but instead are hyperpigmented or gray, then **erythema dyschromicum perstans (EDP)** should be considered. EDP predominantly occurs in darker skinned individuals and presents with hyperpigmented, gray-brown, or blue-gray macules and patches commonly on the face, neck, trunk, or arm.

If lesions are not violaceous or gray, other conditions to consider include secondary syphilis and lichenoid keratosis.

Secondary syphilis is characterized by a diffuse eruption of symmetric pink or reddish-brown papules that can also affect the palms and soles. A history of a painless ulcer (syphilitic chancre) 1 to 3 months prior to the skin eruption may be elicited.

Lichenoid keratosis is typically a solitary lesion that arose from a regressed solar lentigo or seborrheic keratosis. On histology, lichenoid keratosis can be distinguished from LP by the presence of epidermal parakeratosis.

See Appendix 1 for Further Reading and Image References.

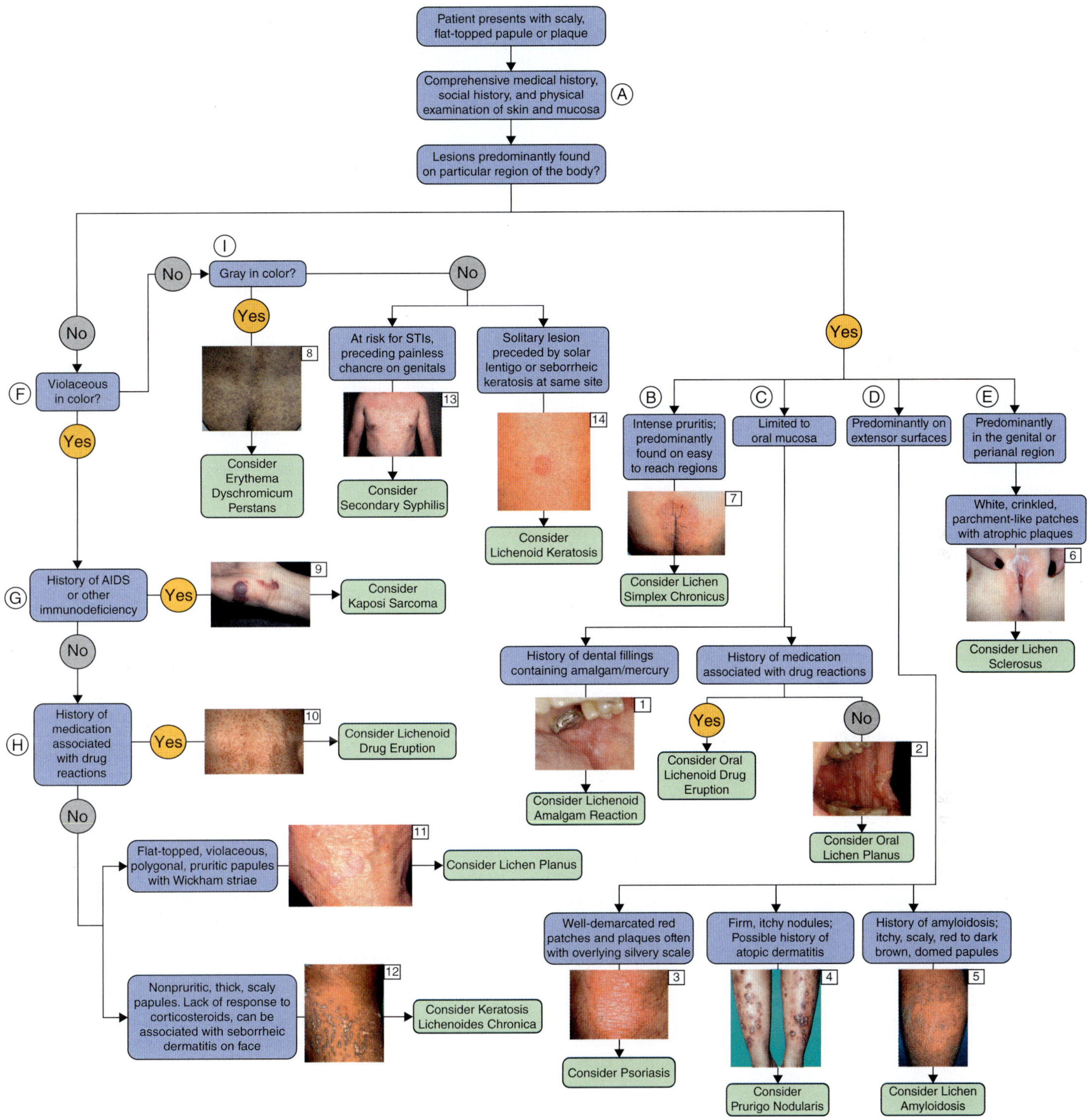
Patient presents with scaly, flat-topped papule or plaque
Comprehensive medical history, social history, and physical examination of skin and mucosa
A
Lesions predominantly found on particular region of the body?
No
Yes
F
Violaceous in color?
No
I
Gray in color?
Yes
8
Consider Erythema Dyschromicum Perstans
No
At risk for STIs, preceding painless chancre on genitals
13
Consider Secondary Syphilis
Solitary lesion preceded by solar lentigo or seborrheic keratosis at same site
14
Consider Lichenoid Keratosis
Yes
G
History of AIDS or other immunodeficiency
Yes
9
Consider Kaposi Sarcoma
No
H
History of medication associated with drug reactions
Yes
10
Consider Lichenoid Drug Eruption
No
Flat-topped, violaceous, polygonal, pruritic papules with Wickham striae
11
Consider Lichen Planus
Nonpruritic, thick, scaly papules. Lack of response to corticosteroids, can be associated with seborrheic dermatitis on face
12
Consider Keratosis Lichenoides Chronica
B
Intense pruritis; predominantly found on easy to reach regions
7
Consider Lichen Simplex Chronicus
C
Limited to oral mucosa
History of dental fillings containing amalgam/mercury
1
Consider Lichenoid Amalgam Reaction
History of medication associated with drug reactions
Yes
Consider Oral Lichenoid Drug Eruption
No
2
Consider Oral Lichen Planus
D
Predominantly on extensor surfaces
Well-demarcated red patches and plaques often with overlying silvery scale
3
Consider Psoriasis
Firm, itchy nodules; Possible history of atopic dermatitis
4
Consider Prurigo Nodularis
History of amyloidosis; itchy, scaly, red to dark brown, domed papules
5
Consider Lichen Amyloidosis
E
Predominantly in the genital or perianal region
White, crinkled, parchment-like patches with atrophic plaques
6
Consider Lichen Sclerosus

39 Eczematous Papules and Plaques

Rachel L. Sadowsky and Peter A. Lio

Eczematous papules and plaques may comprise the cutaneous manifestations of a variety of inflammatory skin conditions. Clinically apparent changes often vary according to the chronicity of the epidermal insult, with acute findings of erythema, swelling, vesiculation, weeping and oozing, and chronic findings of lichenification, hyper- or hypopigmentation, hyperlinearity, and fissuring. Pruritus often accompanies the lesions. Diagnosis of patients presenting with eczematous papules and plaques is often clinical but may require a diagnostic skin biopsy and/or laboratory testing in some cases. A specific diagnosis is not always identified or necessary to initiate treatment, which typically includes a combination of topical corticosteroids, nonsteroidal agents, and/or systemic immunosuppressive and immunomodulating therapies.

A. The initial evaluation of patients presenting with eczematous papules and plaques should involve a thorough history investigating the duration and timeline, provoking and alleviating factors, associated symptoms such as pruritus, burning, or pain, potential sources of contact allergens or irritants, any drug exposures, and any prior treatments. A full-body dermatologic examination should be performed. In more richly pigmented skin, erythema may appear more violaceous or gray in comparison to shades of pink or red in less pigmented skin, and postinflammatory dyspigmentation may be present. Skin biopsy may be nondiagnostic but may demonstrate epidermal changes, including spongiosis and/or acanthosis with perivascular lymphohistiocytic infiltrate and variable eosinophils.

B. **Atopic dermatitis** is commonly seen in childhood but can persist or arise in adulthood. The hallmarks of atopic dermatitis are significant pruritus, involvement of characteristic areas such as the antecubital and popliteal fossae, and a chronic relapsing and remitting course. Many patients with atopic dermatitis have a personal or family history of atopy, including atopic dermatitis, asthma, and/or allergic rhinitis. Patients with atopic dermatitis may also have other characteristic findings on physical examination, including xerosis, ichthyosis, hyperlinear palms, or Dennie-Morgan folds. Skin biopsy is rarely required, as the diagnosis is generally made clinically. Laboratory studies may show an elevated serum immunoglobulin E concentration. Culture may be performed if there is clinical concern for secondary infection.

C. **Irritant contact dermatitis** represents about 80% of cases of contact dermatitis and is caused by direct physical damage to the skin barrier by an irritant. Everyday irritants include water, soaps, and sanitizers, while occupational irritants may include acids, alkalis, detergents, solvents, or adhesives, among others. Acute findings may show well-defined papules or plaques with vesicles or bullae. Chronic exposure to irritants can lead to fissuring or lichenification. Irritant contact dermatitis is commonly localized to the hands but can affect any site of contact with an irritant. Burning and pain are more likely to be seen in irritant contact dermatitis, in contrast to the pruritus seen with atopic dermatitis. If an irritant is identified, protective clothing, use of emollients, or avoidance of the irritant is required for resolution.

D. Eczematous papules and plaques may also be seen in **allergic contact dermatitis**. The rash is caused by a type IV hypersensitivity reaction in which there is a delayed CD4+ T-lymphocyte response to an allergen. Allergens are numerous but commonly include metals, plants, chemicals, cosmetics, and topical medications. Skin findings are often arranged in geometric shapes with well-demarcated borders, but severe reactions can expand beyond the site of contact or progress to erythroderma. If an obvious allergen cannot be identified by history taking, patch testing may be helpful diagnostically.

E. **Asteatotic eczema**, also known as eczema craquelé, is primarily driven by processes that promote xerosis of the skin, including, but not limited to, age, environmental dryness, excessive water or soap exposure, hypothyroidism, malnutrition, or genetic predisposition. Examination can reveal scaly, fissured, reticulated plaques, especially of the shins. Diagnosis is usually made based on the "dry riverbed" clinical appearance.

F. Several dermatoses can present with lesions akin to **nummular eczema**. True nummular eczema involves intensely pruritic, coin-shaped eczematous plaques, usually involving the extremities. Secondary changes similar to those seen in atopic dermatitis, such as weepy vesicles, crusting, or lichenification, are common, although patients with nummular eczema are less likely to possess other features of atopy.

G. Eruption of pruritic, often hyperkeratotic, plaques on the lower legs of patients of middle and older age may indicate **venous stasis dermatitis**. Additional examination findings, such as pitting edema and brawny pigmentation, can support this diagnosis. Chronically, areas of induration, or lipodermatosclerosis, and venous ulcers may develop.

H. Autoeczematization, also known as autosensitization dermatitis or **id reaction**, can present as a secondary dermatitis in response to primary allergic contact or stasis dermatitis, tinea pedis, bacterial or viral infections, or arthropod assault. Typical presentation involves eczematous papulovesicles that can be symmetrically distributed locally or generalized.

I. **Drug-induced eczematous eruptions** should be considered in patients with recent exposure to a variety of medications; this condition is noted frequently after the use of systemic biologics or chemotherapies. The distribution is usually widespread and symmetric. Other commonly implicated medications include antihypertensives, antivirals, and some antibiotics, although an eczematous reaction to any medication may be possible. To confirm this diagnosis, the eczematous eruption should resolve when the drug is discontinued.

J. Eruption of erythematous papules with associated widespread severe pruritus that worsens at night along with secondary excoriations may indicate **scabies infestation**. The dermatitis associated with scabies may be localized to characteristic areas, such as flexural wrists, interdigital spaces, the umbilicus, axillae, or feet, or it can be generalized, although the head and neck are usually spared. Dermoscopy may show visible mites (called the "delta sign") or burrows (gray-edge line), or both (the delta wing jet with contrail). Skin scraping can also aid in diagnosis. A KOH preparation could be done to evaluate for fungal infections, and a scabies preparation can confirm the diagnosis of infestation. A drop of mineral oil is placed on the testing site to aid in sample removal, and the site is then scraped with a 15-blade scalpel. The specimen is placed on a glass slide for subsequent microscopic evaluation of scabies mites, eggs, or feces. Biopsy may be pursued in rare cases when clinical suspicion remains high despite negative dermoscopic and microscopic findings.

See Appendix 1 for Further Reading.

Patient presents with eczematous papules and plaques

(A) Thorough history and full-body dermatology examination including the skin, hair, nails, and mucosa

Does the history reveal a recent initiation of a new medication or supplement?

Yes → Morbilliform, erythematous maculopapules usually distributed symmetrically over the trunk and extremities

3
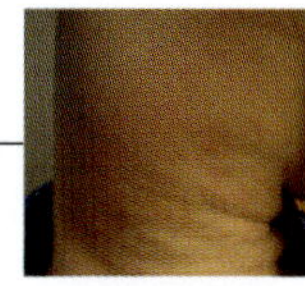

→ Consider Drug-Induced Eczematous Eruption (I)

No → Does the patient have a history of an underlying dermatologic condition?

Yes →

- Personal or family history of asthma, allergic rhinitis, or atopic dermatitis; weepy, crusted, and/or lichenified eczematous plaques characteristically involving the antecubital or popliteal fossae

1
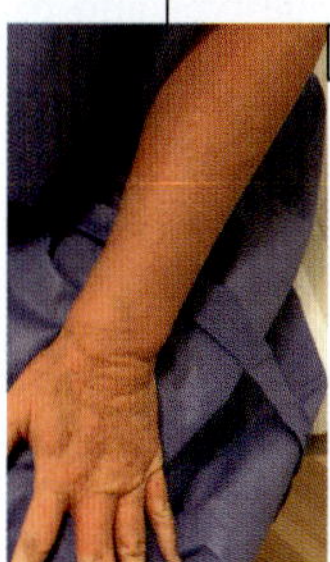

→ Consider Atopic Dermatitis (B)

- Primary dermatitis preceded the current eczematous eruption; focal or generalized symmetrically distributed erythematous papulovesicles

2
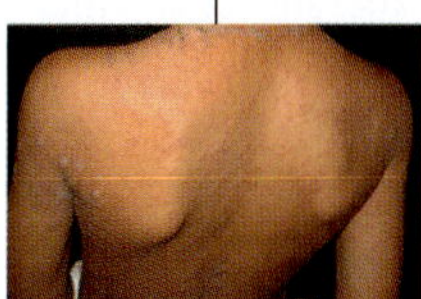

→ Consider Autoeczematization (Id Reaction) (H)

No →

- Occupational exposure to irritants, such as acids, alkalis, solvents, or detergents or repeated exposure to everyday irritants, such as soap, water, and sanitizers; acute well-defined, vesicular papules or plaques and chronic lichenification often involving the hands or any site of contact with the irritant

4
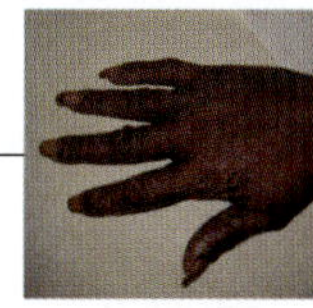

→ Consider Irritant Contact Dermatitis (C)

- History reveals contact with potential allergen(s), or patch testing is diagnostic for hypersensitivity to an allergen; well-demarcated, geometrically shaped erythematous plaques

5
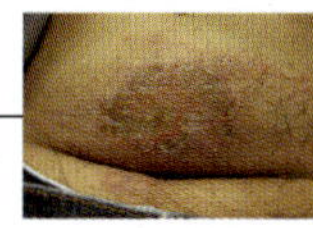

→ Consider Allergic Contact Dermatitis (D)

- Older patient, exposure to environmental dryness or excessive water or soap, or history of hypothyroidism, malnutrition, or family history of asteatotic eczema; scaly, reticulated, fissured plaques with a "dry riverbed" appearance often localized to the shins

6
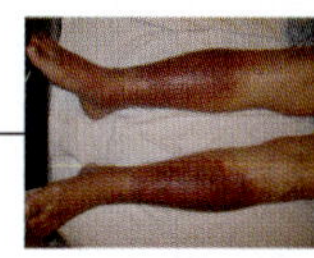

→ Consider Asteatotic Eczema (E)

- Patient usually without a history of atopy presenting with new coin-shaped eczematous plaques; intensely pruritic, coin-shaped eczematous plaques often involving the extremities

7
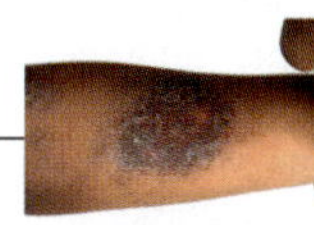

→ Consider Nummular Eczema (F)

- Elderly patient with history of venous insufficiency and lower extremity edema; lower extremities with brown, hyperkeratotic, pruritic plaques with late-stage lipodermatosclerosis and venous ulceration

8
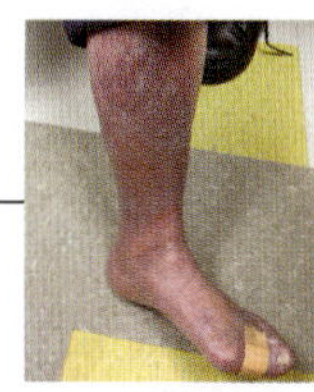

→ Consider Venous Stasis Dermatitis (G)

- Severe pruritus with dermoscopic evidence of mites or burrows, microscopic evidence of mites, eggs, or feces, and/or close contact with similar symptoms; eruption of erythematous papules involving the flexural wrists, interdigital spaces, umbilicus, axillae, or feet with sparing of the head and neck

9
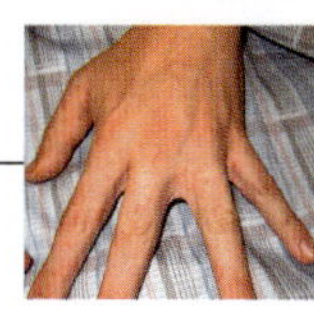

→ Consider Scabies Infestation (J)

40 Psoriasiform Papules and Plaques

Samuel A. Stetkevich and Jason E. Hawkes

A papulosquamous (or "psoriasiform") morphology is a common clinical presentation. Investigative interviewing helps providers work through an extensive differential diagnosis in a stepwise approach.

A. Initial evaluation of papulosquamous papules or plaques begins with the skin distribution pattern.

B. Lesions that appear in a more diffuse, generalized pattern suggest a systemic cause. Poor oral intake or gut absorption, dietary restrictions, substance use, or socioeconomic deprivation may provide clues to a potential nutritional dermatosis. The symptoms of the "4 D's," dermatitis (photosensitive rash), dementia, diarrhea, and death in the setting of poor nutrition, are suggestive of **pellagra (vitamin B_3 deficiency)**. Poor nutrition with a periorificial or acral exfoliating scale or a bullous eruption suggests **acquired acrodermatitis enteropathica (AAE) (zinc deficiency)**. Other symptoms of AAE include glossitis, anemia, and increased infection risk. Lastly, a scaly follicular-based eruption primarily on the extensors in the setting of poor nutrition suggests **phrynoderma (vitamin A deficiency)**.

C. Infectious etiologies are another cause of widespread psoriasiform papules and plaques. Risk factors include recent travel, sick contacts, high-risk sexual behaviors, animal exposure, underlying immunodeficiency, and poor sanitation. Since the skin lesions of **syphilis** mimic a variety of conditions, a psoriasiform papule or plaque in the setting of a high-risk sexual history warrants diagnostic consideration. **Tinea infections** remain in the differential, given their overlapping morphology with many dermatoses. Recent travel, contact with armadillos, or psoriasiform lesions with noted peripheral neuropathy suggest **Hansen's disease (leprosy)**.

D. Any widespread psoriasiform eruption in the setting of a known or suspected malignancy should raise concern for **mycosis fungoides (MF or cutaneous T-cell lymphoma), Paget disease, dermatomyositis, large plaque parapsoriasis, and acrokeratosis paraneoplastica (Bazex syndrome). MF** often presents as a persistent pruritic rash resistant to routine topical treatments and may have a wrinkled surface resembling "cigarette paper." A biopsy with immunophenotyping confirms this diagnosis. **Paget disease** frequently presents with an erythematous, scaly, weeping, and/or bleeding nipple resembling eczema without improvement with topical steroids. **Dermatomyositis** is classically characterized by proximal symmetric myopathy and a violaceous, pruritic, photodistributed cutaneous eruption. **Large plaque parapsoriasis** presents similarly to MF but will lack the classic histopathologic changes of MF. **Acrokeratosis paraneoplastica** will appear as a scaly acral eruption resistant to classic psoriasis therapy. If malignancy is not suspected, consider **pityriasis rubra pilaris (PRP)**, **drug eruption, pityriasis lichenoides et varioliformis acuta (PLEVA), pityriasis lichenoides chronica (PLC), and lymphomatoid papulosis (LyP)**. Coalescing, red-orange, psoriasiform plaques (especially on the trunk and acral skin) with discrete islands of sparing is suggestive of **PRP**. A rash that begins on the trunk, spreads symmetrically, and worsens or improves in conjunction with exposure to a specific medication may represent a **drug eruption**. **PLEVA** and **PLC** present as scattered lesions in multiple stages of healing, although PLEVA is more acute and active while PLC is chronic and indolent. **LyP** is most commonly a self-limiting condition that presents as waxing and waning papulonecrotic skin lesions due to an unclear etiology with large CD30-positive lymphocytes on immunohistochemistry. A subset of patients with LyP may develop T-cell lymphoma.

E. Recurrence of skin lesions at the same location and/or following a specific exposure (e.g., trauma or tattoo placement) is a helpful clue. A history of repetitive trauma to an affected area suggests **lichen simplex chronicus**. Recurrence of violaceous or erythematous psoriasiform papules or plaques in conjunction with the use of a specific medication (e.g., nonsteroidal antiinflammatory drugs, antibiotics) suggests **fixed drug eruption**. Lesions following physical contact with an object or substance (i.e., metal or tattoo ink) indicate **allergic or irritant contact dermatitis**.

F. Involvement of flexural/intertriginous skin includes **tinea cruris, Langerhans cell histiocytosis (LCH), Hailey-Hailey disease, inverse psoriasis, intertrigo**, and **atopic dermatitis (AD). Tinea cruris** usually presents as sharply demarcated scaly plaques with peripheral scale in the groin or buttock region. **LCH** should be considered in recalcitrant diaper rashes in infants or in those with erythematous to brown papules and plaques with concomitant bone pain. **Hailey-Hailey disease** is diagnosed when characteristic linear fissures and furrows appear within whitish plaques of intertriginous skin. Patients with **inverse psoriasis** will often present with sharply demarcated lesions with minimal scale and a history of failing fungal or bacterial treatments. **Intertrigo** occurs in skin folds in overweight or diabetic patients and is exacerbated by heat, moisture, and friction. **AD** is a common diagnosis characterized by poorly demarcated plaques in skin folds with associated pruritus and a personal or family history of allergies or asthma. The plaque-type and papular patterns of AD are more common in darker skin types and children, respectively.

G. Involvement of the face or scalp should prompt consideration of **discoid lupus erythematosus (DLE), seborrheic dermatitis, sarcoidosis**, and **sebopsoriasis. DLE** involves the photodistributed regions of the scalp and face, with the conchal bowl being a characteristic site. Loose greasy scale involving the scalp, eyebrows, glabella, beard, ears, and/or nasolabial folds suggests **seborrheic dermatitis. Sarcoidosis** will often present with asymptomatic, red-brown, dermal papules and plaques that favor the face and neck and show noncaseating granulomas on biopsy. **Sebopsoriasis** will provide a mixed picture of the sharply demarcated erythematous plaques of psoriasis in conjunction with the distribution pattern of seborrheic dermatitis.

H. An acral distribution pattern suggests **tinea pedis, palmoplantar psoriasis, PRP, and secondary syphilis** as possible diagnoses. Sharply demarcated, itchy, scaly plaques with peripheral scale on the hands or feet may suggest **tinea pedis**. Sharply demarcated, scaly plaques with erythema and fissures on the hands and feet may be indicative of **palmoplantar psoriasis**. Orange-red psoriasiform plaques on the hands and feet with discrete islands of skin-sparing suggest **PRP**. Nonpruritic psoriasiform papules with overlying scale or targetoid macules on acral surfaces raise concern for **secondary syphilis**.

Continued

(A) Do the lesions follow a recognizable distribution pattern?

- **No** → **(B) Is there a suspicion of or risk factor for a nutritional deficiency?**
  - **No** → Is there a suspicion of or risk factor for infection?
    - **(C) Yes** →

      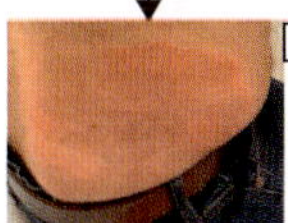

      1 Tinea infection of the trunk

      Consider
      - Tinea Infection
      - Syphilis
      - Hansen's Disease (Leprosy)
    - **No** → **(D) Is there a suspected or known history of malignancy?**
      - **Yes** →

        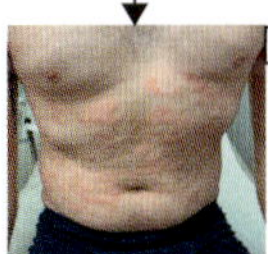

        2 Mycosis Fungoides on the abdomen

        Consider
        - Mycosis Fungoides (Cutaneous T-cell Lymphoma)
        - Paget Disease
        - Dermatomyositis
        - Large Plaque Parapsoriasis
        - Acrokeratosis Paraneoplastica (Bazex Syndrome)
      - **No** →

        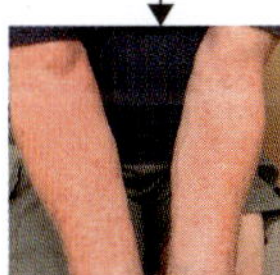

        3 Drug eruption on the bilateral arms

        Consider
        - Drug Eruption
        - Pityriasis Lichenoides et Varioliformis Acuta
        - Pityriasis Lichenoides Chronica
        - Lymphomatoid Papulosis
        - Pityriasis Rubra Pilaris
  - **Yes** →

    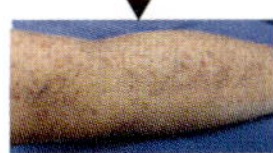

    4 Phrynoderma on the arm

    Consider
    - Phrynoderma
    - Pellagra
    - Acquired Acrodermatitis Enteropathica
- **Yes** → **(E) Do the lesions recur in the same location and/or follow a specific exposure (e.g., tattoo placement)?**
  - **Yes** →

    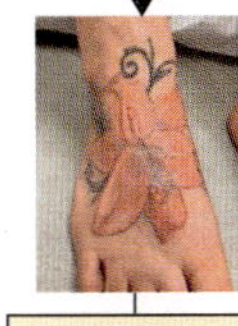

    5 Allergic contact dermatitis on the foot

    Consider
    - Allergic Contact Dermatitis
    - Lichen Simplex Chronicus
    - Fixed Drug Eruption
  - **No** → **(F) Do the lesions appear primarily in flexural/intertriginous areas?**
    - **Yes** →

      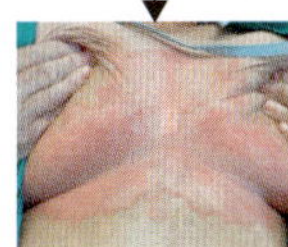

      6 Inverse psoriasis in the mammary region

      Consider
      - Inverse Psoriasis
      - Tinea Cruris
      - Langerhans Cell Histiocytosis
      - Hailey-Hailey
      - Intertrigo
      - Atopic Dermatitis
    - **No** → Do the lesions primarily appear on the face/scalp?
      - **(G) Yes** →

        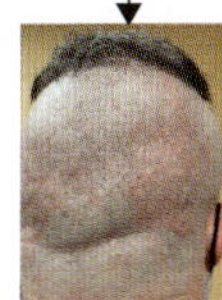

        7 Seborrheic dermatitis of the scalp

        Consider
        - Seborrheic Dermatitis
        - Discoid Lupus Erythematosus
        - Sarcoidosis
        - Sebopsoriasis
      - **No** → Do the lesions appear on acral skin?
        - **(H) Yes** →

          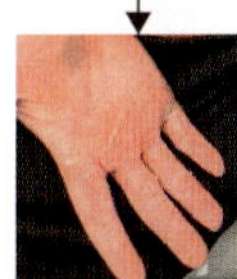

          8 Atopic dermatitis of the hand

          Consider
          - Atopic Dermatitis
          - Tinea Pedis
          - Palmoplantar Psoriasis
          - Pityriasis Rubra Pilaris
          - Secondary Syphilis
        - **No** → **(I) Do the lesions primarily appear on the trunk?**
          - **Yes** →

            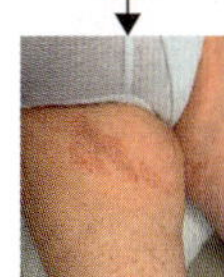

            9 Erythema annulare centrifugum on the leg

            Consider
            - Erythema Annulare Centrifugum
            - Darier Disease
            - Pityriasis Rosea
            - Plaque Psoriasis

I. The differential for the trunk includes **pityriasis rosea (PR), erythema annulare centrifugum (EAC), Darier disease, and plaque psoriasis**. **PR** presents as a rash that begins with a single red, scaly lesion ("herald patch"), followed by smaller lesions along skin tension lines. **EAC** often appears as asymptomatic, annular, psoriasiform plaques on the trunk with central clearing and a trailing scale. **Darier disease** presents as gritty, yellow-brown papules on the trunk with a history of nail chipping, cobblestoning of the hard palate, and family members with similar lesions. **Plaque psoriasis** presents as well-demarcated erythematous plaques with thick white scales common on the trunk, umbilicus, extensor surfaces, gluteal folds, and scalp.

See Appendix 1 for Further Reading.

(A) Do the lesions follow a recognizable distribution pattern?

- **No** → (B) Is there a suspicion of or risk factor for a nutritional deficiency?
  - **No** → Is there a suspicion of or risk factor for infection?
    - (C) **Yes** →

      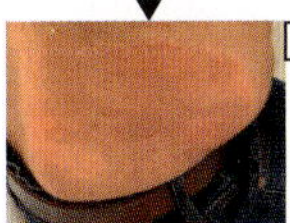

      1 Tinea infection of the trunk

      Consider
      - Tinea Infection
      - Syphilis
      - Hansen's Disease (Leprosy)
    - **No** → (D) Is there a suspected or known history of malignancy?
      - **Yes** →

        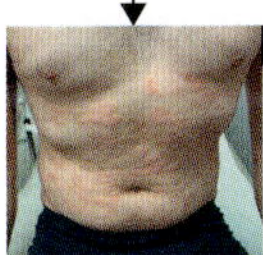

        2 Mycosis Fungoides on the abdomen

        Consider
        - Mycosis Fungoides (Cutaneous T-cell Lymphoma)
        - Paget Disease
        - Dermatomyositis
        - Large Plaque Parapsoriasis
        - Acrokeratosis Paraneoplastica (Bazex Syndrome)
      - **No** →

        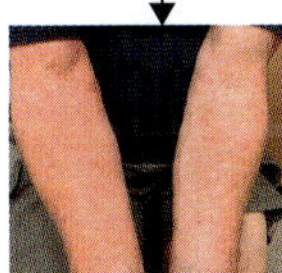

        3 Drug eruption on the bilateral arms

        Consider
        - Drug Eruption
        - Pityriasis Lichenoides et Varioliformis Acuta
        - Pityriasis Lichenoides Chronica
        - Lymphomatoid Papulosis
        - Pityriasis Rubra Pilaris
  - **Yes** →

    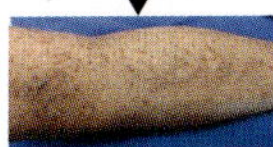

    4 Phrynoderma on the arm

    Consider
    - Phrynoderma
    - Pellagra
    - Acquired Acrodermatitis Enteropathica
- **Yes** → (E) Do the lesions recur in the same location and/or follow a specific exposure (e.g., tattoo placement)?
  - **Yes** →

    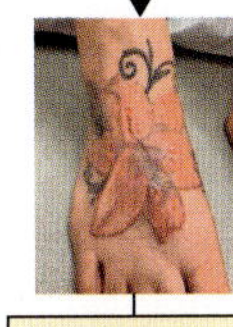

    5 Allergic contact dermatitis on the foot

    Consider
    - Allergic Contact Dermatitis
    - Lichen Simplex Chronicus
    - Fixed Drug Eruption
  - **No** → (F) Do the lesions appear primarily in flexural/intertriginous areas?
    - **Yes** →

      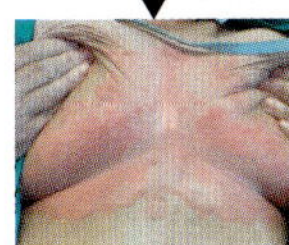

      6 Inverse psoriasis in the mammary region

      Consider
      - Inverse Psoriasis
      - Tinea Cruris
      - Langerhans Cell Histiocytosis
      - Hailey-Hailey
      - Intertrigo
      - Atopic Dermatitis
    - **No** → Do the lesions primarily appear on the face/scalp?
      - (G) **Yes** →

        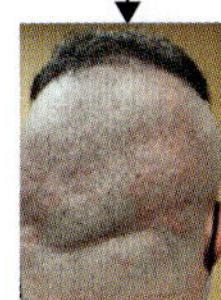

        7 Seborrheic dermatitis of the scalp

        Consider
        - Seborrheic Dermatitis
        - Discoid Lupus Erythematosus
        - Sarcoidosis
        - Sebopsoriasis
      - **No** → Do the lesions appear on acral skin?
        - (H) **Yes** →

          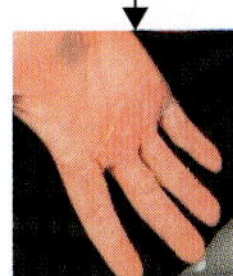

          8 Atopic dermatitis of the hand

          Consider
          - Atopic Dermatitis
          - Tinea Pedis
          - Palmoplantar Psoriasis
          - Pityriasis Rubra Pilaris
          - Secondary Syphilis
        - **No** → (I) Do the lesions primarily appear on the trunk?
          - **Yes** →

            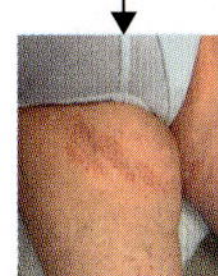

            9 Erythema annulare centrifugum on the leg

            Consider
            - Erythema Annulare Centrifugum
            - Darier Disease
            - Pityriasis Rosea
            - Plaque Psoriasis

41 Morbilliform Rash

Makana D. Williams and Jan M. Smogorzewski

Morbilliform (measles-like) rashes are characterized by erythematous macules and papules symmetrically distributed over the trunk and extremities; they may also be referred to as exanthems or exanthematous rashes.

A. The initial evaluation of a patient with a morbilliform rash begins with a full-body skin and mucous membrane examination (ocular, oral, perianal/genital). Blistering or erosive lesions, mucosal involvement, lesions coalescing into larger patches or plaques, and purpuric lesions are all concerning findings and bring a spectrum of severe, potentially life-threatening diseases into the differential diagnosis. A review of systems should be performed to identify systemic symptoms, including fever, chills, or sore throat. In addition, a thorough drug history must be obtained with careful attention to onset and duration of medication use. Other useful information includes history of drug reactions, recent sick contacts, travel history over the preceding year (particularly international travel), and vaccination history.

B. A morbilliform rash in the setting of hemodynamic instability should raise suspicion for **toxic shock syndrome**, a systemic illness mediated by superantigens from *Staphylococcus* or *Streptococcus* species, which cause widespread T-cell activation and cytokine release. Cutaneous findings include diffuse macular erythema that typically spreads from the trunk to the extremities; the rash may progress to erythroderma. Nikolsky sign is negative.

C. If a patient has a suspicious drug history (recently initiated antimicrobial, anticonvulsant, or nonsteroidal antiinflammatory drug [NSAID], among others), several severe drug reactions should be considered. The early stages of **Stevens-Johnson syndrome/ toxic epidermal necrolysis** may present with a morbilliform rash; patients may have a positive Nikolsky sign, in which slight tangential pressure results in sloughing of the overlying epidermis. Lesions begin as early as 1 to 2 weeks after medication initiation. Other concerning findings include atypical target lesions and oral or ocular pain.

D. Facial edema is a distinguishing feature of **drug reaction with eosinophilia and systemic symptoms (DRESS) syndrome**. The morbilliform rash of DRESS occurs 4 to 6 weeks after initiation of a culprit medication, and laboratory abnormalities are typically present. DRESS is a multisystem drug reaction that may affect the liver, kidneys, lungs, lymph nodes, and heart. Eosinophilia may also be an important clue to clinching the diagnosis.

E. If the skin and mucous membrane examination does not reveal any alarming features, the patient is otherwise well appearing, and a drug culprit is suspected, a simple **exanthematous drug eruption** is most likely. Patients typically present 7 to 10 days after initiation of the culprit medication. The most frequently implicated medications are antibiotics, antiepileptic agents, and NSAIDs. Systemic symptoms and laboratory abnormalities are not seen. Desquamation may be observed 1 to 2 weeks after rash onset.

F. In a patient with underlying hematologic or rheumatologic disease, the development of a morbilliform rash alongside fever, splenomegaly, and laboratory abnormalities including cytopenias should raise suspicion for **hemophagocytic lymphohistiocytosis (HLH)**, a life-threatening state of immune system hyperactivity. HLH must be identified early in the disease course as it can progress rapidly to multisystem organ failure and death. In the appropriate clinical setting, **acute graft-versus-host disease** can present with a morbilliform eruption, abdominal pain, and diarrhea typically 2 to 4 weeks after hematopoietic stem cell transplantation. Palmoplantar involvement is an important clue to the diagnosis. A chronic, waxing and waning course of a morbilliform eruption alongside recurrent, unexplained fevers should raise suspicion for **Still disease**.

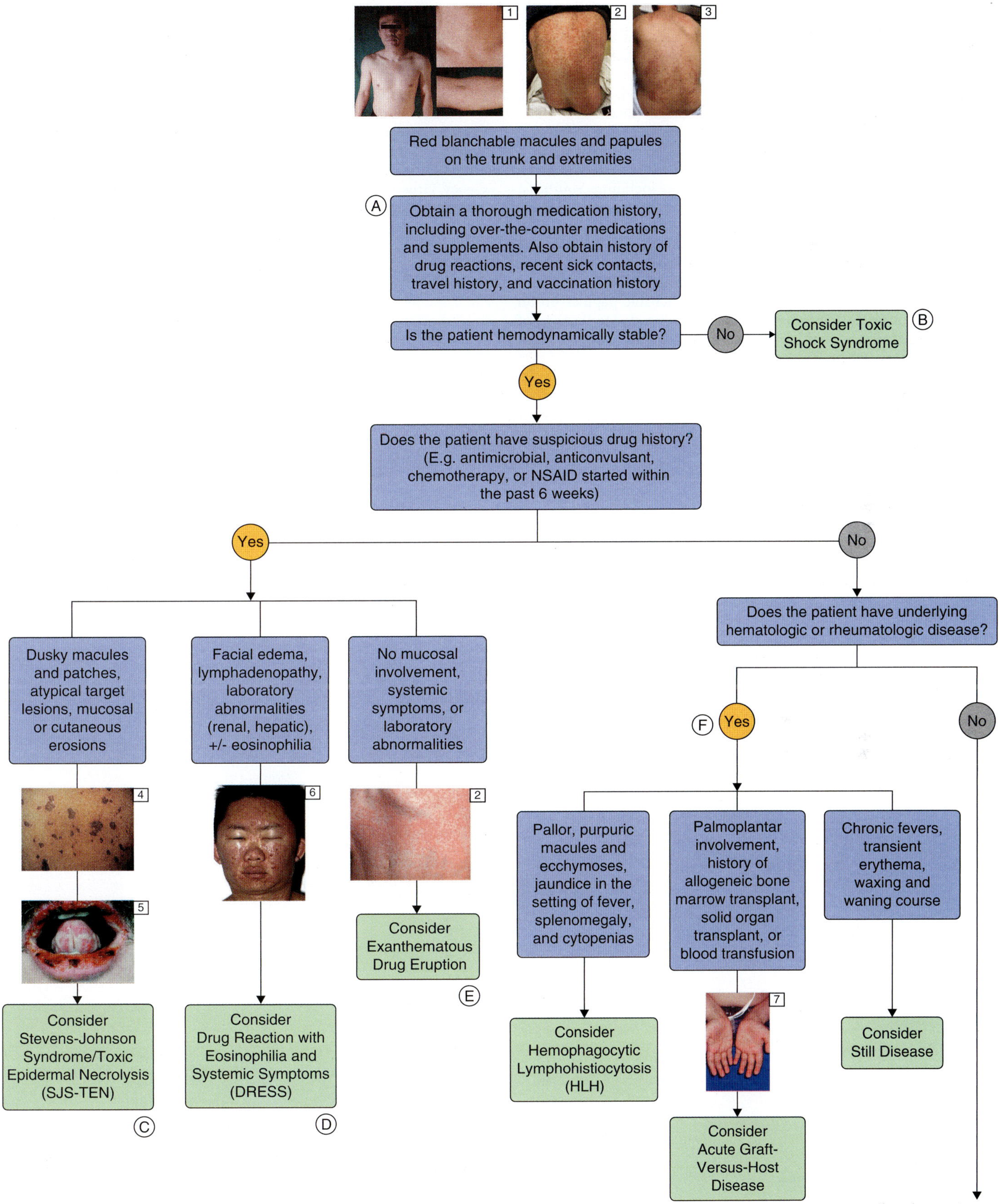

continued on next page

Continued

G. In a patient who reports a fever lasting for greater than 5 days, **Kawasaki disease**, a multisystem vasculitis, should be considered. Bilateral nonexudative conjunctivitis with perilimbal sparing, erythematous or fissured lips, loss of the filiform papillae on the tongue resulting in a "strawberry tongue," and erythema or desquamation of the hands and feet are other important diagnostic clues.

H. There are several infectious etiologies to consider in patients with a morbilliform rash. If a patient has recently traveled to continents where mosquito-borne illnesses are endemic, including Southeast Asia, Africa, and South or Central America, the presence of petechiae on the skin or mucous membranes alongside diffuse macular erythema interspersed with islands of normal skin should raise suspicion for **dengue fever**. **Scarlet fever** classically follows streptococcal pharyngitis or tonsillitis. Examination will reveal a sandpaper-like rash with 1- to 2 mm blanchable papules on an erythematous base. Circumoral pallor can occur due to flushing of the cheeks. Linear petechiae in intertriginous areas (also known as Pastia lines) may be present.

Rubella may present with a physical examination clue of palatal petechiae, also known as Forchheimer spots. Koplik spots, white papules with a halo of erythema on the buccal mucosa, are pathognomonic for **measles**. The rash of measles usually demonstrates craniocaudal spread. Conjunctivitis, cough, and coryza are seen.

Finally, a morbilliform rash may represent a **nonspecific viral exanthem**. Epstein-Barr virus should be considered if the cutaneous eruption occurred 1 to 3 days after the administration of a beta-lactam antibiotic, classically ampicillin. Screening for human immunodeficiency virus should be considered in all patients with a morbilliform rash and pharyngitis, especially those with a history of high-risk sexual activity or intravenous drug use.

See Appendix 1 for Further Reading and Image References.

Are there risk factors or signs of infection?

(G) No

Bilateral conjunctival injection, diffuse erythema of the mucosa ("strawberry tongue"), cervical lymphadenopathy

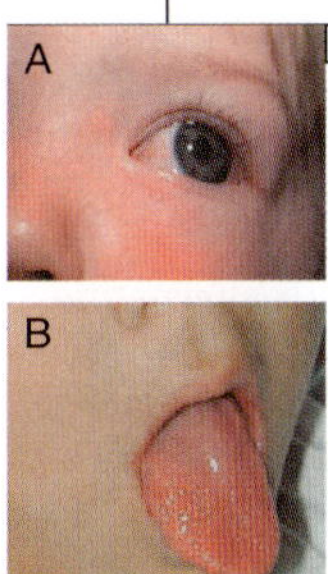

8

Consider Kawasaki Disease

(H) Yes

Diffuse pink patches with islands of normal skin ("islands of white in a sea of red")

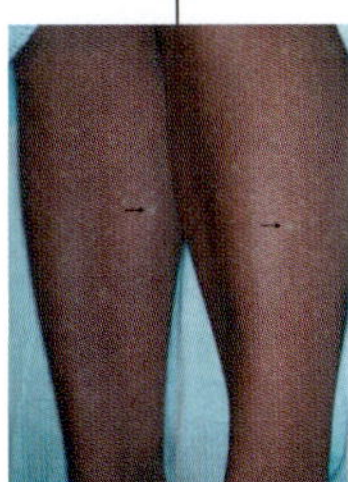

9

Consider Dengue Fever

Sandpaper-like exanthem with minute, blanchable papules on an erythematous base, circumoral pallor and scale, +/- Pastia lines, +/- strawberry tongue

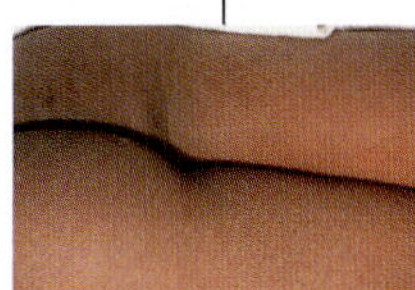

10

Consider Scarlet Fever

Under- or unvaccinated, craniocaudal spread of rash, Forchheimer spots (palatal petechiae), occipital lymphadenopathy

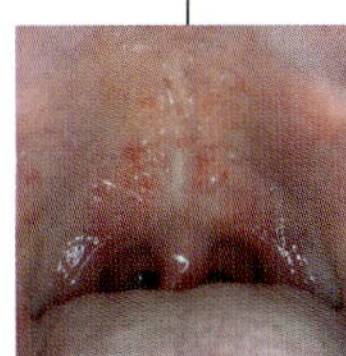

11

Consider Rubella

Koplik spots (white papules on the buccal mucosa), cephalocaudal spread of rash

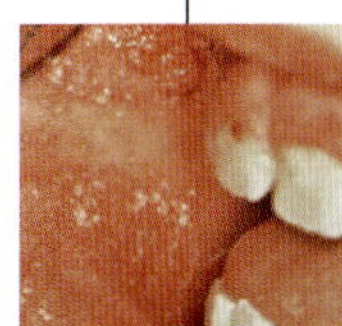

12

Consider Measles

Viral prodrome (fever, malaise, pharyngitis)

Consider Nonspecific Viral Exanthem (HIV, EBV)

42 Erythroderma

Sanmeet Atwal and Scott D. Worswick

Erythroderma, also known as exfoliative dermatitis, is a potentially life-threatening inflammatory reaction presenting with diffuse erythema and scaling involving 90% or more of the body surface area. Due to the increased risk of sepsis and fluid losses, patients with erythroderma are often managed in an inpatient setting for close monitoring and management.

A. The initial evaluation of patients presenting with erythroderma should involve recording a detailed history (particularly a thorough drug history and history of prior dermatosis), asking for photographs of how their rash began, and performing a thorough physical examination (not only of the skin but also of the nails, lymph nodes, and mucosal surfaces). Before becoming erythrodermic, a patient may have had initial blisters (as can be seen in pemphigus foliaceous [PF]), follicular accentuation or initial involvement of the scalp and palms/soles (as can be seen in pityriasis rubra pilaris [PRP]), initial involvement of the scalp (as can be seen in PRP, psoriasis, and seborrheic dermatitis), or a photodistribution of initial lesions (as can be seen in chronic actinic dermatitis or dermatomyositis). Skin biopsy may be useful, although often in acute erythroderma, it shows only irregular psoriasiform hyperplasia.

B. The most commonly reported medications that trigger a **drug-induced erythrodermic reaction** include allopurinol, penicillins-cephalosporins, and antiepileptics. Any drug that has been started in the weeks before the eruption began should be highly suspected. Physical examination clues can include a morbilliform eruption preceding the erythroderma, facial edema, and intractable pruritis. Eosinophilia, hepatitis, and acute interstitial nephritis may be found in patients with drug reaction with eosinophilia and systemic symptoms. Resolution of drug-induced erythroderma often occurs faster than in other etiologies, often over weeks.

C. Erythroderma can also occur in patients with an underlying chronic dermatological rash, most commonly psoriasis or atopic dermatitis, or less commonly due to seborrheic dermatitis or PRP.

Poorly controlled psoriasis, recent cessation of psoriasis medications, or a recent streptococcal infection can trigger **erythrodermic psoriasis**. Physical examination may reveal characteristic nail changes, including onycholysis, nail pitting, or oil spots. Subcorneal pustules and comorbid inflammatory arthritis may also point to psoriasis as the underlying cause.

Atopic dermatitis can also lead to erythroderma and may present with lichenification in flexural areas, intense pruritus, and elevated immunoglobulin E (IgE) levels.

Seborrheic dermatitis often begins on the scalp or head and is characterized by a waxy scale.

PRP often starts with an initial eruption of perifollicular keratotic papules on the head and neck that spread caudally, in association with waxy keratoderma. Of note, any patient with erythroderma will likely have islands of sparing given the extent of the eruption, so this physical examination finding should be interpreted with caution.

D. Older patients presenting with erythroderma, weight loss, and generalized lymphadenopathy (particularly if firm or fixed) should prompt a workup for cutaneous T-cell lymphoma (CTCL). Patients with CTCL may present with chronic signs of erythroderma, including cachexia, ectropion, and diffuse alopecia. Some of these patients will ultimately be diagnosed with **Sézary syndrome (SS)**, which is defined by a triad consisting of erythroderma, generalized lymphadenopathy, and a peripheral blood smear illustrating atypical lymphocytes with a cerebriform nucleus (i.e., Sézary cells). Patients with SS may also have intense pruritus, leonine facies, and palmoplantar hyperkeratosis.

E. In an adult with preexisting flaccid bullae or impetigo-like erosions (especially on the face and upper trunk), consider a diagnosis of **PF**. PF classically spares the mucous membranes. Skin biopsy with direct immunofluorescence may aid in diagnosis as histology reveals linear IgG and C3 deposits in the superficial epidermis along with subcorneal or granular acantholysis.

F. Elderly male patients presenting initially with alternating strips of unaffected skin and polygonal brown papules and plaques on the trunk (the "deck-chair sign") may have an erythroderma from a rare underlying diagnosis of **papuloerythroderma of Ofuji**. Laboratory findings include peripheral eosinophilia, elevated IgE, and elevated levels of thymus- and activation-regulated chemokine.

G. Acute **graft-versus-host disease (GVHD)** can cause erythroderma in patients who have undergone a hematopoietic stem cell transplant (or, more rarely, a solid organ transplantation, or after nonradiated whole blood transfusion or maternal-fetal transfusion in utero). The initial rash in GVHD often includes punctate lesions around hair follicles and small dusky macules on the palms and soles. In acute GVHD, patients may also have associated sloughing and pain of mucosal surfaces, diarrhea due to intestinal involvement, and hepatic dysfunction (leading to elevated alkaline phosphatase and bilirubin).

H. Additional rarer causes of erythroderma include connective tissue disease, chronic actinic dermatitis, contact dermatitis, scabies, and more. Despite extensive workup to uncover the underlying etiology in a patient presenting with erythroderma, about 25% of cases are ultimately categorized as **idiopathic**.

See Appendix 1 for Further Reading and Image References.

Patient presenting with diffuse erythema and scale involving 90% of body surface area

↓

(A) Detailed history and physical examination of the skin, nails, lymph nodes, and mucosal surfaces to discover underlying etiology

↓

Does the history reveal that the patient had a morbilliform eruption preceding erythroderma and recently initiated a new medication or supplement?

- **Yes** → Consider Drug-Induced Erythrodermic Reaction (B)
- **No** → Does the patient have a history of an underlying dermatologic condition?
  - (C) **Yes**
    - Recent cessation of psoriasis medications, recent streptococcal infection, or physical examination findings of onycholysis or nail pitting

      1 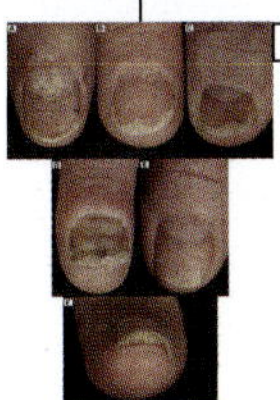

      Nail psoriasis demonstrating nail pitting, onycholysis, red macules or oil spots in the nail plate → Consider Erythrodermic Psoriasis
    - History of AD and physical examination showing lichenification in flexural areas, intense pruritus, and elevated IgE levels

      2 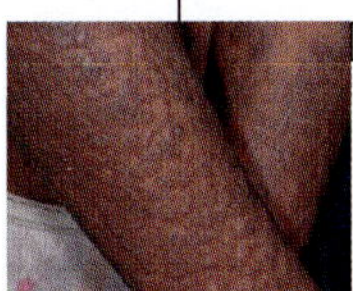

      Lichenification overlying scaly patches and excoriation in the antecubital fossae → Consider Erythrodermic Atopic Dermatitis
    - History of greasy scales and erythema on the scalp, nasolabial folds, or chest prior to erythrodermic eruption

      3 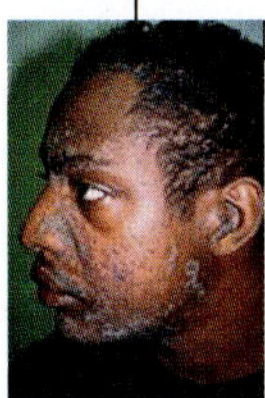

      Scaling violaceous plaques with underlying hypopigmentation surrounding the medial forehead and bilateral nasolabial folds → Consider Erythrodermic Seborrheic Dermatitis
    - Initial eruption of perifollicular keratotic papules on the head and neck, waxy palmoplantar keratoderma, and erythema with islands of sparing

      4 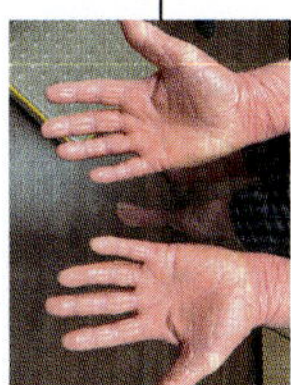

      Excessive thickening or hyperkeratosis of the palms with accompanying fissures → Consider Pityriasis Rubra Pilaris
  - **No**
    - Older patient with weight loss, firm generalized LAD, and peripheral blood smear with atypical lymphocytes → Consider Sézary Syndrome (D)
    - Pre-existing moist lesions on the face and upper trunk, flaccid bullae; Impetigo-like erosions

      5 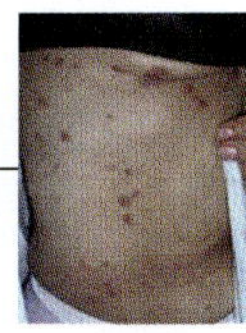

      Impetigo-like erosions overlying erythematous patches with adjacent ruptured bullae → Consider Pemphigus Foliaceous (E)
    - Elderly patient with deck-chair sign, elevated IgE and TARC

      6 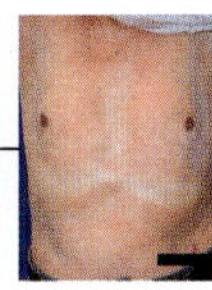

      Coalescing brown-red papules sparing the submammary folds (deck-chair sign) → Consider Papuloerythroderma of Ofuji (F)
    - History of HSCT with keratosis pilaris–like eruption, dusky macules and papules on the palms and soles, hepatic dysfunction and diarrhea

      7 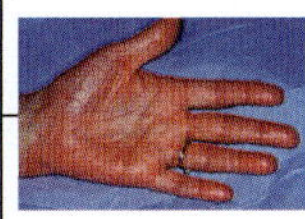

      Dusky erythematous macules and papules on the palms → Consider GVHD (G)
    - Nonspecific physical examination and laboratory findings; unable to identify an underlying etiology with history → Consider Idiopathic or Other Causes of Erythroderma (H)

43 Palmoplantar Papules and Plaques

Franklin R. Blum and Christopher Sayed

Palmoplantar papules and plaques include a variety of benign, infectious, and malignant pathologies. Many of the associated conditions can have significant impact on activities of daily living and quality of life due to acral cutaneous involvement. Depending on the pathology, management can include topical agents, surgical excision, or systemic therapy. Key cutaneous morphological features and careful patient history are essential to narrowing a differential, and biopsy or additional testing may be required in some scenarios.

A. The initial evaluation of palmar or plantar lesions should begin with the physical examination to determine if the lesions are predominantly papules or plaques. The differential diagnosis differs significantly depending on primary lesion morphology, yielding this step essential for clinical decision-making.

B. After determining primary lesion morphology, obtaining a detailed history from the patient can help determine severity and/or urgency of the underlying pathology. For example, if the lesions are primarily papules and a patient reports symptoms consistent with systemic illness (fever, fatigue, shortness of breath, etc.), infectious etiologies should be highest on the differential, such as **meningococcemia**. In someone with high-risk sexual behaviors, disseminated sexually transmitted diseases, such as **gonococcemia** and **syphilis**, should be considered. Similarly, a recent history of herpes simplex infection followed by systemic symptoms and a diffuse targetoid rash would favor **erythema multiforme**. Finally, history of intravenous drug use with systemic symptoms and signs of Janeway lesions or Osler nodes would point to **subacute bacterial endocarditis**. Vital signs and associated physical examination findings can help further provide a clinician with investigational direction.

C. Pruritus is a cutaneous symptom that can prove especially helpful in narrowing down a diagnosis for papules found on the palms and/or soles. For example, when examining papular lesions, pruritus can point a clinician to diagnoses such as **scabies** or **palmoplantar pustulosis**. Although not entirely specific to any one condition, pruritis is also present in the dermatologic manifestations of reactive arthritis, such as keratoderma blennorrhagicum and circinate balanitis/vulvitis.

D. For nonpruritic papules on the palms/soles, a medical history of arthritis or a quick clinical arthritis symptom screening can direct a clinician to consider arthritic-associated cutaneous papules, such as rheumatoid nodules or gouty tophi. Further history and clinical examination can delineate between the two diagnoses. Importantly, although rare, patients presenting with these two pathologies may have no known history of arthritis. If rheumatoid nodules or gouty tophi are favored clinically, further evaluation with laboratory and/or imaging tests may be warranted.

Patient presents with palmoplantar papules and/or plaques

(A) Thorough history and physical examination of the skin, including the palms and soles, to identify underlying etiology and discover any systemic symptoms and signs

(B) Lesion(s) predominantly papules (solitary or multiple)?

- No → continued on next page
- Yes → Does the patient show any of the following signs of systemic illness: fever, sepsis, altered mentation or fatigue?
  - Yes → Consider infectious etiology
    - History of recent herpes infection, prodromal symptoms, fever, arthralgias, fatigue/weakness; circular erythematous papules and/or macules, target lesions on acral surfaces initially, progresses centrally; May have mucosal involvement

      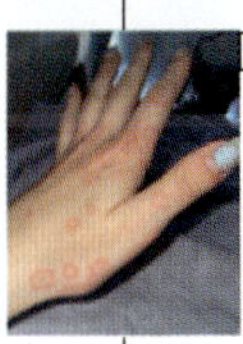
      1

      → Consider Erythema Multiforme
    - IV drug use, recent transcutaneous blood-draw or dental procedure; dyspnea; tender (Osler nodes) or nontender (Janeway lesions); erythematous papules on the palms/soles

      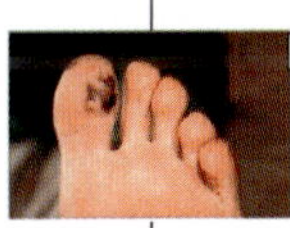
      2

      → Consider Subacute Bacterial Endocarditis
    - History of sexual activity, multiple sexual partners. More common in females. Rapid-onset fever, rash, arthralgias; pustules with a purpuric base and petechiae diffusely and often asymmetrically on acral surfaces

      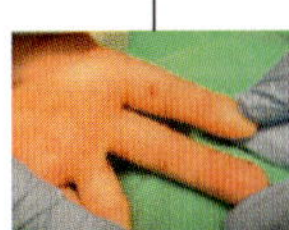
      3

      → Consider Gonococcemia
    - Fever and rapid-onset septic symptoms; violaceous papules and/or macules (petechiae) on the palms/soles, progress to gunmetal gray color

      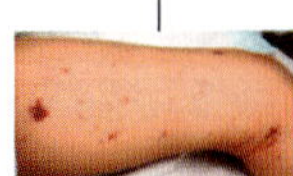
      4

      → Consider Meningococcemia
    - Painless oral or anogenital chancre within past 3–6 months, new sexual partners; erythematous, violaceous, or copper-colored papules with overlying scale +/– tenderness on the palms/soles

      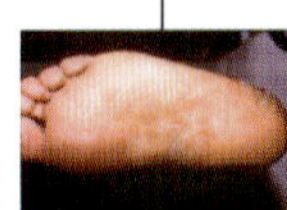
      5

      → Consider Secondary Syphilis
  - No → Pruritus is a significant symptom?
    - (C) Yes
      - Females aged 40–60, smoker, significant life stressors; erythematous, hemorrhagic papules and pustules on the palms/soles

        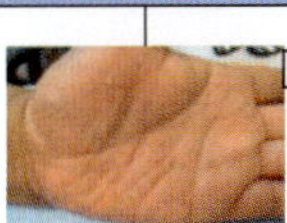
        6

        → Consider Palmoplantar Pustulosis
      - Close interpersonal contact, confined shared living spaces; erythematous, pruritic papules, plaques and "burrows"; favors interdigital web spaces

        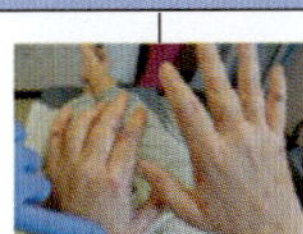
        7

        → Consider Scabies
    - No → History of arthritis?
      - (D) Yes
        - Painful bilateral arthritis, classically worse in morning; firm, nontender, subcutaneous skin-colored nodules primarily on extensor surfaces and/or palms and soles

          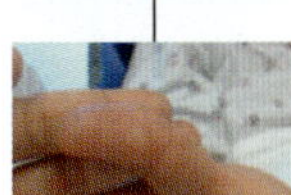
          8

          → Consider Rheumatoid Nodule
        - Chronic flares of painful arthritis +/– kidney disease; erythematous, tender, warm subcutaneous nodule overlying a joint and/or on the palms and soles

          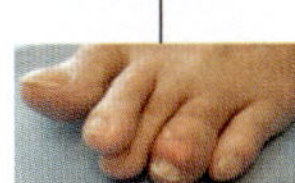
          9

          → Consider Gouty Tophus
      - No → Bleeds easily with manipulation?
        - Yes
          - Usually children or young adults +/– history of trauma; erythematous, friable papule that bleeds easily after trauma +/– ulceration or crusting

            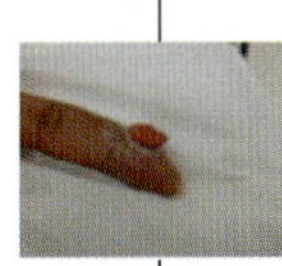
            10

            → Consider Pyogenic Granuloma
          - Usually adults; solitary, slow growing, pink/erythematous, smooth papule +/– easily bleeds with manipulation

            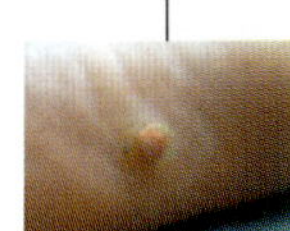
            11

            → Consider Poroma
        - No → continued on next page

Continued

E. A similar approach to Section B above for papules can be followed for plaques. After determining primary lesion morphology, obtaining a detailed history from the patient can help determine severity and/or urgency of the underlying pathology. For example, if the lesions are primarily plaques and the patient reports a history of diffuse pain/itch and widespread cutaneous involvement with thermoregulatory imbalance, **pityriasis rubra pilaris** should be considered. History of gastrointestinal or urinary infection, joint pains, or eye symptoms points toward **reactive arthritis** as a possible diagnosis.

F. Pruritis is also particularly helpful when differentiating plaque-dominant lesions. However, for pruritic plaques, the differential is much broader, so several other clinical correlates are needed to narrow possible diagnoses. The presence of vesicles will help a clinician favor diagnoses, such as **dyshidrotic eczema** and **allergic contact dermatitis** (although not required). Consider swabbing grouped, painful vesicular or pustular lesions for herpes simplex virus polymerase chain reaction testing. Pruritic plaques without the presence of vesicles may be seen in **palmoplantar psoriasis, tinea pedis/manuum**, and **atopic dermatitis**, each of which have differentiating characteristics. Importantly, **allergic contact dermatitis** can present with or without vesicles, so it should remain on the pruritic plaque differential even in the absence of vesicles. **Palmoplantar psoriasis** may present in a patient with psoriasis elsewhere on the body. Psoriatic nail changes such as nail pitting and onycholysis may be present. **Tinea pedis and/or manuum** often involves the finger or toe web spaces and may be annular. **Atopic dermatitis** on the hands and feet may present in individuals with other signs of atopy, such as allergic rhinitis or asthma.

G. Considering the timing and onset of cutaneous palmoplantar plaques is also important. Specifically, childhood-onset should prompt a clinician to consider **congenital palmoplantar keratodermas** (e.g., Vörner disease, pachyonychia congenita).

See Appendix 1 for Further Reading and Image References.

Lesion(s) predominantly papules (solitary or multiple)?

Bleeds easily with manipulation?

No

- Local trauma; firm, skin-colored to erythematous, exophytic, hyperkeratotic papule on a solitary nail or digit

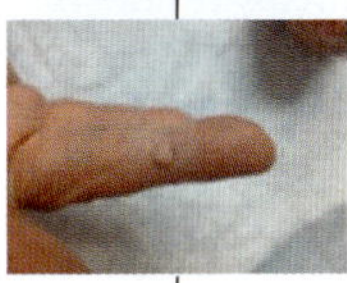

12

Consider Digital Fibrokeratoma

- Often in children, close contacts have similar lesions, public shower use; hyperkeratotic verrucous papules on the hands, feet, or limbs

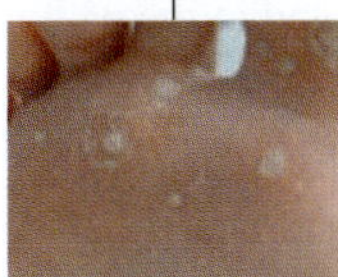

13

Consider Verruca Vulgaris

- Usually in adults, frequent friction over involved area, ill-fitting shoes; indurated, hyperkeratotic papules overlying areas of friction

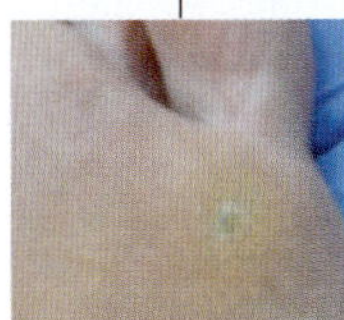

14

Consider Corn

- Progressive growth over weeks to months and may be painful or asymptomatic; May develop scale, ulcer, and/or crust over time

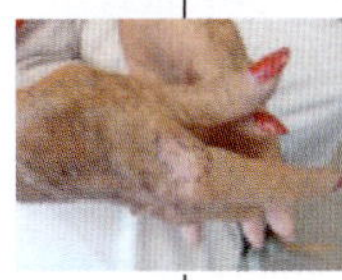

15

Consider Cutaneous Malignancy (Squamous Cell Carcinoma, Digital Papillary Carcinoma)

- Slowly growing, irregular hyperpigmented macule or patch that may form a papule or nodule over time

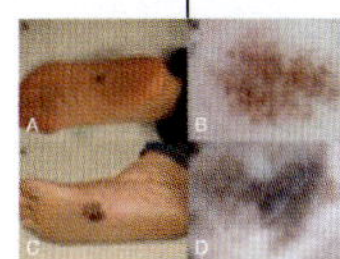

16

Consider Acral Melanoma

No

(E) Lesion(s) predominantly plaque

Does the patient show signs of diffuse illness, including thermoregulatory imbalance, diffuse pain/itch, or erythroderma?

No

(F) Pruritus is a significant symptom?

Yes → Vesicles present?

Yes

- Classic craniocaudal spread; subacute, spreading, scaly, erythematous papules and plaques that become extensive or erythrodermic with islands of sparing. Can involve palms and soles as waxy plaques

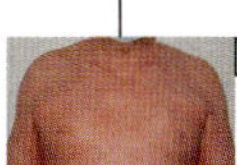

17

Consider Pityriasis Rubra Pilaris

- History of gastrointestinal or urinary infection/ symptoms (diarrhea, urethritis), asymmetric oligoarthritis, and eye pain/ irritation (uveitis); pustules on acral surfaces that progress into scaly, psoriasiform plaques. Also look for circinate balanitis/vulvitis, significant paronychia, and geographic tongue

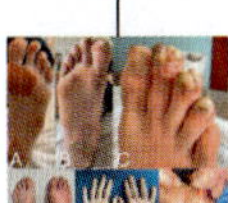

18

Consider Keratoderma Blennorrhagicum

Yes

- Chronic, frequent handwashing, new or harsh soap use; papules and small, tense, clear, fluid-filled vesicles primarily on the medial and/or lateral aspects of the digits on background of erythema

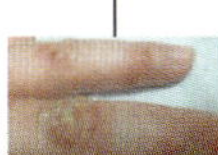

19

Consider Dyshidrotic Eczema

- Recent contact with new soap, metal, cosmetic, or unknown trigger; vesicles or bullae with crusting, fissuring and/or surrounding erythema

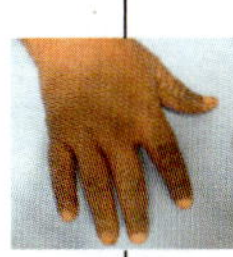

20

Consider Allergic Contact Dermatitis

No

- Possible history of plaque psoriasis; develops over days to weeks and becomes chronic; thick, erythematous scaly plaques on palms/soles; may have painful fissures and nail thickening

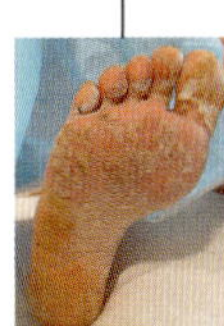

21

Consider Palmoplantar Psoriasis

- Athletes, occlusive footwear, communal showering; erythematous plaques with prominent advancing edge and surrounding powdery white scale; web space predilection

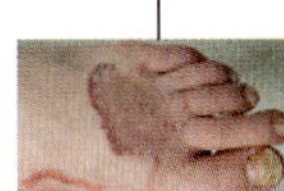

22

Consider Tinea Pedis/ Manuum

- History of eczema, allergic rhinitis, asthma; scaly, erythematous papules and plaques; secondary lichenification or scale

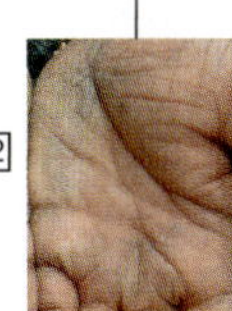

23

Consider Atopic Dermatitis

- Recent contact with new soap, metal, cosmetic, or unknown trigger; erythematous papules, plaques, or bullae with crusting and fissuring

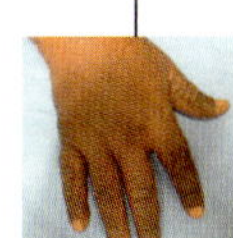

24

Consider Allergic Contact Dermatitis

No

(G) Presented in childhood/ adolescence?

Yes

- Scaly plaques developing in childhood on the palms and soles; family history may be present; thick, scaly plaques, often with erythema and painful fissuring on the palms and soles

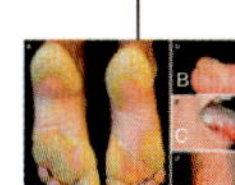

25

Consider Congenital Palmoplantar Keratodermas (e.g., Vörner Disease, Pachyonychia Congenita)

44 Periorificial Papules and Plaques

Peter A. Lio and Cristina M. Foschi

Inflammatory papules or pink, scaly plaques in the perioral, periocular, or perinasal regions—around the orifices of the face—have several etiologies. An eruption in these cosmetically sensitive areas can be emotionally distressing for patients and families. Most diagnoses can be managed with topical regimens, such as nonsteroidal or antimicrobial medications, with a rare need for systemic agents. While initial medical management is important, understanding the etiology is imperative to set expectations and prevent recurrence.

A. The initial evaluation of periorificial papules or plaques involves eliciting prior use of any topical, inhaled, or intranasal products (especially corticosteroids), gaining information (sometimes in the form of photographs) about how the lesions began, and determining recent changes in hygiene products (i.e., toothpaste). Additional significant history details include questioning if this has happened before or if they have a history of a dermatologic condition. A thorough examination of the skin and oral mucosa is critical, noting in particular if the lesions are unilateral or bilateral, present elsewhere on the face or on the mucosa. Symptoms such as burning, pain, or itch should also be noted. While the diagnosis is usually clinical, microscopy or KOH preparation can be useful in some cases. Given the delicate region involved, skin biopsy is generally reserved for those with atypical presentation or a lack of response to treatment.

B. A common diagnosis that presents in this manner is **periorificial dermatitis,** which has multiple environmental exposures associated with it. Most notably, the recent utilization of topical or inhaled steroids, fluoridated toothpastes, or new cosmetic products may induce a flare. Wearing masks, especially for prolonged periods, also seems to be a risk factor in some. Physical examination findings include grouped erythematous papules that are typically bilaterally symmetric surrounding the mouth, eyes, and nose. The vermilion border of the lips is often spared, and patients may report burning or sensitivity to the region. Topical steroids may initially resolve these lesions; however, upon cessation of steroid use, the eruption may return, and sometimes the eruption occurs primarily from steroid use.

C. Periorificial papules and plaques can be seen in those with underlying dermatologic conditions, such as **rosacea, acne**, or **seborrheic dermatitis**.

While periorificial dermatitis is thought by some to be a variant of **rosacea**, those with this condition often have telangiectasias and erythema with intermittent periods of exacerbation and remission. In addition, there may be papules involving the central face, including the nose, as well as baseline flushing.

In young adults with papules clustered in the perioral region, one should consider **acne mechanica** commonly due to friction such as from a helmet or chin strap in football players. **Hormonal acne** may also have papules, pustules, and comedones clustered around the mouth and jawline. This is seen in females or those on hormonal replacement therapy and may notably worsen with menstrual cycles or changing hormones.

Ill-defined erythematous plaques around the mouth with a greasy scale may be indicative of **seborrheic dermatitis**, especially in patients with beards. However, additional regions are also often affected, such as the eyebrows, glabella, nasolabial folds, or scalp.

D. ***Demodex* folliculitis** forms scattered facial and perioral papules and pustules. An increased density of a mite that normally resides on the skin and has been implicated in the pathogenesis of rosacea induces a facial eruption. This should especially be considered in those who may have impaired immunity or recent immunosuppressive use, such as corticosteroids. Diagnosis includes scraping a papule or pustule and viewing the contents under microscopy, which reveals numerous *Demodex* mites.

E. In cases of an isolated, annular plaque, one should consider **tinea faciei**. This is a dermatophytic fungal infection which often presents unilaterally with sharp borders. Hyphae will be seen with KOH preparation and microscopic examination of scale, which confirms the diagnosis.

F. Periorificial papules can also occur in **lupus miliaris disseminatus faciei,** which typically presents in young adults and manifests as reddish-yellow or brown papules. The distribution is bilateral and is typically seen on the central face and eyelids. Skin biopsy can aid in diagnosis, which reveals dermal epithelioid granulomas and lymphohistiocytic infiltrate.

G. In cases of recurrent vesicular or papular lesions on the lips or perioral skin, consider **herpes labialis**. This condition usually begins with a prodrome of burning or tingling and is generally painful once manifested. Herpes appears as grouped lesions or an isolated larger lesion on the lip or corners of the mouth. The lesions are contagious when active, but asymptomatic shedding can also occur.

H. Finally, certain systemic conditions, such as **sarcoidosis**, can manifest with red-brown papules on the periorificial regions of the face. Patients may also have other cutaneous findings, such as nodules on the legs (erythema nodosum). Systemic symptoms such as cough, shortness of breath, or fever may also be present. Skin biopsy is helpful in distinguishing this condition, which would demonstrate noncaseating granulomas.

See Appendix 1 for Further Reading and Image Reference.

- Patient presents with inflammatory papules or pink, scaly plaques around their eyes, mouth, or nose
- (A) Obtain a detailed history (particularly of new exposures/products) and thorough examination of skin and oral mucosal surfaces
  - → Management involves addressing underlying etiology; may use nonsteroidal topicals or antimicrobial medications to affected areas
- Does history indicate recent utilization of steroids or new products?
  - **Yes** → Consider Periorificial Dermatitis (B)
  - **No** → History of an underlying dermatologic condition?
    - **No** →
      - "Treatment-resistant" rosacea, immunosuppressed or on corticosteroids; unroofing lesion demonstrates mite under microscopy

        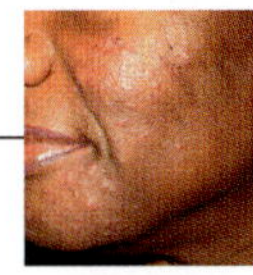
        4

        Inflammatory papules or pustules on the cheeks or perioral region → Consider Demodex Folliculitis (D)
      - Unilateral presentation; hyphae seen on KOH examination of scale

        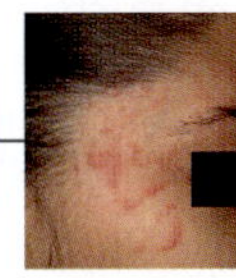
        5

        Annular plaque with sharp, well-demarcated borders and peripheral scale → Consider Tinea Faciei (E)
      - Young adult with lesions localized around periorbital region (bilateral eyelids, central face)

        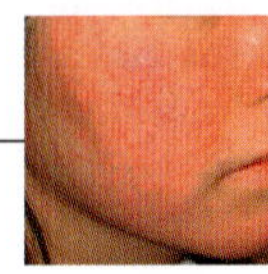
        6

        Discrete red-brown or yellow papules → Consider Lupus Miliaris Disseminatus Faciei (F)
      - Hx of recurrent lesions around the lips, prodrome of burning/tingling

        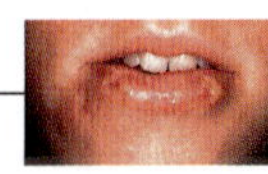
        7

        Multiple grouped or large isolated clear-to-yellow hued vesicles → Consider Herpes Labialis (G)
      - Eruption with other systemic findings such as cough, shortness of breath, or nodules on the legs

        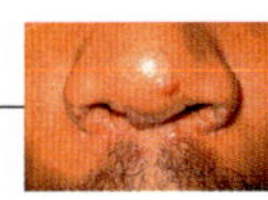
        8

        Red-brown papules or plaques → Consider Sarcoidosis (H)
    - **Yes** (C) →
      - Hx of rosacea, intermittent flares, or baseline flushing

        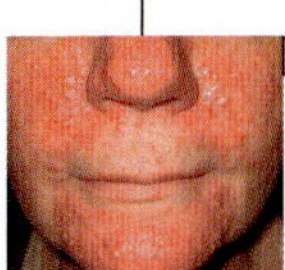
        1

        Telangiectasias and erythema with papules of central face → Consider Rosacea
      - Young adult; Hx of mechanical friction (i.e., chin strap or helmet) or worsens with menstrual cycles

        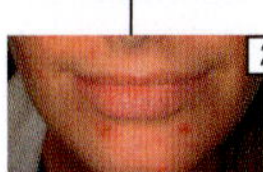
        2

        Papules, pustules, or comedones clustered around the mouth/jawline → Consider Acne Mechanica or Hormonal Acne
      - Hx of seborrheic dermatitis; affecting the eyebrows, glabella, nasolabial folds, or scalp

        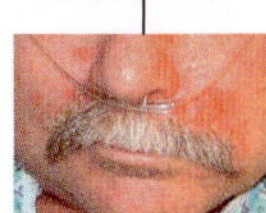
        3

        Ill-defined erythematous plaques with greasy scale → Consider Seborrheic Dermatitis

45 Groin/Genital Papules and Plaques With Scale

Hana Ahmed and Tiffany Mayo

Cutaneous conditions that are present in the groin can be challenging for a practicing dermatologist. Common skin conditions may involve the crural folds and genitalia, but without specific questioning from the clinician, patients may feel hesitant to share their concerns. In addition, patients may have genetically assigned genitalia that do not correspond with the sex they identify by. The authors of this chapter recommend open and direct communication with a nonjudgmental attitude when addressing skin conditions in this anatomical location.

The first step involves identifying the exact anatomical location of involvement, whether this be genitalia (A through F) or inguinal folds (G through K).

A. If psoriasiform plaques are present on the penis, diagnoses to consider include **plaque psoriasis (PsO)** and reactive arthritis with balanitis circinata. The former will often also involve other sites classic for PsO, including the extensor surfaces, scalp, and lower back and may have associated nail findings and psoriatic arthritis.

B. **Balanitis circinata** associated with reactive arthritis is commonly preceded by an infection (e.g., *Chlamydia trachomatis*), and the patient may also have urethritis, conjunctivitis, and arthritis. Notably, nail involvement is absent. A helpful way to distinguish PsO on the penis from balanitis circinata is that the latter localizes to the corona and coronal sulcus.

C. **Lichen planus (LP)** is an inflammatory papulosquamous disease of the skin, mucous membranes, and hair follicles with many clinical variants. Common sites of involvement include the flexor surface of the wrist and forearms, anterior lower legs, and presacral areas. LP on the penis often presents in an annular or figurate pattern, and lesions are typically asymptomatic. Simultaneous involvement of gingival and penile mucosa can occur. When on the vulva, there are several clinical variants, including the classic type, which involves the clitoral hood and labia minora. If a female has genital involvement, the oral mucosa must be examined, as the patient may have vulvovaginal-gingival syndrome and can have long-term sequelae due to scarring.

D. **Scabies** is an infestation caused by *Sarcoptes scabiei* in which the female mite burrows into the stratum corneum to deposit her eggs. The pathognomonic sign is the burrow, which is a wavy, grayish-white linear lesion 1 to 10 mm in length. The most common sites of involvement include the finger web spaces, wrists, axillae, areolae, umbilicus, lower abdomen, genitals, and buttocks. Involvement of both the penis and scrotum is highly characteristic of scabies. A mineral oil preparation of skin scrapings can help with visualization of adult mites, eggs, and/or scybala on microscopy.

E. **Squamous cell carcinoma (SCC)** often develops as a stepwise progression from **squamous cell carcinoma in situ**, and the vast majority of malignancies in the penile and vulvar regions are SCC. The carcinoma is insidious and develops as asymptomatic, indolent, and varied colored plaques. Risk factors include immunosuppression, tobacco use, history of human papillomavirus infection, and long-standing lichen sclerosus et atrophicus. On male genitalia, SCC can appear on the glans, coronal sulcus, or prepuce as ulcers or scaling plaques. A delay in diagnosis may occur in uncircumcised males. On female genitalia, SCC occurs most frequently on the labia and can present as nonhealing ulcers, fissures, nodules, and scaling plaques.

F. **Extramammary Paget disease (EMPD)** is an intraepithelial adenocarcinoma. The vulva, scrotum, and penis are common locations, but it may also involve the perineal and perianal regions. It may be asymptomatic, pruritic, or burning. Clinical presentations include erosions, ulcerations, and lichenification. Up to 29% of patients with genital EMPD are found to have a coexisting internal malignancy. EMPD tends to affect adults between the ages of 65 and 70 years. "Underpants erythema" (or redness involving the entire genital area) may be indicative of widespread lymphatic involvement in the pelvic basin and is a poor prognostic sign. In general, a slowly progressive plaque or patch in the genitalia should raise concern, and the clinician should have a low threshold to biopsy and rule out EMPD and SCC.

G. There are several conditions that cause pink scaling patches and plaques in the inguinal folds and medial thighs. As previously discussed, PsO can present as classic plaque PsO on the genitalia. However, another variant of PsO, **inverse psoriasis**, predominantly involves flexural sites (i.e., axillae, inguinal crease, intergluteal cleft, inframammary region, and retroauricular folds). A localized dermatophyte, candidal, or bacterial infection can be a trigger for flexural psoriasis.

H. **Tinea cruris** is a superficial mycosis caused by dermatophyte infection (most commonly *Trichophyton rubrum*) of the inguinal area, most commonly the medial upper thighs and crural folds. Plaques can extend onto the abdomen and buttocks. The condition is more commonly seen in males, and risk factors include obesity and excessive perspiration. These patients often have preceding tinea pedis and onychomycosis; spread to the crural folds occurs from autoinoculation.

I. **Erythrasma** is caused by *Corynebacterium minutissimum* infection. Hyperpigmented or erythematous patches occur in intertriginous regions. It is more common in the settings of advanced age, diabetes, obesity, and humid environments. Thick yellowish hyperkeratosis of the vulva may be seen in females. Diagnosis is confirmed by a Wood's lamp examination demonstrating characteristic coral pink fluorescence. Patients may rarely present with a triad of erythrasma, pitted keratolysis, and trichomycosis axillaris, which are all caused by the same pathogen.

J. **Seborrheic dermatitis** is a chronic superficial inflammatory disease due in part to *Malassezia furfur*. Sebaceous anatomical regions such as the head and neck, as well as the sternum, axilla, and body folds are favored sites. Involvement of the groin and gluteal crease can mimic tinea cruris and inverse psoriasis. Examining other body sites (nails, scalp, genitalia) as well as utilizing diagnostic tools such as biopsies and KOH preparation tests can help differentiate the entities.

K. **Darier disease** is an autosomal dominant genodermatosis due to a mutation in the ATP2A2 gene, which leads to dysfunction of the endoplasmic reticulum calcium ATPase. Patients present with keratotic, crusted red to brown papules in a seborrheic distribution of the trunk, scalp, and face, as well as in intertriginous sites. The peak age of onset is young adulthood. Patients are at risk for secondary infections (e.g., Kaposi varicelliform eruption). There is a risk of neurological sequelae, including seizure disorder, intellectual disability, and other mental health disorders. Inguinal involvement may be mistaken for Hailey-Hailey disease, necessitating a tissue biopsy. Although histopathology in both diseases shows acantholysis of keratinocytes, Darier disease has pronounced dyskeratosis, which is absent in Hailey-Hailey disease.

See Appendix 1 for Further Reading and Image References.

Adult patient presenting with scaly papules and plaques in the groin

↓

Detailed history with pertinent positives, negatives, and thorough physical examination of the skin, hair, nails, and mucosal surfaces

↓

Do the skin lesions mainly involve the genitalia?

Yes → Does the patient have psoriasiform plaques on the penis?

- **Yes** →
  - Occurs on the penis and scrotum
    +/–Koebner phenomenon
    +/–Nail changes
    +/–Arthritis
    +/–Annulus migrans

    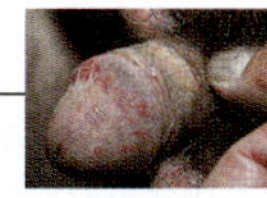
    1

    → Consider Plaque Psoriasis (A)
  - Tends to localize to the corona and coronal sulcus
    Preceded by *Chlamydia, Shigella*, or other infection
    +/–Urethritis
    +/–Arthritis

    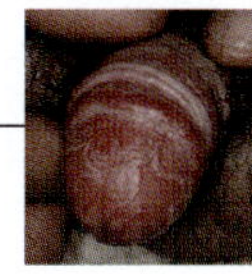
    2

    → Consider Balanitis Circinata (B)
- **No** →
  - Small polygonal violaceous papules and plaques with network of fine white scale, may be annular on the penis
    +/–Mucosal involvement
    +/–Koebner phenomenon
    +/–Hepatitis C

    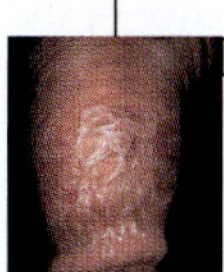
    3

    → Consider Lichen Planus (C)
  - Pruritic papules with scale, crust, nodules, excoriations, burrows; Male: penis and scrotum; Female: areolae, nipples, vulva;
    + extremely pruritic
    +/–Close contact history

    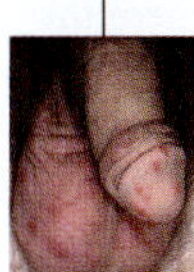
    4

    → Consider Scabies (D)
  - Asymptomatic, indolent, varied colored plaque on the genitals
    Can have varied presentation
    +/–Scale, ulceration
    +/–HPV history
    +/–Long-standing LS&A
    +/–Tobacco use
    +/–Immunosuppression

    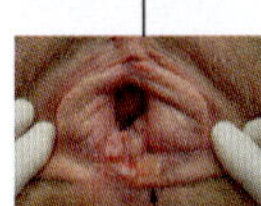
    5

    → Consider Squamous Cell Carcinoma (E)
  - Slowly expanding sharply demarcated erythematous plaque with scale and erosions (strawberries and cream)
    "Underpants erythema" is a poor prognostic sign

    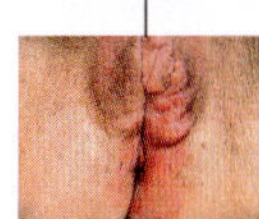
    6

    → Consider Extramammary Paget Disease (F)

No → Does the rash primarily involve the crural folds and medial thighs?

- **Yes** →
  - Shiny pink to red well-demarcated plaques with minimal scale in flexural surfaces
    +/–Central fissure
    +/–Nail changes

    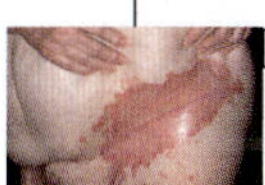
    7

    → Consider Inverse Psoriasis (G)
  - Sharply demarcated erythematous plaques with central clearing, advancing scaly border; scrotum characteristically spared
    +/–Pustules or vesicles
    +/–Onychomycosis

    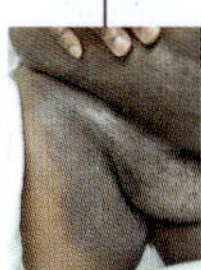
    8

    → Consider Tinea Cruris (H)
  - Sharply delineated red-brown scaly patches in intertriginous regions, humid environment
    + Coral red fluorescence on Wood's lamp

    → Consider Erythrasma (I)
  - Yellow greasy bran-like scale on erythematous base in sebaceous sites and body folds (common in groin folds and gluteal crease); may involve scalp, central chest, alar groove, and eyebrows

    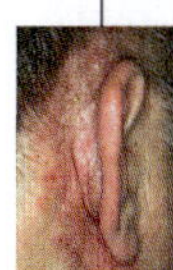
    9

    → Consider Seborrheic Dermatitis (J)
  - Warty crusted red to brown papules and plaques in seborrheic distribution; keratotic palmar papules and pits; oral cobblestoning; nail findings: "V" notching, red and white streaks
    +/–Kaposi varicelliform eruption

    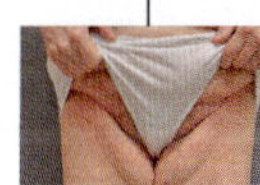
    10

    → Consider Darier Disease (K)

46 Axillary Papule

Katelyn J. Rypka and Noah Goldfarb

The axilla is a unique anatomical site, rich in pilosebaceous units, as well as apocrine and eccrine glands. It is also an intertriginous region, susceptible to friction, increased heat, and moisture. These distinct features make it prone to a variety of skin conditions. Scaly papules and plaques in the axilla can be divided into papulosquamous disorders, eczematous eruptions, infections, and infestations. Axillary eruptions can be solely found in intertriginous regions or present more diffusely. Most axillary eruptions may be diagnosed clinically, although some may require a Wood's lamp or skin scraping with examination using potassium hydroxide (KOH) or mineral oil.

A. Initial evaluation should involve taking a detailed medical history, including lesion duration, associated symptoms, and previous attempted treatments. While performing a thorough evaluation of the skin, one should identify the morphology of the primary lesion(s).

B. Scaly axillary eruptions may present as either discrete scaly papules or scaly papules and plaques coalescing into larger plaques.

C. Discrete scaly papules in the axillary region should prompt consideration of **scabies** or **pityriasis lichenoides**, which may involve regions outside the axilla as well. While these conditions can usually be differentiated clinically based on lesion morphology and the unique anatomic locations affected by scabies, skin scraping and microscopic examination with oil preparation can be used to identify mites, scybala and eggs. Scabies characteristically presents as intensely pruritic papules, involving the web spaces of the hands and feet, nipples, umbilicus, navel, waist, buttocks, and genitals. Short linear burrows are pathognomonic and are the highest yield sites to find mites with skin scraping. Pityriasis lichenoides can be subdivided into acute (**pityriasis lichenoides et varioliformis acuta [PLEVA]**) and chronic (**pityriasis lichenoides chronica [PLC]**) presentations. Pityriasis lichenoides presents as red to brown papules on the trunk, proximal extremities, and skin flexures, typically in children and young adults. Lesions may resolve with postinflammatory hyper- and hypopigmented macules and patches. Compared with PLC, in which the papules develop gradually and develop a wafer-like scale, PLEVA presents acutely, and the papules rapidly progress to papulovesicles with hemorrhagic crust and necrosis.

D. Eruptions comprised of scaly papules and plaques that coalesce into larger plaques can be further differentiated by their configuration and border delineation. A reticular distribution suggests **confluent and reticulated papillomatosis (CARP)**. CARP typically appears during adolescence with scaly, papillomatous, or atrophic brown papules coalescing into reticulated plaques. The eruption classically presents on the central chest, abdomen, and skin folds.

Eczematous processes, also referred to as dermatitis, are characterized by scaly pink papules and plaques with poorly demarcated borders. The different types of dermatitis are differentiated based on their configuration, distribution, and pertinent history.

E. **Seborrheic dermatitis** has a unique distribution involving regions rich in sebaceous glands (e.g., hair-bearing areas on the scalp and face, ears, central chest, and flexural regions) and presents with greasy scale. **Irritant contact dermatitis (ICD)** is more common than **allergic contact dermatitis (ACD)**, especially within intertriginous sites where ICD is triggered by friction, heat, and moisture. ACD may be localized to the axillary vault in cases related to deodorant/antiperspirant or shaving product use, but most cases are more widespread. When the axillary vault is spared, ACD due to clothing or detergents should be suspected. Patch testing may help to differentiate between ACD and ICD.

F. The presence of satellite papules and pustules can help differentiate **candidal intertrigo** from an eczematous process. Candidal intertrigo presents as red, moist, variably circumscribed plaques located in body folds. Maceration is common, and if scale is present, it is typically at the periphery. Papulosquamous disorders and their mimics are characterized by pink-purple scaly papules and plaques with well-demarcated edges.

G. **Pityriasis rubra pilaris (PRP)**, **Darier disease**, and **granular parakeratosis** all present as discrete scaly papules that coalesce into larger plaques.

H. PRP can be differentiated from these other conditions as the papules are follicularly based with follicular plugging. The papules coalesce into well-demarcated scaly plaques with follicular prominence. This condition mostly affects areas outside the axilla, often presenting with erythroderma, alopecia, and waxy-appearing, yellow-orangish, palmoplantar keratoderma. When involving diffuse areas, PRP has a distinctive sparing of normal skin ("islands of sparing"). Age of onset is bimodal with peaks in the first and fifth decades of life.

Darier disease and **granular parakeratosis** present with nonfollicularly based scaly papules that can be distinguished from each other by their unique morphology and distribution. Darier disease typically has distinctive orangish-brownish papules with greasy wart-like scale and crusting in a seborrheic distribution. Darier disease is an autosomal dominant genodermatosis that typically presents during childhood or adolescence, a family history can help confirm the diagnosis. Biopsy of Darier disease demonstrates dyskeratotic acantholysis. Granular parakeratosis has a similar morphology, composed of orangish-brown papules coalescing into plaques, but these lesions are limited to body folds, most commonly the axilla. Spontaneous resolution is common, as is recurrence.

I. The other papulosquamous disorders and mimics that are not comprised of discrete coalescing papules can be clinically distinguished based on the amount and type of scale present. **Inverse psoriasis** presents as symmetric, well-demarcated, flat, moist, shiny, pink to violaceous plaques with minimal or absent scale in intertriginous regions. Associated nail changes (thickening, crumbling, onycholysis, yellow-red discoloration, irregular pits) support the diagnosis.

Erythrasma is typically limited to a single site: interdigital, groin, perianal, or axillary. The morphology of the plaques is also unique, presenting as thin faint plaques, with minimal to absent scale. While it can appear pink, erythrasma is often more hyperpigmented or brown. A coral-red fluorescence under Wood's lamp examination helps differentiate erythrasma from the other axillary eruptions discussed.

Inverse lichen planus (LP) has Wickham striae, a delicate, gray-white, reticular scale. The Wickham striae of inverse LP is more likely to be subtle or absent compared with classic LP. Inverse LP lesions are usually arranged in a linear distribution following skin cleavage lines.

Tinea corporis, a superficial dermatophyte infection of the skin and papulosquamous disorder mimic classically presents as a well-defined annular plaque with central clearing. Classically, plaques of tinea corporis have a collarette of scale at the leading edge.

J. This can typically be differentiated from **inverse pityriasis rosea (PR)** and **erythema annulare centrifugum (EAC)**, which present with "trailing scale," where the scale trails behind the edge of the inflammatory border of the lesion. As tinea corporis can sometimes have variable presentations with different types of scale, a scraping with KOH preparation may help to confirm the diagnosis. Inverse PR is a self-limited eruption composed of more discrete flat papules and some small plaques in flexural regions, including the axilla, face, neck, and extremities, sparing the trunk. It is more common in adolescents and children. In contrast to the acute onset of PR, EAC presents gradually with a chronic course. It is also typically localized to one region and composed primarily of annular plaques with few or absent papules. These plaques expand centrifugally and coalesce into larger arcuate and serpiginous plaques.

See Appendix 1 for Further Reading and Image References.

Patient presenting with axillary papules and/or plaques with scale

(A) Detailed history and physical examination of the skin and mucous membranes

(B) Morphology

(C) Discrete scaly papules

- Mineral oil skin scraping preparation
  - Negative
    - A child, adolescent, or young adult patient presenting with mildly pruritic clusters of ovoid red-brown papules with wafer-like scale or more acutely as papulovesicular and papulonecrotic lesions

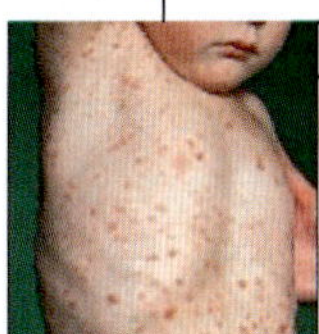
2

→ Consider Pityriasis Lichenoides Chronica (PLC) or Pityriasis Lichenoides et Varioliformis Acuta (PLEVA)

  - Positive
    - Intensely pruritic small scaly papules with pinpoint vesicles and linear burrows often within finger/toe webs, genitals, umbilicus, and flexor surfaces

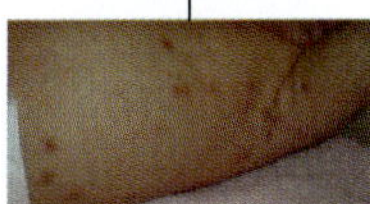
1

→ Consider Scabies

Coalescing scaly papules and plaques

(D) Configuration

- Well-demarcated

(G) Plaques composed of discrete coalescing papules?

- No
  - (I) Evaluate scale
    - Minimal scale
      - Pink to brown, flat, minimally scaly plaques in intertriginous regions; Coral red fluorescence on Wood's lamp exam

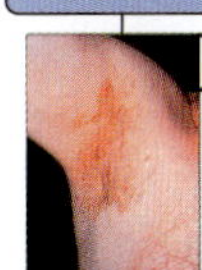
8

→ Consider Erythrasma

      - Shiny pink symmetric plaques in skin folds with minimal scale; May present with chronic plaque psoriasis and/or nail changes

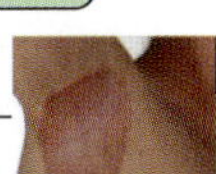
7

→ Consider Inverse Psoriasis

    - Wickham striae
      - Middle-aged patient with purple, planar, polygonal papules and small plaques often following a linear distribution of the skin cleavage lines within intertriginous sites; Often with faint or even absent Wickham striae

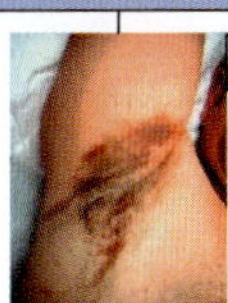
9

→ Consider Inverse Lichen Planus

    - Peripheral scale
      - Trailing scale?
        - (J) Yes
          - Middle-aged adult with onset of a superficial annular/arcuate plaque with trailing edge of scale. Negative KOH

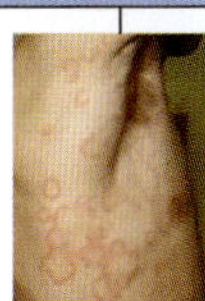
12

→ Consider Erythema Annulare Centrifugum

          - Ovoid, minimally elevated, scaly papules and small plaques in skin folds with a trailing edge of scale behind the inflammatory border of the lesion. Typically distributed within intertriginous sites and on the face

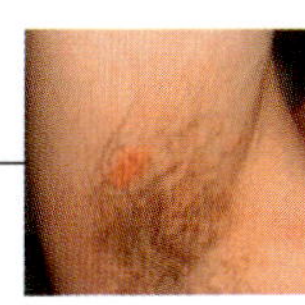
11

→ Consider Inverse Pityriasis Rosea

        - No
          - Classically a plaque with a raised indurated border, central clearing, and leading edge of scale. Positive KOH

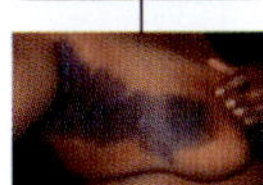
10

→ Consider Tinea Corporis

- Yes
  - (H) Follicular distribution?
    - Yes
      - Hair follicle-based keratotic papules coalescing into pink-orange plaques with "islands of sparing." Often with waxy yellow-orange palmoplantar keratoderma

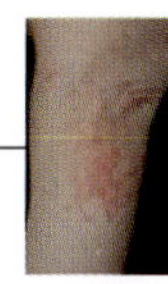
13

→ Consider Pityriasis Rubra Pilaris

    - No
      - Hyperpigmented nonfollicularly-based keratotic papules that coalesce into scaly plaques in the axillae

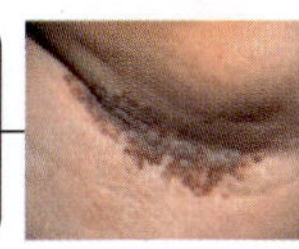
15

→ Consider Granular Parakeratosis

      - Nonfollicularly-based papules coalescing into keratotic plaques in a seborrheic distribution; often accompanied by warty papules on the dorsum of hands (acrokeratosis verruciformis of Hopf), palmar pits, and nail disease (v-nicking, red streaks)

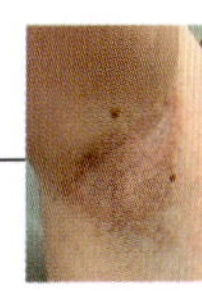
14

→ Consider Darier Disease

- Poor or variable demarcation
  - (E) Seborrheic distribution?*
    - No
      - Satellite papules and pustules?
        - No
          - Presenting as either pink poorly demarcated edematous plaques (acute) or scaly lichenified and hyperpigmented plaques (chronic) following exposure to an allergen or irritant—commonly detergent, deodorant, or clothing

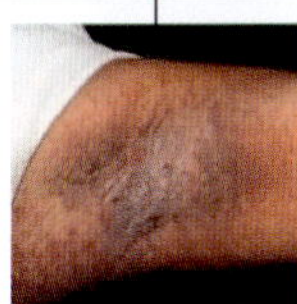
6

→ Consider Allergic (ACD) or Irritant Contact Dermatitis (ICD)

Further work-up with patch testing can help differentiate between ACD and ICD

        - (F) Yes
          - Beefy red plaques with peripheral scale and surrounding satellite papules and/or pustules

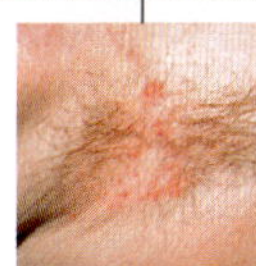
5

→ Consider Candidal Intertrigo

    - Yes
      - Chronic salmon pink plaques with greasy scale on the scalp, eyebrows, glabella, ears, central chest, and less commonly axilla and groin

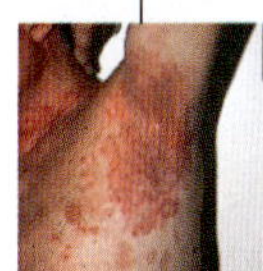
4

→ Consider Seborrheic Dermatitis

- Reticulated
  - Multiple, brown, keratotic, verrucous, thin papules that coalesce into reticulated plaques

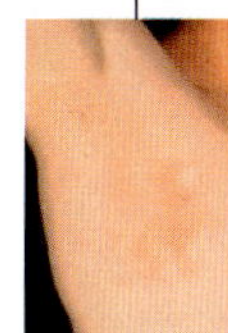
3

→ Consider Confluent and Reticulated Papillomatosis

*Seborrheic distribution: Areas rich in sebaceous glands particularly the scalp, forehead, eyebrows, facial hair, glabella, postauricular area, and skin folds

PART VIII
Pustules

47 Scalp Pustules

Cathryn Sibbald and Chaocheng Liu

Several immunobullous disorders affect the scalp and present as crusted erosions, and they may mimic a pustular eruption, especially if secondarily infected. The three most common are described below (A–C), with a key differentiator being the amount of mucosal involvement clinically.

A. **Pemphigus foliaceus** presents with superficial blisters and crusted erosions in a seborrheic distribution, including the scalp, face, and upper trunk. It is caused by autoantibodies against desmoglein 1 (anti-Dsg1). Patients have minimal mucosal involvement because of intact desmoglein 3 (Dsg3) throughout the mucosal epithelium. Direct immunofluorescence (DIF) of skin biopsy demonstrates intercellular staining of the epidermis with IgG and C3.

B. In contrast, patients with **pemphigus vulgaris**, in addition to flaccid bullae and crusted erosions over the scalp and other skin sites, can have moderate erosive mucosal involvement, typically the oral mucosa. The condition's target antigens are Dsg3 (mucosal-dominant pemphigus) or both Dsg1 and Dsg3 (mucocutaneous pemphigus). DIF staining of intact mucosa and skin demonstrates similar findings as pemphigus foliaceus.

C. In **mucous membrane pemphigoid**, patients develop more severe and extensive erosions most commonly affecting the oral mucosa and conjunctiva. Additionally, blisters and crusted erosions are found on the scalp, face, and neck. Anogenital, laryngeal, and esophageal mucosal surfaces are less commonly affected. Mucous membrane pemphigoid comprises a heterogeneous group of chronic blistering disorders caused by antibodies to several different antigens, including bullous pemphigoid antigen 1/2, laminin-5, laminin-6, and integrin beta-4 subunit of alpha-6-beta-4 integrin.

D. **Erosive pustular dermatosis (EPD)** of the scalp is a rare inflammatory condition that most commonly occurs in elderly patients with lighter skin phototypes and extensive actinic damage. Patients may have a history of actinic keratoses with cryotherapy treatment and/or skin cancer. It presents with superficial sterile pustules and crusted erosions that can lead to weeping and shallow ulcers and ultimately scarring alopecia. Affected areas may be beefy red with atrophy of the surrounding skin. There are no pathognomonic histological findings for EPD. Detailed clinical examination with possible biopsy is important to rule out keratinocytic carcinoma.

E. **Eosinophilic folliculitis (EF)** presents as recurrent crops of pustules on an erythematous base with crusting mostly over the scalp that may spread to the face, neck, and extremities. Prominent pruritus is the hallmark symptom. There are three subtypes of EF that present in distinct demographic groups, including classic eosinophilic pustular folliculitis (Ofuji disease, commonly in the Japanese population in their 30s–40s), immunosuppression-associated EF (most commonly in HIV-positive patients), and neonatal eosinophilic pustular folliculitis. A smear of the central pustule content reveals numerous eosinophils on Wright stain preparations. Skin biopsy demonstrating spongiosis and dense perifollicular mixed infiltrate with eosinophils and lymphocytes is diagnostic.

Infectious folliculitis presents as folliculocentric and erythematous pustules and papules on hair-bearing skin. Assessment of risk factors and associated clinical findings can help delineate the causes and guide investigations.

F. **Staphylococcal folliculitis** is the most common bacterial folliculitis that affects the scalp, face, upper trunk, buttocks, and legs. Risk factors include colonization with *Staphylococcus aureus*, hyperhidrosis, and shaving. It can be diagnosed clinically, but a Gram stain and culture of the contents of a pustule can confirm the species.

G. ***Malassezia* folliculitis**, with common causes being *Malassezia globosa*, *Malassezia sympodialis*, and *Malassezia furfur*, usually presents with monomorphic erythematous papules and pustules with seborrheic distribution and sometimes over the scalp. Patients may have risk factors, including immunosuppression, humid weather, or recent antibiotic use. A KOH preparation, fungal culture, or skin biopsies help with the diagnosis.

H. ***Demodex* folliculitis** is less common and characterized by inflammatory papules and pustules classically over the face and neck. Scalp involvement is rare and may be associated with erythema, scales, and nonscarring alopecia. A KOH preparation of a skin scraping is used to detect *Demodex* mites.

I. **Herpes simplex viruses (HSV)** 1 and 2 can present as tender grouped 2- to 4 mm vesicles, erosions, or pustules on an erythematous base. It can affect anywhere on the body including the scalp. The lesions may progress to punched-out monomorphic circular ulcers. Tzanck preparation demonstrates multinucleate keratinocytes, acantholysis, keratinocyte ballooning, and nuclear margination in herpetic infections but cannot differentiate HSV from varicella zoster virus (VZV). A viral swab of the content of an intact blister or pustule for polymerase chain reaction testing can confirm the diagnosis.

J. **Herpes zoster** can have a similar morphology as HSV but with dermatomal distribution. It is due to the reactivation of VZV in dorsal root ganglia. Patients often report a few days of paresthesia or pain before rash onset. Examination of the eye is critical if the nasal tip is involved, as this indicates involvement of the nasociliary nerve which also innervates the eye. Diagnostic methods are similar to HSV.

K. **Folliculitis decalvans (FD)** presents as perifollicular erythematous papules and pustules in crops on the vertex scalp, most commonly in middle-aged adults. The follicular pustules are often painful, and scarring alopecia can develop if untreated. A characteristic feature is polytrichia when several residual hairs growing out of a single hair follicle ("tufted hairs"). Scalp biopsy of active lesions reveals a suppurative folliculitis with dense, neutrophilic perifollicular inflammation at the upper portion of follicles. *S. aureus* is often isolated when culture of the pustules is performed.

L. **Dissecting cellulitis of the scalp**, also known as perifolliculitis capitis abscedens et suffodiens, is another type of neutrophilic scarring alopecia that often affects both the vertex and occipital scalp, most commonly in young adult Black males. In the early stage, there are boggy or fluctuant pustules and nodules that may exude pus. These may be tender, but marked pain is usually absent. Dermal fibrosis, sinus tracts, and hypertrophic scarring with alopecia occur with disease progression. One should be aware of the risk of squamous cell carcinoma in patients with chronic disease. Skin biopsy and culture can help with the diagnosis. Dissecting cellulitis is part of the follicular occlusion tetrad along with acne conglobata, hidradenitis suppurativa, and pilonidal cyst. Screening for these conditions with a detailed history and physical examination is important.

Continued

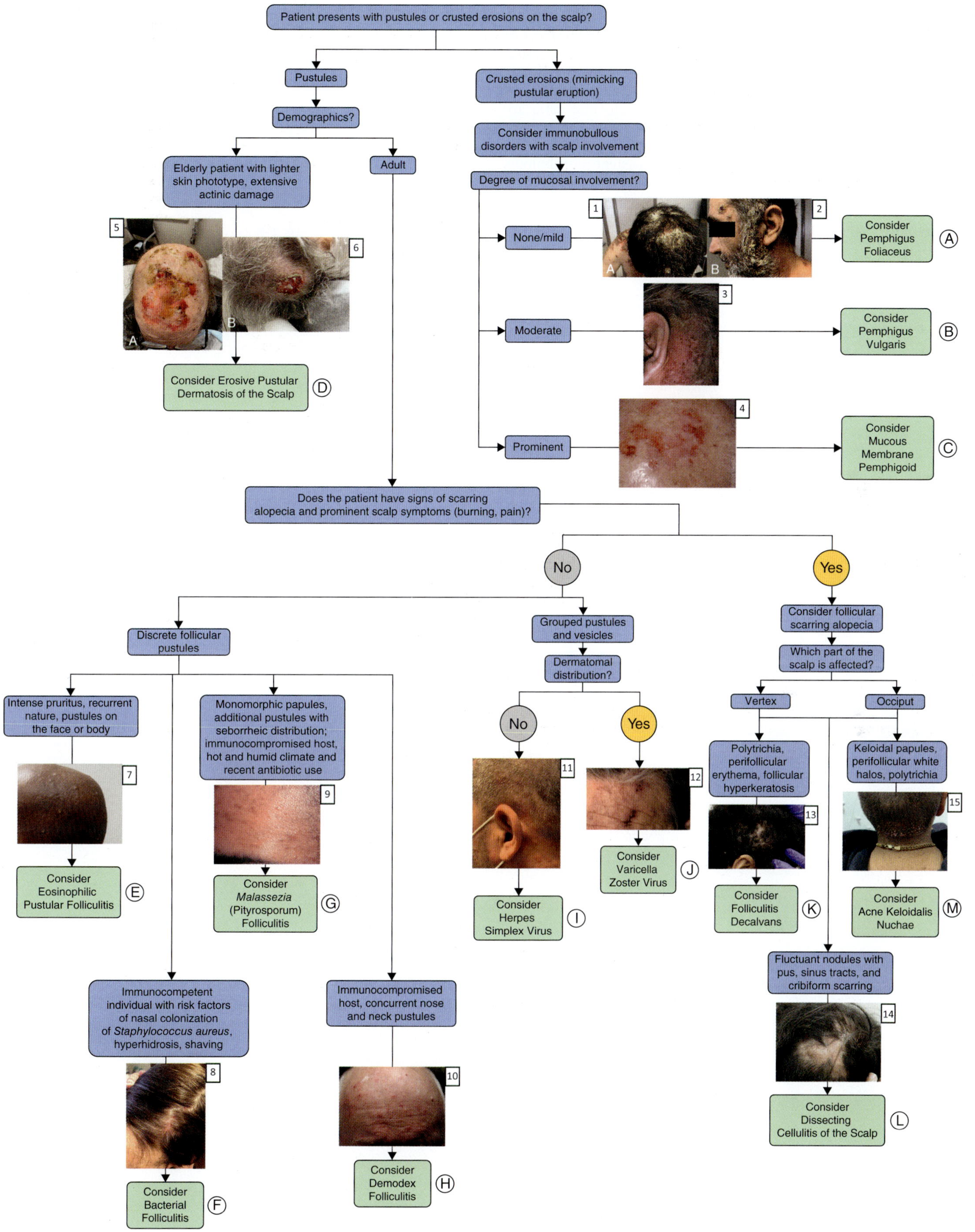
Patient presents with pustules or crusted erosions on the scalp?
Pustules
Demographics?
Elderly patient with lighter skin phototype, extensive actinic damage
5
A
6
B
Consider Erosive Pustular Dermatosis of the Scalp
D
Adult
Crusted erosions (mimicking pustular eruption)
Consider immunobullous disorders with scalp involvement
Degree of mucosal involvement?
None/mild
1
A
B
2
Consider Pemphigus Foliaceus
A
Moderate
3
Consider Pemphigus Vulgaris
B
Prominent
4
Consider Mucous Membrane Pemphigoid
C
Does the patient have signs of scarring alopecia and prominent scalp symptoms (burning, pain)?
No
Yes
Discrete follicular pustules
Intense pruritus, recurrent nature, pustules on the face or body
7
Consider Eosinophilic Pustular Folliculitis
E
Monomorphic papules, additional pustules with seborrheic distribution; immunocompromised host, hot and humid climate and recent antibiotic use
9
Consider *Malassezia* (Pityrosporum) Folliculitis
G
Immunocompetent individual with risk factors of nasal colonization of *Staphylococcus aureus*, hyperhidrosis, shaving
8
Consider Bacterial Folliculitis
F
Immunocompromised host, concurrent nose and neck pustules
10
Consider Demodex Folliculitis
H
Grouped pustules and vesicles
Dermatomal distribution?
No
11
Consider Herpes Simplex Virus
I
Yes
12
Consider Varicella Zoster Virus
J
Consider follicular scarring alopecia
Which part of the scalp is affected?
Vertex
Occiput
Polytrichia, perifollicular erythema, follicular hyperkeratosis
13
Consider Folliculitis Decalvans
K
Keloidal papules, perifollicular white halos, polytrichia
15
Consider Acne Keloidalis Nuchae
M
Fluctuant nodules with pus, sinus tracts, and cribiform scarring
14
Consider Dissecting Cellulitis of the Scalp
L

M. Acne keloidalis nuchae (AKN) most commonly affects Black males in their 20s. It presents with erythematous, indurated follicular papules and pustules without comedones over the occipital scalp, which may coalesce to form keloidal plaques in long-standing disease. AKN may be asymptomatic, or patients may complain of pain and pruritus. Polytrichia and loss of follicular ostia are apparent in the advanced disease under dermoscopy. Concurrent acneiform eruptions and pseudofolliculitis may be present. The diagnosis can be made clinically based on consistent morphology, distribution, and demographics.

See Appendix 1 for Further Reading and Image References.

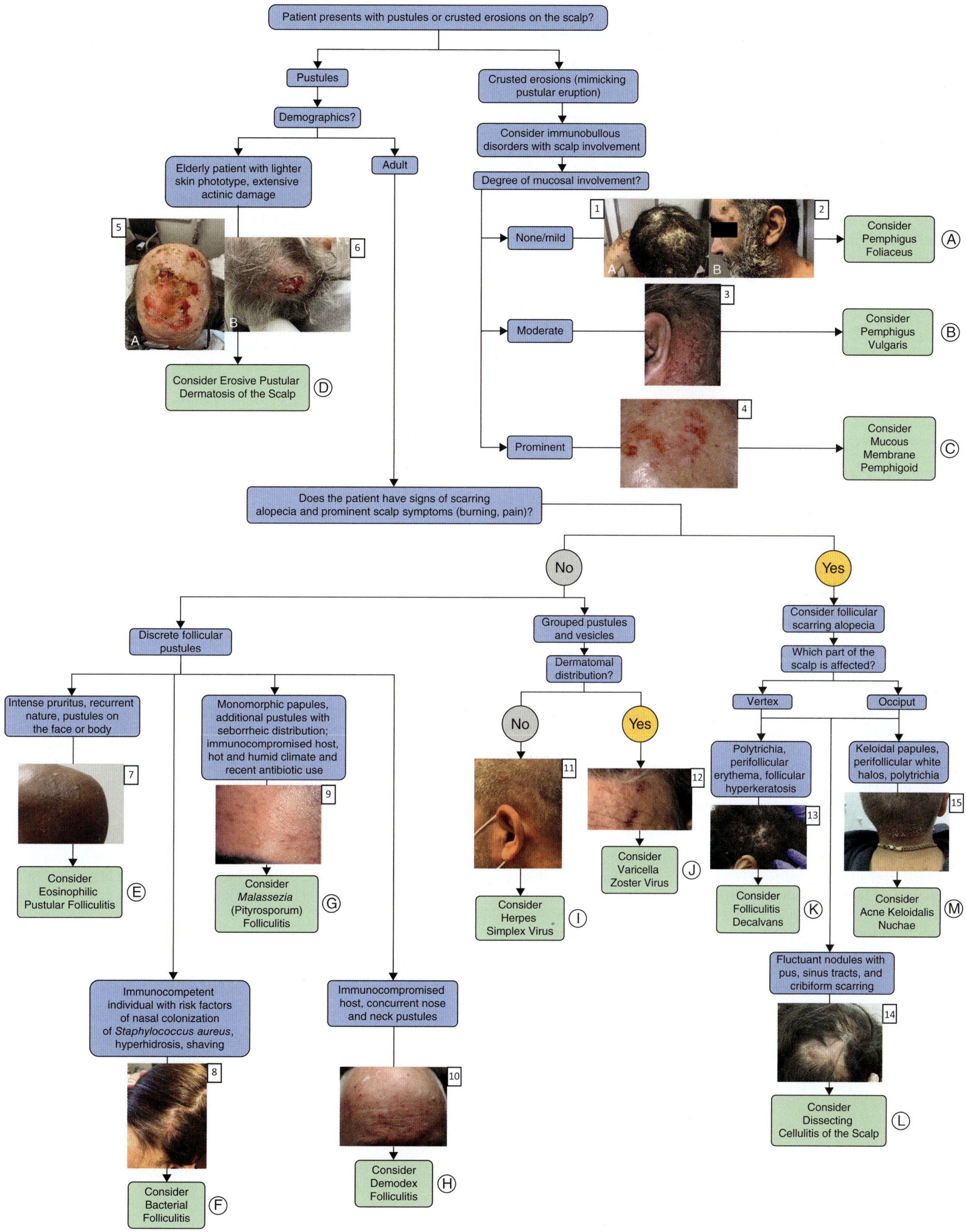
Patient presents with pustules or crusted erosions on the scalp?
Pustules
Demographics?
Elderly patient with lighter skin phototype, extensive actinic damage
5
A
B
6
Consider Erosive Pustular Dermatosis of the Scalp
D
Adult
Crusted erosions (mimicking pustular eruption)
Consider immunobullous disorders with scalp involvement
Degree of mucosal involvement?
None/mild
1
A
B
2
Consider Pemphigus Foliaceus
A
Moderate
3
Consider Pemphigus Vulgaris
B
Prominent
4
Consider Mucous Membrane Pemphigoid
C
Does the patient have signs of scarring alopecia and prominent scalp symptoms (burning, pain)?
No
Discrete follicular pustules
Intense pruritus, recurrent nature, pustules on the face or body
7
Consider Eosinophilic Pustular Folliculitis
E
Monomorphic papules, additional pustules with seborrheic distribution; immunocompromised host, hot and humid climate and recent antibiotic use
9
Consider *Malassezia* (Pityrosporum) Folliculitis
G
Immunocompetent individual with risk factors of nasal colonization of *Staphylococcus aureus*, hyperhidrosis, shaving
8
Consider Bacterial Folliculitis
F
Immunocompromised host, concurrent nose and neck pustules
10
Consider Demodex Folliculitis
H
Grouped pustules and vesicles
Dermatomal distribution?
No
11
Consider Herpes Simplex Virus
I
Yes
12
Consider Varicella Zoster Virus
J
Yes
Consider follicular scarring alopecia
Which part of the scalp is affected?
Vertex
Polytrichia, perifollicular erythema, follicular hyperkeratosis
13
Consider Folliculitis Decalvans
K
Occiput
Keloidal papules, perifollicular white halos, polytrichia
15
Consider Acne Keloidalis Nuchae
M
Fluctuant nodules with pus, sinus tracts, and cribiform scarring
14
Consider Dissecting Cellulitis of the Scalp
L

48 Palmoplantar Pustules

David Croitoru and Cathryn Sibbald

Pustules are formed by collections of granulocytes, often neutrophils, and macrophages in the epidermis. Their presence often prompts investigation for infectious etiology, but many causes are inflammatory, including manifestations of systemic disease, paraneoplastic phenomena, and hypersensitivity reactions. Localization of the eruption, focally or with generalized pustules, along with clinical history helps narrow the differential diagnosis substantially. Management of inflammatory noninfectious entities may include topical and systemic immunosuppressive and immunomodulating therapeutics, whereas antimicrobials and antiparasitic agents are indicated for infectious etiologies.

The clinical approach to palmoplantar pustules relies on a detailed but focused history that includes infectious risk factors, exposure history (e.g., contact allergens, irritants, medications, biologics), and personal/familial medical history of primary inflammatory skin diseases and their associated systemic diseases (e.g., inflammatory bowel disease). Despite presumed localization to acral sites, full-body skin examination should be performed to exclude the involvement of special sites that may point to a specific diagnosis (scalp, concha, nails, and umbilicus for psoriasis; interdigital space for scabies; contiguous dermatomes for secondary varicella-zoster virus). Bacterial and viral swabs of lanced pustules or superficial abscesses should be sent for culture and biopsy for histopathology; biopsy for direct immunofluorescence is rarely required.

Several pustular entities can be localized to the palms and soles.

A. **Blistering dactylitis**, due to *Streptococcus pyogenes* or *Staphylococcus aureus*, presents with acutely painful pustules or blisters localized to a digit with concurrent inflammation and possible paronychia or deeper abscesses. It starts at the distal fat pad of the digit (or toe) but can then spread to the rest of the phalanx. Although it is more common in children, adults can also be affected. Bacterial cultures can confirm the etiology, and viral cultures can rule out mimickers.

B. **Herpes simplex virus** (**HSV**) and **varicella zoster virus** can present as pustules at acral sites, often characterized by a loculated painful cluster of deep pustules, in the same location if recurrent. These pustules may desquamate, leaving monomorphic "punched-out" erosions. Herpetic whitlow, HSV infection of the finger, can occur in healthcare providers such as dentists, whose fingers may be inoculated from active viral particles in a patient's mouth.

C. **Tinea manuum** and **tinea pedis** describe dermatophyte infection, affecting the hands and feet, respectively. These have several morphological forms, including a hyperkeratotic form (most common), interdigital, vesiculobullous, exfoliative, and papular. The vesiculobullous form can present with pustules and tends to concentrate around the interdigital spaces. Less commonly, it may present as an annular plaque with studded pustules. Concurrent onychomycosis may be present. Tinea infections tend to be asymptomatic; scrapings of pustules for KOH and culture can aid in the diagnosis.

D. Dermatitis eruptions that are localized to hands include **contact dermatitis** and **dyshidrotic dermatitis (pompholyx)**. A history of potential allergens suggests contact dermatitis, whereas frequent handwashing and deep monomorphic vesicopustules along the lateral sides of the fingers and thenar eminence are characteristic of dyshidrosis. Dyshidrosis and allergic contact dermatitis are intensely pruritic. Irritant contact dermatitis can present with pustules when secondary to chlorhexidine.

E. **Palmoplantar pustulosis** presents with sterile pustules localized to the hands and feet, often affecting middle-aged patients with a history of smoking and no history of tumor necrosis factor (TNF) inhibitors. Pustules may be localized to smaller areas such as the hypothenar and thenar eminence of the hands and heels of the feet or may affect the entire palmoplantar surface. Pustules may evolve to red-brown macules, and nails may be affected by pustules under the nails. This entity is thought to differ from psoriasis in its involvement of interleukin-36 signaling and resistance to TNF inhibition.

   Paradoxical psoriasis, appearing after initiation of treatments indicated to treat psoriasis, presents in a localized pustular form on the palms and soles in more than 50% of cases in some series. It can look identical to palmoplantar psoriasis, with small deep pustules and red-brown macules within larger psoriasiform plaques. The most common implicated triggers are TNF-alpha inhibitors, with a large range of onset from days to months after drug exposure. History of drug exposure and resolution with discontinuation of the trigger help confirm the diagnosis.

F. If substantial weight loss, rigors, or drenching night sweats are detected on a review of systems, a thorough assessment of age-appropriate malignancy screening and risk factors should be performed. Rarely, **acrokeratosis paraneoplastica (Bazex syndrome)** can present as a pustular palmoplantar eruption, often with the involvement of the helices and nails in the first stage. Keratotic plaques can develop on the palms and soles with more systemic symptoms in the second stage. The most common associated malignancies are squamous cell carcinomas of the aerodigestive tract.

The differential diagnosis for patients who present with palmoplantar pustules is wide. However, an approach that utilizes both regional distribution and etiological distinction with a focused history and physical examination can effectively delineate diagnoses and substantially improve pretest accuracy.

See Appendix 1 for Further Reading.

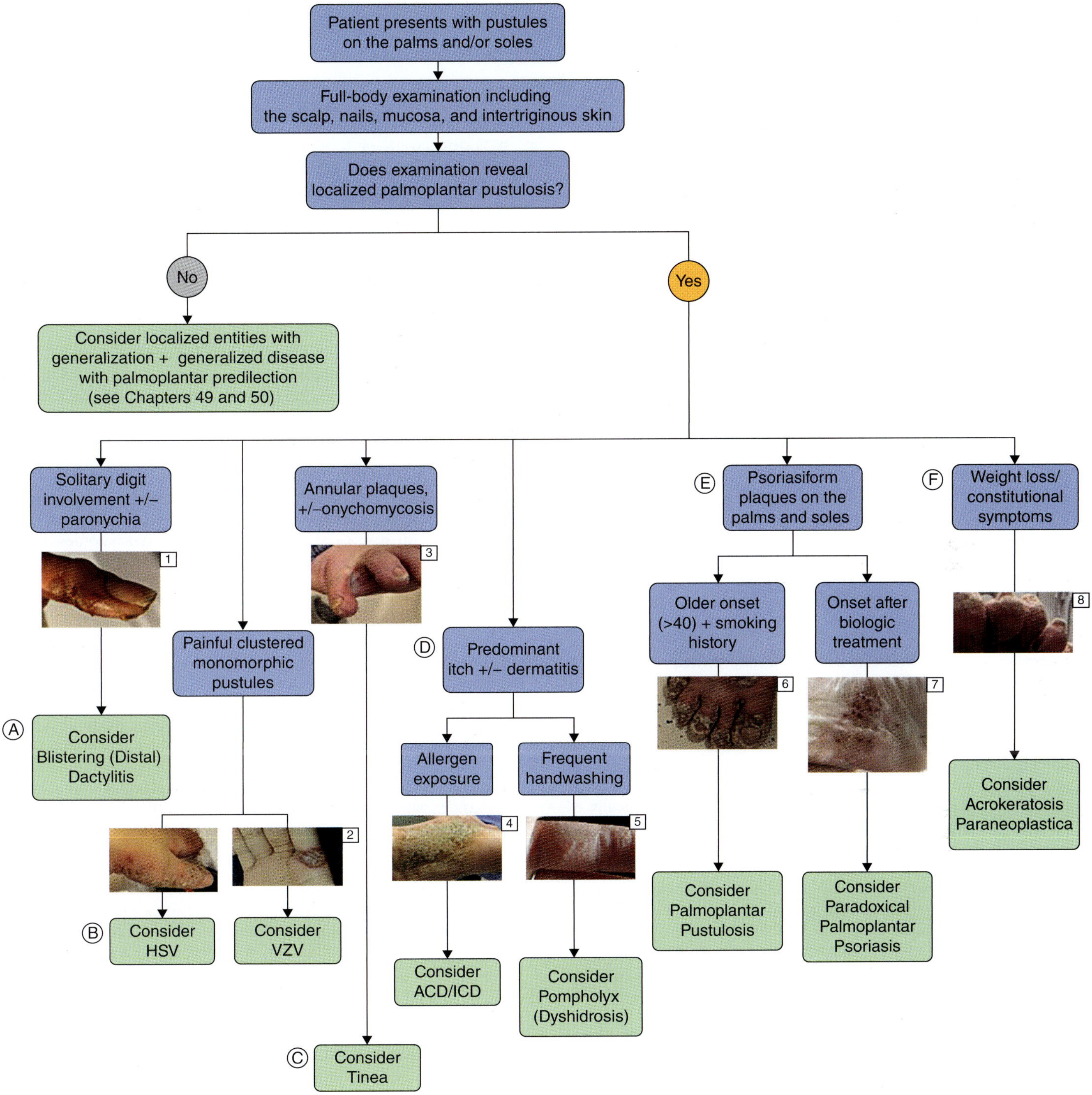
Patient presents with pustules on the palms and/or soles
Full-body examination including the scalp, nails, mucosa, and intertriginous skin
Does examination reveal localized palmoplantar pustulosis?
No
Consider localized entities with generalization + generalized disease with palmoplantar predilection (see Chapters 49 and 50)
Yes
Solitary digit involvement +/− paronychia
1
Ⓐ Consider Blistering (Distal) Dactylitis
Painful clustered monomorphic pustules
2
Ⓑ Consider HSV
Consider VZV
Annular plaques, +/−onychomycosis
3
Ⓒ Consider Tinea
Ⓓ Predominant itch +/− dermatitis
Allergen exposure
4
Consider ACD/ICD
Frequent handwashing
5
Consider Pompholyx (Dyshidrosis)
Ⓔ Psoriasiform plaques on the palms and soles
Older onset (>40) + smoking history
6
Consider Palmoplantar Pustulosis
Onset after biologic treatment
7
Consider Paradoxical Palmoplantar Psoriasis
Ⓕ Weight loss/ constitutional symptoms
8
Consider Acrokeratosis Paraneoplastica

49 Localized Pustules

Evan Alexander Choate and Emily Michelle Altman

Localized pustular dermatoses encompass a broad array of inflammatory and infectious etiologies, defined both by accompanying systemic symptoms and by the contents found within the pustules. Central to their evaluation is the elicitation of the eruption's timeline and evolution, inoculation events, and occupational hazards. Outpatient management usually suffices as these conditions carry a low mortality risk, although careful identification of higher-risk features, including fevers, arthralgias, sepsis, and further dissemination, remains critical. Treatments range from antimicrobials or antineutrophilic agents to supportive therapies and anticipatory guidance. Localized scalp pustules are discussed in Chapter 47. Generalized pustules are discussed in Chapter 50.

A. The following select members of *Poxviridae* cause localized vesiculopustules and can be confirmed by virus-specific real-time polymerase chain reaction (RT-PCR). Live **vaccinia** virus is used for smallpox immunization in the military, first responders, and global health workers. Satellite lesions may arise locally or via Kaposi varicelliform eruption and leave pitted scars. Monkeypox virus (causing mpox), although historically acquired solely by direct inoculation with infected monkey or rodent hosts in Africa, spreads rapidly via human to human transmission. **Cowpox** is acquired via inoculation by an infected bovine or feline host. As such, an inflamed papule emerges at the hand or extremity before evolving into a hemorrhagic vesicle or pustule and later ulcerating.

B. **Impetigo** and **cellulitis** can complicate any primary dermatosis, including posttraumatic, eczematous, and dermatophytic conditions, and thereby promote pustulation. Concomitant symptoms including fevers, lymphadenopathy, arthritis, and sepsis may be present. Bacterial culture and Gram stain will often yield gram-positive cocci, namely *Staphylococcus* or *Streptococcus* species. Animal handlers are at risk for *Listeria monocytogenes* inoculation in particular, which prompts a hemorrhagic pustular or petechial eruption typically of an upper extremity. Diagnosis is achieved with bacterial culture and Gram stain demonstrating gram-positive rods.

C. Flaring **psoriasis** can present with pustules situated in annular configurations or at the leading edge of unstable chronic plaques, often triggered by rapid tapering of oral systemic therapies. Patients may endorse fever, malaise, or inflammatory arthropathy. Biopsy will demonstrate corneal and subcorneal neutrophilic pustules (spongiform pustules of Kogoj) in addition to classic psoriasis characteristics.

D. **Pustular pyoderma gangrenosum (PG)** will demonstrate small, sterile, and occasionally pathergic pustules. Some may represent early lesions that subsequently necrose into classic pyoderma gangrenosum ulcers. It is most commonly associated with inflammatory bowel disease, although inflammatory arthritides (e.g., rheumatoid), autoinflammatory syndromes (e.g., PAPA syndrome), and hematologic disorders (e.g., IgA monoclonal gammopathy) are also linked. Diagnosis requires ruling out infectious etiologies and inquiring about associated conditions; a biopsy may be supportive but typically demonstrates nonspecific neutrophilic infiltrates with early leukocytoclasia. Other neutrophilic dermatoses, including **Behçet syndrome** and **Crohn's disease**, may show nonspecific localized pustules accompanying other disease-specific findings.

E. **Balanitis circinata** is a parainfectious dermatosis triggered by Chlamydia, bacterial gastroenteritis, or HIV. Here, psoriasiform plaques and inflammatory papules and pustules predominate on the penis. This, alongside keratoderma blennorrhagicum, is a common cutaneous sign of reactive arthritis (conjunctivitis, urethritis, polyarthritis). While fevers and gastrointestinal symptoms may resolve by rash onset, supportive diagnostic features include HLA-B27 positivity, elevated ESR, sterile pyuria, positive stool cultures/PCR, or positive chlamydia testing.

F. **Gonococcemia** can exhibit small petechiae, erythematous or hemorrhagic papules, or vesiculopustules overlying large joints. Systemic symptoms include fevers, chills, myalgias, tenosynovitis, and mucopurulent urethritis/cervicitis. Pustule culture is the diagnostic gold standard; however, nucleic acid amplification testing or Gram stain for neutrophils and diplococci may be employed.

G. **Varicella zoster virus (VZV)**, typically in the elderly or immunocompromised, will classically materialize as painful, hyperesthetic "dew drops on rose petals" along the affected dermatomes. Older lesions evolve into pustules and crust over in various stages of healing. There may be a constitutional prodrome or morbidity associated with ocular or otic involvement. Diagnosis is achieved by fresh lesional VZV PCR.

H. **Miliaria pustulosa** represents subcorneal eccrine obstruction secondary to excessive heat or humidity at sites occluded by clothing, dressings, emollients, or dependent positioning. It is clinically evidenced as nonfollicular, minimally erythematous pustules, which may be accompanied by the erythematous papules of miliaria rubra.

I. Scattered inflammatory pustules of the face or other sebaceous areas alongside papulonodules, comedones, postinflammatory dyspigmentation, and scars characterize **acne vulgaris**. Hormonal influences shape disease activity and flares, both physiologically (menses, stress) and pathologically (hyperandrogenism).

J. Acneiform papules and pustules of the central face without scarring typify **papulopustular rosacea**. This morphology may overlap with erythematotelangiectatic, ocular, or phymatous subtypes. Patients may endorse concomitant flushing and burning or observe triggers for their symptoms, including ultraviolet light, spicy food, alcohol, or topical corticosteroids. Variants include predominant periorificial clustering (periorificial dermatitis) and robust reactivity to colonizing mites *(Demodex* folliculitis).

K. **Drug-induced acneiform eruptions** of the head and neck are more monomorphous and occur after 2 to 8 weeks of using topical and systemic corticosteroids, anabolic steroids, progestins, lithium, or occupational halogens.

L. Lastly, any localized vesiculobullous eruption (Chapter 18) over time may acquire pustular morphologies.

See Appendix 1 for Further Reading and Image References.

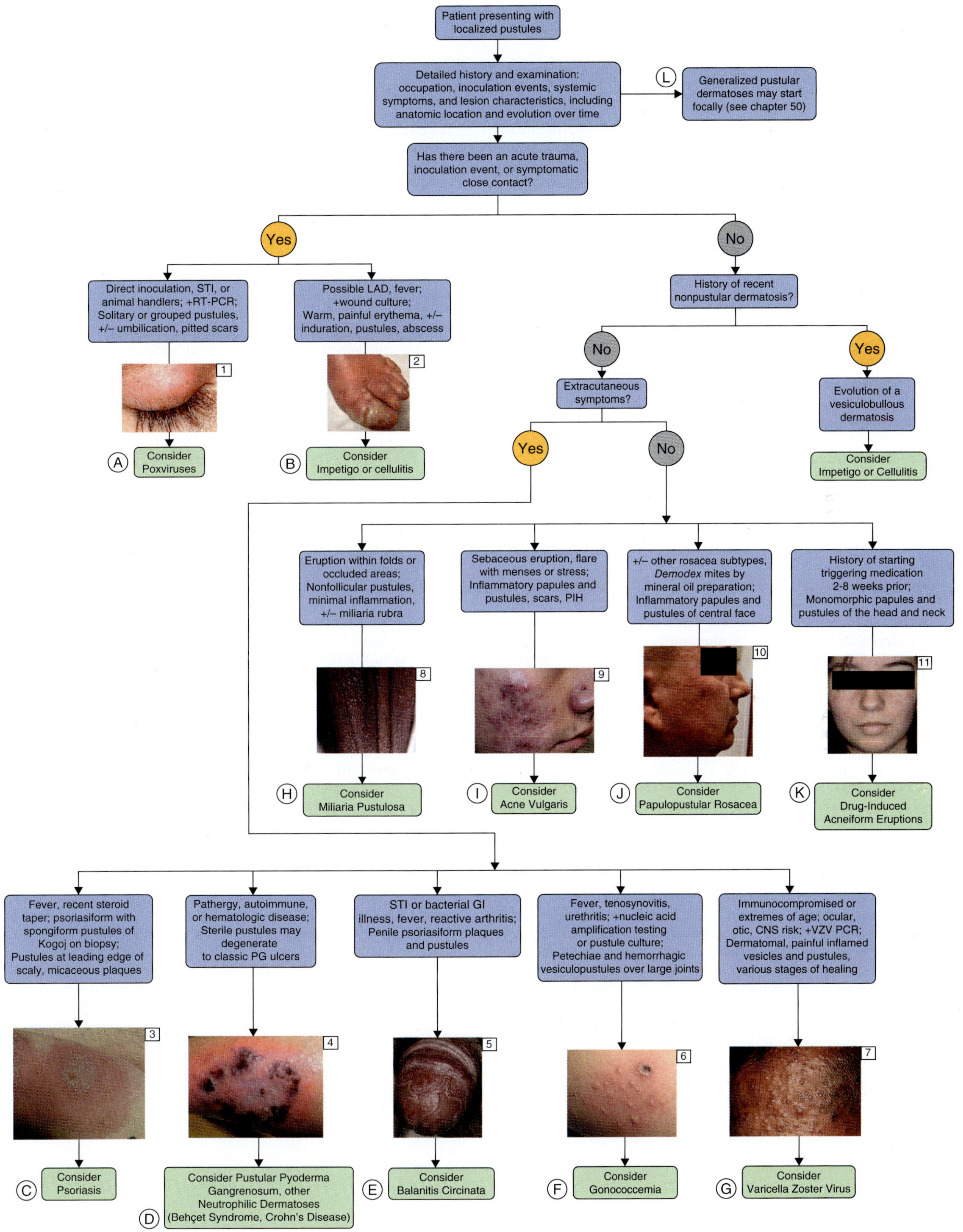
Patient presenting with localized pustules
Detailed history and examination: occupation, inoculation events, systemic symptoms, and lesion characteristics, including anatomic location and evolution over time
L
Generalized pustular dermatoses may start focally (see chapter 50)
Has there been an acute trauma, inoculation event, or symptomatic close contact?
Yes
Direct inoculation, STI, or animal handlers; +RT-PCR; Solitary or grouped pustules, +/– umbilication, pitted scars
1
A
Consider Poxviruses
Possible LAD, fever; +wound culture; Warm, painful erythema, +/– induration, pustules, abscess
2
B
Consider Impetigo or cellulitis
No
History of recent nonpustular dermatosis?
Yes
Evolution of a vesiculobullous dermatosis
Consider Impetigo or Cellulitis
No
Extracutaneous symptoms?
No
Eruption within folds or occluded areas; Nonfollicular pustules, minimal inflammation, +/– miliaria rubra
8
H
Consider Miliaria Pustulosa
Sebaceous eruption, flare with menses or stress; Inflammatory papules and pustules, scars, PIH
9
I
Consider Acne Vulgaris
+/– other rosacea subtypes, Demodex mites by mineral oil preparation; Inflammatory papules and pustules of central face
10
J
Consider Papulopustular Rosacea
History of starting triggering medication 2-8 weeks prior; Monomorphic papules and pustules of the head and neck
11
K
Consider Drug-Induced Acneiform Eruptions
Yes
Fever, recent steroid taper; psoriasiform with spongiform pustules of Kogoj on biopsy; Pustules at leading edge of scaly, micaceous plaques
3
C
Consider Psoriasis
Pathergy, autoimmune, or hematologic disease; Sterile pustules may degenerate to classic PG ulcers
4
D
Consider Pustular Pyoderma Gangrenosum, other Neutrophilic Dermatoses (Behçet Syndrome, Crohn's Disease)
STI or bacterial GI illness, fever, reactive arthritis; Penile psoriasiform plaques and pustules
5
E
Consider Balanitis Circinata
Fever, tenosynovitis, urethritis; +nucleic acid amplification testing or pustule culture; Petechiae and hemorrhagic vesiculopustules over large joints
6
F
Consider Gonococcemia
Immunocompromised or extremes of age; ocular, otic, CNS risk; +VZV PCR; Dermatomal, painful inflamed vesicles and pustules, various stages of healing
7
G
Consider Varicella Zoster Virus

50 Generalized Pustules

Katherine Elizabeth Park and Emily Michelle Altman

Generalized pustular disorders encompass a broad differential of inflammatory and infectious etiologies. The differential also contains multiple disorders with potential systemic involvement that can be life threatening. For accurate diagnosis, it can be critical to have a detailed history, including medication history, thorough infectious workup, evaluation for systemic involvement, and biopsy.

A. **Folliculitis** presents as multiple pruritic follicularly based pustules. Mild systemic symptoms may be present but are uncommon. Common causative microorganisms include bacteria such as *Streptococcus* species, *Staphylococcus aureus*, and *Pseudomonas aeruginosa*, yeasts such as *Malassezia* species, viruses including herpes simplex virus, and less commonly, mites such as *Demodex*. Pustule cultures, viral polymerase chain reaction (PCR), and skin scrapings/KOH preparations can help identify the causative organism.

B. **Disseminated herpes simplex** and **herpes zoster** can present with generalized pustules, especially in immunocompromised patients. Pustules may occur alongside or develop from vesicles, classically grouped and overlying an erythematous base. Punched-out ulcerations may also be present. Systemic symptoms may include fevers, lymphadenopathy, and internal organ involvement such as lung or central nervous system disease. Herpes simplex virus or varicella zoster virus PCR can aid in diagnosis.

C. **Reactive arthritis**, formerly Reiter syndrome, is a typically self-limited syndrome of ocular inflammation, mucosal ulcers, urethritis, arthritis, and psoriasiform skin lesions. It is strongly associated with HLA-B27 but may occur after various infections, including *Chlamydia trachomatis, Shigella flexneri, Yersinia enterocolitica*, and *Campylobacter jejuni,* and in patients with human immunodeficiency virus. Cutaneous lesions often occur on the scalp, dorsal fingers and hands, nails, penis, extensor legs, and soles of the feet. Biopsy is indistinguishable from pustular psoriasis.

D. **Subcorneal pustular dermatosis** (Sneddon-Wilkinson disease) is a neutrophilic dermatosis consisting of recurrent sterile subcorneal pustules predominantly on the trunk and proximal extremities, especially flexural and intertriginous skin. "Half-half" blisters may be noted with clear fluid superiorly and pus inferiorly. Pathology is not specific but consists of subcorneal pustules with neutrophils and occasional eosinophils. Acantholysis may be present on biopsies from older lesions. Lesions generally respond to dapsone. A complete blood count with differential and serum protein electrophoresis with immunofixation should be performed to rule out associated disorders, such as IgA monoclonal gammopathy and multiple myeloma.

E. **Drug reaction with eosinophilia and systemic symptoms (DRESS)** has a pustular variant. Similar to acute generalized exanthematous pustulosis (see section G), DRESS is a drug-induced hypersensitivity syndrome; however, it typically occurs weeks to months after starting the offending drug. The classic presentation includes fevers, facial and hand edema, purpura, and cervical lymphadenopathy. On labs, peripheral leukocytosis, atypical lymphocytes, eosinophilia, as well as elevated transaminases may be observed. Renal, cardiac, and lung involvement can also occur.

F. **Generalized pustular psoriasis** is a rare subtype of psoriasis presenting as a generalized eruption of pustules and erythematous plaques. Episodes may be recurrent with rapid onset and are often present in patients with a history of psoriasis. It is associated with mutations in the *IL36RN* gene encoding an interleukin 36 receptor antagonist. Potential triggering factors include rapid tapering of corticosteroids, certain medications, pregnancy, and infections. Histology demonstrates a psoriasiform dermatosis with epidermal neutrophils and spongiform pustules of Kogoj. It typically lacks the necrotic keratinocytes and eosinophils present in acute generalized exanthematous pustulosis (see section G). There are several described variants of generalized pustular psoriasis. Pustular psoriasis in pregnancy, also known as impetigo herpetiformis, most commonly occurs early in the third trimester, starting in flexural areas and spreading outward with erythematous plaques with peripheral sterile pustules. Leukocytosis, electrolyte abnormalities, cardiac or renal failure, and sepsis have been associated with pustular psoriasis in pregnancy, as well as placental insufficiency leading to fetal growth restriction or miscarriage/stillbirth. The "localized" pattern involves pustules at the periphery of existing psoriatic plaques following application of an irritant, such as tar. The annular pattern demonstrates ringlike lesions with scaling and pustules at the advancing edge with central healing. The exanthematous pattern results in eruptions of small pustules that resolve after a few days, often secondary to medications such as lithium. Finally, the von Zumbusch pattern involves rapid onset of pustules and systemic symptoms ranging from fevers and malaise to life-threatening symptoms, such as sepsis, acute respiratory distress syndrome, neutrophilic pneumonitis, neutrophilic cholangitis, and renal dysfunction. Laboratory workup may reveal leukocytosis, elevated erythrocyte sedimentation rate, electrolyte abnormalities, and elevated antistreptolysin antibody.

G. **Acute generalized exanthematous pustulosis (AGEP)** is a rare, acute, nonfollicular pustular eruption. Medications are thought to trigger approximately 90% of cases, most commonly antimicrobial agents and calcium channel blockers. The eruption is acute, occurring within hours to days of starting the offending medication. AGEP classically occurs as an eruption of sterile pustules on an erythematous base. It typically starts on the face or intertriginous skin before spreading more diffusely. Fevers and leukocytosis with neutrophilia and eosinophilia are often present. Mucous membrane involvement is rare and is typically limited to erosions of the lips. Mild elevation of liver transaminases and creatinine clearance have been reported. Histological features include subcorneal or superficial intraepidermal pustules with adjacent neutrophils, vasculitis, and scattered necrotic keratinocytes. Eosinophils are often present within the pustules or dermis. Skin symptoms usually resolve within a few weeks of discontinuing the offending agent.

See Appendix 1 for Further Reading and Image References.

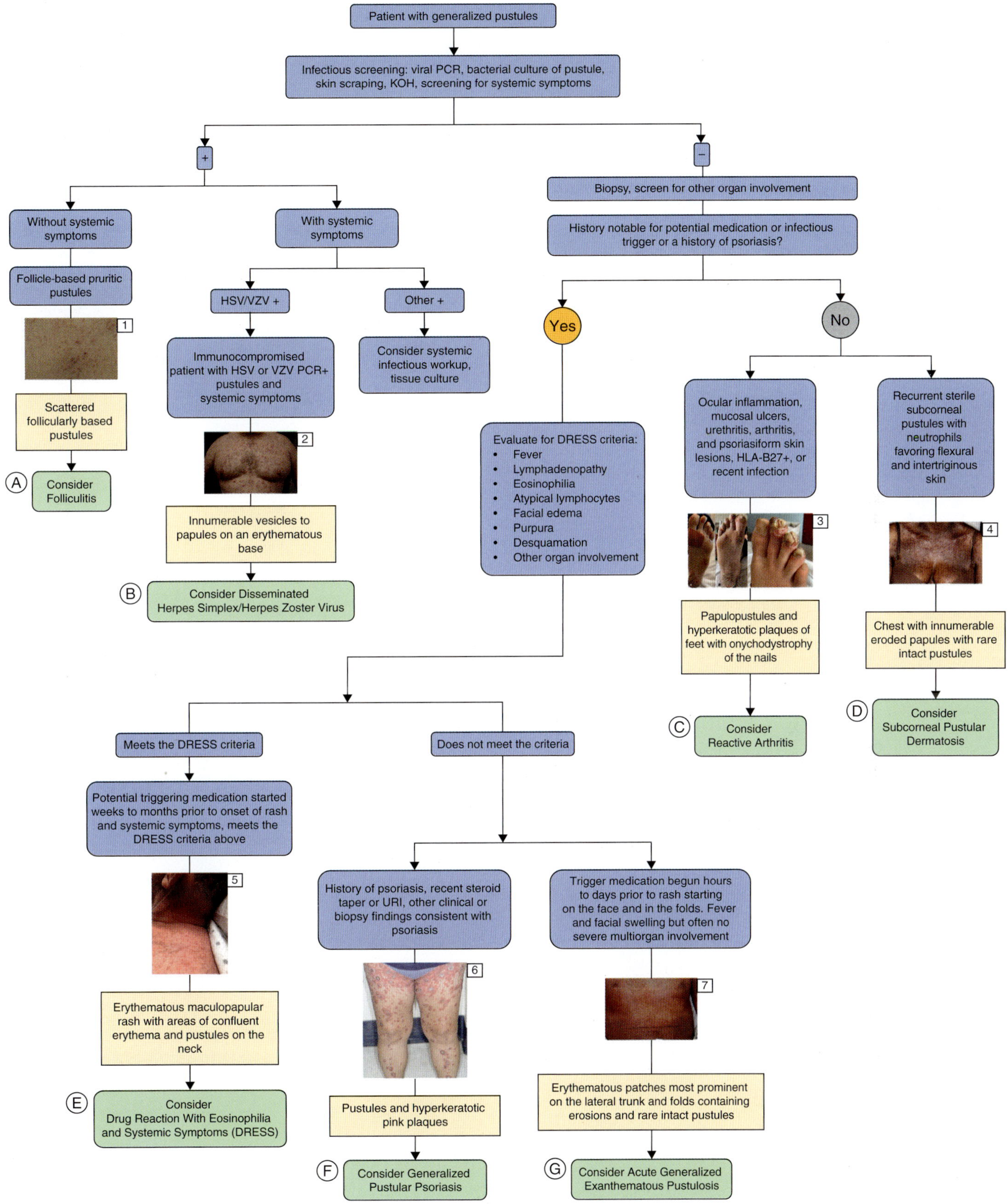
Patient with generalized pustules
Infectious screening: viral PCR, bacterial culture of pustule, skin scraping, KOH, screening for systemic symptoms
+
Without systemic symptoms
Follicle-based pruritic pustules
1
Scattered follicularly based pustules
A
Consider Folliculitis
With systemic symptoms
HSV/VZV +
Immunocompromised patient with HSV or VZV PCR+ pustules and systemic symptoms
2
Innumerable vesicles to papules on an erythematous base
B
Consider Disseminated Herpes Simplex/Herpes Zoster Virus
Other +
Consider systemic infectious workup, tissue culture
–
Biopsy, screen for other organ involvement
History notable for potential medication or infectious trigger or a history of psoriasis?
Yes
Evaluate for DRESS criteria:
• Fever
• Lymphadenopathy
• Eosinophilia
• Atypical lymphocytes
• Facial edema
• Purpura
• Desquamation
• Other organ involvement
Meets the DRESS criteria
Potential triggering medication started weeks to months prior to onset of rash and systemic symptoms, meets the DRESS criteria above
5
Erythematous maculopapular rash with areas of confluent erythema and pustules on the neck
E
Consider Drug Reaction With Eosinophilia and Systemic Symptoms (DRESS)
Does not meet the criteria
History of psoriasis, recent steroid taper or URI, other clinical or biopsy findings consistent with psoriasis
6
Pustules and hyperkeratotic pink plaques
F
Consider Generalized Pustular Psoriasis
Trigger medication begun hours to days prior to rash starting on the face and in the folds. Fever and facial swelling but often no severe multiorgan involvement
7
Erythematous patches most prominent on the lateral trunk and folds containing erosions and rare intact pustules
G
Consider Acute Generalized Exanthematous Pustulosis
No
Ocular inflammation, mucosal ulcers, urethritis, arthritis, and psoriasiform skin lesions, HLA-B27+, or recent infection
3
Papulopustules and hyperkeratotic plaques of feet with onychodystrophy of the nails
C
Consider Reactive Arthritis
Recurrent sterile subcorneal pustules with neutrophils favoring flexural and intertriginous skin
4
Chest with innumerable eroded papules with rare intact pustules
D
Consider Subcorneal Pustular Dermatosis

PART IX
Vascular

51 Telangiectasias

Nikhil Nair and Megan S. Evans

Telangiectasias are vascular lesions representing abnormal persistent dilations of previously established vasculature. Typical presentation is small, blanchable, light red to blue-purple macules or papules on cutaneous or mucocutaneous surfaces. Telangiectasias can be localized or widespread and may be primary or secondary in nature. Lasers, including intense pulsed light or pulsed dye laser, may be used in the treatment of telangiectasias.

A. The initial evaluation of a patient with telangiectasias should include a detailed history and physical examination. This includes determining the duration, location, and extent of the telangiectasias, as well as identifying any related signs or symptoms.

B. Primary localized telangiectasias are restricted to a certain region of the body and are not directly associated with another preexisting disease.

Spider telangiectasia, also known as spider angioma or spider nevus, presents as a small vascular papule with radiating vessels reminiscent of a spider's legs. Spider telangiectasias may present in high estrogen states and tend to favor the face, upper trunk, and hands.

Unilateral nevoid telangiectasia may be congenital or acquired and presents with numerous telangiectasias in an asymmetric dermatomal pattern, most commonly involving the trigeminal, third cervical, or fourth cervical dermatomes. Acquired cases may present during puberty, pregnancy, and other times of estrogen excess.

Angioma serpiginosum is rare condition typically presenting in childhood as numerous punctate telangiectasias localized to one of the lower extremities and grouped into a serpiginous pattern. Slow progression of the telangiectasias may occur over time.

C. Secondary localized telangiectasias are restricted to a certain region of the body and represent only one feature of a larger underlying condition.

Rosacea is a chronic inflammatory condition that may present with facial telangiectasias among other cutaneous and ocular signs and symptoms. **Erythematotelangiectatic rosacea** should be considered when facial telangiectasias are accompanied by periodic flushing, persistent centrofacial erythema, and skin sensitivity. Treatment of erythematotelangiectatic rosacea centers on gentle skin care, avoidance of flushing triggers, as well as various topical and laser treatments.

Localized telangiectasias may develop in response to external factors. **Telangiectatic photoaging** presents with telangiectasias and erythema in sun-exposed sites. **Corticosteroid-induced atrophy** may lead to telangiectasias, atrophy, and striae at the site of chronic corticosteroid application. **Chronic radiation dermatitis** may present with localized telangiectasias, dyschromia, and atrophy at the site of previous radiation therapy.

D. Primary generalized telangiectasias are present in a wide distribution and are not associated with an underlying disease.

Generalized essential telangiectasia (GET) is more common in females and presents with symmetric diffuse involvement of telangiectasias across the legs, eventually spreading upward to the trunk and arms. Skin biopsy reveals dilated capillaries within the papillary dermis.

Cutaneous collagenous vasculopathy (CCV) is seen with equal incidence in males and females and presents with symmetric diffuse involvement of telangiectasias across the trunk and extremities. CCV is clinically identical to GET, and histological examination is necessary to distinguish CCV, which, in contrast to GET, is characterized by the presence of hyalinized vessel walls.

E. Secondary generalized telangiectasias present in a wide distribution and are associated with underlying conditions.

Hereditary hemorrhagic telangiectasia (HHT) is an autosomal dominant disorder characterized by punctate mucocutaneous telangiectasias and visceral arteriovenous malformations. The telangiectasias present during adolescence and increase in number and size over time. Most common locations include the face, palms, soles, and oral and nasal mucosa. Symptoms and complications may include epistaxis, gastrointestinal bleeding, and iron-deficiency anemia, among others. Diagnosis can be confirmed through genetic testing revealing a pathogenic mutation in *ENG* or *ACVRL1*.

Capillary malformation-arteriovenous malformation (CM-AVM) syndrome is an autosomal dominant disorder presenting with multiple pink macules reminiscent of capillary malformations with a surrounding white halo. Patients may have cutaneous and visceral arteriovenous malformations as well as punctate telangiectasias mimicking HHT. These telangiectasias are most common on the face, neck, and acral sites and are seen in increased incidence in CM-AVM2 compared with CM-AVM1. CM-AVM can be distinguished from HHT by genetic testing revealing a pathogenic mutation in *RASA1* (CM-AVM1) or *EPHB4* (CM-AVM2).

Ataxia telangiectasia is a rare autosomal recessive disorder characterized by oculocutaneous telangiectasias, progressive cerebellar ataxia, and premature death due to malignancy or infection. Telangiectasias initially present on the conjunctiva in early childhood and become more widespread with time. The diagnosis can be confirmed through the detection of a pathogenic mutation in *ATM*.

Systemic sclerosis is a rare connective tissue disease characterized by progressive cutaneous and visceral fibrosis. Telangiectasias are matted in appearance and are most common across the hands and face. The diagnosis can be confirmed by serological evaluation to identify associated autoantibodies.

Telangiectasia macularis eruptiva perstans is a rare form of cutaneous mastocytosis presenting with erythematous telangiectatic macules distributed symmetrically across the trunk and extremities. Patients may have pruritus and systemic symptoms related to mast cell activation, such as flushing, diarrhea, and breathing difficulty. Skin biopsy demonstrates dilated capillaries with perivascular mast cells.

See Appendix 1 for Further Reading and Image References.

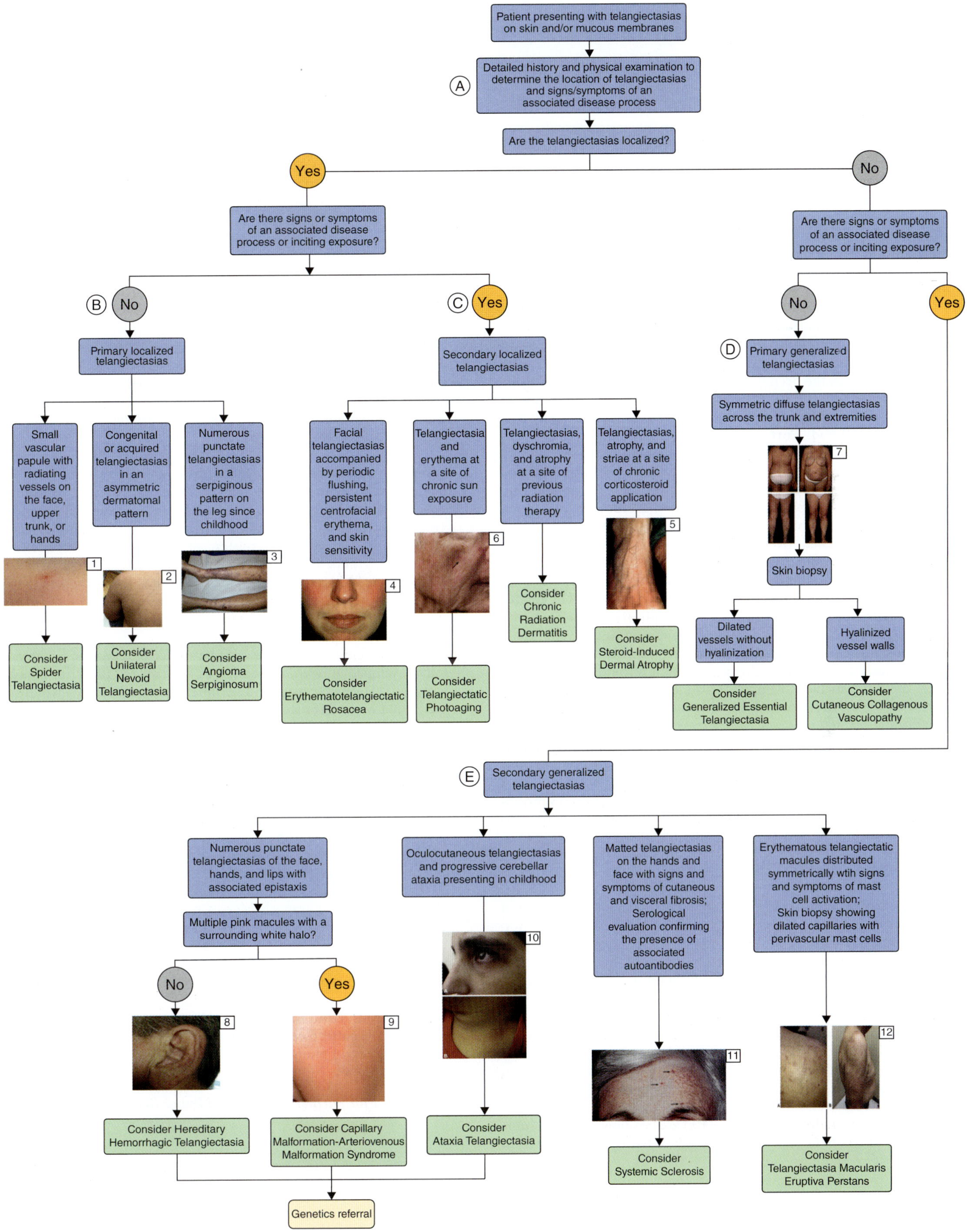
Patient presenting with telangiectasias on skin and/or mucous membranes
A
Detailed history and physical examination to determine the location of telangiectasias and signs/symptoms of an associated disease process
Are the telangiectasias localized?
Yes
No
Are there signs or symptoms of an associated disease process or inciting exposure?
B
No
Primary localized telangiectasias
Small vascular papule with radiating vessels on the face, upper trunk, or hands
1
Consider Spider Telangiectasia
Congenital or acquired telangiectasias in an asymmetric dermatomal pattern
2
Consider Unilateral Nevoid Telangiectasia
Numerous punctate telangiectasias in a serpiginous pattern on the leg since childhood
3
Consider Angioma Serpiginosum
C
Yes
Secondary localized telangiectasias
Facial telangiectasias accompanied by periodic flushing, persistent centrofacial erythema, and skin sensitivity
4
Consider Erythematotelangiectatic Rosacea
Telangiectasia and erythema at a site of chronic sun exposure
6
Consider Telangiectatic Photoaging
Telangiectasias, dyschromia, and atrophy at a site of previous radiation therapy
Consider Chronic Radiation Dermatitis
Telangiectasias, atrophy, and striae at a site of chronic corticosteroid application
5
Consider Steroid-Induced Dermal Atrophy
Are there signs or symptoms of an associated disease process or inciting exposure?
No
D
Primary generalized telangiectasias
Symmetric diffuse telangiectasias across the trunk and extremities
7
Skin biopsy
Dilated vessels without hyalinization
Consider Generalized Essential Telangiectasia
Hyalinized vessel walls
Consider Cutaneous Collagenous Vasculopathy
Yes
E
Secondary generalized telangiectasias
Numerous punctate telangiectasias of the face, hands, and lips with associated epistaxis
Multiple pink macules with a surrounding white halo?
No
8
Consider Hereditary Hemorrhagic Telangiectasia
Yes
9
Consider Capillary Malformation-Arteriovenous Malformation Syndrome
Oculocutaneous telangiectasias and progressive cerebellar ataxia presenting in childhood
10
Consider Ataxia Telangiectasia
Genetics referral
Matted telangiectasias on the hands and face with signs and symptoms of cutaneous and visceral fibrosis; Serological evaluation confirming the presence of associated autoantibodies
11
Consider Systemic Sclerosis
Erythematous telangiectatic macules distributed symmetrically wtih signs and symptoms of mast cell activation; Skin biopsy showing dilated capillaries with perivascular mast cells
12
Consider Telangiectasia Macularis Eruptiva Perstans

52 Vascular Birthmarks

Nikhil Nair and Megan S. Evans

Vascular birthmarks are divided into two main categories: vascular malformations or vascular tumors. These may be isolated or associated with an underlying syndrome. While vascular malformation birthmarks typically persist into adulthood, most vascular tumor birthmarks resolve or improve prior to adulthood.

A. The initial evaluation of an adult with a vascular birthmark should include a thorough history and physical examination to identify the morphologic features of the birthmark and any signs or symptoms of an associated syndrome.

B. **Capillary malformations (CM)** are slow-flow vascular malformations typically presenting as red patches. **Nevus simplex** presents as pink-red macules or patches favoring specific sites on the scalp and face, such as the occipital scalp, eyelids, glabella, and philtrum. Most of these lesions resolve in early childhood, but nevus simplex of the occipital scalp and nape of the neck ("stork bite") may persist into adulthood. **Port-wine birthmark**, also known as nevus flammeus, presents as a red patch with a predilection for the face or extremities. These malformations typically persist into adulthood and may become darker and thicker over time. Treatment with pulsed dye laser can be pursued. Various syndromes may be associated with port-wine birthmarks, including Sturge-Weber Syndrome and PIK3CA-related overgrowth spectrum. **Sturge-Weber syndrome (SWS)** presents with facial CM and leptomeningeal and ocular anomalies. Complications of SWS may include developmental delay, seizures, and early-onset glaucoma. **PIK3CA-related overgrowth spectrum** includes various syndromes associated with somatic PIK3CA mutation, CM, and tissue overgrowth. Treatment depends on the location, extent, and severity of involvement but may include laser therapy, sclerotherapy, excision, sirolimus, or alpelisib. The spectrum includes Klippel-Trénaunay syndrome (KTS), which presents with extremity CM, underlying venous or venolymphatic malformation, and progressive limb overgrowth. Additional complications may include chronic intravascular coagulopathy and internal bleeding. Macrocephaly-capillary malformation syndrome presents with enlarged head circumference, reticulated CM along the trunk or extremities, and neurologic symptoms. A third syndrome within the PIK3CA-related overgrowth spectrum includes CLOVES syndrome, which presents with **C**ongenital **L**ipomatous **O**vergrowth of the trunk, CM, and other slow- or fast-flow **V**ascular malformations, **E**pidermal nevi, and **S**keletal anomalies.

C. **Venous malformation (VM)** is a slow-flow vascular malformation presenting as a compressible bluish mass that fills with dependency. Radiologic evaluation should include magnetic resonance imaging (MRI) with contrast to determine the extent of the malformation, and laboratory evaluation for chronic local intravascular coagulation (LIC) should be considered in patients with large or extensive VM. Treatment depends on the location and extent of the malformation but may include sclerotherapy, excision, low-molecular weight heparin for LIC, and/or sirolimus. Blue rubber bleb nevus syndrome presents with multiple cutaneous and visceral VMs. Gastrointestinal involvement may lead to anemia due to blood loss in the stool.

D. **Arteriovenous malformations (AVMs)** are fast-flow malformations most common on the head or neck. AVMs initially present as a warm red patch with rapid capillary refill and increase in size over time. A thrill may be detected on palpation. Doppler ultrasound may aid in early diagnosis of AVM, while MRI with contrast can determine the extent of involvement. Complications may include ulceration and high-output cardiac failure. Treatment may include surgical modalities such as embolization and excision. AVMs may be isolated or associated with an underlying syndrome. **Capillary malformation-arteriovenous malformation (CM-AVM) syndrome** is an autosomal dominant disorder presenting with multiple pink macules with a surrounding white halo. Patients may have cutaneous and visceral arteriovenous malformations. Genetic testing reveals a pathogenic mutation in RASA1 (CM-AVM1) or EPHB4 (CM-AVM2). **Parkes Weber syndrome** presents with a large red patch on the lower limb with associated limb hypertrophy reminiscent of KTS. However, the limb overgrowth of this syndrome is related to the presence of arteriovenous fistulae. **Cobb syndrome** presents with cutaneous and spinal AVM and may result in severe neurologic complications, including paraplegia, if untreated.

E. **Lymphatic malformations (LM)** are slow-flow vascular malformations most often located on the head and neck. Ultrasound typically shows multilocular anechoic lesions with internal septae. Treatment depends on the extent of involvement and symptoms but may include sclerotherapy, excision, or sirolimus. **Microcystic LM** presents as grouped vesicles containing clear-to-hemorrhagic fluid. **Macrocystic LM** presents as a translucent soft mass and may be associated with various genetic conditions, such as Trisomy 21, Turner syndrome, and Noonan syndrome.

F. Congenital hemangiomas are vascular tumor birthmarks, which are fully developed at birth, presenting as a bluish-red tumor or plaque with course telangiectasias and peripheral pallor. Rapidly involuting congenital hemangiomas do not persist into adulthood, while non-involuting congenital hemangiomas do persist and can be treated with surgical modalities. Congenital hemangiomas are high flow on Doppler ultrasound and can be histologically differentiated from infantile hemangiomas (IH) by the lack of expression of GLUT-1.

G. Tufted angioma (TA) is a rare vascular tumor typically presenting at birth or in early childhood with rare reports of adult-onset TA. TA presents as a violaceous firm nodule or plaque on the trunk or extremity. Histologic findings include groups of capillaries in a "cannonball" distribution throughout the dermis and subcutis. TA can be complicated by Kasabach-Merritt phenomenon with severe and life-threatening thrombocytopenia and consumptive coagulopathy.

H. Kaposiform hemangioendothelioma (KHE) is a rare, locally aggressive vascular tumor typically presenting at birth or in early childhood with rare reports of adult-onset KHE. KHE presents as a violaceous firm mass with continued growth. Histologic examination reveals an infiltrative pattern of spindled endothelial cells. The incidence of Kasabach-Merritt phenomenon is much higher in KHE versus TA.

See Appendix 1 for Further Reading and Image References.

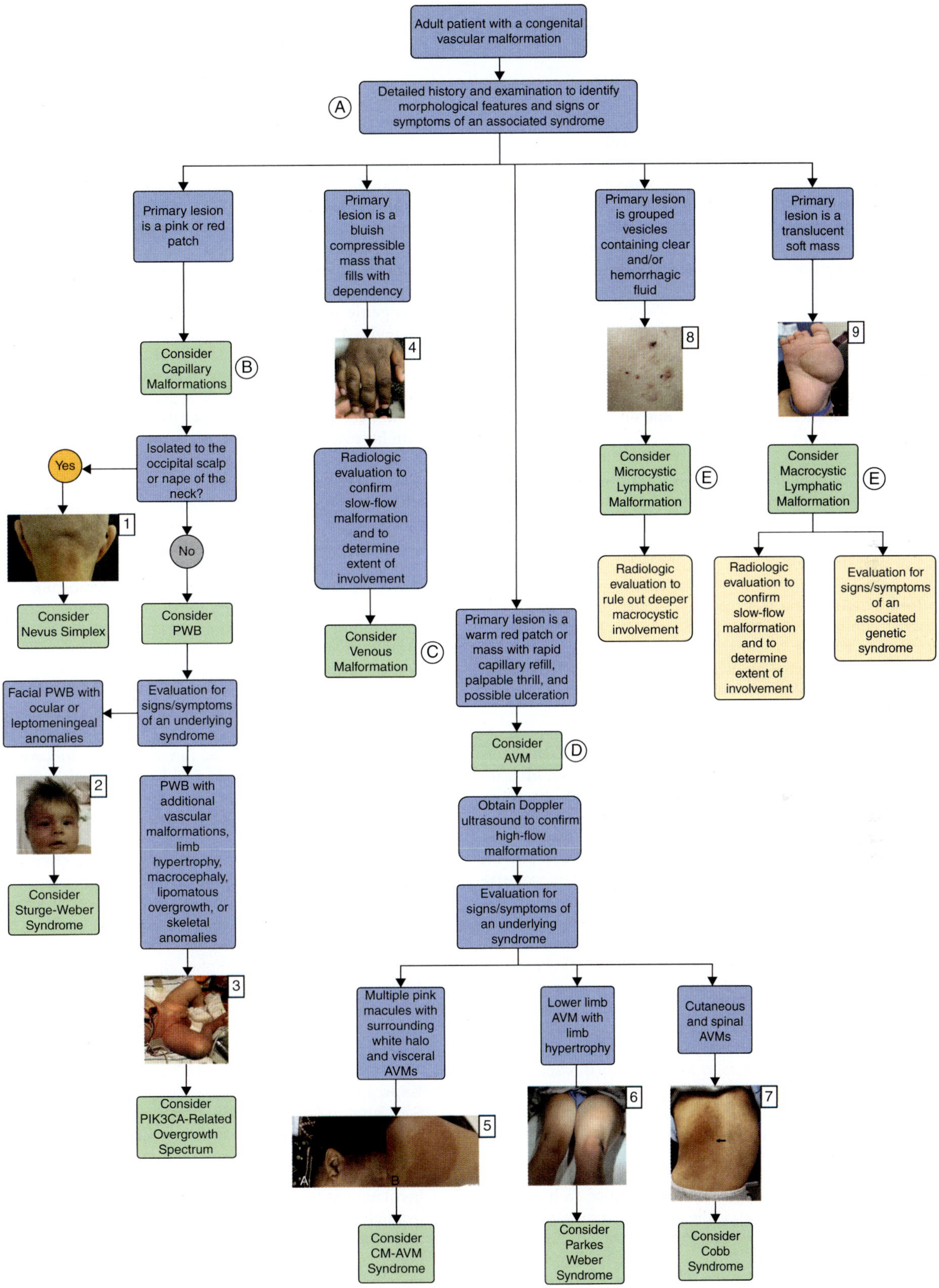
Adult patient with a congenital vascular malformation
A
Detailed history and examination to identify morphological features and signs or symptoms of an associated syndrome
Primary lesion is a pink or red patch
Consider Capillary Malformations
B
Isolated to the occipital scalp or nape of the neck?
Yes
1
Consider Nevus Simplex
No
Consider PWB
Evaluation for signs/symptoms of an underlying syndrome
Facial PWB with ocular or leptomeningeal anomalies
2
Consider Sturge-Weber Syndrome
PWB with additional vascular malformations, limb hypertrophy, macrocephaly, lipomatous overgrowth, or skeletal anomalies
3
Consider PIK3CA-Related Overgrowth Spectrum
Primary lesion is a bluish compressible mass that fills with dependency
4
Radiologic evaluation to confirm slow-flow malformation and to determine extent of involvement
Consider Venous Malformation
C
Primary lesion is a warm red patch or mass with rapid capillary refill, palpable thrill, and possible ulceration
Consider AVM
D
Obtain Doppler ultrasound to confirm high-flow malformation
Evaluation for signs/symptoms of an underlying syndrome
Multiple pink macules with surrounding white halo and visceral AVMs
5
A
B
Consider CM-AVM Syndrome
Lower limb AVM with limb hypertrophy
6
Consider Parkes Weber Syndrome
Cutaneous and spinal AVMs
7
Consider Cobb Syndrome
Primary lesion is grouped vesicles containing clear and/or hemorrhagic fluid
8
Consider Microcystic Lymphatic Malformation
E
Radiologic evaluation to rule out deeper macrocystic involvement
Primary lesion is a translucent soft mass
9
Consider Macrocystic Lymphatic Malformation
E
Radiologic evaluation to confirm slow-flow malformation and to determine extent of involvement
Evaluation for signs/symptoms of an associated genetic syndrome

53 Bright Red Vascular Papule(s)

Nikhil Nair and Megan S. Evans

A variety of conditions may present as bright red vascular papules, ranging from benign vascular proliferations to vascular proliferations secondary to an underlying condition to malignant vascular tumors.

A. The initial evaluation of an adult with one or more red vascular papules should include a history and physical examination to identify the morphological features of the lesions and any indications of an associated syndrome.

B. **Cherry angiomas** are common benign vascular proliferations presenting as small, bright red papules that favor the trunk and upper extremities. These lesions are often numerous, tend to present with advancing age or pregnancy, and are typically an isolated finding. Cosmetic treatment with surgical or laser modalities can be pursued if desired.

C. **Spider angioma** is a type of telangiectasia that presents as a small red-to-purple blanchable papule with radiating vessels. The face and extremities are the most common sites of involvement, and these lesions may develop in the setting of high estrogen states, such as pregnancy or liver disease.

D. **Glomeruloid hemangioma** is a benign vascular proliferation that presents most commonly on the trunk and extremities as multiple red-to-purple papules. These lesions have a distinct histologic appearance, resembling renal glomeruli and are classically appreciated in the setting of POEMS syndrome.

E. **Microvenular hemangioma** is a rare benign vascular tumor presenting as a solitary red-to-purple papule or nodule on the extremities or trunk in young to middle-aged adults. These lesions are characterized by slow growth, and treatment includes surgical excision. Characteristic histologic features include collapsed vascular lumina and pericytes within the vessel linings.

F. **Targetoid hemosiderotic hemangioma** is a rare benign vascular tumor that classically presents as a solitary vascular papule with a targetoid appearance due to the variable presence of peripheral pallor or a surrounding ecchymotic ring. The alternative name, hobnail hemangioma, comes from the characteristic histologic appearance of hobnail-like endothelial cells within the dilated vessels.

G. **Angiofibromas** are benign neoplasms composed of dermal fibroblasts and dilated blood vessels. They may present as skin-colored or red papules, often favoring the face, and are named based on the body region in which they manifest. Fibrous papule refers to a solitary angiofibroma on the face, while multiple penile lesions may be referred to as pearly penile papules. Multiple angiofibromas may be seen in the setting of several conditions, such as tuberous sclerosis (TS), multiple endocrine neoplasia-1, and Birt-Hogg-Dubé syndrome. Multiple facial angiofibromas in the setting of TS have been referred to as adenoma sebaceum, while periungual involvement in the setting of TS may be termed periungual fibroma.

H. **Angiokeratomas** are benign vascular lesions that typically present as red-purple to black papules with hyperkeratosis. The legs, scrotum, and vulva are some of the characteristic sites of involvement. Angiokeratomas may be associated with a variety of inherited metabolic disorders, including Fabry disease, which presents with angiokeratomas in a "bathing trunk" distribution. Histologic evaluation reveals dilated vessels in the superficial dermis with overlying acanthosis and hyperkeratosis. Angiokeratomas can be treated with surgical modalities or laser, if desired.

I. **Pyogenic granulomas** are benign proliferations of blood vessels thought to be reactive in nature and classically associated with trauma and pregnancy. The typical presentation is that of a growing red papule, with a tendency to bleed or ulcerate, in a child or young adult. Surgical modalities are typically pursued, and histologic evaluation reveals a well-circumscribed proliferation of capillaries in a lobular pattern.

J. **Verruga peruana** is characterized by multiple red papules and nodules, resembling pyogenic granulomas, in the setting of *Bartonella bacilliformis* infection. The causative organism may be identified in blood cultures or on a skin biopsy, and treatment is with antibiotics.

K. **Bacillary angiomatosis** presents with polymorphic red-purple papules and nodules secondary to progressive infection with *Bartonella* in an immunosuppressed individual. The causative organism may be visualized on skin biopsy with the use of a silver stain, and treatment is with antibiotics.

L. **Eruptive pseudoangiomatosis (EPA)** is a rare disorder theorized to represent a viral exanthem that presents abruptly with bright red angioma-like papules on the face and trunk following a prodrome. EPA is classically present in children but is also reported in adults. Histologic evaluation reveals blood vessel dilation without vessel proliferation. The cutaneous lesions are self-resolving and do not require treatment.

M. **Angiosarcoma** is a rare aggressive sarcoma of the endothelium, presenting most commonly on the head and neck as a bruise-like patch with the development of violaceous nodules and possible ulceration over time. Angiosarcoma is most common in elderly patients or in the setting of chronic lymphedema or previous radiation therapy. Histopathology reveals vessels in an infiltrative pattern with areas of nuclear pleomorphism and mitoses. Treatment may include excision, chemotherapy, and/or radiotherapy; however, the prognosis is generally poor.

N. **Kaposi sarcoma (KS)** is an angioproliferative disorder associated with human herpesvirus-8 infection. It may be seen in the setting of immunosuppression, such as with acquired immunodeficiency syndrome or organ transplantation. KS may present as red-purple papules, plaques, or nodules, with the most common sites of involvement being the face, lower extremities, or trunk. Histologic evaluation will reveal vascular proliferation with slit-like spaces and without significant mitoses or pleomorphism. Treatment depends on the extent of involvement and course of the disease but may include surgical modalities, cryotherapy, radiation therapy, or chemotherapy.

See Appendix 1 for Further Reading and Image References.

Adult patient with one or more red vascular papules

→ History and examination to identify morphological features of lesions and indications of an associated syndrome (A)

- Multiple small, bright red papules on the trunk and upper extremities in the setting of advanced age or pregnancy

  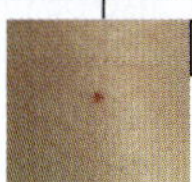
  1

  → Consider Cherry Angioma (B)

- Red papule with radiating vessels on the face or distal extremities

  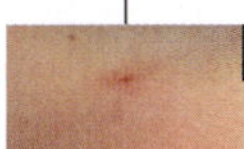
  2

  → Consider Spider Angioma (C)

- Multiple red-to-purple papules on the trunk and extremities in a patient with POEMS syndrome

  → Histological examination: distinct glomeruloid-like appearance

  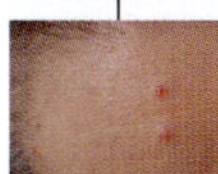
  3

  → Consider Glomeruloid Hemangioma (D)

- Solitary red-to-purple papule or nodule characterized by slow growth on the extremities or trunk of a young to middle-aged adult

  → Histological examination: collapsed vascular lumina and pericytes within vessel linings

  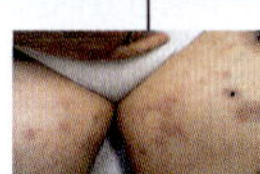
  4

  → Consider Microvenular Hemangioma (E)

- Red papule with a targetoid appearance due to peripheral pallor or a hemosiderotic ring

  → Histological examination to confirm diagnosis: endothelial cells with enlarged nuclei lining dilated blood vessels

  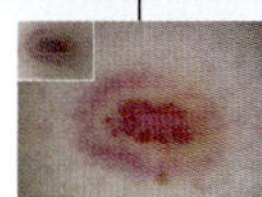
  5

  → Consider Targetoid Hemosiderotic Hemangioma (F)

- Red-to-skin-colored papules favoring the face

  → Histological examination to confirm diagnosis: dermal fibroblasts and dilated blood vessels

  → Consider Angiofibroma (G)

  → If multiple, consider further evaluation for an underlying condition

- Red-purple papule with associated hyperkeratosis

  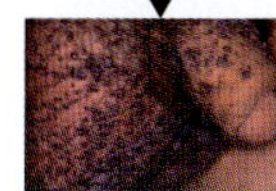
  6

  → Consider Angiokeratoma (H)

  → If multiple lesions in a bathing trunk distribution, consider further evaluation for an underlying condition

- Red papule with tendency to ulcerate or bleed

  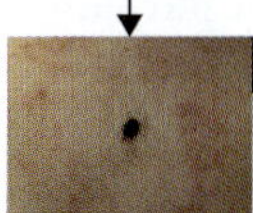
  7

  - Solitary lesion

    → Histological examination to confirm diagnosis: Proliferation of well-circumscribed capillaries in a lobular formation

    → Consider Pyogenic Granuloma (I)

  - Multiple lesions

    → Infectious workup finding *Bartonella bacilliformis* infection

    → Consider Verruga Peruana (J)

- Polymorphic red-purple papules and nodules in an immunosuppressed patient

  → Infectious workup

  - *Bartonella* positive

    → Histological examination: lobules of endothelial cells and vascular proliferation with associated mixed-cellular infiltrate

    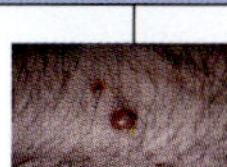
    8

    → Consider Bacillary Angiomatosis (K)

  - HHV-8 positive

    → Histological examination: spindle cell proliferation and formation of slit-like vascular spaces with lymphocytic infiltrate and plasma cells

    → Consider Kaposi Sarcoma (N)

- Abrupt onset of multiple red papules on the face and trunk preceded by systemic symptoms

  → Histological examination: blood vessel dilation without associated vessel proliferation

  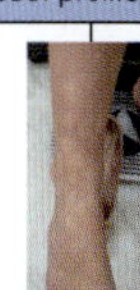
  9

  → Consider Eruptive Pseudoangiomatosis (L)

- Red-purple, bruised patch favoring the head and neck in the setting of advanced age, chronic lymphedema, or radiation dermatitis

  → Histological examination to confirm diagnosis: infiltrative pattern with regions of nuclear pleomorphism and mitoses

  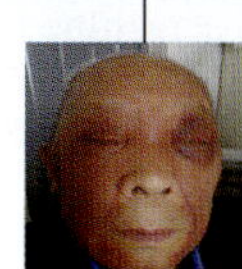
  10

  → Consider Angiosarcoma (M)

54 Petechiae

Alice J. Tan and Daniela Kroshinsky

Petechiae are small (<4 mm) pinpoint, nonblanching, purpuric macules that may present on the skin or mucous membranes and result from extravasation of erythrocytes from small cutaneous vessels into the dermis. Identification of the etiology through detailed history and physical examination is crucial in facilitating prompt diagnosis and treatment. The pathophysiology of petechiae formation typically involves thrombocytopenia or platelet dysfunction. Etiologies range from simple injury or straining to more concerning causes, including infection and malignancy.

A. Initial evaluation of a patient with petechiae involves obtaining an extensive history, including the onset/progression and distribution of petechiae, medication history, recent infections or sick contacts, history of trauma/injury, travel history, insect exposures, and presence of systemic symptoms. Physical examination of the skin, mucous membranes, and lymph nodes should be performed along with assessment for hepatomegaly and splenomegaly. A complete blood count (CBC) with differential, partial thromboplastin time (PTT), prothrombin time (PT), and bleeding time should be ordered.

B. Patients with fever, tachycardia, tachypnea, hypotension, leukocytosis, and/or elevated acute phase reactants should be evaluated for sources of **infection**. Laboratory tests to facilitate diagnosis include blood cultures, skin biopsy and culture, viral serologies, cultures of catheters at insertion sites, and urinalysis. Etiologies may include bacterial sepsis, meningococcemia, Rocky Mountain spotted fever (RMSF), endocarditis, parvovirus B19, streptococcal pharyngitis with scarlet fever, viral exanthems (e.g., rubeola, rubella, Epstein-Barr virus, cytomegalovirus, HIV, togavirus, and herpes viruses), viral hemorrhagic fever (e.g., Ebola, dengue), atypical measles, Queensland tick typhus, or Brazilian purpuric fever.

C. In patients presenting with normal platelet levels and no fever, **mechanical etiologies** may include trauma or causes of increased intravenous pressure. Petechiae due to Valsalva maneuver (straining, childbirth, coughing, forceful vomiting) may appear on the face, neck, and upper trunk, whereas the use of a tourniquet or blood pressure cuff (Rumpel-Leede phenomenon) tends to have a more localized presentation.

D. Different conditions may present as localized petechiae. **Leukocytoclastic vasculitis** is a small-vessel vasculitis that can cause petechiae and palpable purpuric papules characteristically on the lower legs. A lack of systemic symptoms, including fever, lymphadenopathy, myalgias, abdominal pain, hematuria, melena, and hematochezia, can help to rule out systemic vasculitis. Although sometimes idiopathic, various etiologies have been identified, including infection, collagen vascular disease (e.g., scleroderma, systemic lupus erythematosus, rheumatoid arthritis), cryoglobulinemia, medications, and lymphoma. Skin biopsy can be obtained to confirm diagnosis, and screening tests for systemic involvement can be considered.

Pigmented purpuric dermatoses are chronic and benign conditions and should be suspected in patients with pinpoint petechiae ("cayenne pepper") localized primarily to the lower legs, particularly in Schamberg disease. Diagnosis is largely clinical, and laboratory tests examining platelet abnormalities, coagulopathies, and acute phase reactants are expected to be normal.

Vitamin C deficiency may result in scurvy, characterized by perifollicular petechiae with associated bleeding gums, corkscrew hairs, arthralgias, and impaired wound healing. Concomitant nutritional deficiencies, including vitamin B_{12}, folate, and iron, may also be present.

Hypergammaglobulinemic purpura of Waldenström is characterized by recurrent episodes of lower extremity petechiae and purpura, polyclonal hypergammaglobulinemia, elevated erythrocyte sedimentation rate, normal platelet count, and the presence of rheumatoid factor. Young females with autoimmune connective tissue disease, particularly Sjögren's syndrome, are primarily affected. The condition is not considered benign whessn occurring in pregnancy, as circulating anti-SSA antibodies in maternal serum may result in negative fetal and maternal outcomes, such as intrauterine growth restriction, congenital heart block, preeclampsia, and even fetal demise.

E. In patients with generalized petechiae and history of a new medication, consider **medication-induced petechiae** due to altered platelet function or thrombocytopenia. Commonly reported causes include heparin, chemotherapy agents, antibiotics, antiepileptics, quinine, anticoagulants, antiplatelet agents, and steroids.

Petechiae are a major characteristic of thrombocytopenic purpura, and screening tests, including urinalysis and stool guaiac, can help evaluate for sources of bleeding. Patients with petechiae and thrombocytopenia with fever, microangiopathic hemolytic anemia, renal dysfunction, and/or neurologic symptoms should be evaluated for **thrombotic thrombocytopenic purpura**. CBC, peripheral blood smear, and ADAMTS13 activity assay should be ordered to aid in diagnosis.

Petechiae with fever, hypotension, tachycardia, mental status changes, hematuria, oliguria, mucosal bleeding, and retiform purpura should prompt workup for **disseminated intravascular coagulation**, a life-threatening medical emergency. A variety of inciting factors exist, including sepsis, obstetric complications, trauma, and malignancy. In addition to thrombocytopenia and anemia with schistocytes, abnormal laboratory tests may include elevated D-dimer, decreased fibrinogen, and prolonged PT/PTT.

A history of easy bruising with thrombocytopenia, normal platelet morphology, and a positive direct antiglobulin test (Coombs test) may indicate **immune thrombocytopenic purpura**, an autoimmune disease that is frequently idiopathic in etiology but may be triggered by viral infection, systemic autoimmune conditions, pregnancy, or malignancy.

Older patients with weight loss, night sweats, lymphadenopathy, elevated platelet count (>450 x 10^9/L) and/or hepatosplenomegaly should be evaluated for **malignancy**.

See Appendix 1 for Further Reading and Image References.

Patient presenting with petechiae

↓

(A) Detailed history and physical examination of the skin, nails, lymph nodes, and mucosal surfaces

↓

Fever/toxic-appearing?

- **Yes** → (B) Positive blood culture, leukocytosis, elevated ESR and/or CRP
  - Consider Infection:
    - Bacterial Sepsis
    - RMSF
    - Meningococcemia
    - Endocarditis
    - Viral Etiology (Parvovirus B19, Rubeola, Rubella, HIV, CMV)
    - Group A *Streptococcus*
- **No** → History of trauma, tourniquet, blood pressure cuff, or Valsalva (coughing, vomiting, childbirth)?
  - **Yes** →

    1

    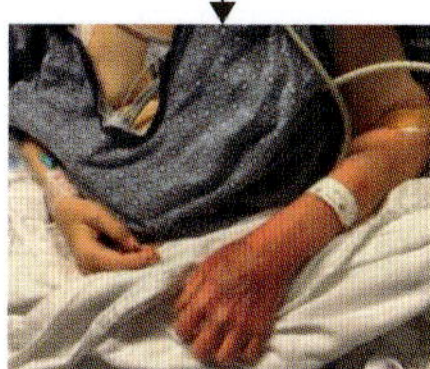

    → (C) Consider Mechanical Etiology
  - **No** → Localized petechiae?
    - (D) **Yes** →
      - Perifollicular petechiae, corkscrew hairs, purpura, and hyperkeratotic papules on the extremities and buttocks

        4

        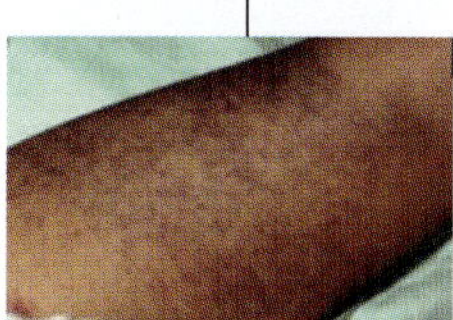

        → Consider Vitamin C Deficiency
      - Petechiae and palpable purpura on the lower legs, normal platelet count

        2

        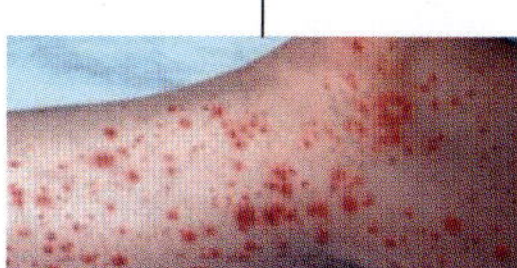

        → Consider Leukocytoclastic Vasculitis
      - Yellow-pink patches with superimposed "cayenne-pepper" petechiae on the lower legs, normal platelet count

        3

        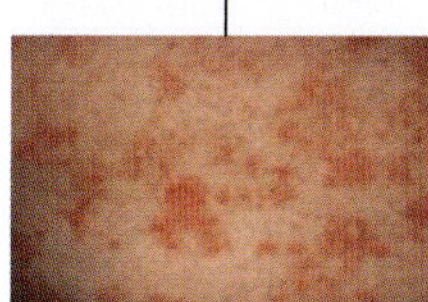

        → Consider Pigmented Purpuric Dermatoses
      - Petechiae typically seen on the dorsal feet and lower legs, with hemosiderin deposition at sites of older lesions, normal platelet count, polyclonal hypergammaglobulinemia

        5

        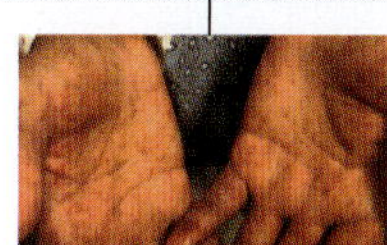

        → Consider Hypergammaglobulinemic Purpura of Waldenström
    - **No** → Generalized (E)
      - Elderly patient, weight loss, lymphadenopathy, night sweats, elevated platelet count → Consider Malignancy
      - History of new medication → Consider Medication-induced Petechiae
      - Gingival bleeding, easy bruising, blood in urine or stool, fever, thrombocytopenia → Consider Thrombotic Thrombocytopenic Purpura, Disseminated Intravascular Coagulation, or Immune Thrombocytopenic Purpura

55 Macular Purpura

Chen Yao and Lindy Fox

Macular purpura is defined by nonblanching purpuric macules or patches that are 5 mm or greater in diameter. The causes of macular purpura include those that cause petechiae (see Chapter 54), such as thrombocytopenia, dysfunctional platelets from a medication or secondary to renal or hepatic dysfunction, anticoagulants, vitamin K deficiency, and scurvy, as well as those that result in tissue fragility (chronic steroid use, amyloidosis, actinic damage, and genetic disorders of connective tissue). Evaluation of a patient with macular purpura should include review of pertinent medical history (e.g., onset, family history, medication exposures), clinical examination, and laboratory studies. Several lab studies can be used to help unveil underlying etiologies and narrow the differential diagnosis, including complete blood count [CBC] to check platelet levels, blood urea nitrogen/creatinine and liver function tests to assess kidney and liver function, and coagulation studies. Skin biopsy should be considered in patients who are systemically ill, including a biopsy for tissue culture if infection is suspected.

A. A thorough history of prescribed anticoagulants, over-the-counter medications, and supplement use should be ascertained. Consider anticoagulant-induced purpura from **warfarin, factor Xa inhibitors, heparins**, or **direct thrombin inhibitors**. Clinicians should also evaluate for use of **aspirin**, **clopidogrel**, **nonsteroidal anti-inflammatory drugs**, or supplements with antiplatelet or anticoagulation properties (e.g., turmeric, fish oil, flaxseed oil, garlic, ginger, *Ginkgo biloba*, feverfew, niacin, vitamin E).

B. If examination reveals distal acral distribution of macular purpura such as lesions on the tips of fingers and/or toes, several processes should be considered. It is important to note, however, that the conditions which will be discussed more commonly present with retiform or palpable purpura than macular purpura. Acral and asymmetric lesions may suggest **emboli** (infection, marantic, fat, cholesterol). Cholesterol emboli should be considered in the setting of a recent procedural intervention, and is also often associated with transient eosinophilia. When macular purpura occurs predominantly on the lower extremities, consider **leukocytoclastic vasculitis (LCV)**, **pigmented purpuric dermatosis**, **hypergammaglobulinemic purpura of Waldenstrom**, and **contact dermatitis**. Skin biopsy can be performed from the center of an involved area to assess for LCV, as this condition can be idiopathic or associated with infections, autoimmune disorders, malignancy, or medications. Serum protein electrophoresis can be used to evaluate for hypergammaglobulinemic purpura of Waldenstrom, which would demonstrate a broad-based peak corresponding to polyclonal hypergammaglobulinemia with predominant increase in IgG.

C. If clinical examination is notable for atrophic or wrinkled skin, suspect conditions characterized by poor dermal support or vascular fragility, including **senile purpura** in an elderly patient, **actinic purpura** in a background of sun-damaged skin, **steroid (topical or systemic)-induced atrophy**, **scurvy**, **amyloidosis**, and inherited connective tissue disorders such as **Ehlers-Danlos syndrome** and **pseudoxanthoma elasticum**. History, physical examination, and other systemic findings can help differentiate between these conditions. Asking about use of topical and systemic corticosteroids should be included in the history taking. Scurvy should be suspected in patients demonstrating classic signs such as perifollicular hemorrhage with corkscrew hair deformity, follicular hyperkeratosis, and gingival bleeding. Periorbital purpura and waxy, translucent, or skin-colored papules and plaques can point to primary systemic amyloidosis. Ehlers-Danlos syndrome is characterized by skin hyperextensibility and fragility with poor wound healing, and is also associated with joint hypermobility and a history of gastrointestinal hemorrhage. Pseudoxanthoma elasticum clinically presents with yellow papules and plaques on the neck and at intertriginous sites.

D. Family history should be obtained for bleeding disorders including hemophilia and congenital platelet function defects, particularly if the patient has had a history of bleeding episodes. If history or physical examination does not reveal a suspected etiology, complete blood count (CBC) can be obtained to evaluate platelet counts. If thrombocytopenia is present, consider thrombocytopenic purpura, and workup for causes of thrombocytopenia such as idiopathic thrombocytopenic purpura, thrombotic thrombocytopenic purpura, disseminated intravascular coagulation (DIC), hemolytic uremic syndrome, drug-induced thrombocytopenia, cirrhosis, and bone marrow failure. In the setting of elevated white blood cell count, consider workup for infectious etiologies that can cause worsening of purpura. Strongyloidiasis can present with periumbilical or upper thigh "thumbprint" purpura in the absence of eosinophilia.

If the platelet count is normal, then proceed to evaluate other coagulation studies including prothrombin time, partial thromboplastin time, international normalized ratio, and bleeding time, as well as fibrinogen and D-dimer if DIC is suspected. If either coagulation studies or bleeding time is abnormal, consider acquired coagulopathies such as **renal or hepatic dysfunction, gammopathy, vitamin K deficiency**, and **DIC**. Uremia secondary to renal insufficiency and elevated immunoglobulins in gammopathies can also interfere with platelet function.

See Appendix 1 for Further Reading and Image References.

Patient presents with purpuric macules or patches 5 mm or greater in diameter

History and physical examination are important to help narrow down the cause of macular purpura. Onset and duration of symptoms, use of medications that may affect platelet function or coagulation, and coexisting medical conditions are important to elicit. Trauma, inflammation, and infection are often underlying contributing factors.

(A) Taking any offending anticoagulants or antiplatelet medications, such as warfarin, rivaroxaban, heparin, aspirin, or NSAIDs?

- Yes → Consider Medication-Associated Purpura
- No → (B) Acral distribution?
  - Yes → Purpuric macules and patches predominantly on the lower extremities

    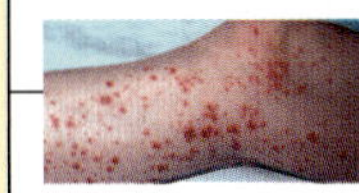

    2

    → Consider Emboli, Leukocytoclastic Vasculitis, Pigmented Purpuric Dermatosis, Hypergammaglobulinemic Purpura of Waldenström
  - No → (D) Family history of bleeding?
    - Yes → Consider Hemophilia, Inherited Platelet Function Disorders
    - (E) No → Signs of poor dermal support or vascular fragility?
      - (C) Yes
        - Older patient with atrophic skin

          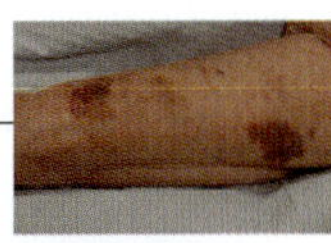

          1

          Purpuric macules and patches on the dorsal forearm → Consider Senile Purpura
        - History of chronic sun exposure with background of sun-damaged skin → Consider Actinic Purpura
        - History of topical or systemic steroid use → Consider Steroid-Induced Atrophy
        - Perifollicular hemorrhage, corkscrew hair deformity, or gingival bleeding → Consider Scurvy
        - Purpuric patches involving the eyelids, weight loss, fatigue, weakness → Consider Amyloidosis
        - Features of joint hypermobility, skin hyperextensibility with poor wound healing → Consider Ehlers-Danlos Syndrome
        - Yellow to skin-colored papules coalescing into reticulated plaques on the neck and flexural areas → Consider Pseudoxanthoma Elasticum
      - No → Consider Platelet Dysfunction, Thrombocytopenia, and Acquired Coagulopathies → Consider checking CBC, BUN/Cr, LFTs, D-dimer, fibrinogen

56 Palpable Purpura

Mohammed Moumen and Lindsay C. Strowd

Leukocytoclastic vasculitis (LCV) is a type of cutaneous small vessel vasculitis that is typically thought to occur in the context of an underlying disease process. LCV classically presents as small nonblanching violaceous or purpuric papules, macules, and plaques with a predilection for the lower extremities. The clinical presentation of LCV reflects destruction of vessel walls with subsequent extravasation of red blood cells into the surrounding tissue. Vessel walls are disrupted by the deposition of complement and a robust inflammatory infiltrate primarily composed of neutrophils, with karyorrhexis. LCV is thought to be a reactive dermatosis with a specific trigger for this inflammatory cascade.

Dermatologists must maintain a broad differential because infectious, inflammatory, autoimmune, and paraneoplastic causes can all result in similar appearing LCV. History should include a detailed timeline of presentation, evolution of skin lesions, and other concurrent symptoms. A complete review of systems can be very helpful in identifying potential underlying causes of LCV. Physical examination should include a complete skin examination to identify all skin areas affected by LCV and to identify additional skin lesions or morphologies. Standard of care for suspected LCV includes a punch biopsy to confirm the diagnosis, as well as a lesional skin biopsy for direct immunofluorescence. Obtain tissue cultures if infectious causes are highly suspected.

A. One of the first steps in working up LCV is determining if the patient has a skin-limited disease process or not. LCV can be idiopathic and limited to the skin with no apparent underlying cause. These patients do not typically have additional symptoms aside from their skin lesions. **Skin-limited LCV** often self-resolves after several weeks with conservative therapy. Examination findings such as fever, arthralgias, arthritis, diarrhea, hematochezia, hemoptysis, lymphadenopathy, or oral ulcerations, would raise concern for an underlying systemic illness.

B. The most common causes of LCV include infectious, paraneoplastic, drug-induced, and autoimmune diseases. **Infectious causes** should be suspected if patients are immunocompromised and display signs of infection such as fever, leukocytosis, leukopenia, cough, diarrhea, or altered mental status. Patients should be queried regarding recent travel, especially travel abroad, recent sick contacts, tick exposure, ingestion of undercooked foods, and occupation. A drug history should also be obtained as intravenous drug use can lead to systemic infections. Diagnostic studies for infectious causes could include chest x-ray or computed tomography scan, complete blood count (CBC) with differential, blood, urine, cerebrospinal fluid, stool, or sputum cultures, echocardiogram, HIV serology, respiratory viral panel, gastrointestinal pathogen panel, QuantiFERON gold, and urinalysis. In some instances, more rare causes of infectious LCV should be considered, such as mycobacterial infections, opportunistic fungal infections, or parasitic infections. Dermatologists can benefit from working closely with infectious disease specialists to help identify the underlying causative agent and choose initial empiric coverage.

C. LCV has been well established as a **paraneoplastic phenomenon**, especially in liquid tumors. LCV may precede the diagnosis of a malignancy, may occur concurrently with diagnosis, or may present with disease progression or relapse. The workup for paraneoplastic LCV includes screening for unintentional weight loss, cachexia, night sweats, fever, and lymphadenopathy. Assessing for family history of malignancy can also be helpful in identifying the risk for certain heritable malignancies. Diagnostic tests that may be helpful include the presence of atypical cells on CBC or peripheral smear, M spike on serum and/or urine protein electrophoresis, abnormal peripheral flow cytometry, abnormal bone marrow biopsy, pancytopenia, elevated lactate dehydrogenase, or other abnormal malignancy screening tests. Patients who have not undergone age-appropriate cancer screening should receive those tests.

D. **Connective tissue or autoimmune diseases** can be present with LCV. Patients with underlying inflammatory bowel disease (IBD) can demonstrate LCV at diagnosis or with subsequent IBD flares. Rheumatologic disorders, including systemic lupus erythematosus, scleroderma, mixed connective tissue disease, dermatomyositis, and others, can also present with LCV. Characterization of extracutaneous symptomology along with serologic studies can aid in correct diagnosis.

E. **IgA vasculitis** is a specific type of LCV where IgA deposits are noted around the dermal vessels on direct immunofluorescence. IgA vasculitis classically presents with arthralgias, abdominal pain, hematochezia, or vomiting in addition to LCV and can be associated with either viral infections or autoimmune conditions.

F. Other causes of LCV include exposure to **medications**, such as diuretics, NSAIDs, antibiotics, or illicit drug exposure to levamisole-contaminated cocaine. A careful medication history including new medications, particularly those initiated within 7 to 10 days of symptom onset, can help determine if this cause is likely.

See Appendix 1 for Further Reading and Image References.

Patient with small, palpable violaceous or deeply erythematous papules, macules, and small plaques. Later lesions can develop central ulceration or become more confluent

↓

Complete skin examination to evaluate all areas of involvement. Mucous membrane and nail evaluation. Detailed history of timeline, medical comorbidities, serological studies, and medications. Consider skin biopsy of lesion along with lesional DIF specimen +/– tissue culture

↓

(A) Does the patient have any systemic symptoms such as fever, leukopenia, leukocytosis, anemia, hemoptysis, arthralgias, oral ulcers, LAD, hematuria, melena, abdominal pain?

No

Typically self-resolves with conservative therapy after several weeks

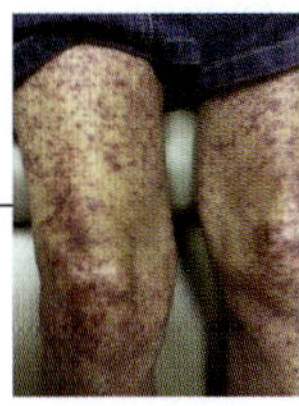

1

→ Consider Skin-Limited LCV

Yes

- (B) Signs and/or symptoms of underlying infection
  - Tick bite exposure → Consider Rocky Mountain Spotted Fever
  - Recent travel, sick contacts, immunocompromised, fever, new heart murmur, + culture, abnormal CXR, HIV+, abnormal RVP or GIP, abnormal urinalysis, neutropenia, leukocytosis → Consider LCV due to Systemic Infection
  - Positive culture for *Neisseria meningitidis* → Consider Meningococcemia
- (C) Signs and/or symptoms of underlying neoplasm
  - LAD, weight loss, cachexia, night sweats, fever, atypical cells on CBC or peripheral smear, M spike on SPEP or UPEP, pancytopenia, elevated LDH, other abnormal malignancy screening tests

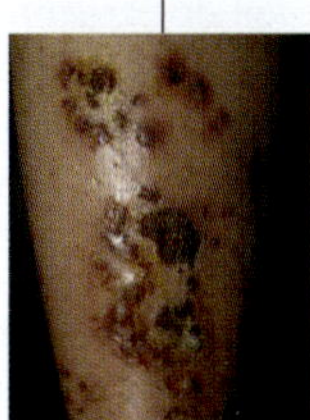

3

  - → Consider LCV as Paraneoplastic Phenomenon
- (D) Signs and/or symptoms of underlying connective tissue disease or autoimmune disease
  - Hemoptysis, hx of IBD, positive ANA, c-ANCA, p-ANCA, RF, anti-Smith, anti-dsDNA, low C3/C4, positive cryoglobulins, synovitis → Consider LCV as part of an underlying Autoimmune Disease
- (E) Hematuria, hematemesis, hematochezia, abdominal pain, arthralgias

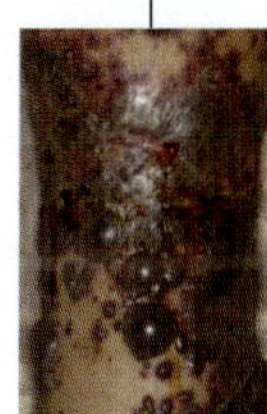

2

  - → Consider IgA Vasculitis (HSP)
- (F) Culprit medications such as diuretics, antibiotics, NSAIDs → Consider Drug-Induced LCV

57 Retiform Purpura

Mohammed Moumen and Lindsay C. Strowd

Retiform purpura (RP) is a distinctive cutaneous sign that often signals a serious underlying pathology. RP is caused by disruption or destruction of the blood vessels that supply the skin and subcutaneous fat, resulting in infarction of tissue and eventual tissue necrosis in all parts of the skin previously nourished by the affected vessels. RP presents clinically as branching or netlike, nonblanching violaceous patches or plaques when found on larger skin surface areas, such as the abdomen or extremities. These branching lesions eventually form an eschar and secondary ulceration. On smaller skin surfaces such as the ears, face, and digits, RP may present as violaceous papules or solid confluent purpura.

RP is not typically a skin finding seen in the outpatient clinic, but rather is found in the inpatient setting, often in the context of a critically ill patient. It is vitally important to take the time to obtain a detailed history of the patient's current illness, as well as their medical comorbidities, prior interventions and medications, and review their current laboratory and imaging studies. A skin biopsy can be helpful in confirming the diagnosis of RP and also helping to guide the final diagnosis. Depositional causes such as calciphylaxis and oxalosis and causes such as cholesterol emboli and intravascular lymphoma can be confirmed by skin biopsy. In contrast, other RP etiologies may require both biopsy and serologic studies.

A. One of the first things to consider when presented with a patient who has RP is whether an infectious process is driving cutaneous findings. Patients with RP from an infectious cause are typically quite ill and display signs of sepsis or multiorgan failure, such as hyperthermia or hypothermia, respiratory and/or kidney failure, cardiovascular compromise requiring pressor support, altered mental status, leukocytosis or leukopenia, and positive culture data. Causes of RP in the setting of systemic infection include **gram-positive and gram-negative bacterial infections, angioinvasive fungal infections**, and rare infections such as **strongyloidiasis**, which tends to involve the periumbilicus. Patients with overwhelming sepsis can also develop disseminated intravascular coagulation (DIC), which can also result in RP formation. Purpura fulminans is a type of RP usually characterized by severe and large areas of RP in the context of systemic bacterial infection. Patients with RP and concern for an underlying infection should have both a skin biopsy and tissue culture performed.

B. If infection is not present or suspected, other types of RP are differentiated with the help of additional medical history and serologic studies. Kidney failure or dialysis with concurrent hyperphosphatemia or hypercalcemia should prompt serious consideration of calciphylaxis. **Calciphylaxis** initially presents as firm, painful subcutaneous nodules and plaques but quickly progresses to RP, followed by ulceration. These lesions are classically located on the pannus, thighs, and legs but are also found on the penis, digits, and breasts. Routine histology reveals calcium lining the arterioles in the deep dermis or deposited among eccrine glands. Calcium stains such as the von Kossa stain can help highlight calcium deposition. Patients with acute leukemia, specifically acute myeloid leukemia (AML), can develop RP as a manifestation of **leukemia cutis** or secondary to AML-associated DIC. **Intravascular lymphoma** is another lymphoproliferative malignancy that can present with RP.

C. Patients with RP should have a thorough clotting history obtained, including a history of deep vein thrombosis, pulmonary embolism, stroke, miscarriage, or spontaneous abortion, to screen for hypercoagulability. Various inherited and acquired hypercoagulable conditions can manifest with RP, including **antiphospholipid antibody syndrome, protein C or S deficiency, antithrombin III deficiency**, and **factor V Leiden**. It may be beneficial to collaborate with a hematologist on a thorough workup for patients who fall into this category.

D. Patients with connective tissue diseases (CTD) can also develop RP, so a history of autoimmune disease and a detailed review of systems should be obtained. CTD most associated with RP includes **antineutrophil cytoplasmic antibody (ANCA)–associated vasculitides, polyarteritis nodosa**, and **rheumatoid vasculitis. Cryoglobulinemia** is somewhat unique in that it can be associated with CTD or malignancy, depending on the subtype.

E. Both heparin and warfarin may induce RP. **Warfarin-induced necrosis** is usually seen when initiating warfarin therapy without concurrent heparin therapy. Initiation of warfarin can lead to a short and transient relative deficiency in Protein C, causing a paradoxical hypercoagulable state resulting in microvascular thrombosis and cutaneous necrosis. The most common patient to develop this is a middle-aged female initiating warfarin therapy within 2 weeks prior to the onset of skin lesions. **Heparin-associated skin necrosis** can appear clinically identical to warfarin necrosis and often occurs initially at the sites of subcutaneous heparin injections.

F. Cocaine contaminated with an antihelminthic agent called **levamisole** has been well documented to result in both vasculopathy and vasculitis, with an unusual distribution of RP that favors the face and ears. This disease process can be associated with agranulocytosis or neutropenia and can recur with the subsequent use of contaminated cocaine. Interestingly, patients with this condition can also express positive autoimmune serologies, such as positive rheumatoid factor, anti-nuclear antibodies (ANA), or ANCA. Levamisole is challenging to detect on serologic studies, so this is often a diagnosis of exclusion. Finally, a recent history of a bone fracture or cardiac, orthopedic, or other surgical procedure should elicit concern for potential **embolism**. RP caused by emboli may be more likely to be acral, with fewer lesions, and possibly unilateral.

See Appendix 1 for Further Reading and Image References.

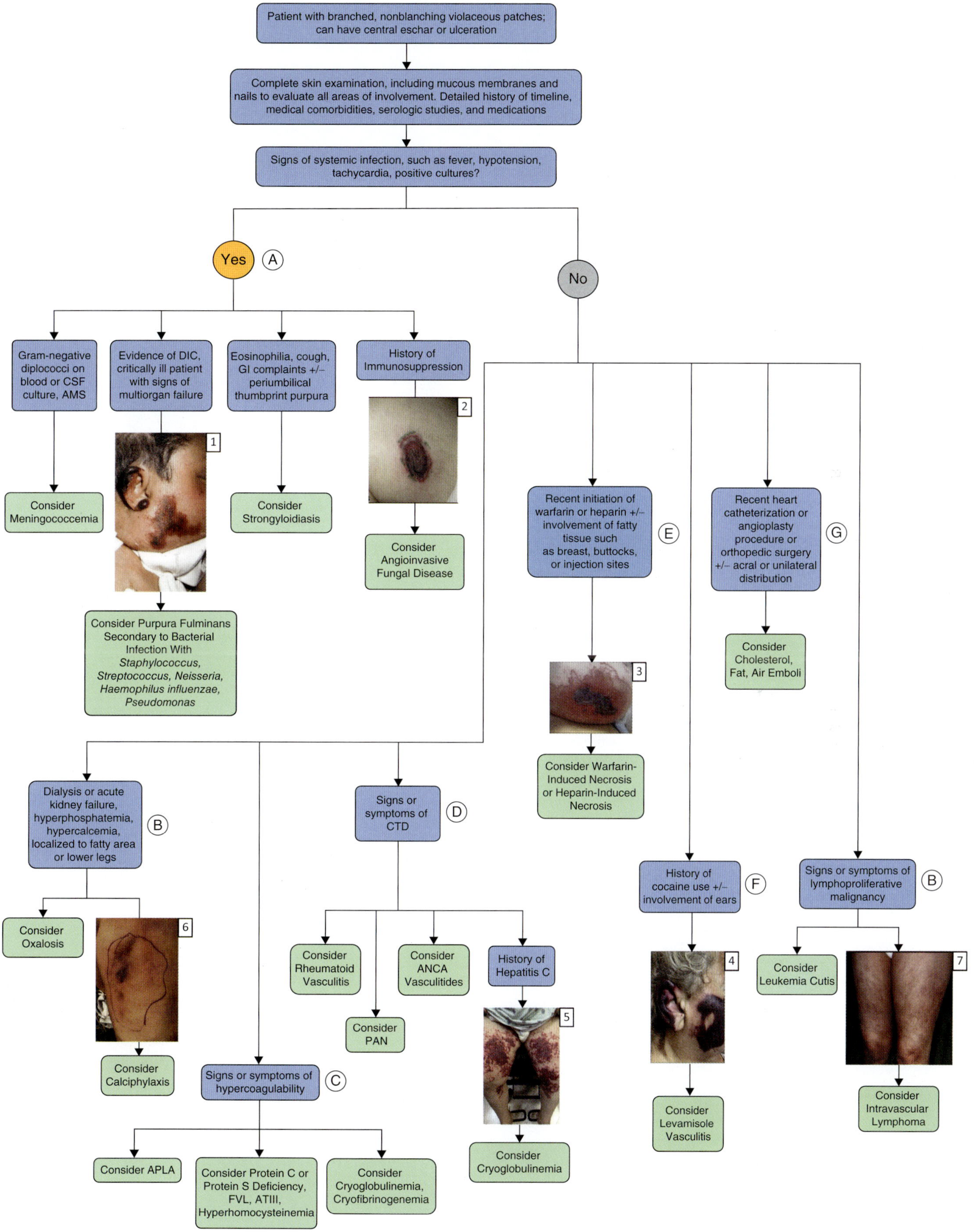
Patient with branched, nonblanching violaceous patches; can have central eschar or ulceration
Complete skin examination, including mucous membranes and nails to evaluate all areas of involvement. Detailed history of timeline, medical comorbidities, serologic studies, and medications
Signs of systemic infection, such as fever, hypotension, tachycardia, positive cultures?
Yes
A
No
Gram-negative diplococci on blood or CSF culture, AMS
Consider Meningococcemia
Evidence of DIC, critically ill patient with signs of multiorgan failure
1
Consider Purpura Fulminans Secondary to Bacterial Infection With *Staphylococcus, Streptococcus, Neisseria, Haemophilus influenzae, Pseudomonas*
Eosinophilia, cough, GI complaints +/– periumbilical thumbprint purpura
Consider Strongyloidiasis
History of Immunosuppression
2
Consider Angioinvasive Fungal Disease
Recent initiation of warfarin or heparin +/– involvement of fatty tissue such as breast, buttocks, or injection sites
E
3
Consider Warfarin-Induced Necrosis or Heparin-Induced Necrosis
Recent heart catheterization or angioplasty procedure or orthopedic surgery +/– acral or unilateral distribution
G
Consider Cholesterol, Fat, Air Emboli
Dialysis or acute kidney failure, hyperphosphatemia, hypercalcemia, localized to fatty area or lower legs
B
Consider Oxalosis
6
Consider Calciphylaxis
Signs or symptoms of hypercoagulability
C
Consider APLA
Consider Protein C or Protein S Deficiency, FVL, ATIII, Hyperhomocysteinemia
Consider Cryoglobulinemia, Cryofibrinogenemia
Signs or symptoms of CTD
D
Consider Rheumatoid Vasculitis
Consider PAN
Consider ANCA Vasculitides
History of Hepatitis C
5
Consider Cryoglobulinemia
History of cocaine use +/– involvement of ears
F
4
Consider Levamisole Vasculitis
Signs or symptoms of lymphoproliferative malignancy
B
Consider Leukemia Cutis
7
Consider Intravascular Lymphoma

PART X
Urticaria

58 Acute Urticaria

Nathan Rojek and Lina Saeed

Urticaria is a term to describe whealing of the skin caused by dermal edema and is often accompanied by angioedema or swelling of the deeper dermis and subcutaneous tissues. Wheals present as pink pruritic dermal swellings that blanch with pressure, and in the case of true urticaria, the individual lesions come and go within 24 hours.

When taking a history of a patient presenting with urticaria, it is helpful to ask about the frequency and duration of flares, associated local and systemic symptoms, previous or current allergies, possible exposure to common triggers (see below), medication history, lifestyle (including hobbies, stress, and smoking habits), other underlying diseases, and psychiatric history. Skin biopsies are of limited utility in the diagnosis and management of urticaria, unless the patient has refractory chronic urticaria (CU), urticarial vasculitis or other urticaria mimickers are being considered, or if the disease is unresponsive to antihistamines.

First-line treatment of urticaria is second-generation antihistamines due to their safety and efficacy profile. Higher than recommended doses may be necessary to attain disease control. To achieve maximal clinical response, once daily dosing is preferred to dosing on an as-needed basis. First-generation antihistamines are less favorable due to their sedative properties.

Urticaria is divided into two main categories: acute and chronic. While all urticarias are acute initially, CU is defined by daily or almost daily wheals or angioedema for more than 6 weeks.

A. In patients with acute urticaria, it is important to evaluate for signs and symptoms of **anaphylaxis** as this is a medical emergency that can ultimately result in hemodynamic instability and death. These include respiratory distress, hemodynamic instability, gastrointestinal stress, and/or neurologic symptoms. Once this has been ruled out and/or adequately managed, a detailed history is imperative to reveal any possible exposures or triggers that may have induced this reaction.

B. In the majority of cases, no trigger is identified despite a detailed history, and the correct diagnosis is acute urticaria.

C. However, there are diagnostic mimics of urticaria that should be considered in any patient presenting with presumed acute urticaria. These mimics are frequently distinguished through a thorough physical examination of the skin alone (although in some cases, direct immunofluorescence or blood work can also be helpful). The presence of bullae on examination in addition to urticaria may point to a diagnosis of **contact dermatitis, arthropod assault reaction,** or **bullous pemphigoid (BP)**. Linear or geometric shapes would be more suggestive of contact dermatitis, while small, red isolated pink papules would suggest an arthropod assault reaction. BP sometimes presents solely with urticarial lesions.

D. Other causes of acute urticaria that may have no systemic symptoms include **urticaria pigmentosa (UP)** and **urticaria multiforme**. These entities may be distinguished by the presence of a positive Darier sign in patients with UP, and the presence of annular, polycyclic, dusky, or targetoid lesions in the case of urticaria multiforme. Other entities that can mimic acute urticaria are discussed in Chapter 59 and include urticarial vasculitis and connective tissue diseases, including Still disease.

E. When the above entities are ruled out, one can more confidently make a diagnosis of acute urticaria. At this point, it is important to determine if there is an eliciting factor. **Infections**, as a whole, comprise 40% of the causes of acute urticaria, with upper respiratory infections (URIs) being the most common trigger. The next most commonly identified triggers are **drugs/medications** and **food**. Nonsteroidal antiinflammatory drugs are a common cause among drugs, so patients with acute urticaria should also be queried not only about chronic medication use, but also about as needed use. In children, the most common urticaria-inducing infections include URIs, *Mycoplasma pneumonia*, and parasitic infections. In adults, viral hepatitis and infectious mononucleosis have been reported in association with acute urticaria.

Generally, no further diagnostic workup is recommended for the evaluation of acute urticaria, but it can be considered if an allergic cause is suspected (see Chapter 59 for further details).

See Appendix 1 for Further Reading and Image References.

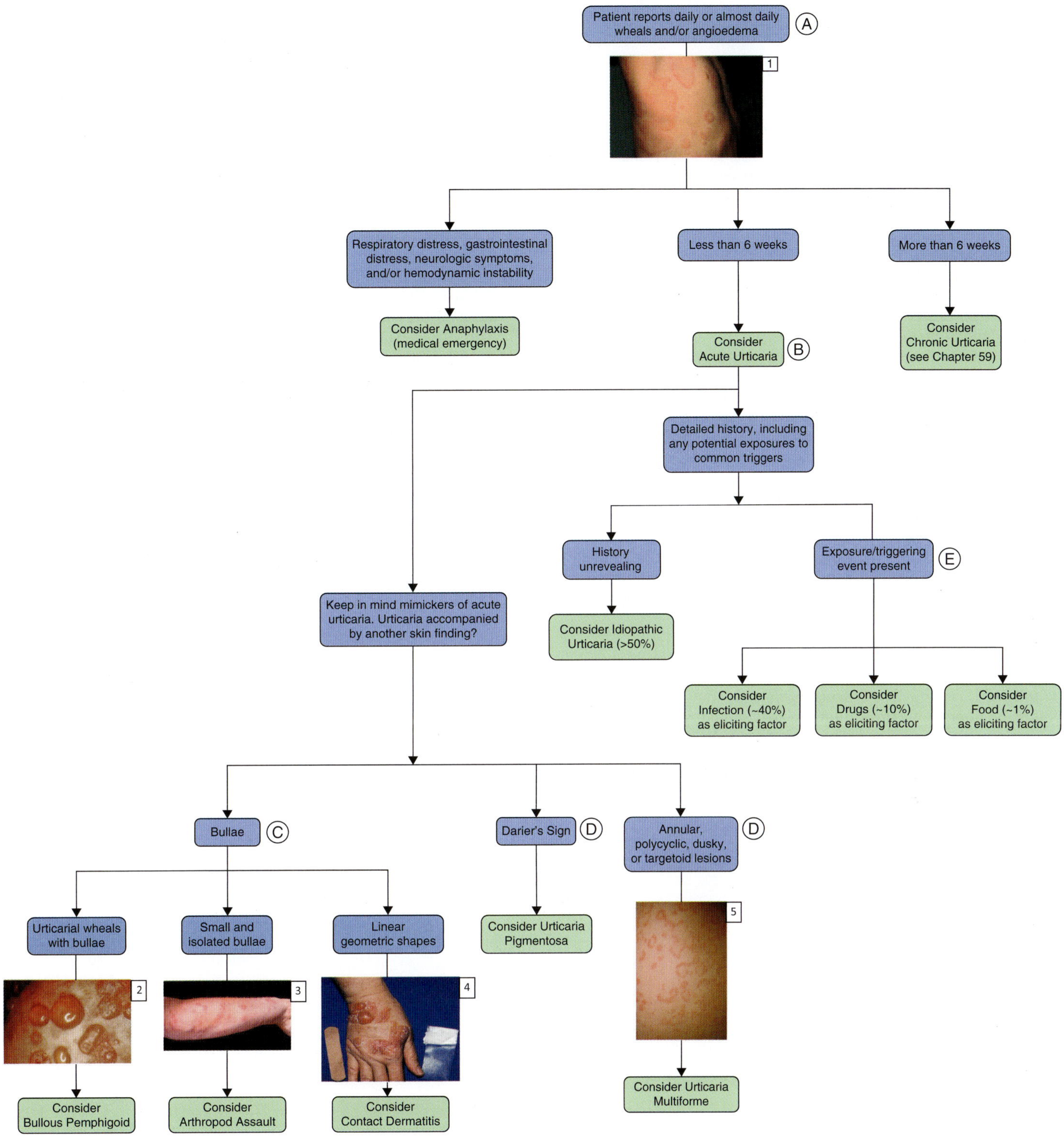
Patient reports daily or almost daily wheals and/or angioedema
A
1
Respiratory distress, gastrointestinal distress, neurologic symptoms, and/or hemodynamic instability
Less than 6 weeks
More than 6 weeks
Consider Anaphylaxis (medical emergency)
Consider Acute Urticaria
B
Consider Chronic Urticaria (see Chapter 59)
Detailed history, including any potential exposures to common triggers
History unrevealing
Exposure/triggering event present
E
Keep in mind mimickers of acute urticaria. Urticaria accompanied by another skin finding?
Consider Idiopathic Urticaria (>50%)
Consider Infection (~40%) as eliciting factor
Consider Drugs (~10%) as eliciting factor
Consider Food (~1%) as eliciting factor
Bullae
C
Darier's Sign
D
Annular, polycyclic, dusky, or targetoid lesions
D
Urticarial wheals with bullae
Small and isolated bullae
Linear geometric shapes
Consider Urticaria Pigmentosa
5
2
3
4
Consider Bullous Pemphigoid
Consider Arthropod Assault
Consider Contact Dermatitis
Consider Urticaria Multiforme

59 Chronic Urticaria

Nathan Rojek and Lina Saeed

In chronic urticaria (CU), wheals still dissipate within 24 hours. However, the overall course of disease persists for longer than 6 weeks. It is important to distinguish this diagnosis from acute urticaria because management can differ dramatically, and the causes are often different.

A. When considering a patient with CU, it is important to ask about potential triggers. Triggers for CU, when identifiable, often fall into one of the following categories: infections, foods, drugs, fluctuations in normal physiology, emotional and/or psychological disturbances, or physical causes. Like acute urticaria, more than one trigger can contribute to a patient's condition.

B. For infections linked to CU, causative agents vary widely according to geographic location and patient population. Various bacteria, parasites, fungi, and viruses may induce urticaria. While food is often reported by patients as a trigger for urticaria, a type I allergy is in fact rarely the cause of CU. However, it should be considered if the patient reports intermittent symptoms and flares occurring within 1 hour of consuming the suspected allergen. Most common food culprits include hazelnut, potato, pork, beef, and seafood. Prick testing and/or IgE serologies can be done to confirm the diagnosis. Angiotensin-converting enzyme inhibitors and nonsteroidal antiinflammatory drugs are the most common culprits of medication-induced urticaria and angioedema. Counseling patients to avoid suspected trigger medications is crucial.

C. **Cholinergic urticaria** is induced by periods of increased core body temperature, for example, during exercise or with consumption of hot foods or liquids. Participating in moderate sustained exercise can be done as a provocation test and should reproduce the rash. Avoiding triggers is the primary treatment. This type of urticaria is characterized by much smaller lesions than other types of urticaria.

D. If urticaria is suspected to be a result of stress, an intradermal injection of epinephrine or norepinephrine can be done as a diagnostic test. A positive result would reproduce the urticarial wheals, supporting the diagnosis of **adrenergic urticaria**. Adrenergic urticaria is best treated by avoiding triggers and using oral beta-blockers, as antihistamines are often ineffective.

E. In **chronic inducible urticaria (CIU)**, lesions often resolve within 2 hours after cessation of stimuli exposure, with the exception of **delayed pressure urticaria**. CIU makes up 20% to 30% of all CU. This diagnosis relies on taking a thorough history and provocation testing, if applicable. There are numerous physical triggers, including the application of shearing forces to the skin (**dermatographism**); exposure to extreme temperatures (**cold and heat urticaria**); application of **pressure**; and exposure to **sunlight, vibration**, or **water** that must all be elicited through history or provocation testing as part of the workup for patients with CU. It is important to ask about each exposure specifically, as patients may not otherwise associate the exposure with their rash.

F. If no trigger is elicited from a thorough history, patients fall under the category of **chronic spontaneous urticaria (CSU)**. When a patient is given the diagnosis of CSU, obtaining a CU index is beneficial to evaluate for autoantibodies that, if elevated, suggest a type IIb autoimmune CSU subtype. This CSU subtype makes up approximately 30% of patients with CSU. Clinical utility of this assay and a positive result remain under scrutiny.

See Appendix 1 for Further Reading and Image References.

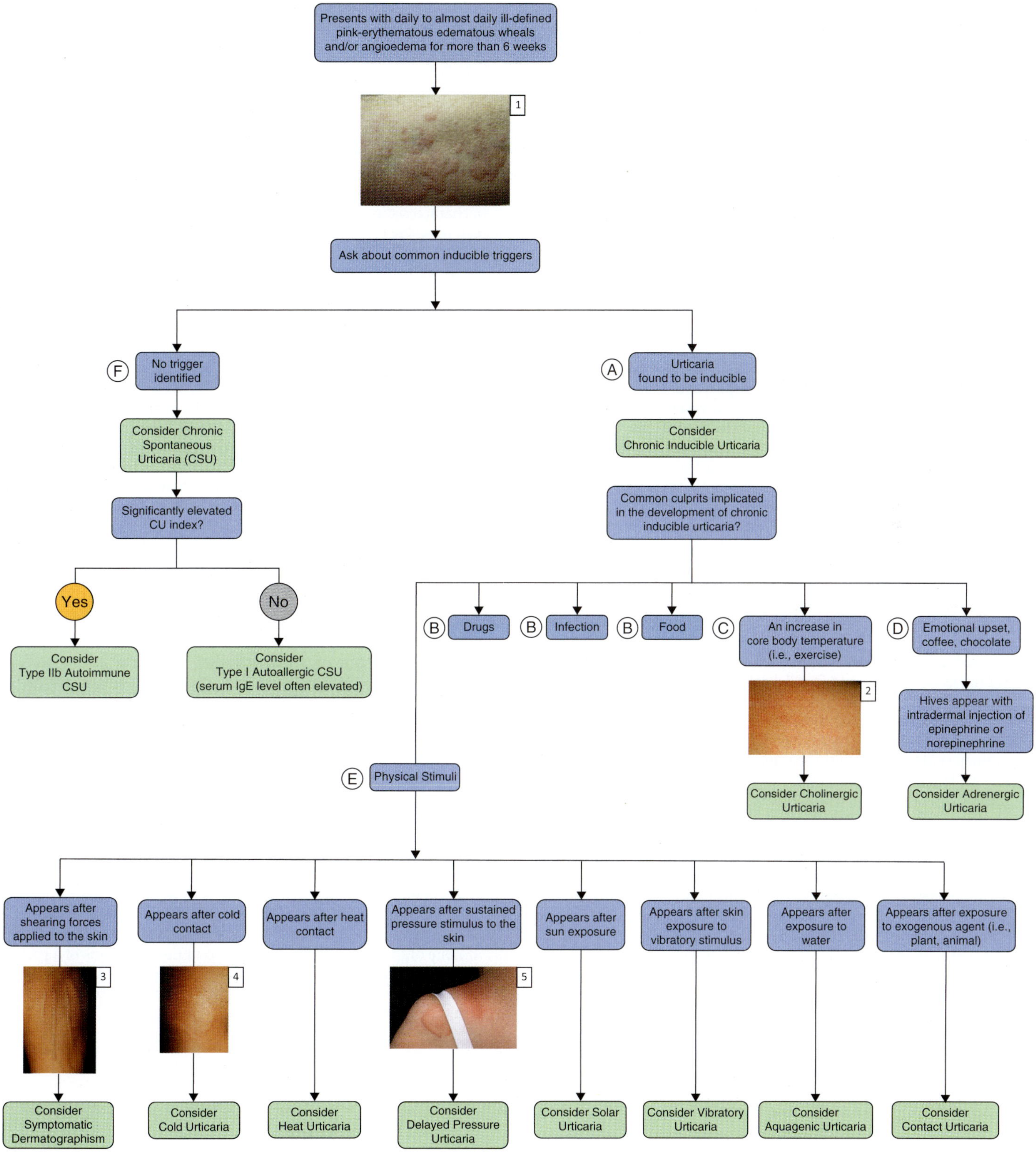
Presents with daily to almost daily ill-defined pink-erythematous edematous wheals and/or angioedema for more than 6 weeks
1
Ask about common inducible triggers
F
No trigger identified
Consider Chronic Spontaneous Urticaria (CSU)
Significantly elevated CU index?
Yes
Consider Type IIb Autoimmune CSU
No
Consider Type I Autoallergic CSU (serum IgE level often elevated)
A
Urticaria found to be inducible
Consider Chronic Inducible Urticaria
Common culprits implicated in the development of chronic inducible urticaria?
B
Drugs
B
Infection
B
Food
C
An increase in core body temperature (i.e., exercise)
2
Consider Cholinergic Urticaria
D
Emotional upset, coffee, chocolate
Hives appear with intradermal injection of epinephrine or norepinephrine
Consider Adrenergic Urticaria
E
Physical Stimuli
Appears after shearing forces applied to the skin
3
Consider Symptomatic Dermatographism
Appears after cold contact
4
Consider Cold Urticaria
Appears after heat contact
Consider Heat Urticaria
Appears after sustained pressure stimulus to the skin
5
Consider Delayed Pressure Urticaria
Appears after sun exposure
Consider Solar Urticaria
Appears after skin exposure to vibratory stimulus
Consider Vibratory Urticaria
Appears after exposure to water
Consider Aquagenic Urticaria
Appears after exposure to exogenous agent (i.e., plant, animal)
Consider Contact Urticaria

60 Urticaria With Other Symptoms

Liat Bainvoll and Scott D. Worswick

Urticaria presents as wheals (erythematous and nonscaly plaques that blanch with pressure); lesions are pruritic and can be associated with angioedema. Although urticaria itself is caused by vasodilation leading to superficial dermal edema, identifying the underlying cause is complex. Isolated urticaria may be acute or chronic and is described in the preceding two chapters. This chapter details a process by which to approach urticaria when it is associated with systemic symptoms.

Initial evaluation should include clarification of the timing of onset, the duration and distribution of wheals, a thorough medical and drug history, an evaluation for a family history of autoimmune conditions, a comprehensive review of systems, and a complete physical examination.

A. Patients with individual urticarial lesions that persist beyond 24 hours and/or resolve with residual purpura or hyperpigmentation should prompt a workup of **urticarial vasculitis.** The urticarial lesions may be painful rather than pruritic. Patients may also present with other symptoms, including fever, arthralgias, abdominal pain, and lymphadenopathy; vasculitis may occur in any organ. Definitive diagnosis requires biopsy that demonstrates evidence of leukocytoclastic vasculitis. A subset of patients will have hypocomplementemic urticarial vasculitis syndrome, so all patients should have antinuclear antibody, complement levels, and antibodies to C1q checked.

B. **Autoinflammatory disorders** are a family of disorders resulting from inappropriate activation of the innate immune system. Generally, patients present with recurrent fevers and various inflammatory symptoms, including arthralgias/arthritis. Urticarial rash is present in cryopyrin-associated periodic syndrome (CAPS), Schnitzler syndrome, and familial cold autoinflammatory syndrome type 2 (FCAS2). CAPS is associated with an NLRP3 mutation and may present with ocular symptoms or sensorineural hearing loss. Schnitzler syndrome occurs later in life and is characterized by laboratory evidence of monoclonal paraproteinemia, particularly IgM, and acute phase reactant elevation. FCAS2 is an autosomal dominant disease associated with a mutation in NLRP12.

C. Alternative diagnoses to consider in patients with urticaria, arthralgias, and persistent fevers are **serum sickness** or **serum sickness-like reaction**. Patients may report a recent exposure to heterologous serum or new drugs or have signs of infection 1 to 2 weeks prior to presentation. Serum sickness often leads to renal dysfunction and sometimes neuropathy. Laboratory tests demonstrate neutropenia, elevated acute phase reactants, and hypocomplementemia.

D. Urticaria is a nonspecific symptom of many **connective tissue diseases.** If a patient presents with symptoms of arthralgias, fever, photosensitivity, or other classic skin findings, investigation of an underlying connective tissue disease is warranted. **Systemic lupus erythematosus, dermatomyositis (DM), Sjögren syndrome**, and **scleroderma** have all been associated with urticaria. Further specification of the disease requires serum autoantibody evaluation and correlation with other symptoms and signs. **Adult-onset Still disease (AOSD)** may similarly present with arthralgias and fevers, but a characteristic evanescent rash may be present. Flagellate erythema can be a clue to either AOSD or DM (see Chapter 8).

E. **Mastocytosis** occurs most frequently in children and can be cutaneous or systemic. It presents with red-brown macules and papules most commonly on the trunk and extremities. Darier sign is pathognomonic for mastocytosis. Biopsy reveals scattered eosinophils and uniformly spaced mast cells infiltrating the papillary dermis, and sometimes the reticular dermis.

F. Evidence suggests an association between urticaria and **autoimmune thyroid disease**, but the causal relationship is still unknown. Patients may present with signs and symptoms of hyperthyroidism, including tachycardia, tremor, palpitations, weight loss, diarrhea, diaphoresis, and exophthalmos; or they may present with signs of hypothyroidism, including fatigue, weight gain, constipation, dry hair, and brittle nails. Laboratory evidence will demonstrate alterations in thyroid function tests, which vary depending on the underlying etiology. When associated with thyroid disease, urticaria will resolve with treatment of the endocrinopathy.

G. **Eosinophilic dermatoses** are a broad category of diseases characterized by eosinophilic infiltration of the skin. Many different eosinophilic dermatoses can manifest with urticaria as well as systemic symptoms, including drug reactions, contrast reactions, and contact dermatitis. It is important to remember that bullous pemphigoid can present with urticarial lesions without bullae; in patients with urticaria and eosinophilic spongiosis, it is therefore also important to consider obtaining a biopsy for direct immunofluorescence. If a patient presents with recurrent episodes of nonallergic angioedema, urticaria, fever, and weight gain, consider Gleich syndrome. Coalescing erythematous plaques resembling urticaria may be due to eosinophilic cellulitis (Wells syndrome). Patients with hypereosinophilia and coexisting organ damage may have hypereosinophilic syndrome. Lastly, patients with hematologic malignancy may also present with urticaria due to eosinophilic infiltration into the skin.

If none of the above diagnoses seem to fit the symptoms of a patient with urticaria, it is possible that the patient is experiencing acute or chronic urticaria in addition to another underlying disease driving their systemic symptoms.

See Appendix 1 for Further Reading and Image References.

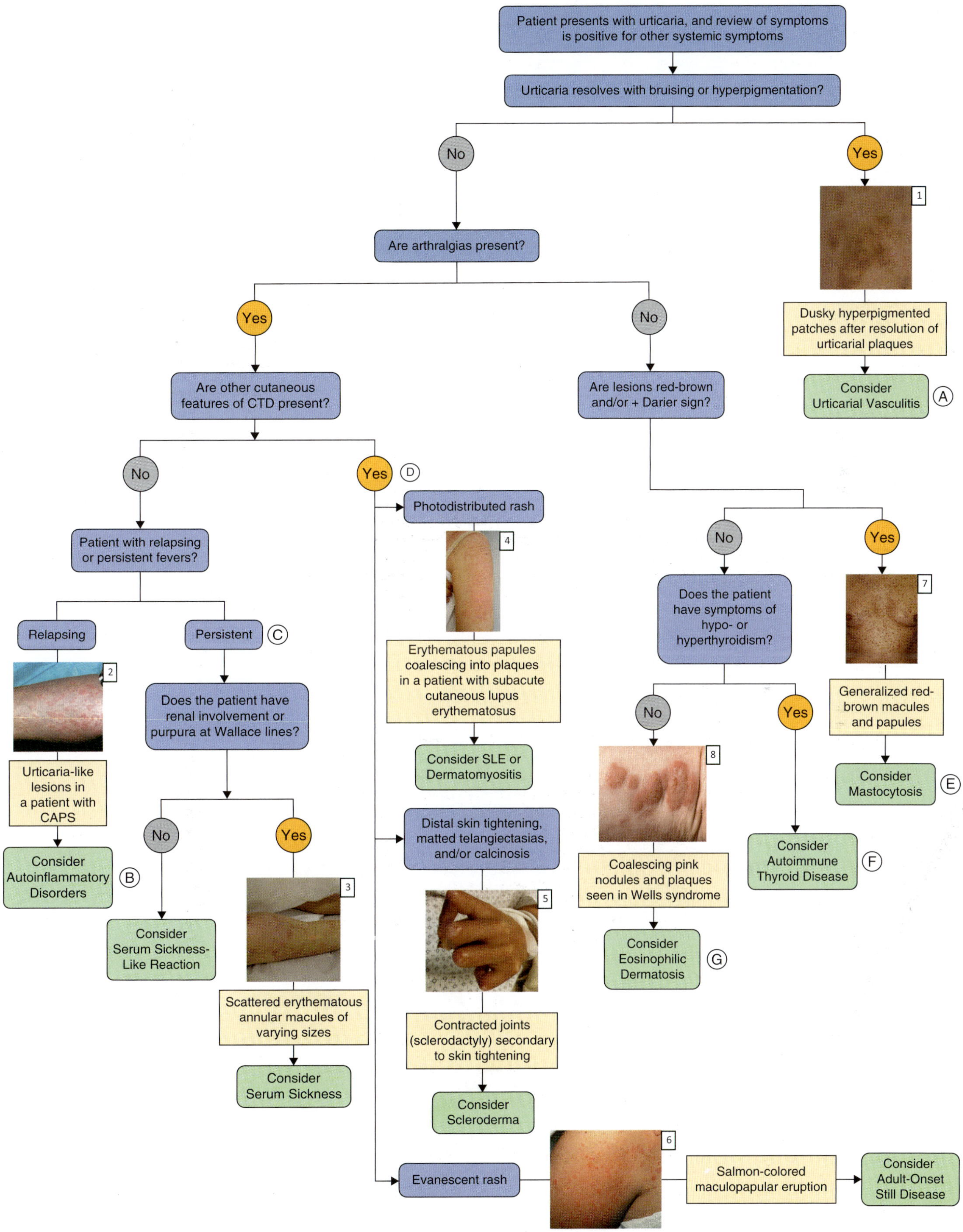
Patient presents with urticaria, and review of symptoms is positive for other systemic symptoms
Urticaria resolves with bruising or hyperpigmentation?
No
Yes
1
Dusky hyperpigmented patches after resolution of urticarial plaques
Consider Urticarial Vasculitis
A
Are arthralgias present?
Yes
No
Are other cutaneous features of CTD present?
Are lesions red-brown and/or + Darier sign?
No
Yes
D
Patient with relapsing or persistent fevers?
Relapsing
Persistent
C
2
Urticaria-like lesions in a patient with CAPS
Consider Autoinflammatory Disorders
B
Does the patient have renal involvement or purpura at Wallace lines?
No
Yes
Consider Serum Sickness-Like Reaction
3
Scattered erythematous annular macules of varying sizes
Consider Serum Sickness
Photodistributed rash
4
Erythematous papules coalescing into plaques in a patient with subacute cutaneous lupus erythematosus
Consider SLE or Dermatomyositis
Distal skin tightening, matted telangiectasias, and/or calcinosis
5
Contracted joints (sclerodactyly) secondary to skin tightening
Consider Scleroderma
Evanescent rash
6
Salmon-colored maculopapular eruption
Consider Adult-Onset Still Disease
No
Yes
Does the patient have symptoms of hypo- or hyperthyroidism?
No
Yes
8
Coalescing pink nodules and plaques seen in Wells syndrome
Consider Eosinophilic Dermatosis
G
Consider Autoimmune Thyroid Disease
F
7
Generalized red-brown macules and papules
Consider Mastocytosis
E

PART XI
Poikiloderma

61 Inherited Poikiloderma

Brandon Andrew Levian and Brandon L. Adler

Poikiloderma is a unique morphology defined as a combination of atrophy, telangiectasia, and hyper- or hypopigmentation. One way of classifying poikiloderma is by inherited versus acquired etiologies. Narrowing the differential diagnosis of an inherited poikiloderma requires a thorough history and physical examination, particularly focusing on the presence or absence of associated photosensitivity. Inherited poikilodermas usually manifest early in life but may go undiagnosed into adulthood. Frequently, genetic testing is necessary to confirm the diagnosis. Prompt diagnosis is essential, as in many cases, poikiloderma precedes internal organ dysfunction.

A. A history of poor growth, short stature, and a photosensitive malar rash should raise concern for **Bloom syndrome (BS)**, an autosomal recessive (AR) disorder caused by mutations in the *BLM (RECQL3)* gene. Facial poikiloderma, cheilitis, and photosensitive bullous eruptions in BS may resemble lupus erythematosus. The characteristic facies are narrow and elongated. Mutational analysis confirms the diagnosis. There is an increased risk for hematologic and solid malignancies as well as basal cell carcinomas (BCC) and squamous cell carcinomas (SCC), which may have early onset.

B. **Rothmund-Thomson syndrome (RTS)**, an AR disorder classically arising between 3 and 6 months of age, manifests with short stature, erythema, and bullae initially involving the face and then the extremities and buttocks, followed by the development of poikiloderma. Further diagnostic clues include the presence of juvenile cataracts, skeletal abnormalities, and sparse scalp, eyebrow, and eyelash hair. Patients with RTS do not exhibit photosensitivity. All patients with RTS have increased risk of developing BCC and SCC; those with type II RTS are also at risk for osteosarcoma. The diagnosis can be confirmed by identifying mutations in *ANAPC1* (type I) or *RECQL4* (type II).

C. A patient with short stature who presents with poikiloderma of the extremities progressing to the face and neck, palmoplantar keratoderma, paronychia, and frequent infections should be evaluated for **Clericuzio-type poikiloderma with neutropenia (PN)**, an AR disorder caused by *USB1* gene mutations. Photosensitivity is sometimes present. Clinical diagnostic criteria for PN have been proposed, but the current gold standard is mutational analysis.

D. A patient presenting with progressive poikiloderma of the face, neck, and dorsal hands, blisters in trauma-prone and acral areas, cutaneous atrophy most prominent on the dorsal hands and feet, and photosensitivity should be evaluated for **Kindler syndrome (KS)**. KS is a distinct subtype of epidermolysis bullosa (EB) caused by an AR mutation in the *FERMT1 (KIND1)* gene. While blistering usually improves with age, the degree of atrophy, photosensitivity, and poikiloderma may worsen. Unlike other types of EB, histopathology of a KS blister demonstrates multiple planes of cleavage at the dermoepidermal junction. The *FERMT1* gene sequencing confirms the diagnosis. Regular dermatologic follow-up is indicated due to the increased risk of nonmelanoma skin cancer.

E. Sun-exposed poikiloderma, photosensitivity, and/or prominent early-onset lentigines are characteristics of **xeroderma pigmentosum (XP)**, an AR disorder that results in ultraviolet-induced DNA damage secondary to impaired nucleotide excision repair. XP is divided into seven complementation groups with variable cutaneous and extracutaneous (including ocular and neurologic) findings, as well as a milder form (XP variant), but any of them may feature poikiloderma. There is a significantly increased risk for BCC, SCC, and melanoma. Mutational analysis confirms the diagnosis.

F. A patient presenting with the constellation of diffuse poikiloderma (most prominent at flexures and bony prominences), linear or reticular hyperkeratotic and sclerotic bands in the axillae, palmar/plantar sclerosis, finger clubbing, and cardiac calcification should prompt suspicion for **hereditary sclerosing poikiloderma (HSP)**. There is no associated photosensitivity. HSP-associated poikiloderma tends to present in previously asymptomatic children aged 2 to 3 years. Diagnosis of this rare autosomal dominant (AD) disorder is purely clinical; no mutations have been identified.

G. The triad of nail dystrophy, oral leukoplakia, and poikiloderma of the chest and/or neck should lead to evaluation for **dyskeratosis congenita (DC)**. DC is caused by AD, AR, or X-linked mutations in a variety of genes involved in telomere maintenance. Photosensitivity is not an accompanying feature. Clinical diagnostic criteria are available, with confirmation by mutational analysis. Given the significantly increased risk of bone marrow failure (BMF), hematologic and solid malignancies, and pulmonary fibrosis, prompt diagnosis is of utmost importance. Furthermore, any patient with BMF who fails to respond to standard immunosuppressive therapy should be evaluated for the possibility of DC.

See Appendix 1 for Further Reading and Image References.

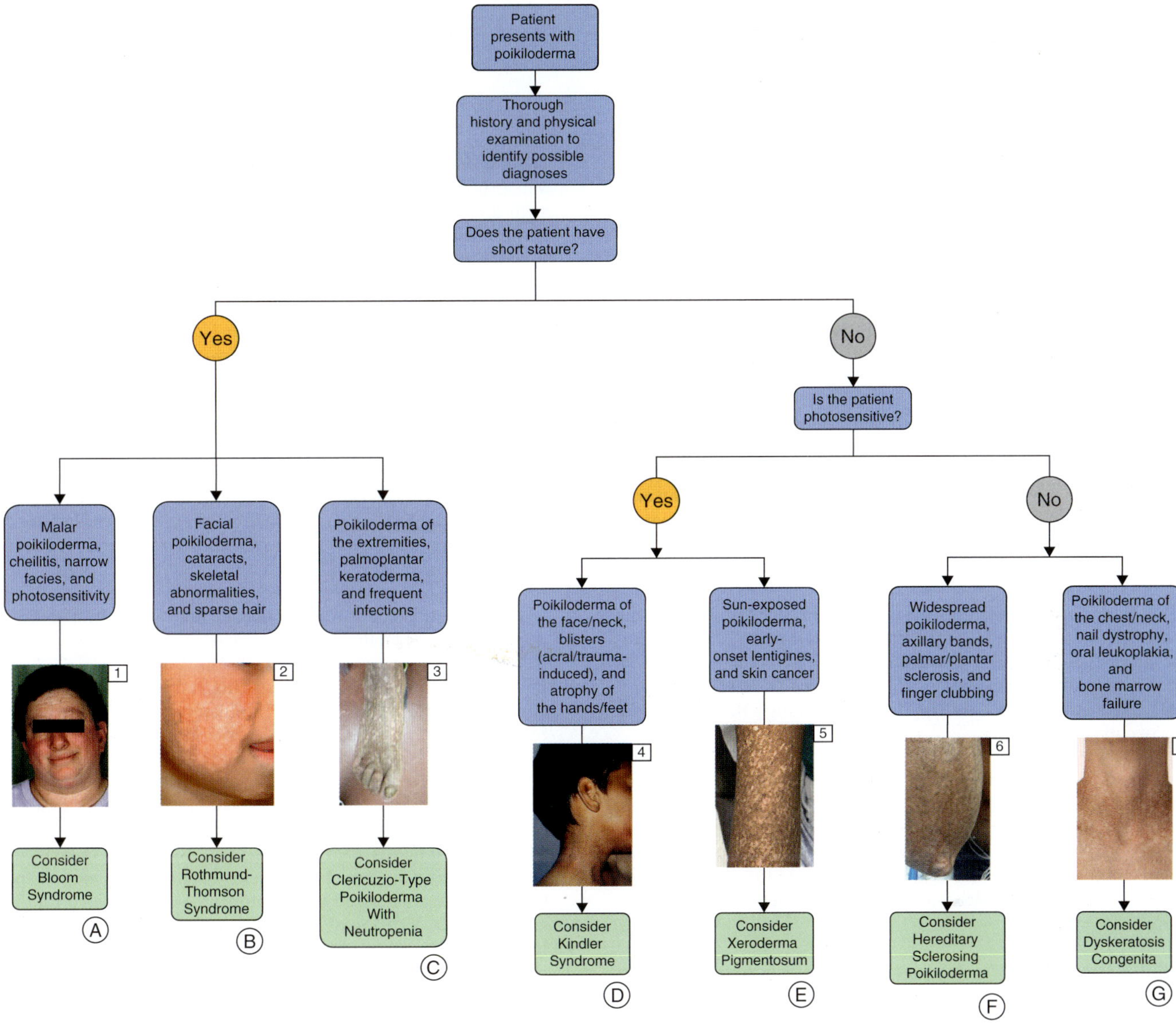
Patient presents with poikiloderma
Thorough history and physical examination to identify possible diagnoses
Does the patient have short stature?
Yes
No
Is the patient photosensitive?
Malar poikiloderma, cheilitis, narrow facies, and photosensitivity
Facial poikiloderma, cataracts, skeletal abnormalities, and sparse hair
Poikiloderma of the extremities, palmoplantar keratoderma, and frequent infections
Yes
No
Poikiloderma of the face/neck, blisters (acral/trauma-induced), and atrophy of the hands/feet
Sun-exposed poikiloderma, early-onset lentigines, and skin cancer
Widespread poikiloderma, axillary bands, palmar/plantar sclerosis, and finger clubbing
Poikiloderma of the chest/neck, nail dystrophy, oral leukoplakia, and bone marrow failure
1
2
3
4
5
6
7
Consider Bloom Syndrome
A
Consider Rothmund-Thomson Syndrome
B
Consider Clericuzio-Type Poikiloderma With Neutropenia
C
Consider Kindler Syndrome
D
Consider Xeroderma Pigmentosum
E
Consider Hereditary Sclerosing Poikiloderma
F
Consider Dyskeratosis Congenita
G

62 Acquired Poikiloderma

Brandon Andrew Levian and Brandon L. Adler

Poikiloderma is a unique morphology defined as a combination of atrophy, telangiectasia, and hyper- or hypopigmentation. One way of classifying poikiloderma is by inherited versus acquired etiologies. The associations of acquired poikiloderma range from benign to (pre) malignant and include potentially life-threatening systemic diseases. The workup of acquired poikiloderma should include a thorough history, detailed physical examination focusing on the distribution and any additional cutaneous findings, and sometimes histopathologic and/or laboratory examination. The treatment must be tailored to the underlying cause.

A. Chronic exposure to infrared heat sources, such as heating pads, space heaters, and laptop computers, may lead to the development of **erythema ab igne (EAI)**, characterized by mottled and reticulated hyperpigmentation with atrophy and telangiectasias. Any anatomic region in frequent close proximity to the heat source may be involved. EAI is usually asymptomatic. Rarely, nonmelanoma skin cancers have been reported to develop within long-standing lesions.

B. In soldiers and refugees, **sulfur mustard–induced poikiloderma** can develop after exposure to chemical warfare agents. Following initial, immediate blistering, poikiloderma can take years to manifest. Ocular and pulmonary complications may also occur. This uncommon diagnosis highlights the importance of taking a thorough social and occupational history.

C. In patients with atopic dermatitis, poikilodermatous changes may be observed on the neck, thought to be the combined result of frictional melanosis, postinflammatory hyperpigmentation, and chronic topical corticosteroid use. This finding may be most common among Asian patients. Historically known as "atopic dirty neck," a less stigmatizing term, **acquired atopic hyperpigmentation** has been proposed.

D. **Poikiloderma of Civatte** is a sign of chronic photodamage, most common in fair-skinned individuals, involving the lateral neck and upper chest. Patients may manifest additional signs of photoaging, including solar purpura, lentigines, cutis rhomboidalis nuchae, Favre-Racouchot syndrome, and actinic keratoses. Photoprotection is essential to prevent skin cancer.

E. An erythematous to violaceous poikilodermatous plaque on the lower extremities or pelvic girdle suggests **poikilodermatous plaque-like hemangioma**, a recently described acquired vascular proliferation with a benign clinical course. Histopathology shows a diffuse band-like vascular proliferation in the papillary and superficial reticular dermis with associated dermal fibrosis/edema, loss of elastic fibers, and frequently overlying acanthosis.

F. The combination of poikiloderma, lichenoid papules, and sometimes blisters on the trunk and limbs is characteristic of **poikiloderma-like cutaneous amyloidosis (PCA)**. There are two forms of PCA: ordinary PCA, which presents around the fifth decade of life, and PCA syndrome, which manifests earlier with associated photosensitivity, short stature, and sometimes palmoplantar keratoderma. Histopathology demonstrates eosinophilic deposits with Congo red staining that display apple-green birefringence under polarized light.

G. Poikiloderma can be associated with autoimmune connective tissue diseases (AI-CTD). In subacute **cutaneous lupus erythematosus**, generalized poikiloderma has been reported, with a predilection for sun-exposed areas. Poikiloderma has also been found in association with discoid lupus, lupus panniculitis, and neonatal lupus. Patients should be assessed for signs of systemic lupus erythematosus (SLE), including malar rash, mucositis, serositis, hematologic disorders, arthritis, and nephritis.

In **dermatomyositis**, poikiloderma may present on the upper back ("shawl sign"), upper chest ("V-neck sign"), and/or lateral thighs ("holster sign"). Other features of dermatomyositis should be sought out, including cutaneous stigmata (e.g., Gottron papules, heliotrope rash, psoriasiform scalp dermatitis), proximal muscle weakness with elevated creatine kinase and/or aldolase (absent in amyopathic cases), and presence of myositis-specific antibodies. Histopathologic findings suggest AI-CTD but cannot reliably distinguish between SLE and dermatomyositis.

Patients taking long-term hydroxyurea can develop **dermatomyositis-like eruptions (hydroxyurea dermopathy)** characterized by photodistributed poikiloderma, without muscle weakness. Leg ulcers are also associated with long-term hydroxyurea therapy and when present, point to the diagnosis. Statins are known to cause drug-induced dermatomyositis as well.

H. Poikiloderma at sites of prior ionizing radiation exposure suggests **chronic radiation dermatitis**. The history should be reviewed for tumor radiotherapy and certain interventional procedures (e.g., fluoroscopy). The development of chronic radiation dermatitis may relate to an imbalance between proinflammatory and profibrotic cytokines.

I. **Chronic cutaneous graft-versus-host disease (cGVHD)** usually develops within 3 years of allogeneic hematopoietic cell transplantation and is characterized by poikiloderma concentrated on the face and trunk. cGVHD may also present with lichenoid or sclerodermoid skin changes, as well as ocular, mucosal, and gastrointestinal complications.

J. **Poikilodermatous mycosis fungoides (pMF)** is a cutaneous T-cell lymphoma that presents with poikiloderma that can be localized (favoring flexural sun-protected sites), generalized, or mixed with other forms of mycosis fungoides (MF). Histopathology displays stage-dependent MF findings, and immunophenotyping favors a CD4+ phenotype. It can be challenging to distinguish pMF from poikilodermatous parapsoriasis, a controversial entity.

K. In a patient with a history of Lyme disease or exposure to tick-infested areas, the development of poikiloderma on the extensor extremities should prompt evaluation for **acrodermatitis chronica atrophicans (ACA)**. ACA is a late cutaneous manifestation of Lyme disease associated with *Borrelia afzelii* infection in Europe and Asia and is very rarely encountered in North America. Months to years after the initial infection, affected patients develop erythematous plaques and nodules, followed by poikilodermatous, atrophic, and fibrotic skin changes. Histopathology reveals a plasma cell dermal infiltrate, fibrosis, and destruction of epidermal appendages. Lyme serologies, tissue polymerase chain reaction, and Warthin-Starry staining on histology are also helpful diagnostic tools.

See Appendix 1 for Further Reading and Image References.

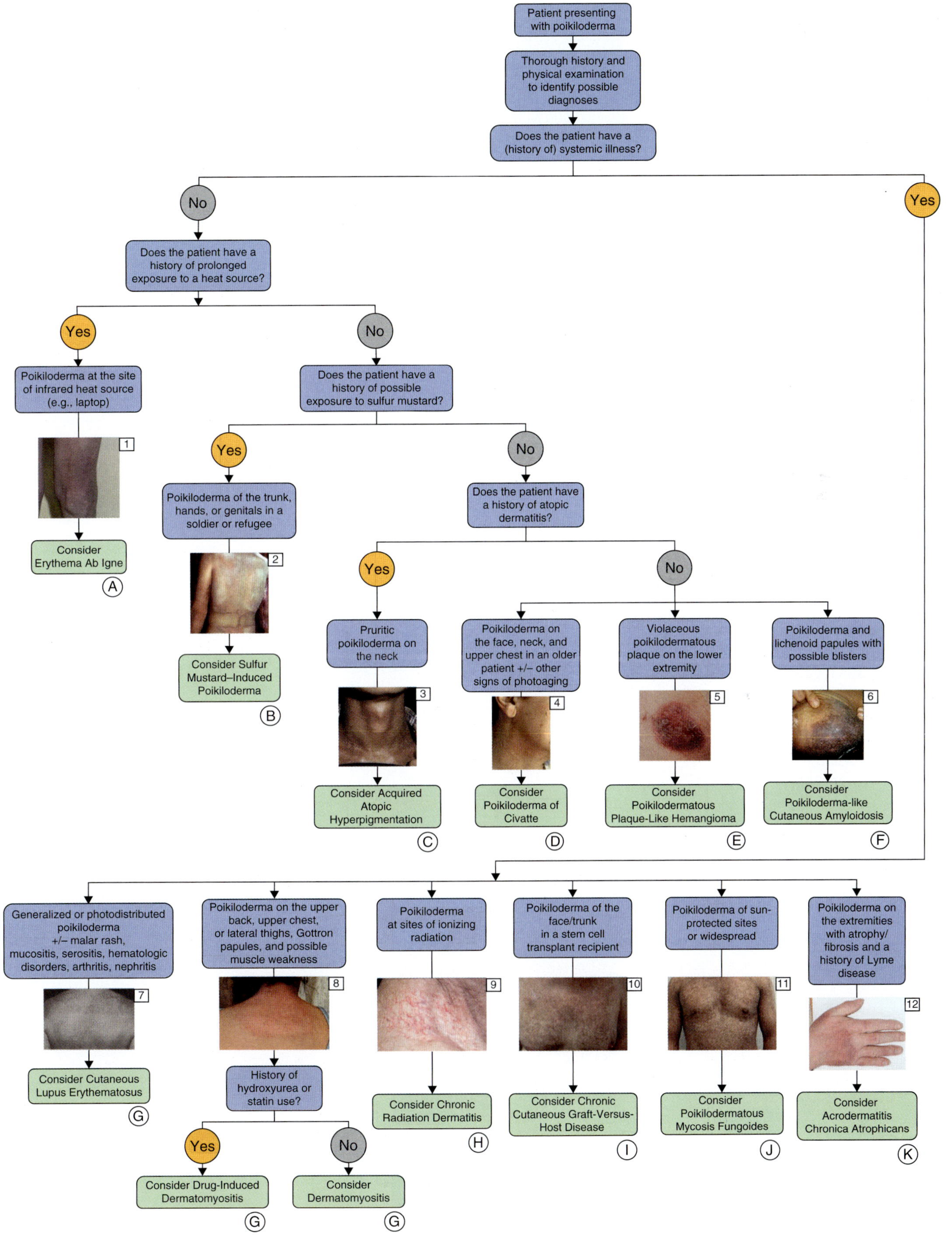
Patient presenting with poikiloderma
Thorough history and physical examination to identify possible diagnoses
Does the patient have a (history of) systemic illness?
No
Does the patient have a history of prolonged exposure to a heat source?
Yes
Poikiloderma at the site of infrared heat source (e.g., laptop)
1
Consider Erythema Ab Igne
A
No
Does the patient have a history of possible exposure to sulfur mustard?
Yes
Poikiloderma of the trunk, hands, or genitals in a soldier or refugee
2
Consider Sulfur Mustard–Induced Poikiloderma
B
No
Does the patient have a history of atopic dermatitis?
Yes
Pruritic poikiloderma on the neck
3
Consider Acquired Atopic Hyperpigmentation
C
No
Poikiloderma on the face, neck, and upper chest in an older patient +/– other signs of photoaging
4
Consider Poikiloderma of Civatte
D
Violaceous poikilodermatous plaque on the lower extremity
5
Consider Poikilodermatous Plaque-Like Hemangioma
E
Poikiloderma and lichenoid papules with possible blisters
6
Consider Poikiloderma-like Cutaneous Amyloidosis
F
Yes
Generalized or photodistributed poikiloderma +/– malar rash, mucositis, serositis, hematologic disorders, arthritis, nephritis
7
Consider Cutaneous Lupus Erythematosus
G
Poikiloderma on the upper back, upper chest, or lateral thighs, Gottron papules, and possible muscle weakness
8
History of hydroxyurea or statin use?
Yes
Consider Drug-Induced Dermatomyositis
G
No
Consider Dermatomyositis
G
Poikiloderma at sites of ionizing radiation
9
Consider Chronic Radiation Dermatitis
H
Poikiloderma of the face/trunk in a stem cell transplant recipient
10
Consider Chronic Cutaneous Graft-Versus-Host Disease
I
Poikiloderma of sun-protected sites or widespread
11
Consider Poikilodermatous Mycosis Fungoides
J
Poikiloderma on the extremities with atrophy/ fibrosis and a history of Lyme disease
12
Consider Acrodermatitis Chronica Atrophicans
K

PART XII
Atrophy

63 Epidermal Atrophy

William Lewis and Robert G. Micheletti

Epidermal atrophy may be seen as a sequela of numerous inflammatory and neoplastic dermopathies and presents clinically as thin wrinkled skin. Other features, such as pigmentary change, purpura, or poikiloderma, may be present depending on the etiology of the atrophy. Histologically, thinning of the epidermis and loss of rete ridges may be observed. Epidermal atrophy can be seen in isolation or in combination with dermal atrophy or lipoatrophy.

Poikiloderma is a frequently encountered combination of epidermal atrophy, telangiectasis, and mottled hyper- and hypopigmentation.

A. When poikiloderma is seen in a geometric pattern, consider **radiation exposure** as the etiology. When present in the flexures or on the trunk, consider **poikilodermatous mycosis fungoides**, a predominantly CD8+/CD4 variant of mycosis fungoides (MF) more commonly seen in males.

B. If the patient has any prior history or physical findings of connective tissue disease, **cutaneous lupus**, **dermatomyositis**, **scleroderma**, and **antiphospholipid antibody syndrome** should be considered in the differential diagnosis.

C. In the absence of signs or symptoms of connective tissue disease, advanced **age** or significant sun exposure (**dermatoheliosis**) can produce photodistributed atrophy of the epidermis, which may be accompanied by actinic purpura. Within a background of significant sun damage, a small focus of atrophy may represent **atrophic actinic keratosis**. If the patient's skin appears poikilodermatous but old age and a sun exposure history are lacking, consider inherited **disorders of photosensitivity. Kindler syndrome** may present at birth with acrally distributed blisters; by later childhood, patients develop widespread poikiloderma and atrophy. **Chronic graft-versus-host disease** should be considered in patients with a history of stem cell transplantation.

Many disorders associated with epidermal atrophy will also produce pigmentary alteration in the skin.

D. **Erythema ab igne, pityriasis rotunda**, and **lichen planus pigmentosus** produce reticulated, circular, and patchy areas of hyperpigmentation, respectively. **Nutritional deficiencies** may show atrophy in conjunction with hyperpigmentation. When atrophy is present along with scaly hypo- or hyperpigmented patches or plaques, consider **parapsoriasis** and **MF**.

E. Epidermal atrophy in conjunction with hypopigmentation is commonly seen in **lichen sclerosus et atrophicus**, most often found on the genitals but also occurring extragenitally. Follicular plugging may be a clinical and histologic clue to the diagnosis of this entity. When occurring in a reticulated pattern on the lower leg, atrophy in conjunction with hypopigmentation may represent **atrophie blanche**, a sequela of livedoid vasculopathy. A "porcelain" appearance with atrophy and papular morphology may occur in the rare entity **Degos disease**, also known as **malignant atrophic papulosis**, a skin-limited or systemic vasculopathy of unknown etiology. **Late-stage pinta**, caused by the spirochete *Treponema carateum* in Mexico, Central America, and South America, may also produce atrophic lesions with hypopigmentation. **Corticosteroid-induced atrophy** should be suspected in any patient receiving topical corticosteroids or glucocorticoid injections for arthritis, especially if the atrophy is found overlying the spine or a joint space.

When epidermal atrophy is not significantly associated with poikiloderma or pigmentary change, it is useful to exclude common causes that may be readily identified by distinctive morphologic features.

F. External trauma leading to **scarring** is the most common cause of localized epidermal atrophy.

G. Clinically, **striae** appear as linear bands of atrophy perpendicular to lines of skin tension in areas of rapid and significant expansion of underlying tissue volume. Associated conditions include normal adolescent growth, pregnancy, weight fluctuation, and endocrine disorders of glucocorticoid excess.

H. For sharply circumscribed solitary areas of skin wrinkling, consider **anetoderma**, which occurs due to the loss of elastin fibers. When epidermal atrophy is present and the patient reports a history of self-resolving lesion at the site, consider the diagnosis of spontaneously involuting **juvenile xanthogranuloma** or **infantile hemangioma**. **Aplasia cutis congenita** is present at birth and may manifest anywhere on the body, although it is most often seen on the vertex scalp as a small, hairless, atrophic area. It is often syndromic, although it has also been described in isolation. Workup for underlying tissue defects may be warranted.

Finally, distribution may provide clues to the etiology of skin atrophy.

I. Atrophic lesions on the lower legs with a yellow hue may represent **necrobiosis lipoidica**. When other lesions suggestive of lichen planus are present, consider a diagnosis of **lichen planus atrophicus**.

J. Acrally distributed atrophy of the skin is seen in **acrodermatitis chronica atrophicans**, which occurs as a late stage of a Lyme-like infection with *Borrelia afzelii*. Although previously described only in Europe, cases have been reported elsewhere, including Mexico.

K. Diffuse atrophy may be seen in patients with **progeria**, who are usually clinically normal at birth. By age 1 to 2 years, they begin to show dermatologic signs of the condition, such as skin atrophy and xerosis, prominent superficial veins, alopecia, nail dystrophy, and sclerodermoid changes, most commonly on the lower extremities and abdomen.

See Appendix 1 for Further Reading.

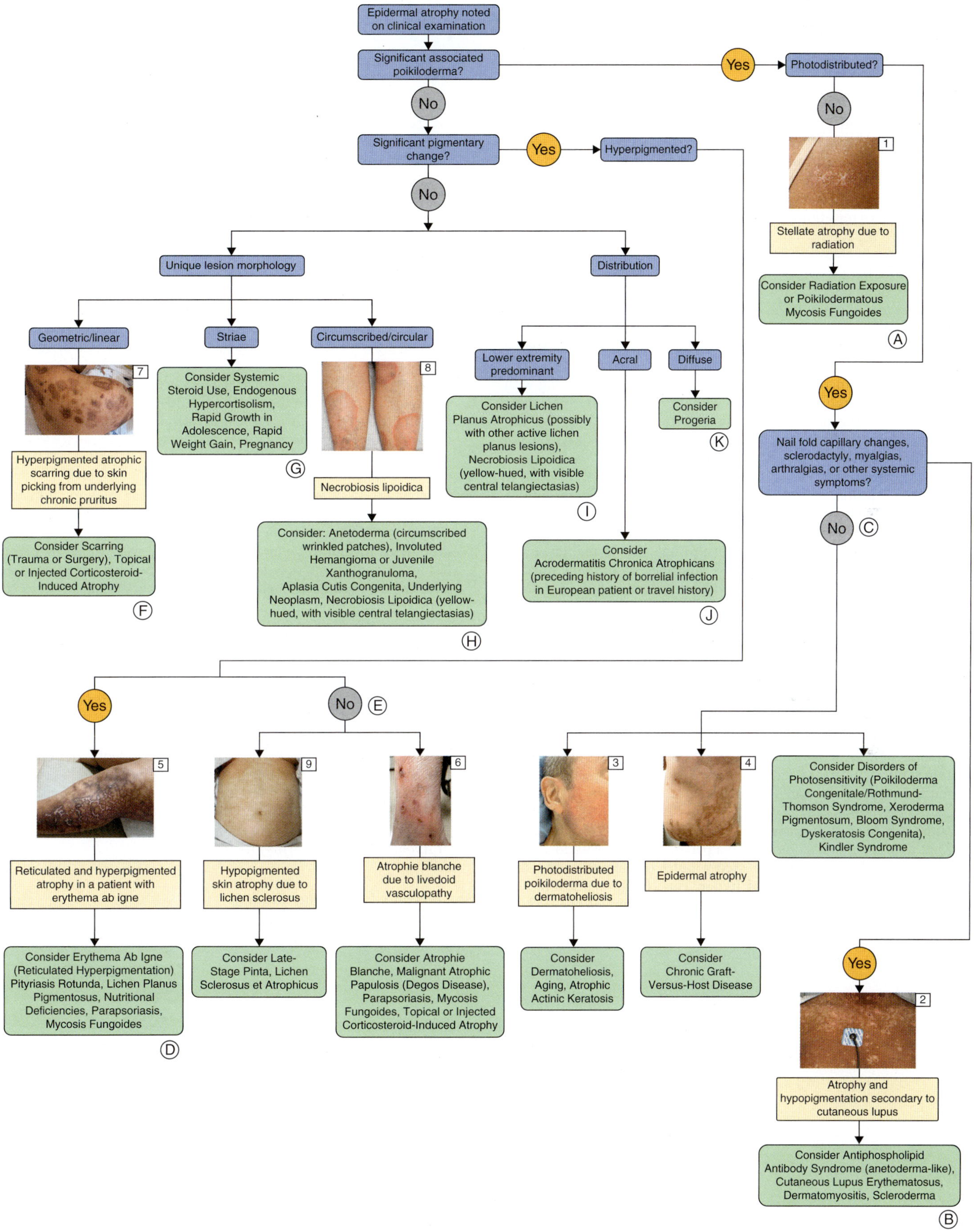
Epidermal atrophy noted on clinical examination
Significant associated poikiloderma?
Yes
Photodistributed?
No
1
Stellate atrophy due to radiation
Consider Radiation Exposure or Poikilodermatous Mycosis Fungoides
A
Yes
Nail fold capillary changes, sclerodactyly, myalgias, arthralgias, or other systemic symptoms?
No
C
No
Significant pigmentary change?
Yes
Hyperpigmented?
No
Unique lesion morphology
Distribution
Geometric/linear
7
Hyperpigmented atrophic scarring due to skin picking from underlying chronic pruritus
Consider Scarring (Trauma or Surgery), Topical or Injected Corticosteroid-Induced Atrophy
F
Striae
Consider Systemic Steroid Use, Endogenous Hypercortisolism, Rapid Growth in Adolescence, Rapid Weight Gain, Pregnancy
G
Circumscribed/circular
8
Necrobiosis lipoidica
Consider: Anetoderma (circumscribed wrinkled patches), Involuted Hemangioma or Juvenile Xanthogranuloma, Aplasia Cutis Congenita, Underlying Neoplasm, Necrobiosis Lipoidica (yellow-hued, with visible central telangiectasias)
H
Lower extremity predominant
Consider Lichen Planus Atrophicus (possibly with other active lichen planus lesions), Necrobiosis Lipoidica (yellow-hued, with visible central telangiectasias)
I
Acral
Consider Acrodermatitis Chronica Atrophicans (preceding history of borrelial infection in European patient or travel history)
J
Diffuse
Consider Progeria
K
Yes
5
Reticulated and hyperpigmented atrophy in a patient with erythema ab igne
Consider Erythema Ab Igne (Reticulated Hyperpigmentation) Pityriasis Rotunda, Lichen Planus Pigmentosus, Nutritional Deficiencies, Parapsoriasis, Mycosis Fungoides
D
No
E
9
Hypopigmented skin atrophy due to lichen sclerosus
Consider Late-Stage Pinta, Lichen Sclerosus et Atrophicus
6
Atrophie blanche due to livedoid vasculopathy
Consider Atrophie Blanche, Malignant Atrophic Papulosis (Degos Disease), Parapsoriasis, Mycosis Fungoides, Topical or Injected Corticosteroid-Induced Atrophy
3
Photodistributed poikiloderma due to dermatoheliosis
Consider Dermatoheliosis, Aging, Atrophic Actinic Keratosis
4
Epidermal atrophy
Consider Chronic Graft-Versus-Host Disease
Consider Disorders of Photosensitivity (Poikiloderma Congenitale/Rothmund-Thomson Syndrome, Xeroderma Pigmentosum, Bloom Syndrome, Dyskeratosis Congenita), Kindler Syndrome
Yes
2
Atrophy and hypopigmentation secondary to cutaneous lupus
Consider Antiphospholipid Antibody Syndrome (anetoderma-like), Cutaneous Lupus Erythematosus, Dermatomyositis, Scleroderma
B

64 Dermal Atrophy and Lipoatrophy

William Lewis and Robert G. Micheletti

Dermal atrophy and lipoatrophy are associated with a wide range of medical and dermatologic conditions and typically present clinically as an indentation of the skin with or without overlying epidermal change. Histologically, loss of the dermis or subcutaneous fat may be seen, with or without other accompanying features, such as inflammation, depending on the underlying etiology of the atrophy.

A. The first step in assessing dermal atrophy or lipoatrophy is determining whether the process is diffuse or focal. Widespread lipoatrophy may present as part of a lipodystrophy syndrome in which adipose stores are lost in parts of the body, such as **familial partial lipodystrophy, acquired partial lipodystrophy**, or **generalized lipodystrophy** (either congenital or acquired). Mutations in the LMNA gene are associated with both familial partial lipodystrophy and **progeria**, which may also manifest with generalized lipodystrophy, along with other systemic findings. In patients with HIV, **antiretrovirals**—most notably stavudine, but also protease inhibitors and didanosine—can produce lipodystrophy associated with the loss of fat pads on the face, limbs, and buttocks.

B. Most focal lesions of dermal atrophy constitute indentations or depressions in the skin, but those of **nevus lipomatosus**, in which fat is admixed with the dermis, and **piezogenic pedal papules**, which represent a herniation of fat through the dermal layer, are exceptions. Clinically, these can be identified as outpouchings of soft fatty tissue. Piezogenic pedal papules are distinguished by their location on the feet.

C. When assessing focal and depressed papules or plaques, first ask if there has been prior trauma or a procedure at the site of atrophy. If yes, consider **scarring** or **injection** with **insulin, corticosteroids**, or other medications as the most likely cause. Interferons injected for multiple sclerosis have been associated with the development of granulomatous dermal lesions responsible for focal atrophy. Prolonged pressure may produce lipoatrophy as well, as in **lipoatrophia semicircularis**, a localized lipoatrophy appearing on the thighs of office workers associated with prolonged sitting.

D. Without a history of trauma or injection, morphologic clues can point to a specific diagnosis when a patient presents with focal dermal atrophy. Reticulated depressed papules or plaques in the skin may be seen in **focal dermal hypoplasia** (**Goltz syndrome**), an X-linked dominant condition in which punched-out lesions are seen on the skin, usually associated with abnormalities of the hair, nails, and teeth. Reticulated depressions are also seen on the face in **atrophoderma vermiculatum**.

E. **Keratosis pilaris atrophicans** presents with atrophic pits on the cheeks and face of children and may be associated with other genetic disorders. Pitted atrophy may be seen in **follicular atrophoderma** associated with Bazex-Dupré-Christol syndrome and other syndromes.

F. Blaschkoid or linear depressed plaques occur in **linear morphea, moulin atrophoderma linearis, Goltz syndrome**, and (when sternal clefting is present) overlying the sternum in **PHACE syndrome**.

G. When no specific morphological clues are present, location alone can sometimes point to the correct diagnosis. **Aplasia cutis congenita** can produce loss of the fat and dermis and typically presents as a focal atrophic plaque on the vertex of the scalp (although it can occur elsewhere) that has been present since birth.

H. **Morphea** is an inflammatory disease of unclear etiology; it may be seen in association with autoantibodies and in families with a significant autoimmune history. Various types of morphea have been described, including generalized morphea, with more than four lesions present in multiple locations on the body; en coup de sabre, affecting the midline forehead and scalp and producing alopecia; circumscribed morphea in an oval or round configuration on the trunk; and linear morphea in a band over the head, neck, or extremities. Lesions of morphea typically begin as erythematous patches with violaceous borders, progressing to indurated hyper- or hypopigmented depressed plaques. **Atrophoderma of Pasini and Pierini**, which may be a variant of morphea, is notable for areas of depressed skin with "cliff-drop borders."

I. Dermal atrophy accompanied by epidermal atrophy of acral sites is seen in **acrodermatitis chronica atrophicans**, which occurs as a late stage of a Lyme-like infection seen in Europe due to infection with *Borrelia afzelii*. **Lipoatrophic panniculitis**, which is a rare disorder predominantly seen in children, may also produce bands of lipoatrophy on the arms and legs.

See Appendix 1 for Further Reading.

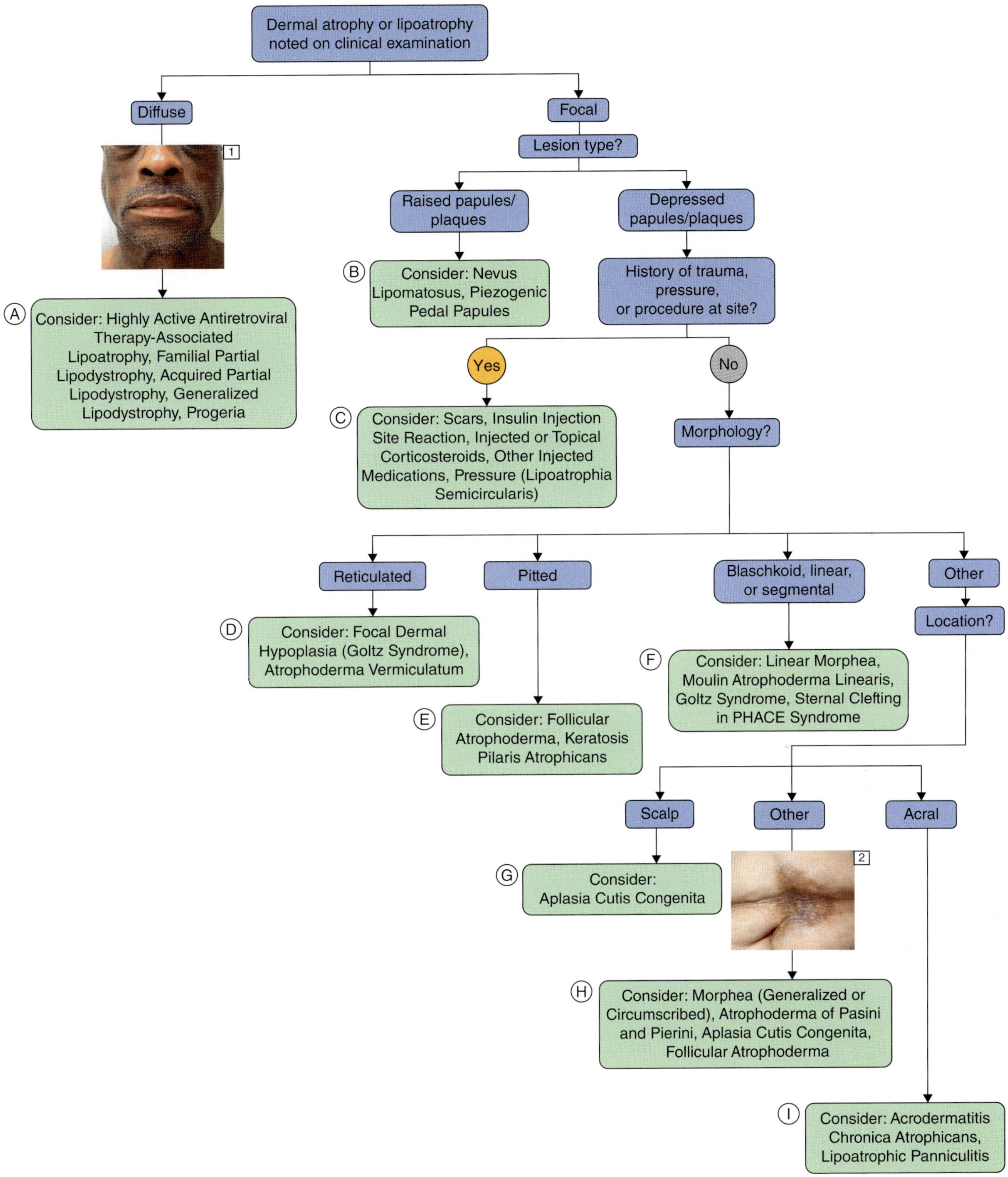
Dermal atrophy or lipoatrophy noted on clinical examination
Diffuse
1
A
Consider: Highly Active Antiretroviral Therapy-Associated Lipoatrophy, Familial Partial Lipodystrophy, Acquired Partial Lipodystrophy, Generalized Lipodystrophy, Progeria
Focal
Lesion type?
Raised papules/ plaques
B
Consider: Nevus Lipomatosus, Piezogenic Pedal Papules
Depressed papules/plaques
History of trauma, pressure, or procedure at site?
Yes
C
Consider: Scars, Insulin Injection Site Reaction, Injected or Topical Corticosteroids, Other Injected Medications, Pressure (Lipoatrophia Semicircularis)
No
Morphology?
Reticulated
D
Consider: Focal Dermal Hypoplasia (Goltz Syndrome), Atrophoderma Vermiculatum
Pitted
E
Consider: Follicular Atrophoderma, Keratosis Pilaris Atrophicans
Blaschkoid, linear, or segmental
F
Consider: Linear Morphea, Moulin Atrophoderma Linearis, Goltz Syndrome, Sternal Clefting in PHACE Syndrome
Other
Location?
Scalp
G
Consider: Aplasia Cutis Congenita
Other
2
H
Consider: Morphea (Generalized or Circumscribed), Atrophoderma of Pasini and Pierini, Aplasia Cutis Congenita, Follicular Atrophoderma
Acral
I
Consider: Acrodermatitis Chronica Atrophicans, Lipoatrophic Panniculitis

PART XIII
Pigment Disorders

65 Facial Hyperpigmentation

Sarah Gonzalez and Nada Elbuluk

Facial hyperpigmentation is the process by which darkening of the face occurs secondary to a change in the distribution of melanin, increased melanin production, and/or increased number of melanocytes. It can vary in color from light to dark brown, gray, black, bronze, and even red-brown. Many disorders of pigmentation have overlapping clinical presentations, which can create a diagnostic challenge. Despite being common and often benign in nature, facial hyperpigmentation can have a profound negative emotional impact on individuals and their quality of life. Genetics, hormones, drugs, the presence of disease(s), and/or the environment may contribute to hyperpigmentation. Clinical presentation and history along with physical examination can often provide sufficient information to make a diagnosis. In cases of uncertainty, histopathology can be helpful. Pigmentation can be epidermal, dermal, or mixed according to the location of pigmentation deposition. Epidermal hyperpigmentation tends to be light to dark brown, whereas dermal pigmentation can have a darker blue-gray color.

At the initial consultation, important elements of the history to acquire include the duration and distribution of the condition, associated symptoms, medical history and medications, social history, possible environmental and/or chemical exposures, prior workup, and treatment options. The clinical examination should include an evaluation of the condition in good lighting. Photographic documentation can be useful to monitor the condition over time. Tools such as a Wood's lamp and dermoscopy can provide additional useful information related to the depth of the pigment and the pigment pattern, which can aid in diagnosis and treatment efficacy over time. In cases where the diagnosis remains unclear with clinical examination and history alone, laboratory workup and tissue biopsy can be useful in determining the final diagnosis.

A. **Erythromelanosis follicularis faciei et colli** is a rare condition presenting with well-demarcated red-brown patches with overlapping follicular papules on the face and upper neck. There can be alopecia of the vellus hairs in these locations. It is more common in adult males and those of Asian descent with a possible autosomal recessive inheritance pattern.

B. **Erythema dyschromicum perstans (EDP) or ashy dermatosis** tends to occur in those of Hispanic origin with no gender predilection. EDP appears as oval to round blue-gray patches typically on nonphotoexposed sites, although in some cases, it can appear on the neck and parts of the face. In earlier stages the macules and patches may have a raised erythematous border. EDP has been associated with ammonium nitrate ingestion, oral contrast media, benzodiazepines, penicillin, pesticides, thyroid disease, whipworm infection, HIV, and HLA-DR4.

C. **Lichen planus pigmentosus (LPP)** has many clinical overlaps with EDP, and many consider them to exist on the same disease spectrum. Some authors classify this spectrum of disorders as being part of acquired dermal macular hyperpigmentation. LPP more commonly affects females of darker skin types in the third to fifth decade of life. In LPP, macules and patches appear brown to gray-brown in photoexposed areas, including on the forehead, temples, neck, and extremities. Historically, LPP has been considered a variant of lichen planus, with classic lichen planus occurring in conjunction only a small percentage of the time. LPP has also been associated with exposures to the application of mustard oil, amla oil, and other potential photosensitizing agents. Typically, both conditions are asymptomatic but can be pruritic.

D. **Argyria** is a blue-gray pigmentation in photoexposed areas secondary to silver exposure with possible involvement of the nails and sclera.

E. **Chrysiasis** is a blue to slate gray pigmentation occurring secondary to gold salt exposure on photoexposed areas, particularly the periorbital region.

F. **Melasma** is a benign pigmentary condition with a complex pathogenesis occurring due to a combination of genetics, hormonal exposures, and light exposure. It is also sensitive to heat. The three main distributions on the face include centrofacial, malar, or mandibular. It tends to be light to dark brown symmetric reticulated patches. It is more common in females of color. The pigment can be epidermal, dermal, or more commonly mixed.

G. **Ephelides** and **lentigines** are light brown well-circumscribed macules in photoexposed areas occurring more commonly in those with lighter skin. Lentigines occur secondary to excess sun exposure. Ephelides may have a genetic component and exist with variants of *MC1R* gene mutation. They tend to intensify in summer and fade in winter.

H. **Drug-induced pigmentation** has been associated with up to 20% of acquired pigmentary disorders. Many different drug classes are implicated, including alkylating agents, antiarrhythmics, anticoagulants, antiepileptics, antibiotics, antimalarials, and psychotropics. The pigmentation can persist for months after insult or have a delayed onset. Anatomic distribution of the pigmentation along with the color of the pigmentation may help narrow the diagnosis. Cessation of the possible offending agents paired with sun protection can sometimes help lead to resolution.

I. **Riehl melanosis** presents as brown-gray to brown-black patches typically on the face and neck and can occasionally include the dorsal hands and forearms. Facial presentation tends to include the forehead and temple with increased darkening of the lateral face. Scale is rarely seen. It is considered a form of pigmented contact dermatitis associated with exposure to cosmetics, fragrances, and/or plants.

J. **Postinflammatory hyperpigmentation (PIH)** appears as light to dark brown macules and patches in sites of previous or ongoing trauma or inflammation. It occurs more commonly in those with skin of color (SOC).

K. **Actinic lichen planus** tends to occur in adults of Middle Eastern and Asian origin emerging as dark brown patches, papules, and/or annular plaques with central hyperpigmentation and a hypopigmented border occurring in photoexposed areas.

L. Prolonged use of hydroquinone of any strength can paradoxically cause **ochronosis**, appearing as blue, brown, and/or black macules, papules, patches, plaques, or nodules in sites of prior application.

M. **Nevus of Ota**, a form of dermal melanocytosis, appears as blue-gray macules and patches on the face in the distribution of the trigeminal nerve. Bilateral discoloration and involvement of the oral mucosa/sclera have been observed. Nevus of Ota may have genetic involvement and is rarely associated with melanoma. It is more common in females of Asian descent.

N. **Hori nevi**, also a form of dermal melanocytosis, presents as brown to brown-gray or blue-gray macules with bilateral malar involvement. It is more common in Asian females.

O. **Periorbital melanosis** refers to medium-to-dark brown darkening of the lower and/or upper eyelids more commonly seen in SOC. It is a common condition with multifactorial etiologies, including genetics, PIH, edema, excess vascularity, friction, and infraorbital hollowing.

P. **Maturational hyperpigmentation** appears as hyperpigmented dark brown to black patches with ill-defined borders on the lateral temples, manifesting in the fourth to fifth decade of life in Fitzpatrick skin types IV–V. Sun exposure, obesity, and diabetes are associated.

See Appendix 1 for Further Reading and Image References.

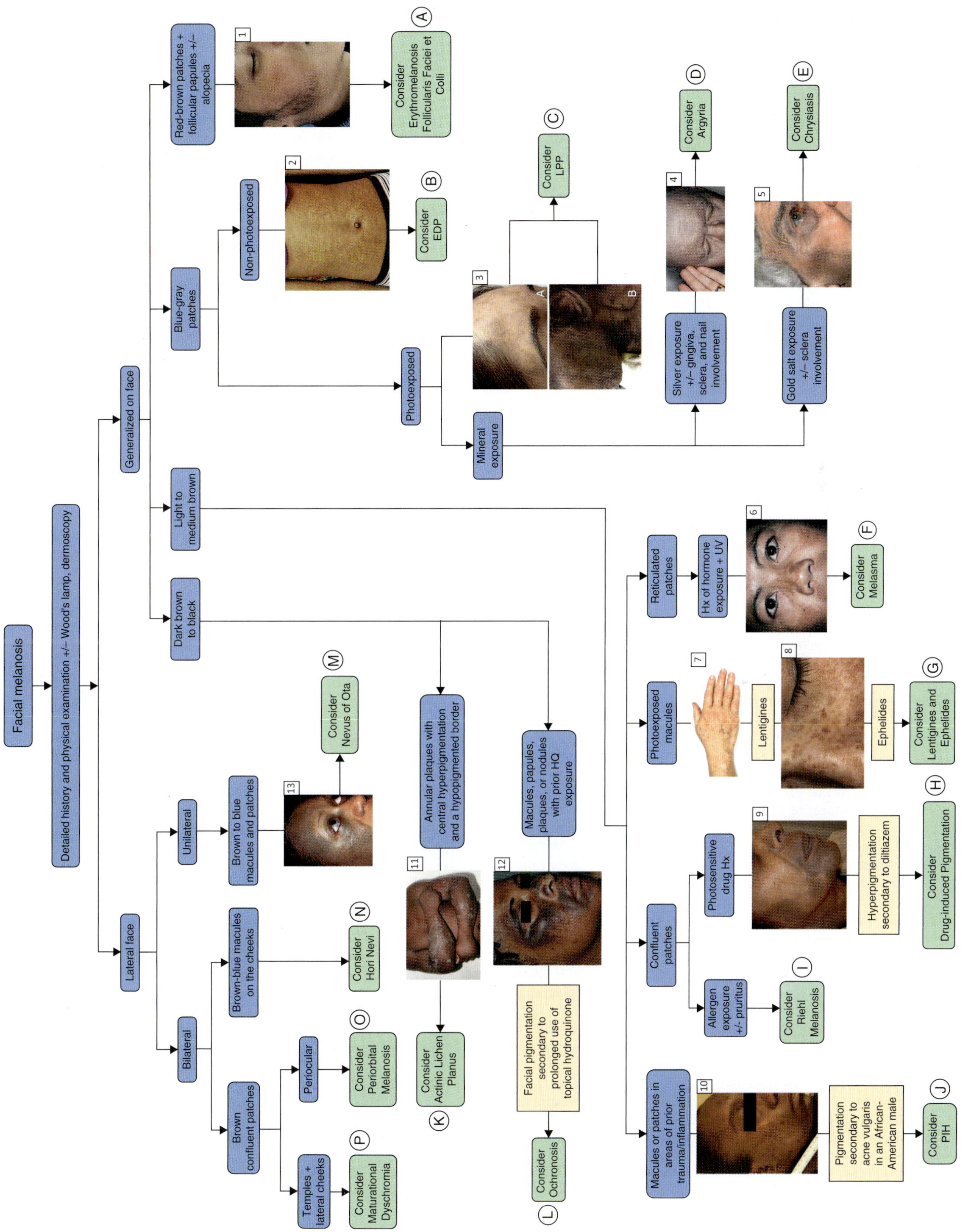
Facial melanosis
Detailed history and physical examination +/− Wood's lamp, dermoscopy
Generalized on face
Red-brown patches + follicular papules +/− alopecia
1
Consider Erythromelanosis Follicularis Faciei et Colli
A
Blue-gray patches
Non-photoexposed
2
Consider EDP
B
Photoexposed
3
A
B
Consider LPP
C
Mineral exposure
Silver exposure +/− gingiva, sclera, and nail involvement
4
Consider Argyria
D
Gold salt exposure +/− sclera involvement
5
Consider Chrysiasis
E
Light to medium brown
Reticulated patches
Hx of hormone exposure + UV
6
Consider Melasma
F
Photoexposed macules
7
Lentigines
8
Ephelides
Consider Lentigines and Ephelides
G
Confluent patches
Photosensitive drug Hx
9
Hyperpigmentation secondary to diltiazem
Consider Drug-induced Pigmentation
H
Allergen exposure +/- pruritus
Consider Riehl Melanosis
I
Macules or patches in areas of prior trauma/inflammation
10
Pigmentation secondary to acne vulgaris in an African-American male
Consider PIH
J
Dark brown to black
Annular plaques with central hyperpigmentation and a hypopigmented border
11
Consider Actinic Lichen Planus
K
Macules, papules, plaques, or nodules with prior HQ exposure
12
Facial pigmentation secondary to prolonged use of topical hydroquinone
Consider Ochronosis
L
Lateral face
Unilateral
Brown to blue macules and patches
13
Consider Nevus of Ota
M
Bilateral
Brown-blue macules on the cheeks
Consider Hori Nevi
N
Brown confluent patches
Periocular
Consider Periorbital Melanosis
O
Temples + lateral cheeks
Consider Maturational Dyschromia
P

66 Other Localized Hyperpigmentation

Chidubem A. V. Okeke, Janyla A. Seltzer and Angel S. Byrd

Hyperpigmentation results from increased pigment in certain areas of the skin as a result of increased melanin production. Melanin is produced by cells in the epidermis called melanocytes. The affected areas of the skin will appear darker in color in comparison to an individual's natural skin tone. The etiologies of hyperpigmentation include underlying health conditions, hormonal changes, injury to the skin, acne, and sun exposure.

The evaluation of a patient with hyperpigmentation should begin with a detailed history and a thorough physical examination. The detailed history should include demographic information, drug history, onset of hyperpigmentation, and history of traumatic events to the skin or preexisting skin conditions. The physical examination should particularly focus on the location on the body, color, size, borders, and distribution. The history and physical examination will inform decisions around diagnosis and treatment of hyperpigmentation.

A. There are several etiologies resulting in circumscribed hyperpigmentation. Commonly reported medications that cause **drug-induced hyperpigmentation (DIH)** include anticonvulsants, antipsychotics, antimalarials, amiodarone, cytotoxic drugs, tetracyclines, NSAIDs, and heavy metals. It is imperative that the clinician takes a detailed medical history and is mindful of the chronological timeline of each medication. The presentation of DIH is variable depending on the causative agent; however, it is more prominent in sun-exposed areas and can also include the mucous membranes. Onset is usually insidious and worsens over months to years. Diagnosis can only be confirmed by the fading of the abnormal pigmentation after cessation of the suspected drug.

Postinflammatory hyperpigmentation (PIH) is an acquired excess of melanin that occurs after injury or inflammation and resolves slowly. In Fitzpatrick skin types III to VI, hyperpigmentation is more severe. PIH is characterized by asymptomatic hyperpigmented macules and/or patches that range in color from tan to dark brown or gray blue to gray brown. PIH is diagnosed clinically, and management includes treatment of the underlying inflammatory disorder, ultraviolet (UV) protection, and topical lightening therapies.

Primary cutaneous amyloidosis is a rare condition in which clumps of abnormal proteins called amyloid accumulate in the skin. The clinical features of this condition are determined by the specific form of cutaneous amyloidosis. Lichen amyloidosis typically presents as pruritic hyperpigmented patches on the extensor surfaces of the lower extremities. Macular amyloidosis is characterized by mildly itchy, dark brown patches on the upper back in either a uniform or reticulated/rippled pattern. Another form of amyloidosis is nodular amyloidosis, which presents with firm, pink-brown nodules on the face, torso, extremities, or genitals. The etiology of cutaneous amyloidosis is poorly understood, but genetic and environmental factors, such as repetitive friction, may play a role in the pathogenesis of this disease.

Acanthosis nigricans presents with hyperpigmented plaques with a velvety or papillomatous appearance. The most common locations are the posterior neck and axillae, but it can also present in other flexural and extensor areas. In many cases, acanthosis nigricans is a sign of insulin resistance. However, it can also be a presenting sign of internal malignancy, particularly malignancies of the gastrointestinal or genitourinary tracts. Currently, there is no reliably effective treatment for acanthosis nigricans itself, but by addressing the underlying insulin resistance or malignancy, the hyperpigmentation may improve.

B. Confluent and reticulated papillomatosis is characterized by asymptomatic, reticulated, hyperpigmented, hyperkeratotic papules and plaques. The lesions can be velvety or scaly and are frequently located on the upper trunk, neck, and flexural areas.

Conditions causing reticulate hyperpigmentation can be acquired or congenital and clinically present as netlike arrangements of brown or pink to red macules or papules.

Long-term repeated exposure to low levels of infrared heat can lead to **erythema ab igne (EAI)**, which presents as an area of reticulated erythema and subsequent hyperpigmentation in the size and shape of the heat source. The chronic use of an external heat source may also predispose to musculoskeletal injury or malignancy and should prompt a thorough history and review of symptoms. Occupational exposures to heat should also be identified. There is a potential risk for the development of squamous cell carcinoma or Merkel cell carcinoma within long-standing lesions of EAI.

Extrafacial melasma presents on body parts excluding the face and tends to display symmetrically distributed brown hyperpigmented patches with irregular borders. It is most commonly seen in postmenopausal females in their 50's.

Prurigo pigmentosa is characterized by pruritic erythematous papules on the trunk and neck with a mottled, reticulated hyperpigmentation. Prurigo pigmentosa has been associated with restricted diets and bariatric surgery. Dietary changes as well as minocycline are the most common treatment options.

C. **Linear hyperpigmentation (LH)** is an uncommon pathology in dermatology, and there is currently no consensus on its classification. Diagnosis of LH can be challenging due to its multitude of causes, involvement of several organ systems, and a lack of specific diagnostic tools.

Pigment demarcation lines (PDLs) are abrupt transitions in skin color, varying from hyper- to hypopigmentation, seen on the limbs, face, and sometimes the trunk. These lines of demarcation occur bilaterally between the ventral and dorsal surfaces. They are more easily appreciated on darker pigmented skin. Currently, there are eight types of PDLs (Groups A–E) that represent different anatomic locations and orientations.

Serpentine supravenous hyperpigmentation presents as linear streaks of hyperpigmentation along superficial veins that occur hours to weeks after intravenous chemotherapy. The hyperpigmentation can resolve within 1 to 3 months after discontinuation of the agent. While 5-fluorouracil is well known to cause this eruption, patients undergoing treatment for HIV, leprosy, and autoimmune hemolytic anemia have also been reported to develop serpentine supravenous hyperpigmentation.

Linea nigra, a strip of increased pigmentation, typically emerges in the second or third trimester of pregnancy. It appears on the abdomen, extending vertically from the pubic area to the xiphoid process. This line is particularly prominent on darker skin tones, but can also be present, to a lesser degree, in males and nonpregnant females.

Phytophotodermatitis is a phototoxic reaction to light-sensitive substances combined with UV-A radiation. It typically occurs in summer and spring after contact with certain plants or plant products and then subsequent exposure to sunlight. The clinical manifestations typically appear approximately 24 hours following exposure and peak in intensity within 48 to 72 hours. The primary clinical presentation includes a burning erythema accompanied by blistering and striking PIH that may persist for weeks to months.

Incontinentia pigmenti is an X-linked condition noticed at birth or within the first few weeks of life. It has four stages, the first starting in infancy. Stage 3 exhibits hyperpigmented linear and whorled bands, which may be accompanied by atrophy. The lesions occur along Blaschko lines and tend to involve the trunk and extremities. Incontinentia pigmenti can present until adulthood; however, the hyperpigmentation usually begins to fade in adolescence.

Continued

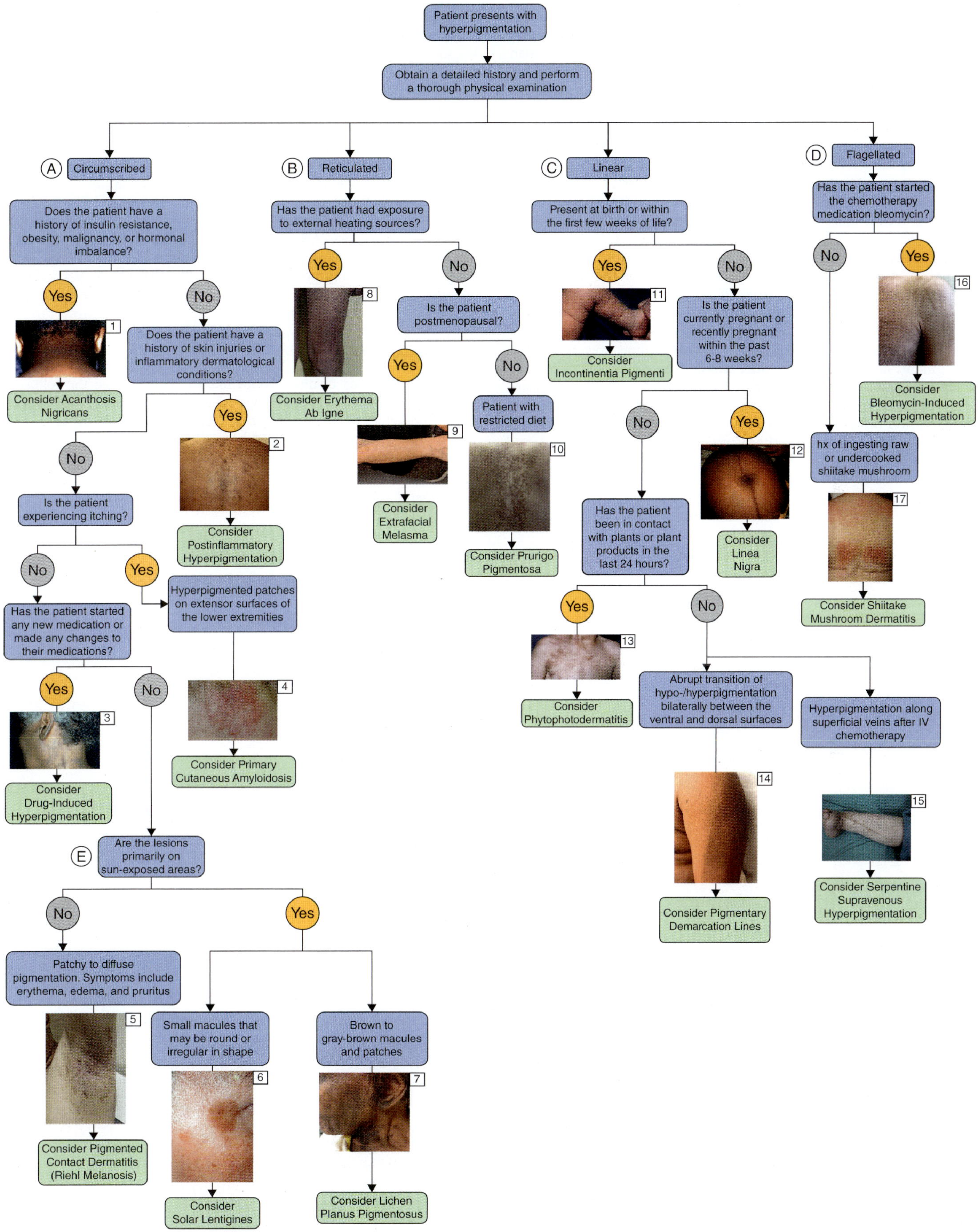
Patient presents with hyperpigmentation
Obtain a detailed history and perform a thorough physical examination
A Circumscribed
Does the patient have a history of insulin resistance, obesity, malignancy, or hormonal imbalance?
Yes
1
Consider Acanthosis Nigricans
No
Does the patient have a history of skin injuries or inflammatory dermatological conditions?
Yes
2
Consider Postinflammatory Hyperpigmentation
No
Is the patient experiencing itching?
Yes
Hyperpigmented patches on extensor surfaces of the lower extremities
4
Consider Primary Cutaneous Amyloidosis
No
Has the patient started any new medication or made any changes to their medications?
Yes
3
Consider Drug-Induced Hyperpigmentation
No
E
Are the lesions primarily on sun-exposed areas?
No
Patchy to diffuse pigmentation. Symptoms include erythema, edema, and pruritus
5
Consider Pigmented Contact Dermatitis (Riehl Melanosis)
Yes
Small macules that may be round or irregular in shape
6
Consider Solar Lentigines
Brown to gray-brown macules and patches
7
Consider Lichen Planus Pigmentosus
B Reticulated
Has the patient had exposure to external heating sources?
Yes
8
Consider Erythema Ab Igne
No
Is the patient postmenopausal?
Yes
9
Consider Extrafacial Melasma
No
Patient with restricted diet
10
Consider Prurigo Pigmentosa
C Linear
Present at birth or within the first few weeks of life?
Yes
11
Consider Incontinentia Pigmenti
No
Is the patient currently pregnant or recently pregnant within the past 6-8 weeks?
Yes
12
Consider Linea Nigra
No
Has the patient been in contact with plants or plant products in the last 24 hours?
Yes
13
Consider Phytophotodermatitis
No
Abrupt transition of hypo-/hyperpigmentation bilaterally between the ventral and dorsal surfaces
14
Consider Pigmentary Demarcation Lines
Hyperpigmentation along superficial veins after IV chemotherapy
15
Consider Serpentine Supravenous Hyperpigmentation
D Flagellated
Has the patient started the chemotherapy medication bleomycin?
Yes
16
Consider Bleomycin-Induced Hyperpigmentation
No
hx of ingesting raw or undercooked shiitake mushroom
17
Consider Shiitake Mushroom Dermatitis

D. Erythema or hyperpigmentation may also present in a flagellate pattern. **Bleomycin-associated hyperpigmentation** is most often seen on the back and chest. It can present as diffuse, circumscribed, or flagellated. The course of flagellate hyperpigmentation varies as it can take up to 9 weeks to appear after administration of the drug. Physical examination shows brown hyperpigmented linear bands or streaks that may also be pruritic.

Shiitake mushroom dermatitis occurs in individuals who have ingested raw or undercooked shiitake mushrooms. The symptoms usually appear within 24 to 48 hours of ingestion. Clinically, it appears as flagellate streaks of erythematous papules or petechiae. Affected individuals may experience pruritus in the affected areas.

E. In patients with newly acquired hyperpigmentation with a recent change in cosmetics use or fragrances, consider the diagnosis of **pigmented contact dermatitis (PCD)**, also known as **Riehl melanosis**. PCD is an acquired low-grade allergic contact dermatitis to fragrance and other cosmetic products that largely affects individuals of Asian descent. Products include aniline dyes, red-yellow pigment, chromium hydroxide, carbanilides, ricinoleic acid, hair dyes, henna, kumkum, perfumes, textile allergens, and occupational allergens. Physical examination shows patchy to diffuse hyperpigmentation favoring the area where the product was applied. Areas of involvement depend on the allergen responsible, but the face and neck are usually affected. Symptoms can include edema, pruritus, and erythema. Diagnosis is clinical, but patch testing is recommended to elucidate the responsible allergen.

Older patients who have had sun exposure tend to develop small hyperpigmented macules called **solar lentigines**. They are most common on sun-exposed regions, including the face, arms, and shoulders, and tend to be darker than ephelides (freckles). UV exposure over time causes hyperproliferation of melanocytes resulting in these patches. They may be round or irregular in shape, so while lentigines are most commonly diagnosed clinically, occasionally a biopsy is warranted to rule out melanoma.

Lichen planus pigmentosus (LPP) is an acquired disorder of dermal hyperpigmentation typically presenting as brown to gray-brown macules and patches in sun-exposed areas. Locations include the forehead, temples, ears, cheeks, and neck. The etiology is unknown, but sunlight is a suspected cause. This condition is chronic in nature and tends to wax and wane. It most commonly affects females of darker skin tones and is frequently resistant to treatment. The hyperpigmentation may be reticulate, blotchy, diffuse, or perifollicular with a generally symmetrical distribution. Of note, LPP is a distinct entity from lichen planus.

Acknowledgments

The authors of this chapter would like to acknowledge the following contributors: Ginette Okoye, David Mcadoo, Nia James, Jordan Young, and Chiemelum Amechi (Howard University College of Medicine), Nikita Wong (Henry Ford Health), and Cheryl Burgess (Center for Dermatology and Dermatologic Surgery).

See Appendix 1 for References and Image References.

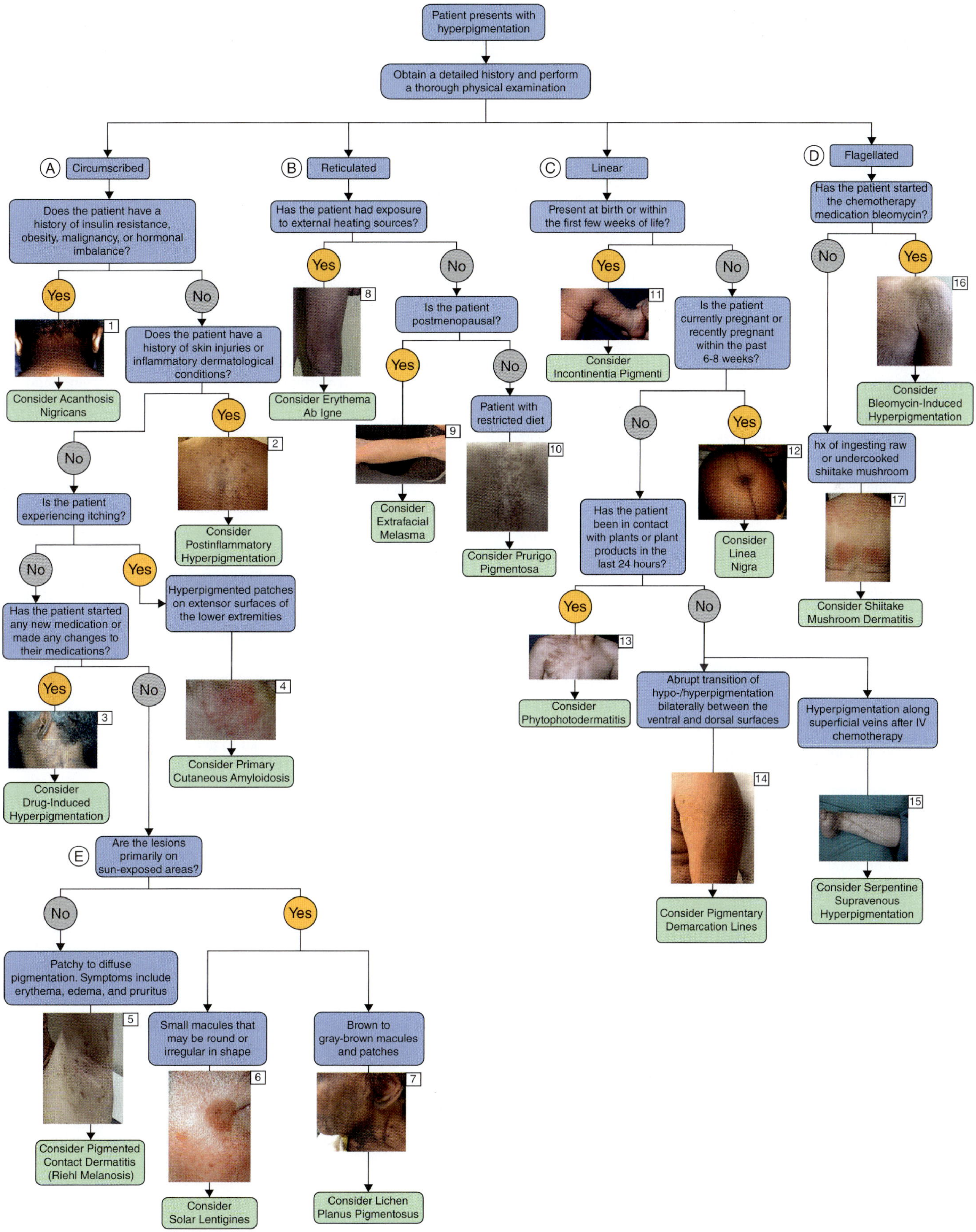
Patient presents with hyperpigmentation
Obtain a detailed history and perform a thorough physical examination
A
Circumscribed
Does the patient have a history of insulin resistance, obesity, malignancy, or hormonal imbalance?
Yes
1
Consider Acanthosis Nigricans
No
Does the patient have a history of skin injuries or inflammatory dermatological conditions?
Yes
2
Consider Postinflammatory Hyperpigmentation
No
Is the patient experiencing itching?
Yes
Hyperpigmented patches on extensor surfaces of the lower extremities
4
Consider Primary Cutaneous Amyloidosis
No
Has the patient started any new medication or made any changes to their medications?
Yes
3
Consider Drug-Induced Hyperpigmentation
No
E
Are the lesions primarily on sun-exposed areas?
No
Patchy to diffuse pigmentation. Symptoms include erythema, edema, and pruritus
5
Consider Pigmented Contact Dermatitis (Riehl Melanosis)
Yes
Small macules that may be round or irregular in shape
6
Consider Solar Lentigines
Brown to gray-brown macules and patches
7
Consider Lichen Planus Pigmentosus
B
Reticulated
Has the patient had exposure to external heating sources?
Yes
8
Consider Erythema Ab Igne
No
Is the patient postmenopausal?
Yes
9
Consider Extrafacial Melasma
No
Patient with restricted diet
10
Consider Prurigo Pigmentosa
C
Linear
Present at birth or within the first few weeks of life?
Yes
11
Consider Incontinentia Pigmenti
No
Is the patient currently pregnant or recently pregnant within the past 6-8 weeks?
Yes
12
Consider Linea Nigra
No
Has the patient been in contact with plants or plant products in the last 24 hours?
Yes
13
Consider Phytophotodermatitis
No
Abrupt transition of hypo-/hyperpigmentation bilaterally between the ventral and dorsal surfaces
14
Consider Pigmentary Demarcation Lines
Hyperpigmentation along superficial veins after IV chemotherapy
15
Consider Serpentine Supravenous Hyperpigmentation
D
Flagellated
Has the patient started the chemotherapy medication bleomycin?
Yes
16
Consider Bleomycin-Induced Hyperpigmentation
No
hx of ingesting raw or undercooked shiitake mushroom
17
Consider Shiitake Mushroom Dermatitis

67 Generalized Hyperpigmentation

Sarah Gonzalez and Nada Elbuluk

Disorders of hyperpigmentation are common and can occur from a variety of etiologies. These conditions are often distressing with profound effects on quality of life. Overlapping clinical presentations can make these conditions challenging to diagnose. Accurate diagnosis requires a thorough medical history, including onset and timeline of the condition along with a physical examination assessing size, distribution, color, and shape of the pigmentation. Please see Chapter 65 (Facial Hyperpigmentation) for further discussion of important elements in the clinical examination. Disorders of hyperpigmentation can have a variety of presentations, including linear, reticulate, circumscribed, flagellate, or diffuse.

However, a multitude of conditions may present with diffuse hyperpigmentation.

A. **Porphyria cutanea tarda** is a condition in which patients have increased photosensitivity, skin fragility, bullae, erosions, crusts, milia, and scars in sun-exposed skin. Other cutaneous findings include hypertrichosis, scarring alopecia, and sclerodermoid skin changes, as well as postinflammatory hyperpigmentation ranging from tan or brown to black.

B. **Hemochromatosis,** also known as bronze diabetes, typically presents in males with a generalized metallic gray, brown discoloration.

C. Endocrinopathies can also produce diffuse hyperpigmentation. **Addison disease** presents with a "muddy," diffuse, orange-brown pigmentation in photoexposed areas, as well as in the perineum, axillae, areolae, palms, and soles with onset during adulthood. Mucous membranes may be involved with blue, brown, or black macules termed "slate spots" in the mouth. Patients will typically have elevated adrenocorticotropic hormone (ACTH) and melanocyte-stimulating hormone levels. Systemic disorders such as Cushing syndrome, hyperthyroidism, Nelson syndrome, ectopic ACTH, pheochromocytoma, and carcinoid tumor may also develop addisonian-like diffuse hyperpigmentation of photoexposed skin.

D. **Deficiency of vitamins B_9 and B_{12}** may present with localized or widespread dark brown pigmentation of the dorsal hands and diffuse or striated melanonychia. Pellagra involves a deficiency of niacin and **vitamin B_3**, presenting with the classic tetrad of dermatitis, diarrhea, dementia, and death. The dermatitis includes dark brown photodistributed plaques of the neck. Other cutaneous findings include painful fissures on acral skin, cheilitis, atrophic glossitis, and ulcerated vaginitis.

E. **Lichen planus pigmentosus:** Please refer to Chapter 65.

F. **Kwashiorkor** is a disease of protein malnutrition presenting with multiple cutaneous findings including hypopigmented macules secondary to ulcerations and abrasions on the thighs or in a diaper distribution. There can also be dark brown macules in areas of trauma on the lower back and abdomen. In mild cases, superficial desquamation termed "enamel paint spots" are seen, whereas in severe disease, larger areas are eroded and can be referred to as "flaky paint dermatosis." Dry, thin "lanugo" hairs, petechiae, purpura, soft, thin nails, cheilitis, vulvovagnitis, and ecchymoses are other cutaneous findings.

G. **Drug-induced hyperpigmentation** may be due to numerous medications and can vary in color from yellow-brown to blue-gray, to brown-black. Distribution may be localized to mucous membranes, teeth, nails, acral skin, joints, sun-exposed distribution, or generalized.

H. **Erythema dyschromicum perstans:** Please refer to Chapter 65.

I. **Idiopathic eruptive macular pigmentation** is an acquired, idiopathic dermal hyperpigmentation found primarily in children and adolescents. It presents as discrete, small, brown macules and patches on the face, neck, trunk, and proximal extremities. Children and adolescents are primarily affected.

J. **Systemic sclerosis** has multiple cutaneous findings, including hyperpigmentation of photoexposed skin and leukoderma of the upper trunk and face giving rise to the "salt and pepper" sign.

K. Dyschromia secondary to **arsenic** has a significant dose-response relationship and can emerge 1 to 20 years after exposure. Affected skin of the axillae, groin, palms, soles, nipples, and pressure points exhibit bronze hyperpigmentation overlapping with guttate hypopigmentation termed "raindrops on a dusty road".

L. **Pinta** is caused by an infection of *Treponema carateum* and has three stages. The second stage of pinta emerges as discrete, scaly red papules coalescing into larger slate blue, brown, gray, or black psoriasiform plaques. The final stage of pinta has vitiligo-like atrophic or hyperkeratotic plaques.

M. **Genodermatoses** may also lead to generalized hyperpigmentation. **Dyschromatosis universalis hereditaria** is an uncommon disorder with both hypo- and hyperpigmented macules in a generalized distribution. **Familial progressive hyperpigmentation** is an inherited disorder where dark brown patches are observed in numerous anatomical locations, including the palms, soles, lips, and conjunctiva. The patches emerge during infancy, becoming larger, more numerous, and confluent with age. **Dyschromatosis symmetrica hereditaria** also known as reticulate acropigmentation of Dohi is characterized by symmetric hyper- and hypopigmented macules, favoring the distal extremities, especially the dorsal hands and feet, and emerges in early childhood. The palms, soles, and mucous membranes are spared. The dark brown macules increase in number and size and stabilize during young adulthood.

See Appendix 1 for Further Reading and Image References.

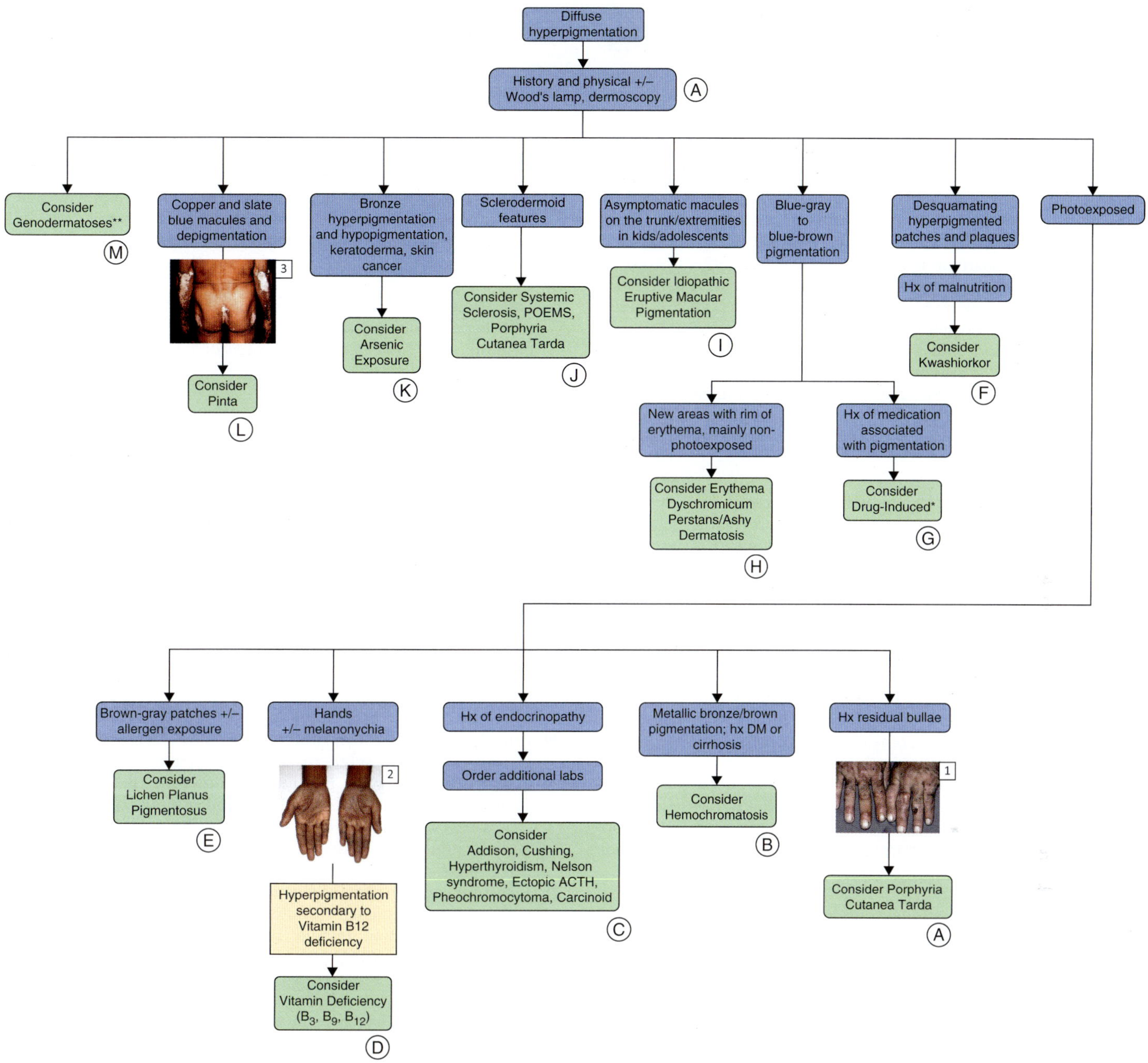

*Common drugs: bleomycin, busulfan, cyclophosphamide, dactinomycin, daunorubicin, 5-fluorouracil, hydroxyurea, nitrogen mustards, methotrexate, hydroxychloroquine, bismuth, gold, iron, lead, mercury, silver, arsenic, oral contraceptives, amiodarone, minocycline, clofazimine, diltiazem, dioxins, ezogabine, hydroquinone, imatinib, zidovudine, psoralens, and psychotropic medications

**Consider Dyschromatosis Hereditaria Universalis (Familial Progressive Hyperpigmentation and Hypopigmentation), Dyschromatosis Symmetrica Hereditaria (Reticulate Acropigmentation of Dohi), Familial Progressive Hyperpigmentation with or without Hypopigmentation.

68 Hypopigmented Macules

Callie M. Roberts and Victor Huang

Hypopigmented macules are flat, light spots marked by pigmentary dilution as opposed to a complete absence of pigment characteristic of depigmented lesions. In the initial evaluation of hypopigmentation, evaluation with a Wood's lamp can be immensely helpful in distinguishing hypopigmentation versus depigmentation and delineating the extent of involvement, particularly in fairer skin types. Depigmented lesions are marked by stark autofluorescence of collagen in light areas contrasting with the surrounding skin. A detailed history and assessment of family history, onset, and associated symptoms can further divide hypopigmented skin conditions into congenital versus acquired conditions.

A. Congenital hypomelanoses that affect the development or distribution of melanocytes or melanosomes lead to generalized hypomelanosis. Genetic testing is indicated when this well-defined set of syndromes is considered.

B. **Oculocutaneous albinism** represents a congenital decrease or lack of pigment due to aberrations in the melanin synthesis pathway. While depigmentation is noted in the most severe types, diffuse hypopigmentation can be seen in more mild variants.

C. Pigmentary dilution in **Hermansky-Pudlak syndrome** is due to derangements in key complexes required for lysosome-related organelle development. The melanosome, as member of this class of organelles, is affected leading to pigmentary dilution of the skin, hair, and eyes. Systemic manifestations of organelle dysfunction include bleeding diathesis (platelet dysfunction), immune deficiencies, pulmonary fibrosis, and granulomatous colitis.

D. **Griscelli syndrome** develops as a consequence of deranged melanosome transport. The inability to transport melanosomes to keratinocytes leads to pigmentary dilution and silvery gray hair. Trichoscopy characteristically demonstrates melanocyte clumping in the hair shafts.

E. **Tuberous sclerosis** should be considered in an infant with three or more hypopigmented macules at birth with lance-ovate hypomelanotic macules being pathognomonic. Classically associated with a triad of adenoma sebaceum, seizures, and intellectual delay, tuberous sclerosis usually presents with hypomelanotic macules on the trunk. Wood's lamp examination may be required to observe these lesions in lighter skinned individuals.

F. **Nevus depigmentosus** (i.e., nevus achromicus) is a congenital disorder characterized by a nonprogressive, well-circumscribed hypopigmented macule or patch that remains stable in shape and distribution throughout life, but typically grows in proportion to body growth. Most patients have just one macule or patch. There are no sites of predilection, no associated systemic abnormalities, and no malignant potential. Hairs within the nevus typically maintain pigment.

G. **Futcher lines** (i.e., pigmentary demarcation lines, Voigt lines) are benign, sharply demarcated marks that separate darker and light regions of the skin, often separating dorsal and ventral aspects of the body. They are common in people with darker skin, found in approximately 50% of Black females and 33% of Black males. Futcher lines are often present at birth or appear in early childhood.

H. **Nevus anemicus (NA)** usually presents at birth on the chest or back as a solitary apparently hypopigmented macule or patch often with surrounding smaller satellite macules. NA is not a pigmentary disorder, however. It is a localized area of vasoconstriction in the skin due to increased sympathetic supply. NA can occur in several syndromes, including neurofibromatosis (up to 4% of cases). Diagnosis is clinical; diascopy results in blanching of the peripheral skin, rendering the lesion indistinguishable from surroundings.

I. **Late-stage pinta** can present with hypomelanotic macules or patches with hyperpigmented brown borders, most commonly over bony prominences. These are usually preceded by mottle hyper- and hypopigmented pintids.

J. **Bejel**, another nonvenereal treponematosis, is marked by hypopigmented patches commonly distributed on the extremities, genitalia, areolae, and trunk. Lesions are often speckled with admixed pigmented macules.

K. **Post-kala-azar leishmaniasis** is associated with visceral leishmaniasis endemic in East Africa and India. It presents with pinpoint macules on the trunk and extremities.

L. **Secondary syphilis** can also present with hypopigmented macules on a hyperpigmented base, particularly on the lateral neck within the first 3 to 4 months of infection. Hypopigmented macules and patches can also develop over areas of previous inflammatory lesions favoring the neck, groin, axillae, upper trunk, and abdomen.

M. Anesthesia or anhidrosis of affected lesions is suggestive of lepromatous (ill-defined subtle macules), tuberculoid (discrete macules or patches that may be infiltrative), borderline (plaques or annular lesions admixed with hypopigmented macules and patches in a "Swiss-cheese" manner), or indeterminate **leprosy** (hypomelanotic, erythematous macules favoring exposed areas).

N. **Kwashiorkor** represents severe protein malnutrition associated with a generalized pigmentary dilution that resolves with dietary protein supplementation. Initially, red-brown to erythematous patches develop with desquamation resolving to hyper- and hypopigmented dyspigmentation.

O. **Phenylketonuria** can present as generalized pigmentary dilution secondary to a relative deficiency in tyrosine secondary to the accumulation of phenylalanine.

P. Dermal papules or plaques with associated hypopigmentation are suggestive of **sarcoidosis**. Associated systemic symptoms (e.g., fever, weight loss, lymphadenopathy, cough, or dyspnea) are suggestive.

Q. **Bier spots** (i.e., physiologic anemic macules, angiospastic macules) are apparently hypopigmented; however, they are actually due to vascular abnormalities as opposed to an alteration in melanin content. They are most often present in young adults aged 20 to 40 years and distributed symmetrically along the extensor surfaces of extremities. When the extremities are elevated or pressure is applied to the surrounding skin, Bier spots will disappear.

R. **Idiopathic guttate hypomelanosis** is an acquired condition, presenting as discrete, scattered 3- to 5 mm hypopigmented macules on chronically sun-exposed skin, commonly on the extensor arms and shins.

Continued

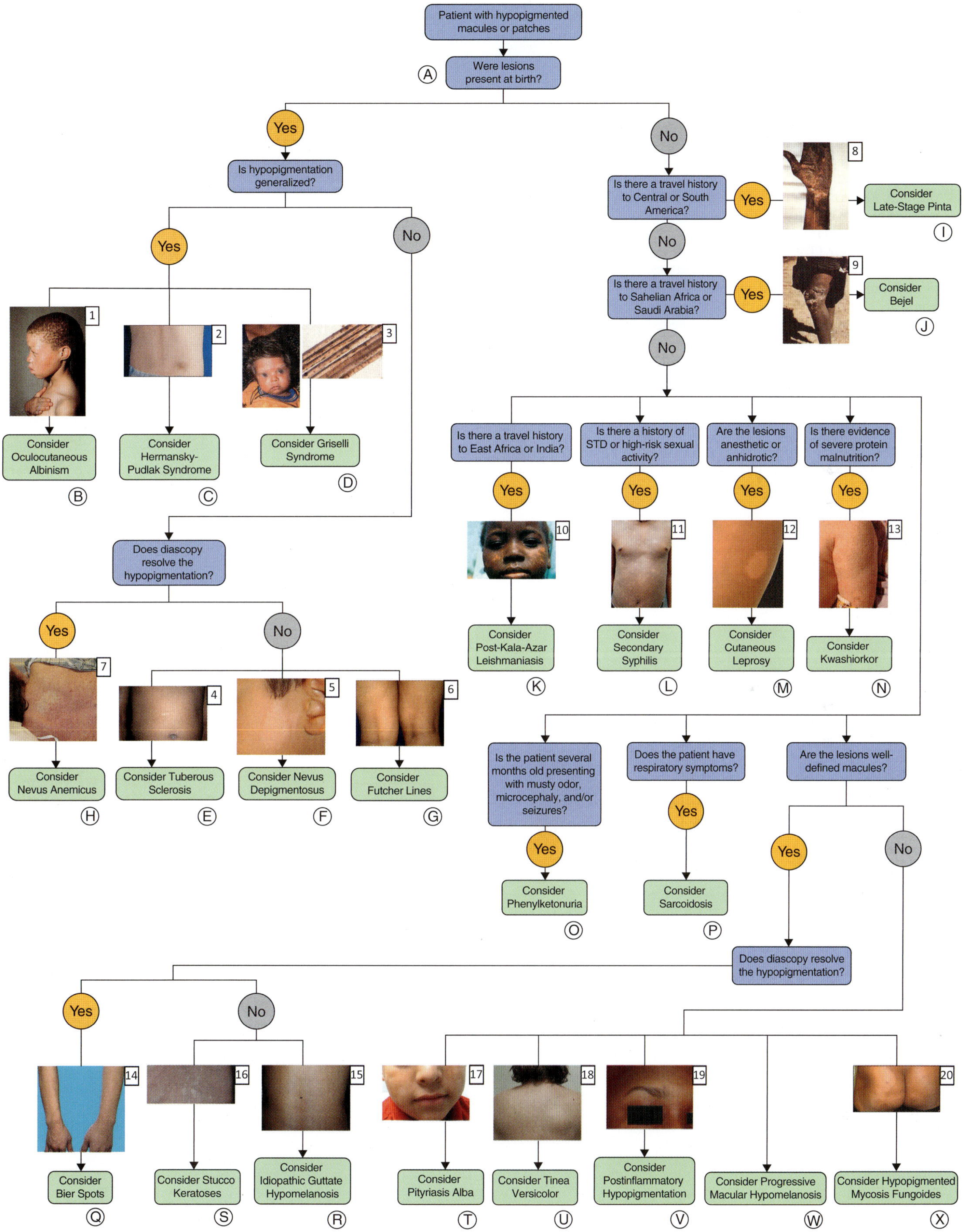
Patient with hypopigmented macules or patches
A
Were lesions present at birth?
Yes
Is hypopigmentation generalized?
Yes
1
2
3
Consider Oculocutaneous Albinism
B
Consider Hermansky-Pudlak Syndrome
C
Consider Griselli Syndrome
D
No
Does diascopy resolve the hypopigmentation?
Yes
7
Consider Nevus Anemicus
H
No
4
Consider Tuberous Sclerosis
E
5
Consider Nevus Depigmentosus
F
6
Consider Futcher Lines
G
No
Is there a travel history to Central or South America?
Yes
8
Consider Late-Stage Pinta
I
No
Is there a travel history to Sahelian Africa or Saudi Arabia?
Yes
9
Consider Bejel
J
No
Is there a travel history to East Africa or India?
Yes
10
Consider Post-Kala-Azar Leishmaniasis
K
Is there a history of STD or high-risk sexual activity?
Yes
11
Consider Secondary Syphilis
L
Are the lesions anesthetic or anhidrotic?
Yes
12
Consider Cutaneous Leprosy
M
Is there evidence of severe protein malnutrition?
Yes
13
Consider Kwashiorkor
N
Is the patient several months old presenting with musty odor, microcephaly, and/or seizures?
Yes
Consider Phenylketonuria
O
Does the patient have respiratory symptoms?
Yes
Consider Sarcoidosis
P
Are the lesions well-defined macules?
Yes
Does diascopy resolve the hypopigmentation?
Yes
14
Consider Bier Spots
Q
No
16
Consider Stucco Keratoses
S
15
Consider Idiopathic Guttate Hypomelanosis
R
No
17
Consider Pityriasis Alba
T
18
Consider Tinea Versicolor
U
19
Consider Postinflammatory Hypopigmentation
V
Consider Progressive Macular Hypomelanosis
W
20
Consider Hypopigmented Mycosis Fungoides
X

S. **Stucco keratoses** are benign, white, or gray scaly papules that classically appear in large numbers on the dorsal feet and lower legs in patients of Northern European descent older than 40 years. Males are about four times more likely to have these than females.

T. **Pityriasis alba (PA)** presents as hypopigmented macules or patches on the face or upper arms. PA may be asymptomatic or pruritic. A fine powdery scale is often associated and more readily observed with gentle scraping of the skin. PA usually affects children aged 3 to 16 years with an atopic diathesis (atopic dermatitis, asthma, allergic rhinitis). PA often has a relapsing-remitting course and may spontaneously resolve before adulthood.

U. **Tinea versicolor (TV)** is a benign, superficial fungal infection due to dimorphic yeast of the *Malassezia* genus. It can appear as macules, papules, patches, and plaques of varying pigmentation with fine scale similar to PA. Gentle scraping may be necessary to evoke the scale. TV often presents in a seborrheic distribution favoring the upper trunk, arms, neck, and face. It commonly affects young adults due to increased sebaceous gland activity. Wood's lamp examination shows fluorescence due to the fluorochrome pityrialactone. To confirm diagnosis, KOH preparation of the scale has a "spaghetti and meatball" appearance (hyphae and spores).

V. **Postinflammatory hypopigmentation (PIH)** is the partial or total loss of pigmentation that occurs after resolution of inflammatory skin diseases (e.g., atopic dermatitis, seborrheic dermatitis, psoriasis, discoid lupus erythematosus), infections (e.g., zoster, pityriasis versicolor, impetigo), procedures (e.g., chemical peels, laser, dermabrasion), and burns. PIH can appear as hypopigmented macules in the same distribution as the primary lesions.

W. **Progressive macular hypomelanosis** (i.e., cutis trunci variata, idiopathic multiple large-macule hypomelanosis) presents as ill-defined, nummular, hypopigmented macules and patches primarily in the lumbar region and abdomen, most often in young adults, particularly females, without history of preceding infection, inflammation, or injury. Wood's lamp examination characteristically shows follicular red fluorescence due to porphyrins in *Cutibacterium acnes*. It may last for years but usually resolves before age 40.

X. **Hypopigmented mycosis fungoides** is a subtype of mycosis fungoides, a form of cutaneous T-cell lymphoma. It typically presents as hypopigmented macules in young patients with dark skin but can be confused with early presentations of vitiligo. It is included herein so as not to be missed when considering the differential of pigmentary disorders.

See Appendix 1 for Further Reading and Image References.

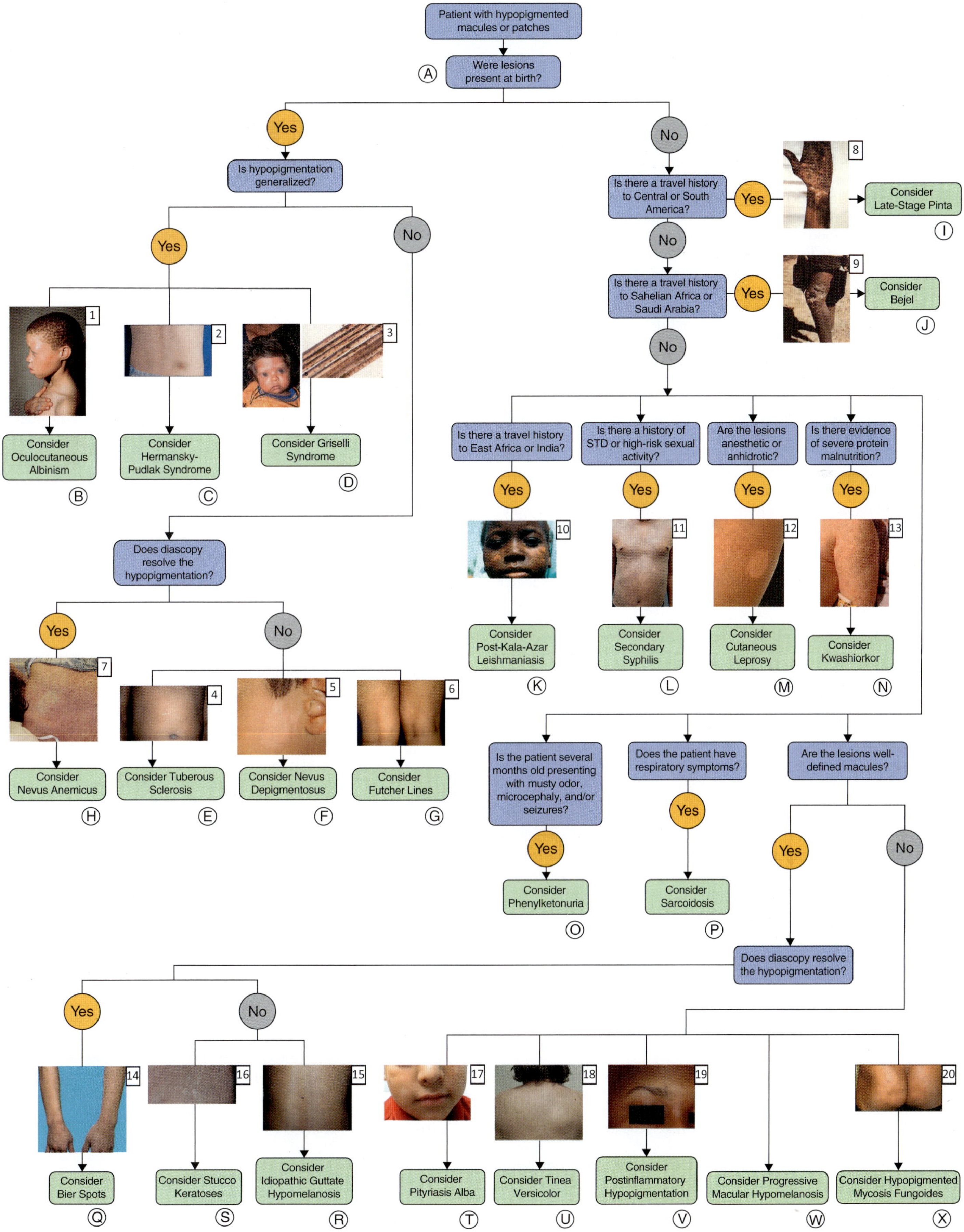
Patient with hypopigmented macules or patches
A
Were lesions present at birth?
Yes
Is hypopigmentation generalized?
Yes
1
Consider Oculocutaneous Albinism
B
2
Consider Hermansky-Pudlak Syndrome
C
3
Consider Griselli Syndrome
D
No
Does diascopy resolve the hypopigmentation?
Yes
7
Consider Nevus Anemicus
H
No
4
Consider Tuberous Sclerosis
E
5
Consider Nevus Depigmentosus
F
6
Consider Futcher Lines
G
No
Is there a travel history to Central or South America?
Yes
8
Consider Late-Stage Pinta
I
No
Is there a travel history to Sahelian Africa or Saudi Arabia?
Yes
9
Consider Bejel
J
No
Is there a travel history to East Africa or India?
Yes
10
Consider Post-Kala-Azar Leishmaniasis
K
Is there a history of STD or high-risk sexual activity?
Yes
11
Consider Secondary Syphilis
L
Are the lesions anesthetic or anhidrotic?
Yes
12
Consider Cutaneous Leprosy
M
Is there evidence of severe protein malnutrition?
Yes
13
Consider Kwashiorkor
N
Is the patient several months old presenting with musty odor, microcephaly, and/or seizures?
Yes
Consider Phenylketonuria
O
Does the patient have respiratory symptoms?
Yes
Consider Sarcoidosis
P
Are the lesions well-defined macules?
Yes
Does diascopy resolve the hypopigmentation?
Yes
14
Consider Bier Spots
Q
No
16
Consider Stucco Keratoses
S
15
Consider Idiopathic Guttate Hypomelanosis
R
No
17
Consider Pityriasis Alba
T
18
Consider Tinea Versicolor
U
19
Consider Postinflammatory Hypopigmentation
V
Consider Progressive Macular Hypomelanosis
W
20
Consider Hypopigmented Mycosis Fungoides
X

69 Depigmented Skin

Xochitl A. Green and Victor Huang

Depigmentation disorders are the result of an absence of melanocytes or the inability of melanocytes to produce and transport melanosomes. Pathologically, depigmentation can be differentiated from hypopigmentation in that depigmentation results in a complete loss of pigmentation as opposed to a decrease in pigmentation (see Chapter 68 on Hypopigmented Macules). In the initial evaluation of depigmentation, evaluation with a Wood's lamp can be immensely helpful in distinguishing hypopigmentation versus depigmentation and delineating the extent of involvement particularly in fairer skin types. Depigmented lesions are marked by stark autofluorescence of collagen in light areas contrasting with the surrounding skin. Depigmentation disorders can be further divided into congenital versus acquired conditions.

A. Congenital depigmentation can present as individual lesions or diffusely.

B. Generalized hereditary hypomelanoses are a diverse and well-defined set of syndromes affecting the function or distribution of melanocytes. In their most severe manifestations, patients can present with generalized depigmentation. **Oculocutaneous albinism** and **Waardenburg syndrome** are classic examples of consequences of disturbing melanin synthesis and melanocyte differentiation and migration, respectively.

C. **Oculocutaneous albinism** may be associated with translucent irises, photophobia, strabismus, and nystagmus in proportion to the degree of reduction in melanin pigment.

D. **Waardenburg syndrome** can be associated with deafness, heterochromia irides, confluent eyebrows, and dystopia canthorum in certain variants.

E. **Piebaldism** is an autosomal dominant genetic disorder in which a mutation of the KIT gene causes reduced or absent melanocytes. It presents as depigmented patches favoring the ventral trunk, face, and mid-extremities sparing the midline back. Most strikingly, the mid-forehead and frontal scalp are often involved, resulting in a white forelock.

F. **Nevus anemicus (NA)** usually presents at birth on the chest or back as a solitary hypopigmented macule or patch often with surrounding smaller satellite macules. NA is not a pigmentary disorder, but a localized area of vasoconstriction in the skin due to increased sympathetic supply. NA can occur in several syndromes, including neurofibromatosis (up to 4% of cases). Diagnosis is clinical; diascopy results in blanching of the peripheral skin, rendering the lesion indistinguishable from surroundings.

G. Acquired depigmentation comprises a varied number of pathologies. Initial evaluation of acquired depigmentation includes consideration of unique symptoms or history.

H. Travel history to areas endemic for diseases can raise the suspicion of **onchocerciasis**, marked by the development of hypomelanotic macules on the anterior shin that progress to amelanotic patches with follicular retention of pigment described as "leopard skin."

I. A history of exposures to phenols and catechols can lead to **chemical leukoderma**. The tyrosinase inhibiting and melanotoxic properties of these chemicals have been exploited in hydroquinone-containing preparations to treat hyperpigmentation, although related molecules have been associated with developing vitiligo. Paraphenylene diamine has been implicated in occupational exposures in industries involving contact with black rubber or in hair dye-associated vitiligo.

J. **Vitiligo** is marked by an immune-mediated destruction of melanocytes. Vitiligo affects between 0.5% and 2% of the world population, and the average age of onset is 20 to 25 years. Vitiligo can broadly be divided into segmental and nonsegmental subtypes, with nonsegmental lesions presenting symmetrically on the face, hands, forearms, neck, genitalia, body folds, and periorificial region. Characteristic patterns of presentation have been described, which aid in clinical diagnosis. Some common patterns include mucosal vitiligo involving the lips, inner nose, and genital areas; acrofacial vitiligo involving the face and hands and ventral wrists; "lip-tip" variants involving the lip vermillion, perioral area, and tips of the fingers. Segmental vitiligo often presents at an earlier age. Vogt-Koyanagi-Harada syndrome is a variation of vitiligo that presents with aseptic meningitis, uveitis, and hearing impairment.

K. **Traumatic leukoderma** can occur in the setting of trauma that leads to melanocyte death. This damage may be in the setting of physical trauma (including excoriation), postsurgical scars, cryotherapy, or as a result of profound inflammation.

L. **Discoid lupus** and associated scarring is one example of an inflammatory pathology leading to melanocyte death and depigmentation secondary to intense inflammatory damage. A hyperpigmented rim often accompanies the depigmented lesions. Facial lesions or involvement of the conchal bowl of the ears is common. **Scleroderma** and related sclerotic disorders often present with depigmented patches involving both sclerotic and nonsclerotic areas with a characteristic supravenous retention of pigment.

M. **Idiopathic guttate hypomelanosis** is common across all races and skin types. It presents as white, discrete small macules most commonly across the distal extremities that are stable over time and asymptomatic. While the cause has not been determined, the distribution favoring extremities and increased incidence with age is suggestive of cumulative sun exposure involvement. **Stucco keratoses** are a variant of seborrheic keratoses that favor the lower extremities presenting as stuck-on 1- to 5 mm white hyperkeratotic papules. **Verruca plana** are a manifestation of human papillomavirus (HPV) infection presenting as skin-colored to hypopigmented flat-topped papules that are often white in color with minimal epidermal change. HPV strains 3, 10, 28, and 49 are often implicated.

N. Finally, a collection of pathologies related to coagulopathy can present with white, scar-like lesions described as atrophie blanche-like. **Livedoid vasculopathy** presents with painful, persistent, punched-out erosions favoring the lower extremities with white round scars, often with surrounding telangiectasias. **Degos disease**, to be distinguished from Dowling-Degos disease, is a vasoocclusive disorder leading to small porcelain-white scar-like papules on the trunk and extremities. Bowel involvement can be fatal.

See Appendix 1 for Further Reading and Image References.

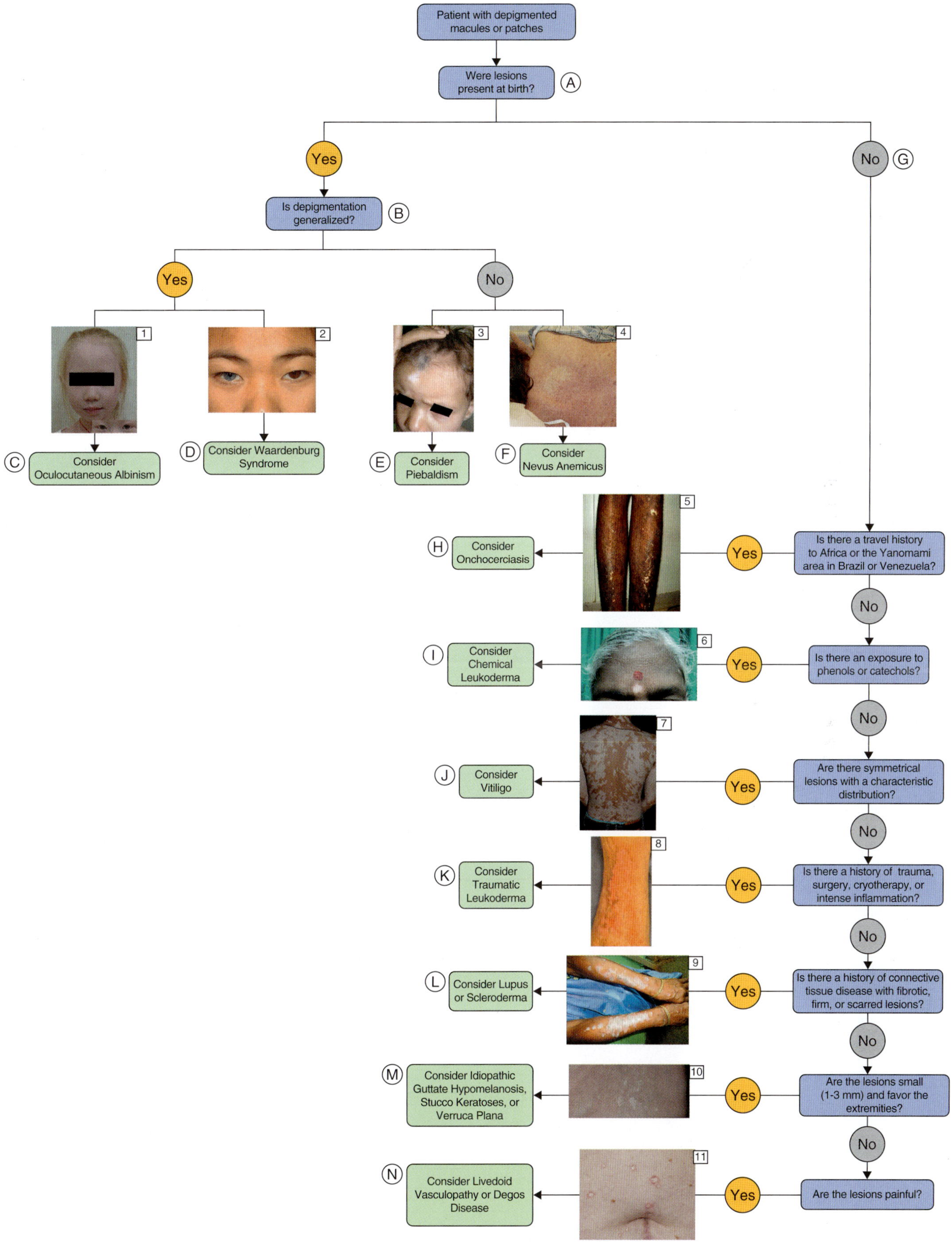
Patient with depigmented macules or patches
Were lesions present at birth?
A
Yes
Is depigmentation generalized?
B
Yes
No
1
2
3
4
C
Consider Oculocutaneous Albinism
D
Consider Waardenburg Syndrome
E
Consider Piebaldism
F
Consider Nevus Anemicus
No
G
Is there a travel history to Africa or the Yanomami area in Brazil or Venezuela?
Yes
5
H
Consider Onchocerciasis
No
Is there an exposure to phenols or catechols?
Yes
6
I
Consider Chemical Leukoderma
No
Are there symmetrical lesions with a characteristic distribution?
Yes
7
J
Consider Vitiligo
No
Is there a history of trauma, surgery, cryotherapy, or intense inflammation?
Yes
8
K
Consider Traumatic Leukoderma
No
Is there a history of connective tissue disease with fibrotic, firm, or scarred lesions?
Yes
9
L
Consider Lupus or Scleroderma
No
Are the lesions small (1-3 mm) and favor the extremities?
Yes
10
M
Consider Idiopathic Guttate Hypomelanosis, Stucco Keratoses, or Verruca Plana
No
Are the lesions painful?
Yes
11
N
Consider Livedoid Vasculopathy or Degos Disease

PART XIV

Colorful Isolated Lesions

70 Black Lesions

Claudia Quarshie and Jenny C. Hu

Individuals may acquire a wide variety of black lesions over the course of a lifetime. The initial evaluation of patients presenting with black lesions should involve obtaining a detailed history of the specific lesion in question and a total body skin examination. Additional support for the diagnosis may be needed, including the use of a dermatoscope and biopsy for histopathologic confirmation.

A. Raised black lesions include **melanoma** in the differential. Any suspicion of melanoma requires a biopsy. Risk factors include a personal or family history of cutaneous melanoma, fair skin that burns easily, chronic sun exposure, and multiple melanocytic nevi, and/or solar lentigines. Although melanomas most often occur in fair-skinned patients, skin of color patients are also at risk of developing melanomas. The ABCDEs of melanoma, which are concerning signs for malignancy in a pigmented lesion, include *a*symmetry, irregular *b*orders, color variation, *d*iameter larger than 6 mm, and *e*volving (i.e., changes in size, shape, or color).

Melanoma may present as flat or raised. **Nodular melanomas** typically present as raised and may be ulcerated or bleeding. Flat melanomas include superficial spreading, lentigo maligna, and acral lentiginous melanomas. **Superficial spreading melanomas**, the most common type, can arise de novo or in a preexisting nevus. **Lentigo maligna (in situ)** or **lentigo maligna melanoma (invasive)** develop within chronically sun-damaged skin. **Acral lentiginous melanomas** are more frequently seen in skin of color patients and occur on the palms, soles, or around the nail apparatus. Histopathology is the gold standard for melanoma diagnosis, and there is an excellent prognosis when diagnosed early.

Patients presenting with a flat or raised black pigmented macule or papule may have a nevus. Clinically, a junctional nevus is flat while an intradermal or compound nevus is raised. A **benign nevus** has smooth borders and a uniform shade of color, which can be black, brown, pink, or skin colored. These nevi should be monitored closely for possible atypical or malignant changes. An **atypical nevus** is usually greater than 5 mm, is often slightly variably pigmented, and can have minimally irregular borders. It is commonly present on the trunk and limbs but can be found on any location of the body.

Pigmented basal cell carcinoma (BCC) may have varying degrees of pigmentation and may clinically resemble cutaneous melanoma. However, a glassy translucency with characteristic dermoscopic features such as arborizing telangiectasias and multiple blue-gray ovoid globules point to the diagnosis of pigmented BCC.

Pigmented seborrheic keratoses usually appear in the fifth decade of life, equally in males and females. They classically present as a crusty, greasy plaque above the skin surface adhering to the epidermis and can be pruritic or irritated. They are usually brown but can have darker pigmentation and thus may mimic other pigmented lesions such as melanomas. Dermoscopic examination may give clues for this diagnosis, including fissures and ridges, loop vessels with white halo, comedo-like openings, and milia-like cysts.

B. Flat black macules or patches include the earlier discussed melanocytic lesions such as melanoma, benign nevus, and atypical nevus, as well as pigmented Spitz nevus and blue nevus. **Pigmented Spitz nevus** presents as a homogeneous black, well-circumscribed macule or patch, which presents mainly in children and adolescents but may be observed in adults as well. It is a rare and benign nevus that may present anywhere on the body but favors the head and neck region in children. These nevi may necessitate a biopsy to evaluate for atypia or potential malignancy.

Patients presenting in childhood or early adulthood with a uniformly pigmented macule, papule, plaque, or nodule with dark bluish or blue-black coloration may have a **blue nevus**. They are usually solitary and appear mostly on the extremities. Most blue nevi can be diagnosed easily by clinical examination (characteristic blue hue) or with the help of dermoscopy.

C. In a patient with a history of radiation therapy for malignancy, consider the diagnosis of a radiation **tattoo**. These small blue or black ink tattoos, usually a few millimeters in size, may mimic metastases of malignant melanoma and other melanocytic neoplasms on clinical and dermoscopic examination given their histologic similarities to dermal pigmentation.

D. A patient presenting with bluish-black macules or patch associated with overlying callosity on their heel may have **talon noir** or traumatic calcaneal petechiae. This classically occurs from repeated lateral shearing forces, creating intraepidermal microhemorrhages. A more severe manifestation of this condition may mimic melanoma, but paring the stratum corneum of the area with a scalpel can readily verify the diagnosis through the removal of the microhemorrhages within the stratum corneum.

E. Patients presenting with a homogeneous black macule with an irregular outline that is reticulated in shape and most resembles a spot of ink on the skin may have **ink spot lentigo**, also known as reticulated black solar lentigo. It is commonly described in fair-skinned individuals on sun-exposed areas of the body.

See Appendix 1 for Further Reading and Image References.

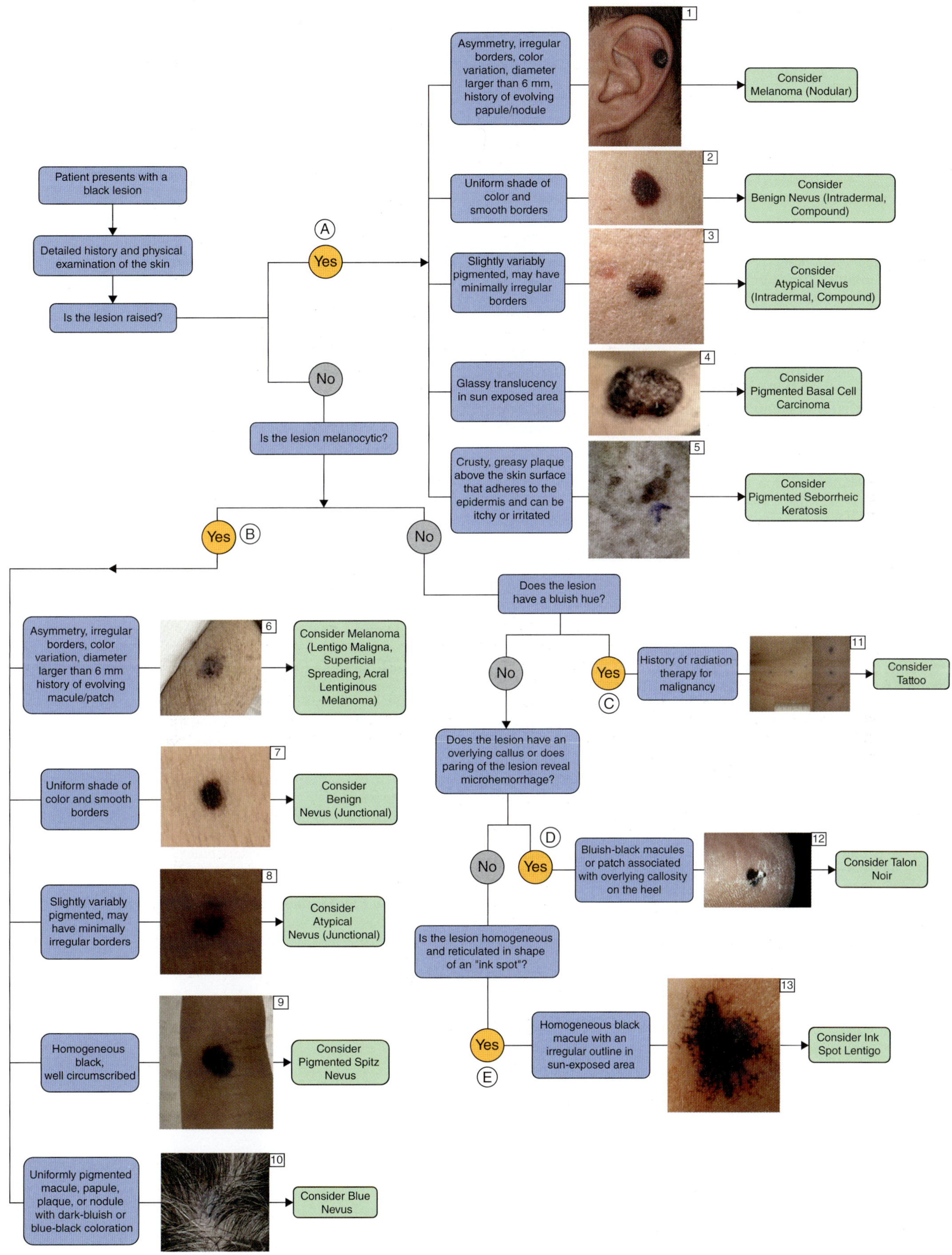
Patient presents with a black lesion
Detailed history and physical examination of the skin
Is the lesion raised?
A
Yes
Asymmetry, irregular borders, color variation, diameter larger than 6 mm, history of evolving papule/nodule
1
Consider Melanoma (Nodular)
Uniform shade of color and smooth borders
2
Consider Benign Nevus (Intradermal, Compound)
Slightly variably pigmented, may have minimally irregular borders
3
Consider Atypical Nevus (Intradermal, Compound)
Glassy translucency in sun exposed area
4
Consider Pigmented Basal Cell Carcinoma
Crusty, greasy plaque above the skin surface that adheres to the epidermis and can be itchy or irritated
5
Consider Pigmented Seborrheic Keratosis
No
Is the lesion melanocytic?
Yes
B
Asymmetry, irregular borders, color variation, diameter larger than 6 mm history of evolving macule/patch
6
Consider Melanoma (Lentigo Maligna, Superficial Spreading, Acral Lentiginous Melanoma)
Uniform shade of color and smooth borders
7
Consider Benign Nevus (Junctional)
Slightly variably pigmented, may have minimally irregular borders
8
Consider Atypical Nevus (Junctional)
Homogeneous black, well circumscribed
9
Consider Pigmented Spitz Nevus
Uniformly pigmented macule, papule, plaque, or nodule with dark-bluish or blue-black coloration
10
Consider Blue Nevus
No
Does the lesion have a bluish hue?
Yes
C
History of radiation therapy for malignancy
11
Consider Tattoo
No
Does the lesion have an overlying callus or does paring of the lesion reveal microhemorrhage?
Yes
D
Bluish-black macules or patch associated with overlying callosity on the heel
12
Consider Talon Noir
No
Is the lesion homogeneous and reticulated in shape of an "ink spot"?
Yes
E
Homogeneous black macule with an irregular outline in sun-exposed area
13
Consider Ink Spot Lentigo

71 Blue Lesions

Elaine J. Ma and Jennifer L. Hsiao

Blue lesions may represent a wide variety of different cutaneous conditions. Careful history and examination of the lesion will aid in diagnosis, and a biopsy may be required if the clinical examination does not rule out malignancy.

A. The initial evaluation of blue lesions should include a detailed history and physical examination. Evaluate the lesions for color variegation, distribution, tenderness, and compressibility. Determine the number of lesions and anatomic areas of involvement.

B. A history of immunodeficiency should be elicited. HIV or human T-lymphotropic virus 1–associated adult T-cell leukemia are common underlying conditions in patients with **Kaposi sarcoma (KS)**. Classic KS is an indolent growth that typically affects older males of Mediterranean or Ashkenazi Jewish descent, while nonclassic KS presents in severely immunocompromised patients as multiple reddish-purple or bluish macules, papules, and nodules. Endemic KS primarily affects young males living in equatorial Africa.

C. Patients who have radiation therapy or a history of trauma with a graphite pencil likely have an **exogenous tattoo**, which presents as a homogeneous bluish macule. Amalgam tattoos may be present in the oral cavity from dental procedures.

Various forms of dermal melanocytosis present with bluish-gray patches. Nevus of Ota, Ito, and Hori can be distinguished based on the time of presentation and anatomic location of the lesion. **Nevus of Ota** frequently presents in infancy or childhood and follows the dermatomes of the first two branches of the trigeminal nerve, resulting in a unilateral distribution on the forehead and ocular region. Nevus of Ota typically occurs in association with other pigmented lesions (i.e., nevus spilus) and presents with ocular manifestations in two-thirds of patients. In contrast, **Nevus of Ito** typically occurs on the side of the neck and shoulder. Similar to nevus of Ota, nevus of Ito appears at birth or during puberty and hormonal changes. In rare instances, melanoma has been reported to arise in association with these conditions. **Nevus of Hori** does not present at birth. It typically occurs on the face bilaterally around the lower eyelids, temples, and nose.

Blue nevi may present as a homogeneous blue macule or noncompressible papule. The lesions are characteristically well-demarcated. Blue nevi have an increased prevalence in Asian females. An agminated blue nevus is a localized cluster of blue nevi.

D. **Blue rubber bleb nevus** and **venous lake** are benign blue lesions that are raised and compressible on palpation. Blue rubber bleb nevus is a venous malformation that is typically seen in patients of European descent at birth or early childhood. It presents with focal areas of overlying hyperhidrosis, may swell in gravity-dependent positions, and may be tender. Venous malformations can also be seen in the gastrointestinal tract, liver, spleen, heart, eyes, and central nervous system. In contrast, venous lakes are associated with aging and are typically found on the lips, ears, and face of older males who have frequent outdoor exposure. They are dark blue to violaceous dilations of preexisting vessels that may bleed if traumatized.

E. If a blue nodule is visible through the fingernail plate or in the subungual area, consider **glomus tumor**. Patients may present with a triad of symptoms, including point tenderness, paroxysmal pain, and hypersensitivity to cold.

F. If the lesion is multicolored, malignancy should be considered and a history of sun exposure queried. The characteristic clinical findings of **pigmented basal cell carcinoma** include a shiny, pearly papule or nodule with telangiectasias and varying degrees of blue, brown, gray, or black pigment. **Melanoma** presents with asymmetry and frequently has color variegation. Blue color is often admixed with white or black structures, creating irregular streaks and abrupt edges.

G. **Apocrine hidrocystoma** is a benign cystic tumor of apocrine sweat glands that presents as an asymptomatic translucent or semitransparent bluish or skin-colored papule or nodule, typically along the eyelid margin. It is moderately firm with some mobility with palpation and is usually solitary.

H. Blue nevi, dermatofibromas, and angiokeratomas may present as bluish papules. **Blue nevi** were discussed in section E.

Dermatofibromas, firm hyperpigmented papules that rarely have blue pigment, are found at sites where the skin may have undergone minor trauma, such as an insect bite. They may have a central, white scar-like area. A dimple can form with the pinch test (squeezing the lesion on the sides).

Angiokeratomas may present in different anatomic locations but are often found on the lower extremities or genitals. Lesions typically present as red, violaceous, or dark blue papules or verrucous plaques.

See Appendix 1 for Further Reading and Image References.

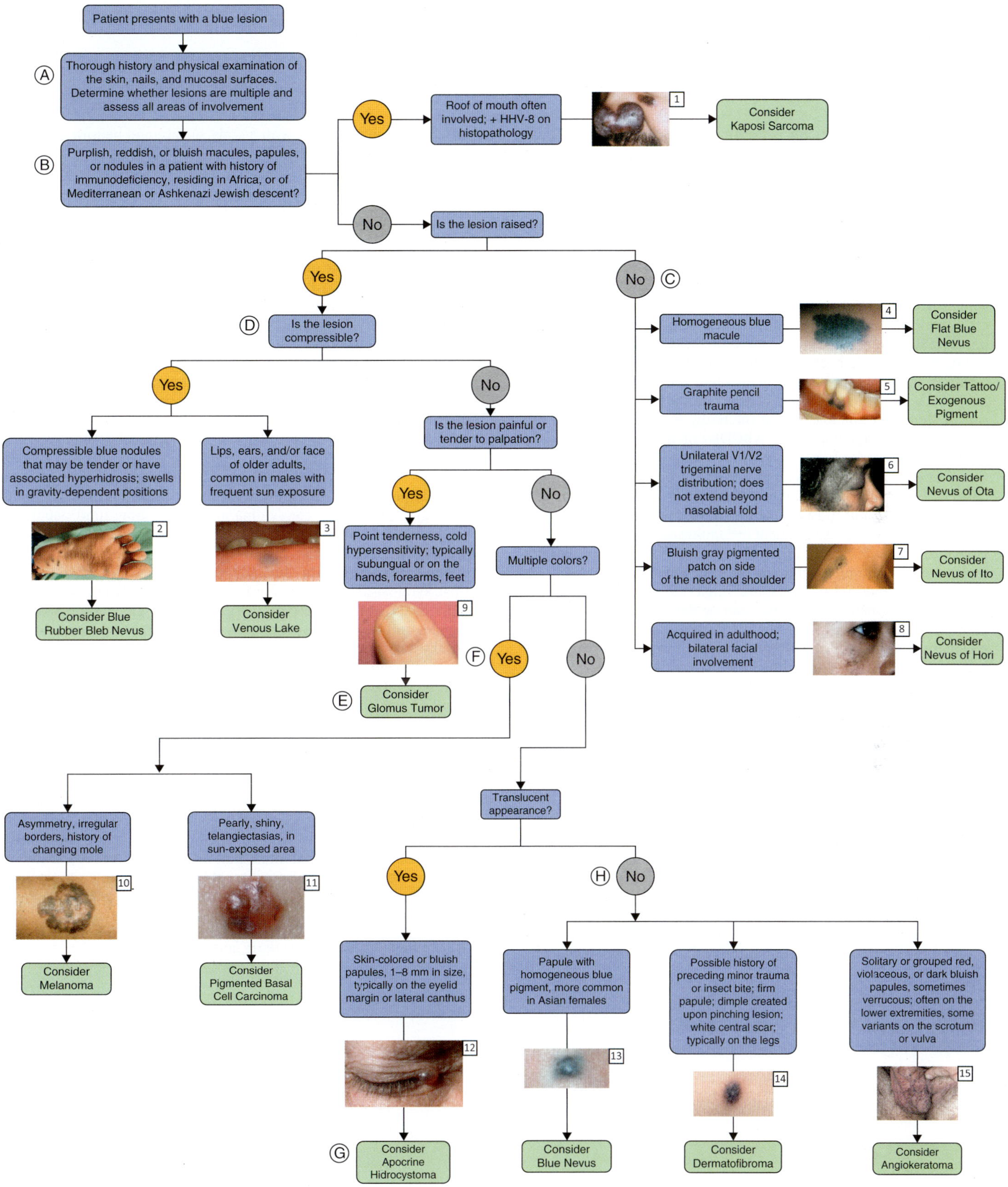
Patient presents with a blue lesion
Ⓐ Thorough history and physical examination of the skin, nails, and mucosal surfaces. Determine whether lesions are multiple and assess all areas of involvement
Ⓑ Purplish, reddish, or bluish macules, papules, or nodules in a patient with history of immunodeficiency, residing in Africa, or of Mediterranean or Ashkenazi Jewish descent?
Yes
Roof of mouth often involved; + HHV-8 on histopathology
1
Consider Kaposi Sarcoma
No
Is the lesion raised?
Yes
Ⓓ Is the lesion compressible?
Yes
Compressible blue nodules that may be tender or have associated hyperhidrosis; swells in gravity-dependent positions
2
Consider Blue Rubber Bleb Nevus
Lips, ears, and/or face of older adults, common in males with frequent sun exposure
3
Consider Venous Lake
No
Is the lesion painful or tender to palpation?
Yes
Point tenderness, cold hypersensitivity; typically subungual or on the hands, forearms, feet
9
Ⓔ Consider Glomus Tumor
No
Multiple colors?
Ⓕ Yes
Asymmetry, irregular borders, history of changing mole
10
Consider Melanoma
Pearly, shiny, telangiectasias, in sun-exposed area
11
Consider Pigmented Basal Cell Carcinoma
No
Translucent appearance?
Yes
Skin-colored or bluish papules, 1–8 mm in size, typically on the eyelid margin or lateral canthus
12
Ⓖ Consider Apocrine Hidrocystoma
Ⓗ No
Papule with homogeneous blue pigment, more common in Asian females
13
Consider Blue Nevus
Possible history of preceding minor trauma or insect bite; firm papule; dimple created upon pinching lesion; white central scar; typically on the legs
14
Consider Dermatofibroma
Solitary or grouped red, violaceous, or dark bluish papules, sometimes verrucous; often on the lower extremities, some variants on the scrotum or vulva
15
Consider Angiokeratoma
No Ⓒ
Homogeneous blue macule
4
Consider Flat Blue Nevus
Graphite pencil trauma
5
Consider Tattoo/ Exogenous Pigment
Unilateral V1/V2 trigeminal nerve distribution; does not extend beyond nasolabial fold
6
Consider Nevus of Ota
Bluish gray pigmented patch on side of the neck and shoulder
7
Consider Nevus of Ito
Acquired in adulthood; bilateral facial involvement
8
Consider Nevus of Hori

72 Brown Lesions

Claudia Quarshie and Jenny C. Hu

The initial evaluation of patients presenting with brown lesions should involve obtaining a detailed history of the specific lesion in question and a total body skin examination. Additional support for the diagnosis may be needed, including the use of a dermatoscope and biopsy for histopathologic confirmation.

A. Patients presenting with a brown melanocytic lesion may have a benign nevus, an atypical nevus, melanoma, or a less common pigmented Spitz nevus. A **benign nevus** may be present at birth or appear later in childhood or adulthood. It has a uniform shade of color, which can be brown, skin colored, or pink, and has smooth borders. These lesions should be monitored closely for possible atypical or malignant changes. An **atypical nevus** is usually greater than 5 mm, is often slightly variably pigmented, and can have minimally irregular borders. It commonly presents on the trunk and limbs but can be found on any location of the body. A nevus that has more atypical features known as the ABCDEs of **melanoma**, including **a**symmetry, irregular **b**orders, **c**olor variation, **d**iameter larger than 6 mm, or **e**volving (i.e., changes in size, shape, or color), should raise concern for malignancy. Of note, melanoma is less common in skin of color patients, but most frequently develops on acral sites or nail units in these patients. A variant of melanoma on chronically sun-exposed skin includes **lentigo maligna** (in situ) and **lentigo maligna melanoma** (invasive). A **pigmented Spitz nevus** typically appears during childhood and presents as a single homogeneous, well-circumscribed pigmented lesion that can be flat or raised. It may also clinically have atypical features and sometimes be concerning for a melanoma. A biopsy is needed when it is unclear whether a melanocytic lesion is benign or if malignancy is suspected.

B. Older patients presenting with well-circumscribed, round, oval, or irregularly shaped, even-colored, brown nonscaly macules on chronically sun-exposed sites (e.g., face, neck, upper trunk, dorsal hands and forearms, shins) may have **solar lentigines**. They almost always present as multiple lesions varying in diameter from 1 to 3 mm and sometimes up to 1 cm.

C. Patients presenting with a brown lesion with scaly surface on sun-exposed skin may have a pigmented actinic keratosis, pigmented squamous cell carcinoma in situ, or pigmented invasive squamous cell carcinoma. **Pigmented actinic keratosis** often lacks associated erythema and has a hyperpigmented appearance with overlying hyperkeratosis. **Pigmented squamous cell carcinomas in situ** are typically flat, and **pigmented invasive squamous cell carcinomas** are usually raised. Both may present with a scaly surface and be mistaken for a seborrheic keratosis.

D. **Seborrheic keratoses** usually appear in the fifth decade of life, arising equally in males and females. They classically present as a crusty, greasy plaque on the skin surface adhering to the epidermis. They are typically brown but may have darker pigmentation and may thus closely resemble other pigmented lesions.

E. In an adult with a firm, minimally elevated to dome-shaped hyperpigmented papule on the lower extremity, consider the diagnosis of a **dermatofibroma**. They usually measure several millimeters in size. Lesions that are nearing 1 cm in size or greater warrant excisional biopsy to rule out atypia or a malignant lesion. On palpation, gently pinching the lesion usually results in a downward movement of the tumor, known as the "dimple sign." Dermatofibromas may occur as an abnormal response to trauma, such as an insect bite, and are often pruritic.

F. Patients presenting with brown lesions in the anogenital or inguinal regions may have condyloma acuminata, Bowenoid papulosis, squamous cell carcinoma in situ, or invasive squamous cell carcinoma, which are associated with the human papillomavirus (HPV). **Condyloma acuminata** clinically and histologically mimic seborrheic keratosis but differ in that it most frequently occurs in younger individuals. Lesions are typically discrete, sessile, smooth-surfaced papules and may be brown or skin colored. **Bowenoid papulosis** is usually associated with HPV genotypes 16 and 18 and demonstrates histopathologic changes of squamous cell carcinoma in situ found within genital warts. The clinical appearance is usually multiple small brown, pink, or skin-colored papules. **Squamous cell carcinoma in situ** and **invasive squamous cell carcinoma** of the genital areas usually appear as brown or pink patches or plaques that can sometimes be ulcerated.

G. **Tinea nigra** most commonly presents as an asymptomatic, single, sharply marginated, brown to gray macule or patch that can be velvety or have mild scale. The advancing border of the lesion may also be more darkly pigmented than its center. There are usually no predisposing factors. Although most frequently seen on the palms, tinea nigra can also appear on the soles, neck, and trunk.

See Appendix 1 for Further Reading and Image References.

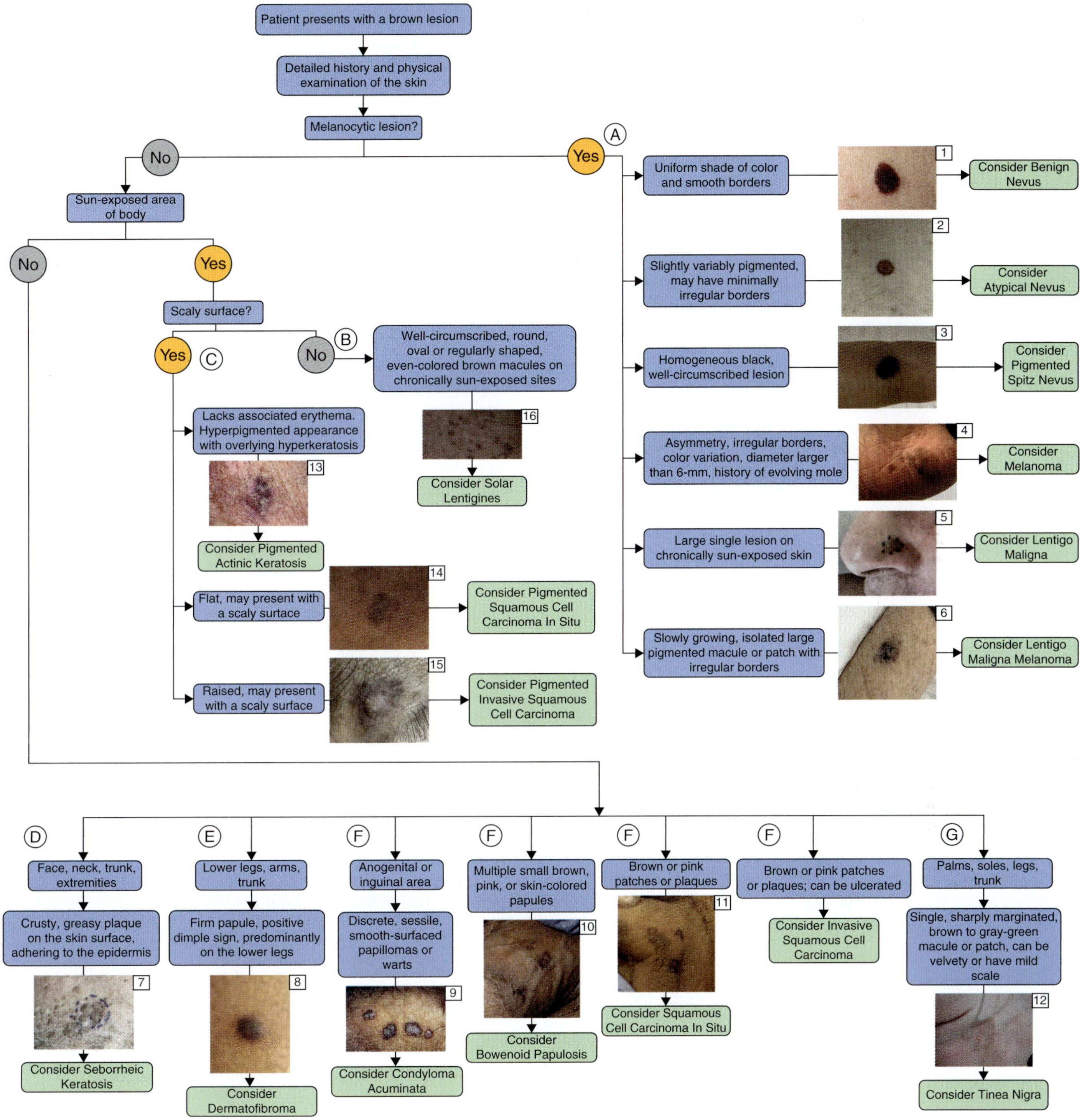
Patient presents with a brown lesion
Detailed history and physical examination of the skin
Melanocytic lesion?
No
Yes
A
Sun-exposed area of body
No
Yes
Scaly surface?
Yes
C
No
B
Well-circumscribed, round, oval or regularly shaped, even-colored brown macules on chronically sun-exposed sites
16
Consider Solar Lentigines
Lacks associated erythema. Hyperpigmented appearance with overlying hyperkeratosis
13
Consider Pigmented Actinic Keratosis
Flat, may present with a scaly surface
14
Consider Pigmented Squamous Cell Carcinoma In Situ
Raised, may present with a scaly surface
15
Consider Pigmented Invasive Squamous Cell Carcinoma
Uniform shade of color and smooth borders
1
Consider Benign Nevus
Slightly variably pigmented, may have minimally irregular borders
2
Consider Atypical Nevus
Homogeneous black, well-circumscribed lesion
3
Consider Pigmented Spitz Nevus
Asymmetry, irregular borders, color variation, diameter larger than 6-mm, history of evolving mole
4
Consider Melanoma
Large single lesion on chronically sun-exposed skin
5
Consider Lentigo Maligna
Slowly growing, isolated large pigmented macule or patch with irregular borders
6
Consider Lentigo Maligna Melanoma
D
Face, neck, trunk, extremities
Crusty, greasy plaque on the skin surface, adhering to the epidermis
7
Consider Seborrheic Keratosis
E
Lower legs, arms, trunk
Firm papule, positive dimple sign, predominantly on the lower legs
8
Consider Dermatofibroma
F
Anogenital or inguinal area
Discrete, sessile, smooth-surfaced papillomas or warts
9
Consider Condyloma Acuminata
F
Multiple small brown, pink, or skin-colored papules
10
Consider Bowenoid Papulosis
F
Brown or pink patches or plaques
11
Consider Squamous Cell Carcinoma In Situ
F
Brown or pink patches or plaques; can be ulcerated
Consider Invasive Squamous Cell Carcinoma
G
Palms, soles, legs, trunk
Single, sharply marginated, brown to gray-green macule or patch, can be velvety or have mild scale
12
Consider Tinea Nigra

73 Pink Lesions

Audrey Hao and Jenny C. Hu

Pink lesions represent a variety of pathologies, from benign to malignant, most of which can be better visualized with the aid of dermoscopy. While dermoscopy may narrow a differential, histopathology should confirm a diagnosis when it is unclear, or help rule out malignancy if it is suspected.

A. Many skin malignancies can present in sun-exposed areas. **Actinic keratoses (AKs)** are typically on sun-damaged skin of the head, neck, upper trunk, and extremities and present as small rough papules that may be erythematous or hyperkeratotic. The importance of treating AKs early is to prevent their potential malignant transformation to **squamous cell carcinoma (SCC)**, which often presents as a rough papule or nodule that can grow quickly and occasionally be painful. **Basal cell carcinoma (BCC)** often presents as a pearly nodule with overlying telangiectasias and can ulcerate and have an elevated rolled border. **Amelanotic melanoma** can present as an asymmetric, skin-colored to light pink nodule that can sometimes be mistaken for a verruca, SCC, or BCC. **Microcystic adnexal carcinoma** is a slow-growing, locally aggressive eccrine/apocrine gland tumor that typically presents as a smooth skin-colored or pink nodule or plaque on the head and neck, particularly the central face. **Merkel cell carcinoma** is a rare neuroendocrine malignancy with high risk for metastasis, which often presents in the elderly as a pink or bluish, firm, dome-shaped nodule that can grow rapidly and ulcerate.

B. Less common skin malignancies can also present as pink lesions on non–sun-exposed skin. **Dermatofibrosarcoma protuberans (DFSP)** is a soft tissue sarcoma that most commonly presents in young to middle-aged adults on the trunk as a firm pinkish to reddish-brown nodule that measures one to several centimeters in diameter and feels attached to subcutaneous tissue. These can be mistaken for keloids. **Sebaceous carcinoma** is an adenocarcinoma with sebaceous differentiation that presents as erythematous and slightly yellow plaques or nodules that may be ulcerated or crusted. **Cutaneous leiomyosarcoma** is a smooth muscle tumor that can arise anywhere on the body and commonly presents as pink nodules that may be painful. **Porocarcinoma** is an eccrine carcinoma with high metastatic potential, often developing on the acral regions and lower limbs in the elderly as pink or erythematous verrucous plaques or polypoid nodules that may bleed with minor trauma.

C. **Supernumerary nipples** are congenital and often occur along the midclavicular line several centimeters below the breast nipple. They may have an area of central elevation and hair growth, and they may grow or swell during puberty.

D. While nevi typically do not present as pink lesions, a rare subtype, **Spitz nevus**, usually presents in childhood or adolescence as a fast-growing, symmetric, pink to dark brown-black dome-shaped papule, often on the lower extremities or face.

E. Multiple red to purple homogeneous small papules may be indicative of **angiomas**. They are commonly found on the neck, trunk, and upper extremities and can usually be diagnosed clinically.

F. Consider a **hypertrophic scar** or **keloid** in anatomical sites with a known prior injury. Hypertrophic scars are raised smooth plaques confined to the wound margin, but keloids tend to be more elevated and extend beyond the boundary of the original wound. If there is no history of known trauma, a biopsy should be performed to rule out DFSP (see section B).

G. **Inflamed cysts** are common, can occur anywhere on the skin, and are typically painful. Diagnosis can usually be made clinically, although lack of improvement after treatment should warrant a biopsy to rule out malignancy, including SCC with cystic features.

H. Rare benign neoplasms of sebaceous, eccrine, and apocrine glands can also appear as pink lesions. **Syringocystadenomas** (from apocrine sweat glands) present as small, pink, red, or purple papules/plaques on the face and scalp or as slowly growing fleshy plaques that sometimes ooze fluid and blood. **Poromas** (from eccrine and apocrine glands) are papules or nodules that are usually found on the palms and soles. They range in color from skin colored to red and pink, and in texture from smooth, verrucous, to ulcerated. **Cylindromas** (from eccrine glands) are typically found on the scalp, where they can coalesce and form dense groups of nodules. **Spiradenomas** appear as painful pink, purple, blue, or gray nodules, most commonly located on the head, neck, and trunk. **Clear cell acanthomas** are rare neoplasms often found on the lower extremities of the elderly. They can present as a slowly enlarging, red or red-brown, dome-shaped papule or nodule with a peripheral wafer–like scale.

I. **Fibrous papules** are benign, asymptomatic, and typically solitary skin-colored papules that commonly appear on the face, especially on or around the nose.

J. **Lichenoid keratosis/lichen planus-like keratosis** present as a pink erythematous or hyperpigmented papule or plaque, usually found on the trunk and upper extremities. They may appear verrucous or scaly.

K. **Dermatofibromas**, most commonly found on the lower extremities, are benign, typically asymptomatic, and present as firm papules.

See Appendix 1 for Further Reading and Image References.

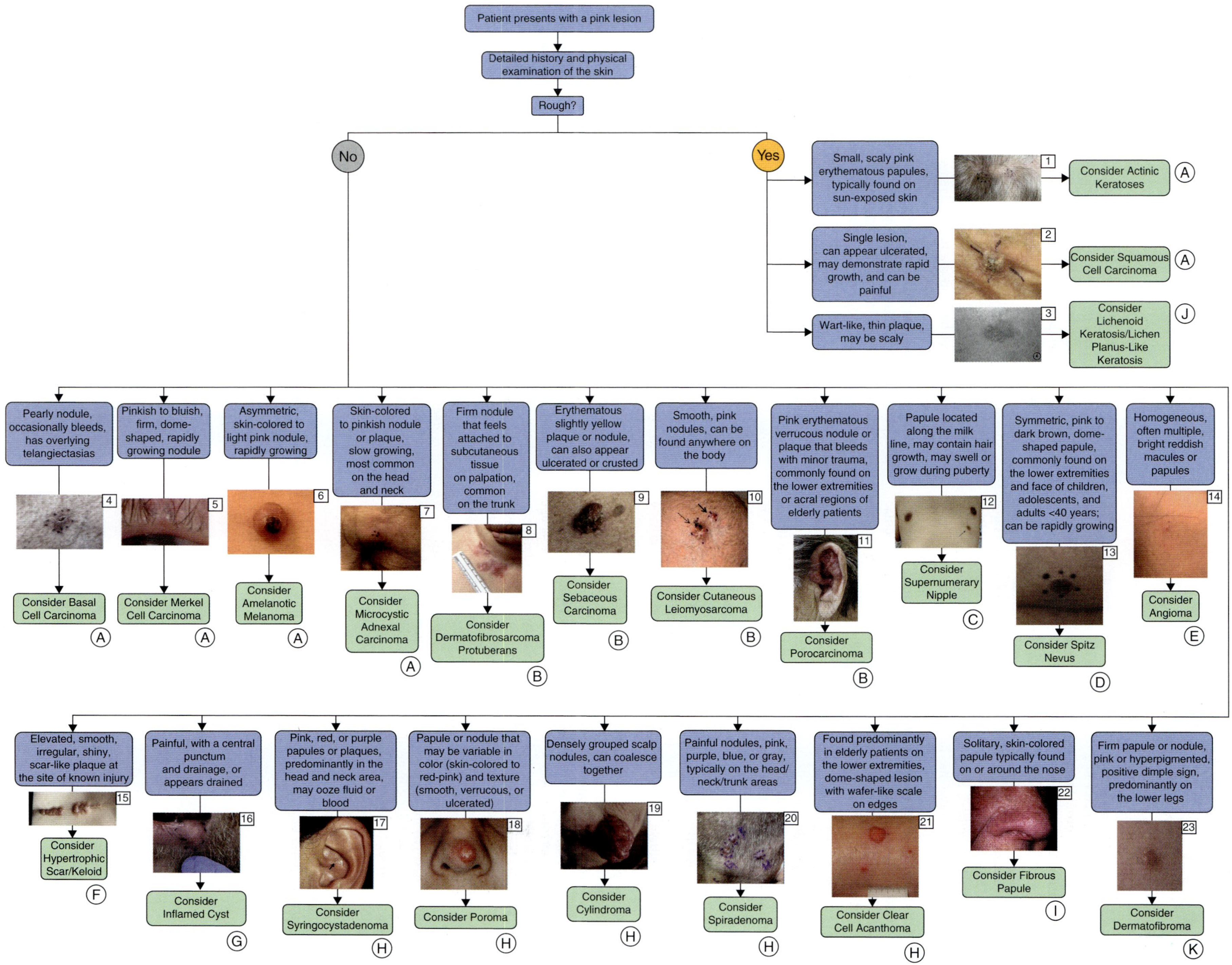
Patient presents with a pink lesion
Detailed history and physical examination of the skin
Rough?
Yes
Small, scaly pink erythematous papules, typically found on sun-exposed skin
1
Consider Actinic Keratoses
A
Single lesion, can appear ulcerated, may demonstrate rapid growth, and can be painful
2
Consider Squamous Cell Carcinoma
A
Wart-like, thin plaque, may be scaly
3
Consider Lichenoid Keratosis/Lichen Planus-Like Keratosis
J
No
Pearly nodule, occasionally bleeds, has overlying telangiectasias
4
Consider Basal Cell Carcinoma
A
Pinkish to bluish, firm, dome-shaped, rapidly growing nodule
5
Consider Merkel Cell Carcinoma
A
Asymmetric, skin-colored to light pink nodule, rapidly growing
6
Consider Amelanotic Melanoma
A
Skin-colored to pinkish nodule or plaque, slow growing, most common on the head and neck
7
Consider Microcystic Adnexal Carcinoma
A
Firm nodule that feels attached to subcutaneous tissue on palpation, common on the trunk
8
Consider Dermatofibrosarcoma Protuberans
B
Erythematous slightly yellow plaque or nodule, can also appear ulcerated or crusted
9
Consider Sebaceous Carcinoma
B
Smooth, pink nodules, can be found anywhere on the body
10
Consider Cutaneous Leiomyosarcoma
B
Pink erythematous verrucous nodule or plaque that bleeds with minor trauma, commonly found on the lower extremities or acral regions of elderly patients
11
Consider Porocarcinoma
B
Papule located along the milk line, may contain hair growth, may swell or grow during puberty
12
Consider Supernumerary Nipple
C
Symmetric, pink to dark brown, dome-shaped papule, commonly found on the lower extremities and face of children, adolescents, and adults <40 years; can be rapidly growing
13
Consider Spitz Nevus
D
Homogeneous, often multiple, bright reddish macules or papules
14
Consider Angioma
E
Elevated, smooth, irregular, shiny, scar-like plaque at the site of known injury
15
Consider Hypertrophic Scar/Keloid
F
Painful, with a central punctum and drainage, or appears drained
16
Consider Inflamed Cyst
G
Pink, red, or purple papules or plaques, predominantly in the head and neck area, may ooze fluid or blood
17
Consider Syringocystadenoma
H
Papule or nodule that may be variable in color (skin-colored to red-pink) and texture (smooth, verrucous, or ulcerated)
18
Consider Poroma
H
Densely grouped scalp nodules, can coalesce together
19
Consider Cylindroma
H
Painful nodules, pink, purple, blue, or gray, typically on the head/neck/trunk areas
20
Consider Spiradenoma
H
Found predominantly in elderly patients on the lower extremities, dome-shaped lesion with wafer-like scale on edges
21
Consider Clear Cell Acanthoma
H
Solitary, skin-colored papule typically found on or around the nose
22
Consider Fibrous Papule
I
Firm papule or nodule, pink or hyperpigmented, positive dimple sign, predominantly on the lower legs
23
Consider Dermatofibroma
K

74 Yellow Lesions

Neha Parvathala and Jennifer L. Hsiao

Yellow lesions represent a diverse set of cutaneous lesions. They can be idiopathic or secondary to a systemic condition; thus, obtaining a detailed history of chronic medical conditions will help inform the differential diagnosis.

A. The initial evaluation of a yellow lesion should include a complete history (including medication history) and a thorough physical examination. Lesion characteristics such as size, whether the lesion is firm or tender, distribution, and anatomic location will aid in diagnosis. Dermoscopy and biopsy may be needed to confirm clinical findings.

B. If the lesion is flat, consider **lichen aureus**. Lichen aureus is characterized by a golden-brown patch, sometimes with speckled petechiae within, typically located on the lower extremities. A lichenoid lymphoid infiltrate on histology can confirm the diagnosis.

C. If the lesion is raised, firm, and predominantly located on the head and neck, possible diagnoses include oral verruciform xanthoma, sebaceous hyperplasia, and sebaceous adenoma. **Oral verruciform xanthoma** is a benign mucosal growth that most commonly occurs in the oral cavity, gingiva, and alveolar ridge and may be associated with a history of trauma. It presents as a slightly raised yellow, pinkish, or whitish papule or plaque.

Sebaceous hyperplasia and **sebaceous adenoma** are benign proliferations of sebaceous glands. Sebaceous hyperplasia presents as single or multiple umbilicated yellow papules, often with overlying telangiectasias. Sebaceous adenoma presents as well-circumscribed yellow papules, less likely to have umbilication or telangiectasia than sebaceous hyperplasia, usually in older adults. Sebaceous adenomas may also be found in individuals with Muir-Torre syndrome.

Nevus sebaceous is a benign hamartoma that typically presents at birth as a verrucous yellow-orange plaque with a crescentic shape and velvety surface on the scalp, face, preauricular area, and neck.

Milia are benign, keratinous, yellow-whitish, or translucent cysts typically smaller than 3 mm in size. Milia commonly appear on the face, but may also occur elsewhere on the body, such as on the genitals, and may also occur within scars.

D. Raised, firm yellow lesions that are not localized to the head and neck include nodular cutaneous amyloidosis, colloid milium, eruptive xanthoma, and necrobiosis lipoidica.

Nodular cutaneous amyloidosis presents as nonpruritic firm nodules on the face, trunk, extremities, and/or genitalia. Middle-aged to elderly adults are most frequently affected, and they must be monitored for progression to systemic amyloidosis. Diagnosis usually requires biopsy.

Colloid milium occurs in sun-exposed areas, such as the face and dorsal forearms. It presents as yellowish amber, translucent, dome-shaped papules that coalesce into plaques.

Abrupt onset of multiple monomorphic, raised, firm yellowish red papules should raise concern for **eruptive xanthomas**. If the patient does not already have a diagnosis of hyperlipidemia or diabetes, appropriate workup for these conditions should be done. Hypertriglyceridemia is the most common underlying abnormality. The papules commonly appear on extensor surfaces of the arms and legs but may present anywhere on the body. Management of the underlying metabolic condition is key.

Necrobiosis lipoidica typically occurs on the lower extremities in patients with diabetes. It manifests as well-circumscribed atrophic yellow-orange plaques with a waxy smooth surface and telangiectasias. The plaques may be asymptomatic or become itchy or painful and may ulcerate. Treatment of the patient's underlying diabetes does not resolve the skin condition.

E. If the raised yellow lesion is not firm on palpation, anatomic location is an important distinguishing characteristic for diagnosis. **Xanthelasma** presents as progressive yellow flat-topped plaques typically on the medial eyelids in a symmetric distribution. The peak incidence is in adults aged 30 to 50 years. Xanthelasma is associated with hyperlipidemia, however, may also occur in patients with a normal cholesterol profile.

Syringomas typically present on the face as multiple asymptomatic yellow- or skin-colored papules in a symmetric distribution. The incidence is highest in patients with African and Asian descent and postpubertal females, but prepubertal and eruptive subtypes with more diffuse distributions also occur.

Pseudoxanthoma elasticum (PXE) is associated with a mutation in the ABCC6 gene that causes progressive degradation of elastic fibers. Skin findings include soft yellowish papules that coalesce into plaques with a cobblestoned appearance, typically on the neck and in skin folds. PXE presents in childhood with a higher female incidence (2:1) and requires cutaneous, ocular, and genetic findings for diagnosis.

Nevus lipomatosus is a nevoid fatty growth usually found in the pelvic girdle or on the buttocks. It presents as a single yellow soft papule or as multiple yellow soft papules that coalesce into plaques with a cerebriform surface. The most common form of nevus lipomatosus presents at birth or within the first two to three decades of life.

See Appendix 1 for Further Reading and Image References.

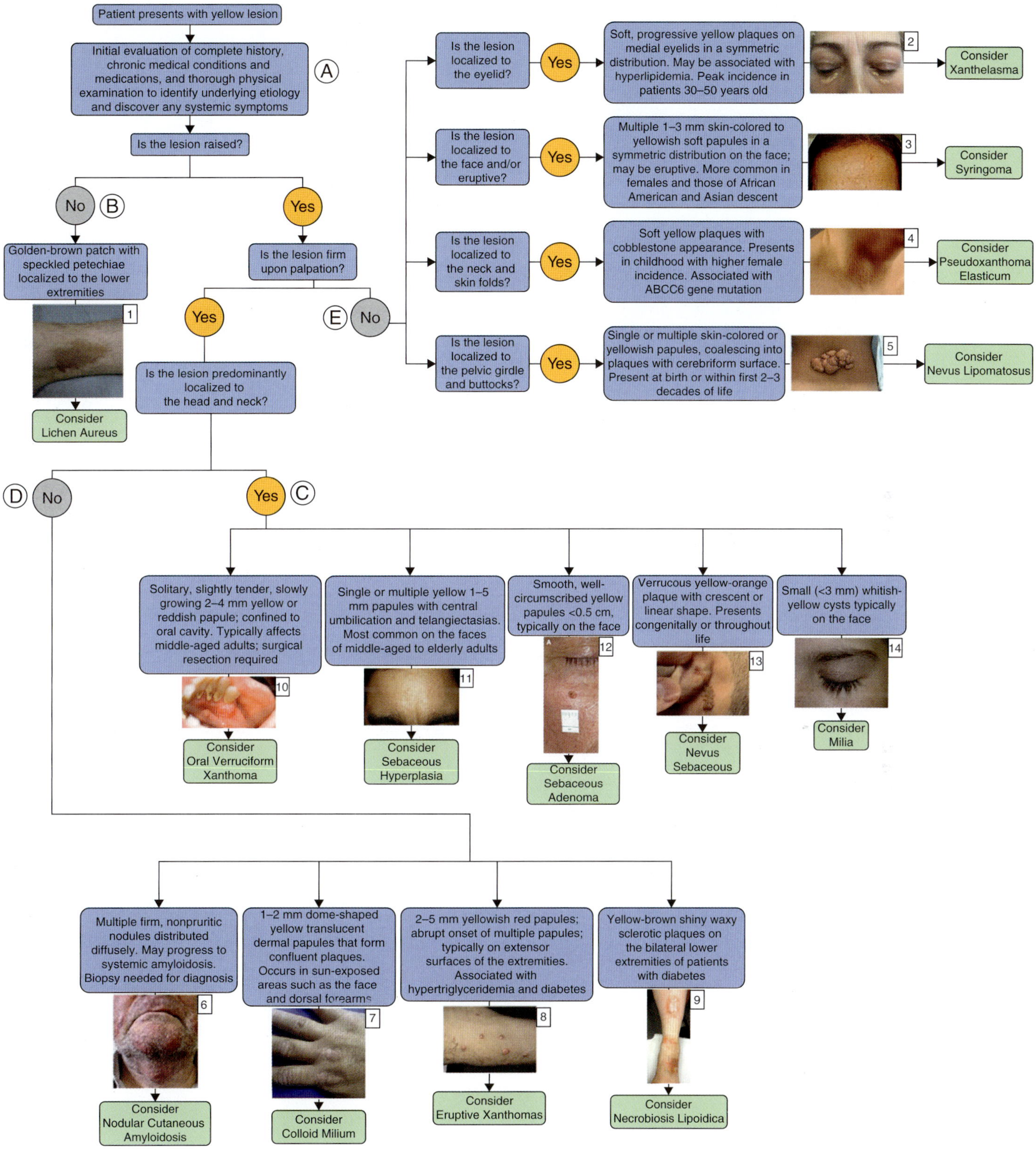
Patient presents with yellow lesion
Initial evaluation of complete history, chronic medical conditions and medications, and thorough physical examination to identify underlying etiology and discover any systemic symptoms
A
Is the lesion raised?
No
B
Golden-brown patch with speckled petechiae localized to the lower extremities
1
Consider Lichen Aureus
Yes
Is the lesion firm upon palpation?
Yes
Is the lesion predominantly localized to the head and neck?
E
No
Is the lesion localized to the eyelid?
Yes
Soft, progressive yellow plaques on medial eyelids in a symmetric distribution. May be associated with hyperlipidemia. Peak incidence in patients 30–50 years old
2
Consider Xanthelasma
Is the lesion localized to the face and/or eruptive?
Yes
Multiple 1–3 mm skin-colored to yellowish soft papules in a symmetric distribution on the face; may be eruptive. More common in females and those of African American and Asian descent
3
Consider Syringoma
Is the lesion localized to the neck and skin folds?
Yes
Soft yellow plaques with cobblestone appearance. Presents in childhood with higher female incidence. Associated with ABCC6 gene mutation
4
Consider Pseudoxanthoma Elasticum
Is the lesion localized to the pelvic girdle and buttocks?
Yes
Single or multiple skin-colored or yellowish papules, coalescing into plaques with cerebriform surface. Present at birth or within first 2–3 decades of life
5
Consider Nevus Lipomatosus
D
No
Yes
C
Solitary, slightly tender, slowly growing 2–4 mm yellow or reddish papule; confined to oral cavity. Typically affects middle-aged adults; surgical resection required
10
Consider Oral Verruciform Xanthoma
Single or multiple yellow 1–5 mm papules with central umbilication and telangiectasias. Most common on the faces of middle-aged to elderly adults
11
Consider Sebaceous Hyperplasia
Smooth, well-circumscribed yellow papules <0.5 cm, typically on the face
12
Consider Sebaceous Adenoma
Verrucous yellow-orange plaque with crescent or linear shape. Presents congenitally or throughout life
13
Consider Nevus Sebaceous
Small (<3 mm) whitish-yellow cysts typically on the face
14
Consider Milia
Multiple firm, nonpruritic nodules distributed diffusely. May progress to systemic amyloidosis. Biopsy needed for diagnosis
6
Consider Nodular Cutaneous Amyloidosis
1–2 mm dome-shaped yellow translucent dermal papules that form confluent plaques. Occurs in sun-exposed areas such as the face and dorsal forearms
7
Consider Colloid Milium
2–5 mm yellowish red papules; abrupt onset of multiple papules; typically on extensor surfaces of the extremities. Associated with hypertriglyceridemia and diabetes
8
Consider Eruptive Xanthomas
Yellow-brown shiny waxy sclerotic plaques on the bilateral lower extremities of patients with diabetes
9
Consider Necrobiosis Lipoidica

PART XV
Pruritus (without primary findings)

75 Scalp Pruritus

Teresa Ju and Gil Yosipovitch

Scalp pruritus is a frequent complaint in the clinical setting and prevalent in 25% of the general population. The scalp is highly innervated, making it more susceptible to itch. Branches of the trigeminal nerve, cervical plexus, and dorsal rami of the cervical nerves innervate the scalp. Hair follicles are highly innervated with free nerve endings, lanceolate nerve endings, Merkel nerve endings, and pilo-Ruffini corpuscles. The scalp also has many blood vessels and a variability in nerve fiber density. Scalp pruritus can be found in patients both with and without dermatologic problems and arise from a variety of conditions, including dermatologic, neuropathic, systemic, and psychogenic causes. This can make scalp pruritus particularly hard to diagnose and manage, particularly in those with no visible manifestations. Until the cause is identified, management can broadly focus on ameliorating itch through topical antipruritic agents.

A. The initial evaluation of patients presenting with scalp pruritus should involve recording a detailed past medical history (particularly of medical, neurologic, psychiatric, and dermatologic comorbidities, surgeries, infections, and injuries) and social history (i.e., living circumstances, job occupation). For physical examination, we recommend the five steps proposed by Shapiro and Otberg for evaluation of hair loss: listen, look, touch, magnify, and sample while focusing on scalp itch. Evaluation of other parts of the body beyond the scalp may be useful in diagnosing dermatologic causes of scalp itch. The most common causes of scalp itch are seborrheic dermatitis, psoriasis, and folliculitis.

B. The first step in physical examination of patients with scalp pruritus is to examine for hair loss. Patients with active **alopecia areata** may complain of mild pruritus preceding the development of new patches.

C. The most common types of scarring alopecias with associated itch are **lichen planopilaris (LPP), frontal fibrosing alopecia (FFA), discoid lupus, central centrifugal cicatricial alopecia (CCCA)**, and **folliculitis decalvans (FD)**.

LPP is commonly seen in middle-aged females with scalp tenderness and whitish atrophic or scarring patches with the loss of follicular openings.

FFA primarily affects postmenopausal females and presents with progressive frontotemporal hairline recession.

Discoid lupus is more common in young to middle-aged females and presents with erythematous patches of alopecia, follicular hyperkeratosis, hyper- or hypopigmentation, and telangiectasias.

CCCA is the most common cause of hair loss in African-American females and presents with flesh-colored, noninflammatory cicatricial alopecia of the central scalp.

FD occurs in young adults and presents with follicular pustules, crusts, and tufted hairs.

D. If alopecia is not identified, the next step is to examine for cutaneous signs, including pustules (indicative of a diagnosis of **folliculitis**), **nits (lice)**, or scale. Location and character of the scale and the patient's history can help elucidate whether the cause is **seborrheic dermatitis, psoriasis, contact dermatitis, red scalp syndrome, tinea capitis**, or **dermatomyositis**.

E. Neuropathic itch is related to pathology located at any point of the afferent pathway of the nervous system. Patients experience neuropathic itch in the absence of, or out of proportion to, external stimuli. In many cases, pruritus is also accompanied by paresthesia, hyperesthesia, and hypoesthesia. Causes of neuropathic itch are **postherpetic neuralgia (PHN), trigeminal trophic syndrome (TTS), cervical spinal disease, small fiber neuropathy in diabetics, brain tumors, multiple sclerosis, stroke, cosmetic procedures, temporal arteritis**, and **post-COVID-19 infection trichodynia**.

PHN often causes damage to the trigeminal nerve and its sensory pathway resulting in the classic triad of trigeminal anesthesia, paresthesia, and self-manipulated facial ulceration (TTS) and predominantly affects females.

History, with a focus on other symptoms and history of procedures, can reveal diagnoses of cervical spinal disease, nerve injury due to cosmetic procedure, temporal arteritis, and other neuropathic itch.

F. Patients with a history of **mental health disease** may have localized (or generalized) pruritus due to underlying depression or anxiety. This itch tends to respond to psychiatric medication and may wax and wane with the symptoms of depression or anxiety.

G. Patients with **internal causes of pruritus** typically have generalized itching but can also have more localized itch. For discussion of these causes, please see Chapter 77 for more details.

H. Despite an extensive workup, many patients will have chronic pruritus of unknown origin. **Older patients** are more likely to have diseases that predispose them to itch, and other age-related neuropathic changes and decay of inhibitory fibers.

See Appendix 1 for Further Reading and Image References.

Patient presenting with scalp pruritus

(A) Detailed history and physical examination of the scalp, hair, face, and body

Does examination reveal primary skin lesions?

Yes

What type of primary lesions? (D)

- Folliculocentric, inflamed papules and/or pustules → Consider Folliculitis
- Presence of live louse or nits on scalp or hair shaft, bumps, lymphadenopathy

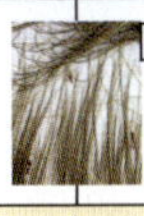

1

Louse feeding on scalp visualized with dermatoscopy → Consider Pediculosis

- Alopecic patches → Presence of scarring?
  - No → Consider Nonscarring Alopecias (i.e., Alopecia Areata) (B)
  - Yes

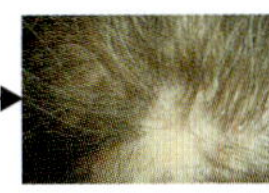

7

White atrophic patch of alopecia on scalp in patient with lichen planopilaris → Consider Scarring Alopecias (Lichen Planopilaris, Frontal Fibrosing Alopecia, Discoid Lupus, Central Centrifugal Cicatricial Alopecia, Folliculitis Decalvans, Keloids, Burn Scars) (C)

- Scaling, erythema
  - Flaking on scalp, midface, or upper chest; pruritus decreases after shampooing. Trichoscopy: arborizing vessels

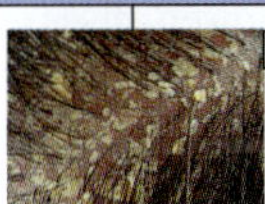

2

Severe scaling on the scalp → Consider Seborrheic Dermatitis

  - History of psoriasis; symmetric, well-defined red, scaly plaques on examination, particularly on extensor surfaces. Trichoscopy: red dots and globules

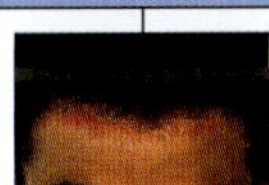

3

Erythema with overlying lamellar, dense scale on the scalp → Consider Scalp Psoriasis

  - History of new hair products (i.e., hair dyes, shampoos, hairstyling products) or allergies to nickel, rubber, or plastic → Consider Contact Dermatitis
  - Presence of papules, pustules, and telangiectasias; may be associated with androgenetic alopecia; resistant to topical steroids and responds to oral tetracyclines

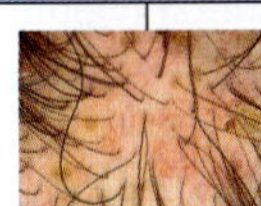

4

Trichoscopy findings → Consider Red Scalp Syndrome

  - Exposure to tinea in close contact or pet; tinea in other body parts; Wood's lamp shows green fluorescence

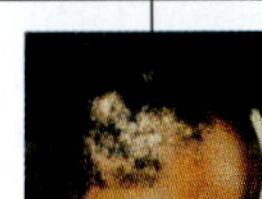

5

Patches of alopecia in a female patient → Consider Tinea Capitis

  - History of dermatomyositis; examination reveals proximal muscle weakness, heliotrope rash, Gottron papules, V-neck sign, and shawl sign. Dermatoscopy: enlarged polymorphous interfollicular vessels

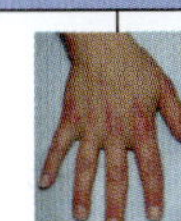

6

Gottron papules: pink, flat-topped papules present over the MCP, PIP, and DIP joints → Consider Dermatomyositis

No

(E)

- Trigeminal distribution of itch and anesthesia, along with unilateral facial ulceration (particularly of the nasal ala). May have history of herpes zoster

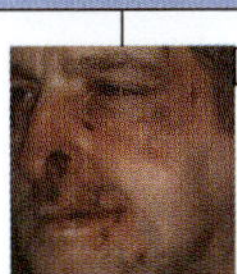

8

Unilateral perioral and nasal ala ulcerations → Consider Postherpetic Neuralgia (or Trigeminal Trophic Syndrome)

- History of cervical spine disease/ cervical neck pain → Consider Cervical Spine Disease
- History of facial or brow lift → Consider Local Nerve Injury From Cosmetic Procedures
- Coexisting headaches in the temporal region, jaw claudication, and elevated erythrocyte sedimentation rate → Consider Temporal Arteritis
- History of diabetes, stroke, brain tumors, multiple sclerosis, or post-COVID-19 scalp dysesthesia → Consider Other Neuropathic Itch
- History of depression, anxiety, and other psychiatric disorders. Stress exacerbates and antidepressants improve itch symptoms → Consider Psychogenic Itch (F)
- History of systemic diseases (diabetes, hyperthyroidism, ESRD, cholestatic liver) with itching that is not limited to the scalp → Consider Systemic Disease Associated Pruritus (G)
- History of hematologic disease, aquagenic pruritus, and abnormal CBC → Consider Myeloproliferative Neoplasms or Lymphoma (G)
- Nonspecific history, physical examination, and laboratory findings in older patient → Consider Old Age Scalp Itch (H)

76 Anogenital Pruritus

Ashley Vander Does and Gil Yosipovitch

Anogenital pruritus can be an extremely bothersome symptom due to inflammatory dermatoses, infections, malignancy, systemic diseases, benign anogenital diseases, or neuropathic causes. As the anogenital area is a sensitive area for patients, they often present to the physician in later stages with atypical manifestations or secondary lesions due to scratching (i.e., lichenification and depigmentation). Patients often try various over-the-counter topical remedies, including steroids, which may result in skin atrophy and striae.

A. A thorough history should be obtained from the patient, including questions about the itch (e.g., quality, severity, timing, and history of itch in the past), relieving/exacerbating factors (including previous treatments and their efficacy), current and past skin care regimen, sexual history (including exposures, contraception, lubrication, and relation to coitus and menstruation), contact with other people or pets, travel history, past medical history (including history of rashes), and a medication history. A proper clinical examination should be performed, and additional diagnostic tests should be considered (including scraping for fungus or mites, performing a skin biopsy, and/or patch testing).

B. When a patient does have primary genital lesions or a rash associated with itch, the next step in refining the differential diagnosis is to assess the type and color of primary lesions/rash. White areas suggest either lichen planus or lichen sclerosus. Genital **lichen planus** occurs most commonly on the penis or the vulvae. In patients with vulvar lichen planus, about 47% will have oral lichen planus and 20% will have other skin involvement. **Lichen sclerosus** can involve other body parts, but is typically localized to the anogenital region. An examination showing white areas admixed with erythema and epidermal atrophy is characteristic. Both lichen planus and lichen sclerosus disproportionately affect females and carry a risk for transformation into squamous cell carcinoma.

C. **Pediculosis pubis** and **scabies** are often transmitted sexually, so a sexual history is imperative, including whether sexual partners are experiencing symptoms. Lice will be visible in the case of pediculosis pubis, and in the case of scabies, examination should reveal burrows and/or scabietic nodules in the anogenital region and elsewhere.

D. The presence of vesicles or erosions on examination can be suggestive of either a herpes infection or contact dermatitis. **Contact dermatitis** tends to present not only with vesicular or eczematous lesions but also in a geometric or linear manner. Irritating agents that have the potential to evoke an eczematous or irritant contact dermatitis include harsh soaps, fragrances, sprays, deodorants, douches, topical anesthetic agents, rubber accelerators, lanolin-based formulations, and propylene glycol-containing products. Further, an irritant contact dermatitis may be instigated by sweat, urine, and feces. **Herpes** can be painful and typically presents as grouped vesicles with an erythematous base, although in the anogenital region, lesions can be diffuse or sometimes even verrucous.

E. If primary scale is present on examination, the diagnoses of tinea, psoriasis, and seborrheic dermatitis should be considered. **Tinea cruris** presents as erythematous, scaly, annular plaques with an elevated leading edge and central clearing. A bedside KOH test can establish the diagnosis. The scrotum is often spared in males. **Psoriasis** is one of the most common causes of anogenital pruritus, and although it occurs predominately in patients with generalized plaque psoriasis, it occurs exclusively in the anogenital region 2% to 5% of the time. While classically scaly, psoriasis in the anogenital region can be simply erythematous. It affects predominantly the folds. **Seborrheic dermatitis** typically affects sebaceous-rich areas of the face and scalp, but is common in the diaper area of infants and can also occur in this region in adults. The rash is erythematous, scaly, and poorly demarcated, resembling other dermatitides such as irritant diaper dermatitis and atopic dermatitis. The scale of seborrheic dermatitis is more yellow, and the rash does involve the intertriginous areas, which is spared in diaper dermatitis.

F. There are many causes of anogenital pruritus associated with erythema without scale. When localized exclusively to the perianal region, consideration should be given to **pinworm infestation** (*Enterobius vermicularis*) and **perianal cellulitis** (often from beta-hemolytic streptococci), both of which are more common in children than in adults. Other causes of chronic anogenital pruritus include **atrophic vulvovaginitis**, malignancies such as **extramammary Paget** or **Bowen disease**, and red scrotum syndrome. **Red scrotum syndrome** typically manifests as well-demarcated, nonscaly erythema of the anterior scrotum associated with pain/burning sensations. **Bacterial vaginosis** can present with pruritus, but the patient will likely also have a frothy vaginal discharge, while **contact dermatitis** can also present in the anogenital region without vesicles, so a good history asking about potential exposures is important in any patient presenting with itch and erythema in the anogenital region.

G. Lichen simplex chronicus and neuropathic itch should be highly suspected if there is no primary rash, but significant itching exists in the anogenital region. **Lichen simplex chronicus** occurs due to the thickening of skin from scratching, so lichenification is the main clue to this diagnosis on examination. Patients with **neuropathic itch** may also present with lichenification due to scratching but more commonly have no findings on examination. Neuropathic causes include lumbosacral stenosis, arthritis, and spinal injuries or surgeries, as well as postherpetic neuralgia and diabetic neuropathy.

See Appendix 1 for Further Reading and Image References.

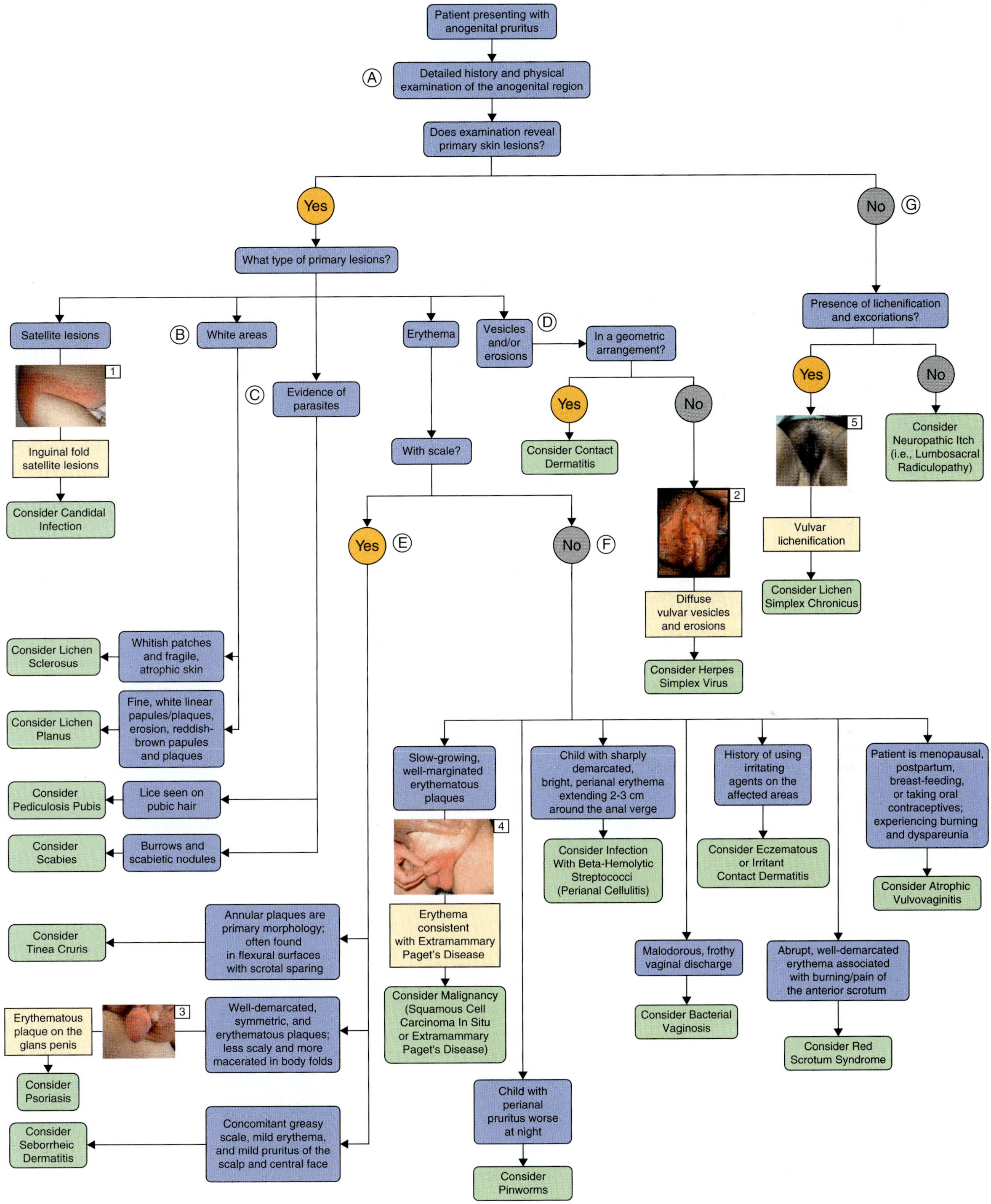
Patient presenting with anogenital pruritus
A
Detailed history and physical examination of the anogenital region
Does examination reveal primary skin lesions?
Yes
What type of primary lesions?
Satellite lesions
1
Inguinal fold satellite lesions
Consider Candidal Infection
B
White areas
Whitish patches and fragile, atrophic skin
Consider Lichen Sclerosus
Fine, white linear papules/plaques, erosion, reddish-brown papules and plaques
Consider Lichen Planus
C
Evidence of parasites
Lice seen on pubic hair
Consider Pediculosis Pubis
Burrows and scabietic nodules
Consider Scabies
Erythema
With scale?
Yes
E
Annular plaques are primary morphology; often found in flexural surfaces with scrotal sparing
Consider Tinea Cruris
Well-demarcated, symmetric, and erythematous plaques; less scaly and more macerated in body folds
3
Erythematous plaque on the glans penis
Consider Psoriasis
Concomitant greasy scale, mild erythema, and mild pruritus of the scalp and central face
Consider Seborrheic Dermatitis
No
F
Slow-growing, well-marginated erythematous plaques
4
Erythema consistent with Extramammary Paget's Disease
Consider Malignancy (Squamous Cell Carcinoma In Situ or Extramammary Paget's Disease)
Child with perianal pruritus worse at night
Consider Pinworms
Child with sharply demarcated, bright, perianal erythema extending 2-3 cm around the anal verge
Consider Infection With Beta-Hemolytic Streptococci (Perianal Cellulitis)
Malodorous, frothy vaginal discharge
Consider Bacterial Vaginosis
History of using irritating agents on the affected areas
Consider Eczematous or Irritant Contact Dermatitis
Abrupt, well-demarcated erythema associated with burning/pain of the anterior scrotum
Consider Red Scrotum Syndrome
Patient is menopausal, postpartum, breast-feeding, or taking oral contraceptives; experiencing burning and dyspareunia
Consider Atrophic Vulvovaginitis
Vesicles and/or erosions
D
In a geometric arrangement?
Yes
Consider Contact Dermatitis
No
2
Diffuse vulvar vesicles and erosions
Consider Herpes Simplex Virus
No
G
Presence of lichenification and excoriations?
Yes
5
Vulvar lichenification
Consider Lichen Simplex Chronicus
No
Consider Neuropathic Itch (i.e., Lumbosacral Radiculopathy)

77 Other Localized Pruritus

Angelina Labib and Gil Yosipovitch

Localized pruritus (apart from the scalp as described in Chapter 75, or the anogenital region as described in Chapter 76) can be due to many different causes, including cutaneous, systemic, and neurologic reasons. This chapter examines the clues that may be present on physical examination that can point the clinician toward the underlying cause of a patient's localized pruritus.

A. The initial evaluation of a patient with localized pruritus consists of obtaining a thorough history and physical examination. A detailed history should elucidate information on prior dermatoses, other medical conditions, history of trauma, history of recent illness, and the presentation of the localized pruritus. Physical examination should include the skin and palmoplantar surfaces, nails, scalp, lymph nodes, and mucosa.

B. Many causes of localized pruritus will be of neurologic origin, and these patients will not present with any primary cutaneous manifestations. Determining the appropriate diagnosis in these patients primarily rests on knowing the location of the itch. **Brachioradial pruritus** will present with unilateral or bilateral itch on the lateral arms and occasionally the shoulder and/or neck region. It can be due to cervical spinal nerve injury or inflammation and is often worse with sun exposure. **Notalgia paresthetica** often presents as unilateral itch on the upper back or posterior shoulder; it is associated with nerve dysfunction in the thoracic spine. **Meralgia paresthetica** most commonly presents on the lateral thighs. **Small fiber neuropathy**, seen in patients with diabetes, primarily affects the distal extremities. **Postherpetic neuralgia** will present unilaterally in a dermatomal distribution following a herpes zoster episode.

C. If a patient does have a primary cutaneous rash/lesion, the clinician should examine the patient closely for the presence of bullae and/or vesicles. Blisters with underlying erythema or geographic shapes could suggest **contact dermatitis**. Tense bullae with no other features present on examination would suggest **bullous pemphigoid**. Bullae with milia in a sun-exposed distribution might suggest **porphyria cutanea tarda** or **pseudoporphyria** due to a drug. Localized and clustered vesicles suggest a diagnosis of **herpes simplex virus** or if dermatomal, a diagnosis of **shingles** (varicella zoster virus [VZV]). Diffuse pruritic vesicles are suggestive of **arthropod bites** or **varicella (VZV)**. Vesicles localized to the palmar and plantar surfaces may be due to **hand-foot-and-mouth disease**.

D. When instead of blisters, the primary rash is hyperkeratotic, a diagnosis of **keratoderma** can be considered if the itching and thickening occur predominantly on the palmoplantar surfaces. **Lichen simplex chronicus (LSC)** is another dermatologic condition that presents with intense itching in areas of hyperkeratotic, thickened, leathery-appearing skin, but is not usually confined to palmoplantar surfaces. **Lichen amyloidosis** can occur in association with LSC or on its own and is a type of cutaneous amyloidosis due to scratching. It appears as hyperkeratotic brown and gray papules, whereas **lichen planus** tends to be purple. Well-demarcated, silvery, scaly, erythematous plaques (especially on extensor regions) suggest **psoriasis.** Lastly, **cutaneous T-cell lymphoma** can take on any morphology but in some instances can be localized and pruritic.

E. In patients with scale and localized itch with primary rash, history, distribution, and morphology are especially helpful. For example, a patient with hand or flexural itching and a history of atopic dermatitis likely has a flare of **atopic dermatitis.** Likewise, patients with **seborrheic dermatitis** often develop itch in involved areas of the central face, chest, and scalp. When lichenification, erythema, and scale are present, atopic dermatitis should be suspected; if the scale is greasy, then seborrheic dermatitis should be considered.

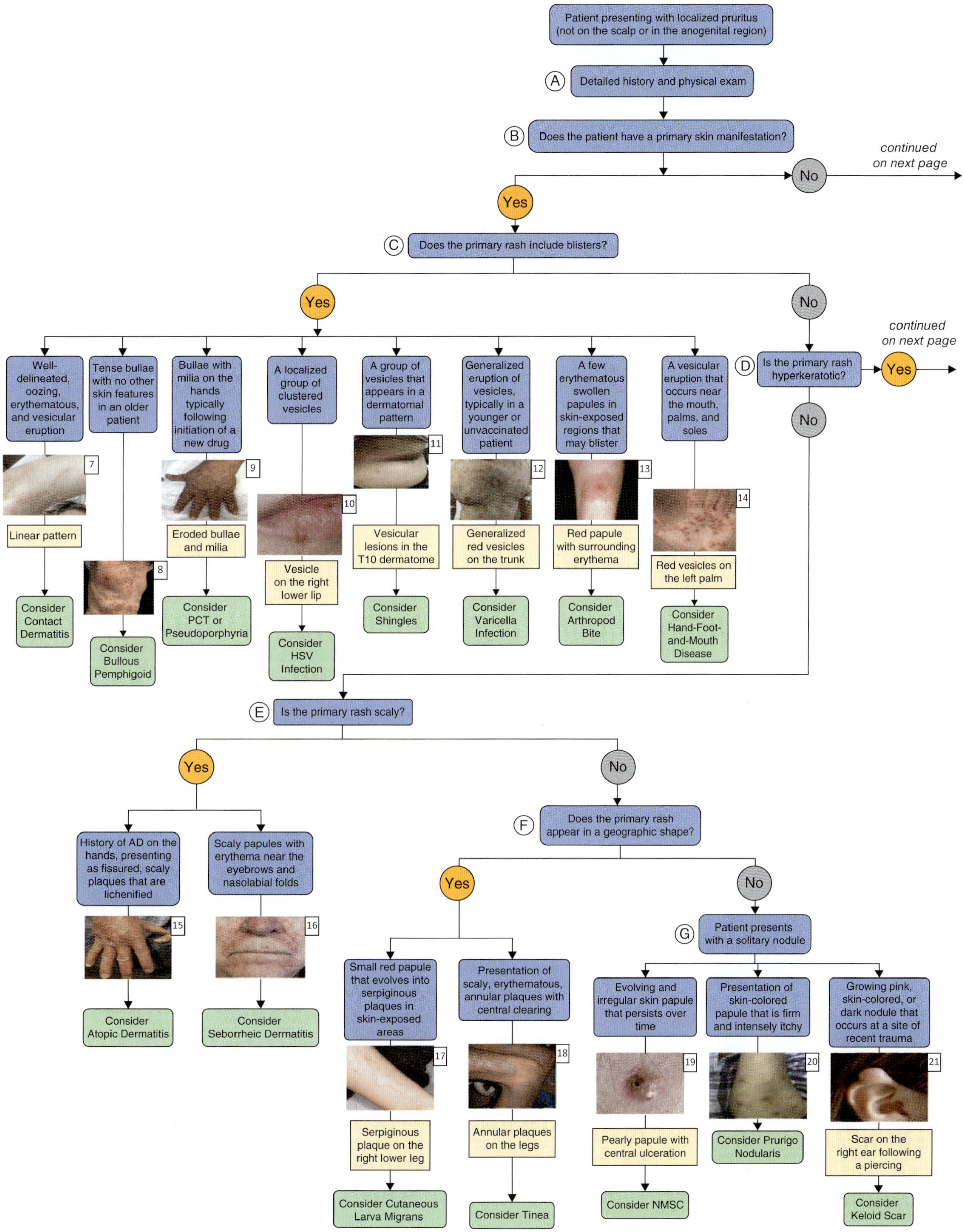
Patient presenting with localized pruritus (not on the scalp or in the anogenital region)
A
Detailed history and physical exam
B
Does the patient have a primary skin manifestation?
No
continued on next page
Yes
C
Does the primary rash include blisters?
Yes
Well-delineated, oozing, erythematous, and vesicular eruption
7
Linear pattern
Consider Contact Dermatitis
Tense bullae with no other skin features in an older patient
8
Consider Bullous Pemphigoid
Bullae with milia on the hands typically following initiation of a new drug
9
Eroded bullae and milia
Consider PCT or Pseudoporphyria
A localized group of clustered vesicles
10
Vesicle on the right lower lip
Consider HSV Infection
A group of vesicles that appears in a dermatomal pattern
11
Vesicular lesions in the T10 dermatome
Consider Shingles
Generalized eruption of vesicles, typically in a younger or unvaccinated patient
12
Generalized red vesicles on the trunk
Consider Varicella Infection
A few erythematous swollen papules in skin-exposed regions that may blister
13
Red papule with surrounding erythema
Consider Arthropod Bite
A vesicular eruption that occurs near the mouth, palms, and soles
14
Red vesicles on the left palm
Consider Hand-Foot-and-Mouth Disease
No
D
Is the primary rash hyperkeratotic?
Yes
continued on next page
No
E
Is the primary rash scaly?
Yes
History of AD on the hands, presenting as fissured, scaly plaques that are lichenified
15
Consider Atopic Dermatitis
Scaly papules with erythema near the eyebrows and nasolabial folds
16
Consider Seborrheic Dermatitis
No
F
Does the primary rash appear in a geographic shape?
Yes
Small red papule that evolves into serpiginous plaques in skin-exposed areas
17
Serpiginous plaque on the right lower leg
Consider Cutaneous Larva Migrans
Presentation of scaly, erythematous, annular plaques with central clearing
18
Annular plaques on the legs
Consider Tinea
No
G
Patient presents with a solitary nodule
Evolving and irregular skin papule that persists over time
19
Pearly papule with central ulceration
Consider NMSC
Presentation of skin-colored papule that is firm and intensely itchy
20
Consider Prurigo Nodularis
Growing pink, skin-colored, or dark nodule that occurs at a site of recent trauma
21
Scar on the right ear following a piercing
Consider Keloid Scar

Continued

F. Three specific diagnoses should come to mind when a patient has a serpiginous, annular, or geographic shape to their rash. **Cutaneous larva migrans** occurs most commonly on the feet in the form of a serpiginous plaque and is due to the infestation of hookworm larvae into the epidermis. **Tinea** presents as itchy, scaly, erythematous, annular plaques. As noted previously, **contact dermatitis** often presents with geographic shapes due to exogenous exposure.

G. Lastly, if a patient has a solitary papule or plaque that is evolving in a sun-exposed region, a diagnosis of **nonmelanoma skin cancer** should be considered. A solitary and firm skin-colored nodule can be suggestive of **prurigo nodularis**, although, more commonly, numerous prurigo nodules will be present on examination. Lastly, a pink, skin-colored, or dark nodule at the site of previous trauma can be indicative of a **keloid scar**.

See Appendix 1 for Further Reading and Image References.

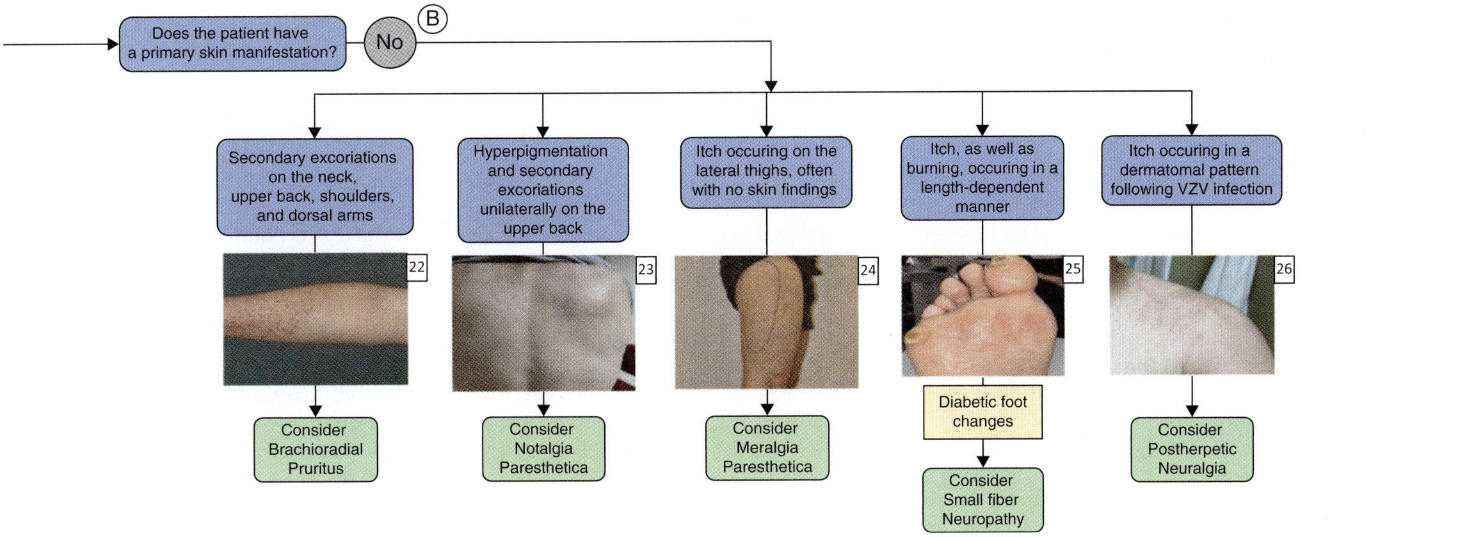
Does the patient have a primary skin manifestation?
No
B
Secondary excoriations on the neck, upper back, shoulders, and dorsal arms
22
Consider Brachioradial Pruritus
Hyperpigmentation and secondary excoriations unilaterally on the upper back
23
Consider Notalgia Paresthetica
Itch occuring on the lateral thighs, often with no skin findings
24
Consider Meralgia Paresthetica
Itch, as well as burning, occuring in a length-dependent manner
25
Diabetic foot changes
Consider Small fiber Neuropathy
Itch occuring in a dermatomal pattern following VZV infection
26
Consider Postherpetic Neuralgia

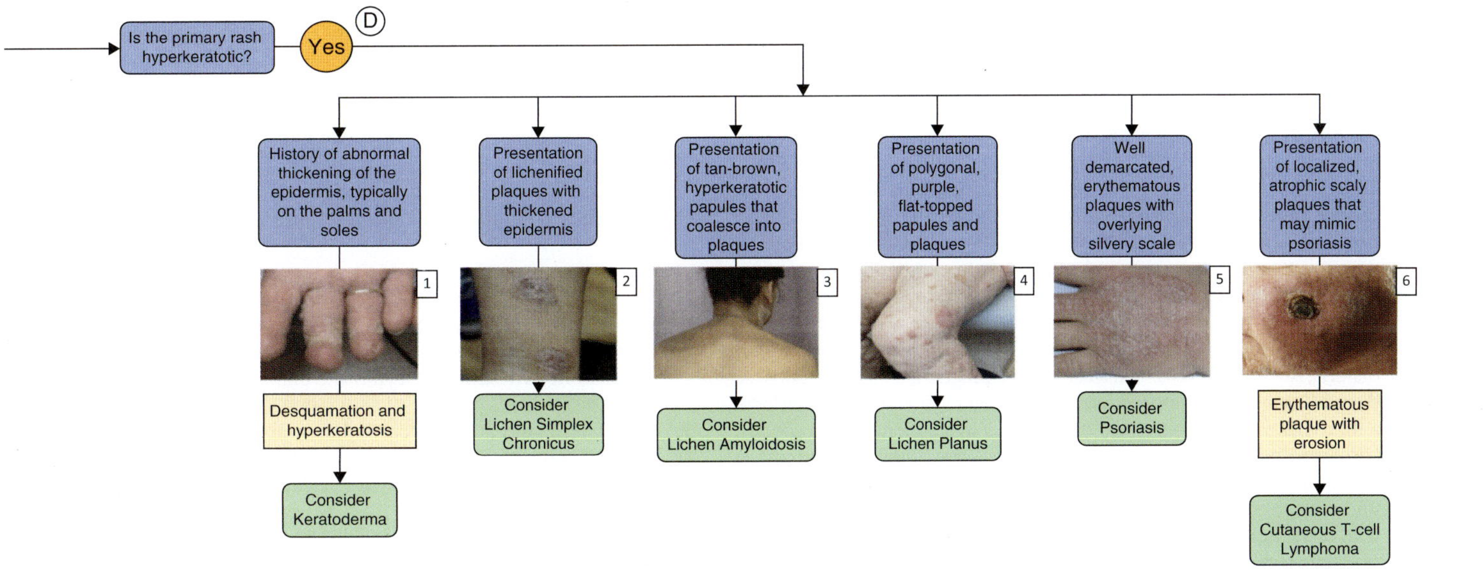
Is the primary rash hyperkeratotic?
Yes
D
History of abnormal thickening of the epidermis, typically on the palms and soles
1
Desquamation and hyperkeratosis
Consider Keratoderma
Presentation of lichenified plaques with thickened epidermis
2
Consider Lichen Simplex Chronicus
Presentation of tan-brown, hyperkeratotic papules that coalesce into plaques
3
Consider Lichen Amyloidosis
Presentation of polygonal, purple, flat-topped papules and plaques
4
Consider Lichen Planus
Well demarcated, erythematous plaques with overlying silvery scale
5
Consider Psoriasis
Presentation of localized, atrophic scaly plaques that may mimic psoriasis
6
Erythematous plaque with erosion
Consider Cutaneous T-cell Lymphoma

78 General Pruritus

Danielle E. Novack and Scott D. Worswick

Pruritus is one of the most common chief complaints of patients presenting to a dermatologist. Generalized pruritus (GP) has been shown to have a lifetime prevalence of up to 22% in some populations and is thought to be as high as 50% in elderly populations. While many older individuals may only have idiopathic pruritus of the elderly, determining the underlying etiology of pruritus with no primary rash is important, as it is a symptom of an underlying systemic disease in up to 50% of cases. This algorithm is intended to help guide the physician or student in how to look for physical examination clues (as well as use laboratory and imaging studies) to determine the cause of GP in select patients. It is not intended to be a comprehensive list of causes of GP.

A. The initial evaluation of a patient with GP requires a thorough physical examination to rule out any associated rashes that can cause GP, such as bullous pemphigoid, scabies infestation, or atopic dermatitis. Additionally, a thorough medication and allergy history should be obtained in any patient with GP in order to rule out a medication-induced cause of GP or another allergic cause such as contact dermatitis.

A detailed history (including medical history and complete review of systems) and physical examination not just of the skin but also of the nails, scalp, and hair, oral mucosa, and lymph nodes are appropriate for any patient with GP, particularly because more than one cause of pruritus may exist in a given patient. Given the most common causes of GP, the initial laboratory workup for a patient presenting with pruritus without specific signs on physical examination should include a complete blood count and complete metabolic panel. A chest x-ray, erythrocyte sedimentation rate, C-reactive protein, lactate dehydrogenase, fasting glucose, thyroid-stimulating hormone, vitamin D, human immunodeficiency virus, and immunoglobulin levels may be included as the next steps in a patient with GP of unknown cause. In selected patients, screening for malaria, strongyloidiasis, schistosomiasis, pregnancy, and hepatitis A, B, and C may also be appropriate. The physician should always perform a thorough examination of all lymph nodes in a patient with suspected GP. Firm, nonmobile lymphadenopathy is concerning for underlying malignancy. If history and physical examination raise concern for an underlying malignancy, consider additionally a computed tomographic scan of the head, neck, chest, abdomen, and/or pelvis, and/or a magnetic resonance imaging of the brain and spinal cord. The majority of patients with GP will have no localizing physical examination signs, and in these patients, the above workup may be warranted.

B. In addition to the examination of the skin for any primary rash as detailed in section A, a thorough examination must also look for specific findings in the skin that can point to an underlying cause of GP. Uremic frost is a clue for **kidney failure**; jaundice and palmar erythema indicate **hepatic disease**; xerosis may signify thyroid dysfunction; and ecchymoses may point toward a potential **hematologic or malignant cause** of GP.

C. There are select patients who will have physical examination clues outside the skin that can help guide the clinician to the underlying diagnosis and appropriate workup. After the skin itself, the next appropriate place to look is at the nails, as they may indicate renal or hepatic dysfunction as the cause of GP. Lindsay nails indicate an underlying renal pathology, while Muehrcke lines and Terry's nails are more strongly associated with an underlying hepatic pathology. Mees lines may be associated with GP when they are due to Hodgkin lymphoma or acute renal failure. Koilonychia (spoon nails) can be due to both iron deficiency anemia and hemochromatosis. For a more detailed description of each of these changes, please see Chapter 92.

D. Clues may also exist in a patient's hair, including in patients with brittle hair (hyperthyroidism), dry hair (hypothyroidism), or shedding/thinning of hair (either type of **thyroid dysfunction**). Notably thinning/shedding of hair may also occur due to medications, anemia, and malignancy, all of which are other potential underlying causes of GP.

E. The oral mucosa should be closely examined. Macroglossia may indicate amyloidosis, while chloroma of the tongue may indicate leukemia. In addition to **malignancy**, the oral mucosa may also provide a clue to **hepatic dysfunction** if the patient has sublingual jaundice.

F. As with the oral mucosa, careful examination of the eyes may show scleral icterus, thereby indicating an underlying **hepatic pathology**. The presence of exophthalmos indicates **hyperthyroidism**.

See Appendix 1 for Further Reading and Image References.

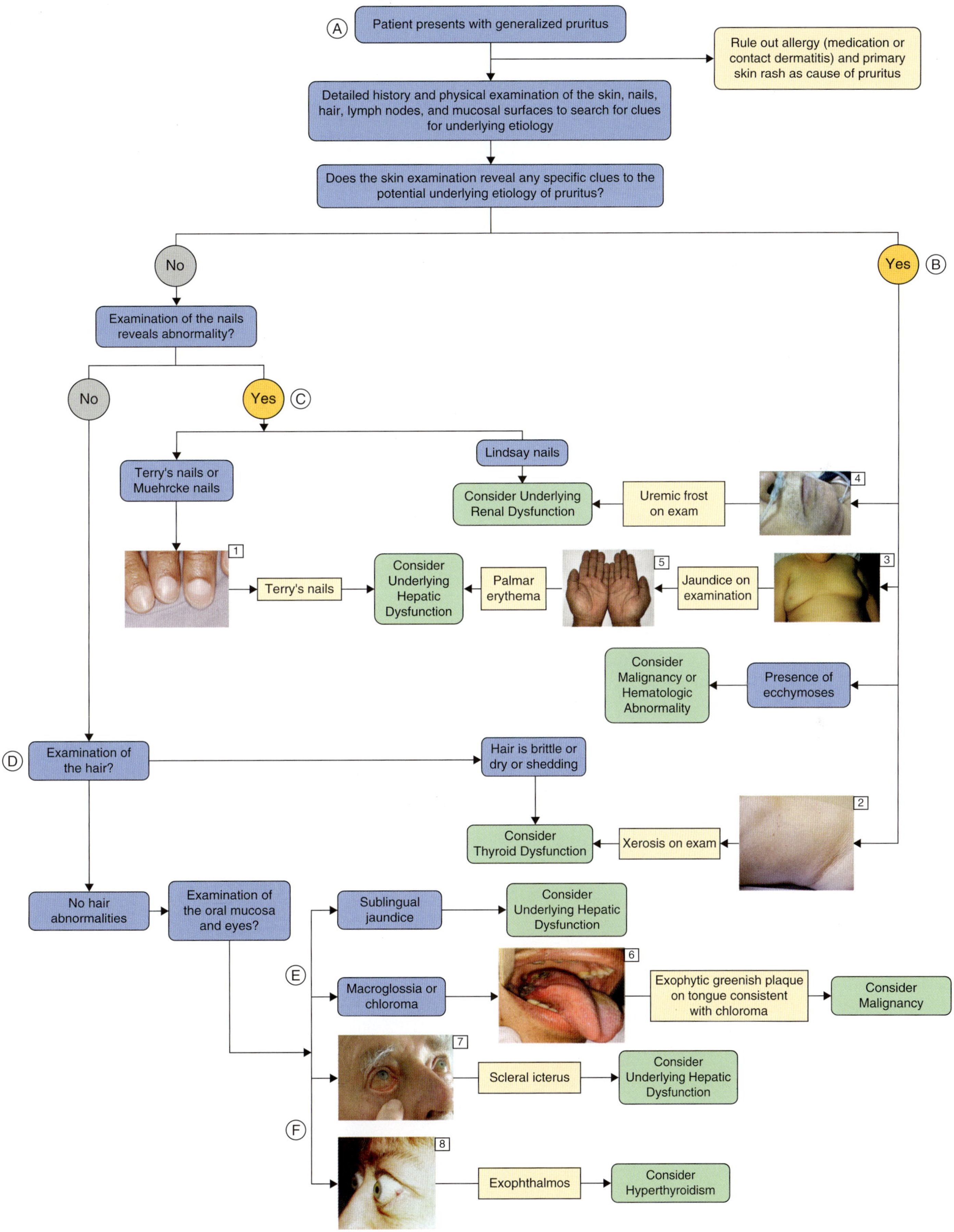
A
Patient presents with generalized pruritus
Rule out allergy (medication or contact dermatitis) and primary skin rash as cause of pruritus
Detailed history and physical examination of the skin, nails, hair, lymph nodes, and mucosal surfaces to search for clues for underlying etiology
Does the skin examination reveal any specific clues to the potential underlying etiology of pruritus?
No
Examination of the nails reveals abnormality?
No
Yes
C
Terry's nails or Muehrcke nails
Lindsay nails
Consider Underlying Renal Dysfunction
Uremic frost on exam
4
1
Terry's nails
Consider Underlying Hepatic Dysfunction
Palmar erythema
5
Jundice on examination
3
Consider Malignancy or Hematologic Abnormality
Presence of ecchymoses
Yes
B
D
Examination of the hair?
Hair is brittle or dry or shedding
2
Consider Thyroid Dysfunction
Xerosis on exam
No hair abnormalities
Examination of the oral mucosa and eyes?
Sublingual jaundice
Consider Underlying Hepatic Dysfunction
E
Macroglossia or chloroma
6
Exophytic greenish plaque on tongue consistent with chloroma
Consider Malignancy
7
Scleral icterus
Consider Underlying Hepatic Dysfunction
F
8
Exophthalmos
Consider Hyperthyroidism

PART XVI
Photodistributed Rash

79 Acute Photodistributed Rash

Nayha Shetty and Henry W. Lim

Photodermatoses are characterized by the development of a cutaneous eruption after exposure to ultraviolet radiation (UVR), and less commonly, to visible light. They commonly present as a photodistributed eruption affecting the forehead, cheeks, neck, upper chest, upper back, and extensor arms with sparing of the nasolabial folds, upper eyelids, submental chin, and postauricular area. Photodermatoses can be broadly classified as immunologically-mediated, secondary to exogenous and endogenous agents, and photoaggravated dermatoses. Management is centered around photoprotection, including the use of sunscreens and physical barriers (e.g., clothing, hat).

A. The initial evaluation of patients with an acute photodistributed rash should involve recording a detailed history and a thorough physical examination of the skin, nails, and mucosal surfaces while paying special attention to distribution and morphology. A detailed history should include timing of onset of rash after light exposure, whether flares occur after exposure to natural or artificial light, duration of eruption, history of dermatoses, topical and systemic (both prescription and over-the-counter) medications, exposure to topical photosensitizing agents (e.g., foods, soaps, plants), occupation, diet (e.g., malnutrition), and family history. Laboratory evaluation may involve skin biopsy, serum studies for autoimmune antibodies, plasma porphyrins, phototesting, or photopatch testing.

B. Photosensitivity induced by exogenous agents can be divided into phototoxic and photoallergic reactions. **Phototoxicity** results when exposure to a phototoxic agent and UVR causes direct tissue and cellular injury in the skin, typically within minutes to hours of exposure. Most often, UVA radiation is responsible for triggering drug-induced phototoxic reactions, but visible light can also be implicated. Systemic medications are more commonly implicated than topicals. Common phototoxic agents include antiarrhythmics, nonsteroidal anti-inflammatory drugs (NSAIDs), tetracyclines, fluoroquinolones, calcium channel blockers, and oncologic medications. Examples of phototoxicity due to topical agents include topical tar and phytophotodermatitis caused by furocoumarins. Phototoxicity does not require prior sensitization and can theoretically occur in any individual. Clues to the diagnosis include an exaggerated sunburn-like reaction in sun-exposed areas within minutes to hours of exposure to light in a patient exposed to a known phototoxic agent. While diagnosis is often clinical, systemic phototoxicity can be confirmed by phototesting, which reveals decreased minimal erythema dose (MED) values. Resolution occurs after the discontinuation of the precipitating drug.

C. **Photoallergy** occurs due to a cell-mediated immune response in a process identical to that of allergic contact dermatitis (ACD), but with the requirement of the presence of a photoallergen and UVR. In sensitized individuals, onset typically occurs 24 to 48 hours after light exposure. Common photoallergens include topical agents such as fragrances and organic UV filters in sunscreens (e.g., oxybenzone), as well as systemic agents such as antiarrhythmics, antimalarials, antifungals, and NSAIDs. In contrast to phototoxicity, photoallergy requires prior exposure and sensitization to the offending agent. Classically, physical examination clues include a pruritic eczematous eruption resembling ACD; however, photoallergy can often be clinically difficult to distinguish from phototoxicity based on morphology alone. Photoallergy can be confirmed by photopatch testing. Resolution occurs after discontinuation of the implicated agent.

D. In a young or middle-aged patient, particularly female, with the onset of an urticarial and pruritic eruption within minutes of sun exposure or history of "sun sensitivity," consider a diagnosis of **solar urticaria**. Angioedema and systemic symptoms such as headache, nausea, dizziness, and wheezing may be present. The action spectrum can be in the UVA, UVB, or visible light range. Physical examination may reveal urticarial papules and plaques, although patients may lack a visible eruption at the time of examination. Phototesting reveals urticaria induction within minutes and normal MED values. Individual lesions resolve within 24 hours of stopping sun exposure.

E. In a patient with the onset of papules, vesicles, or plaques within hours of sun exposure, consider **polymorphous light eruption**. Patients will typically present in spring and summer or after a trip to sunny locations. Physical examination may reveal a symmetric, patchy distribution of polymorphous, erythematous, mildly pruritic lesions with predilection for the upper chest, outer arms, and dorsal hands, although patients may lack a visible eruption at the time of examination. In dark-skinned individuals, the most common morphology is pinhead-sized papules. A "hardening" phenomenon may occur with repeat exposures. Lesions appear 4 to 6 hours after exposure and persist for days to weeks. Phototesting typically demonstrates normal MED.

See Appendix 1 for Further Reading and Image References.

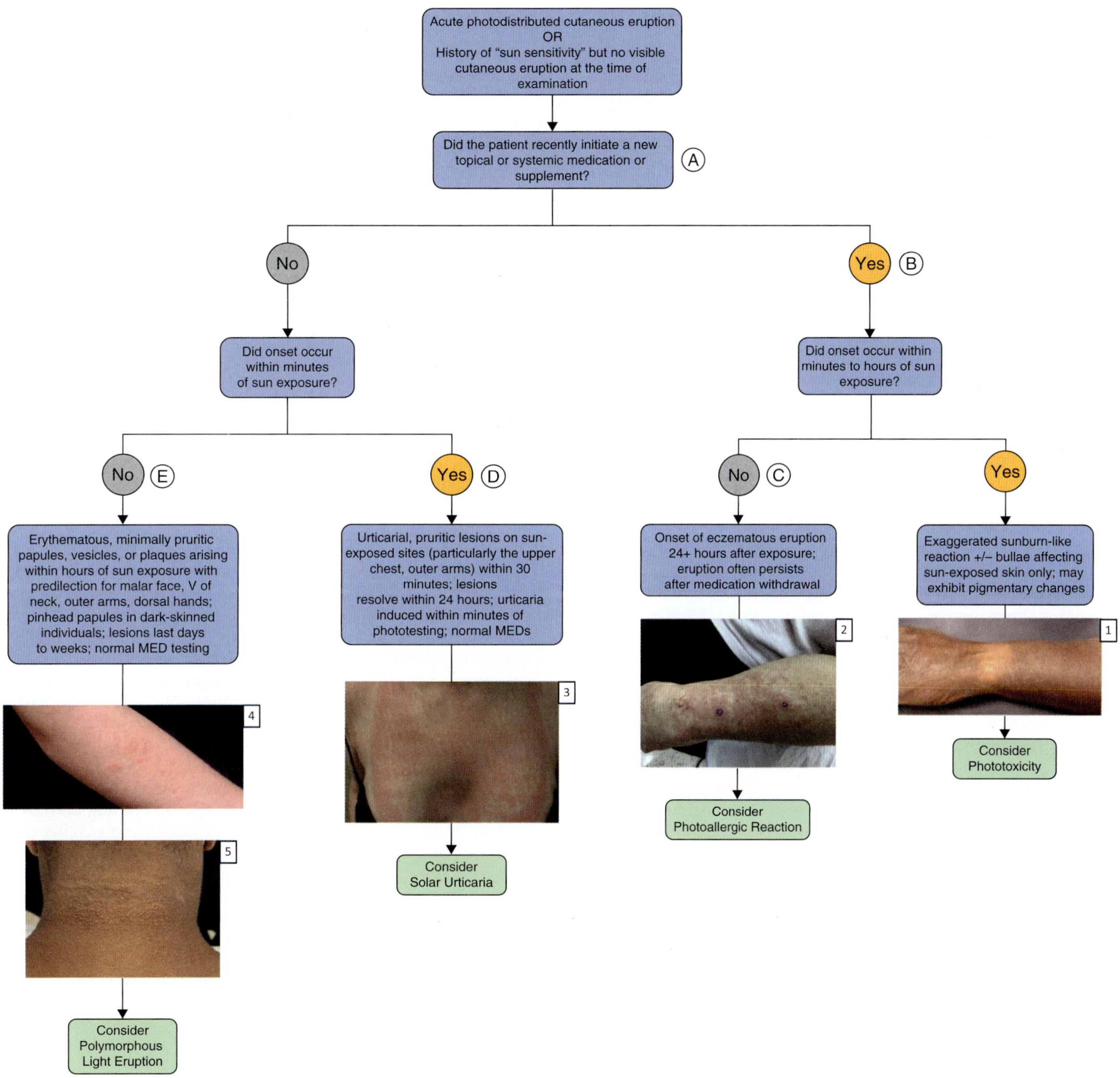
Acute photodistributed cutaneous eruption
OR
History of "sun sensitivity" but no visible cutaneous eruption at the time of examination
Did the patient recently initiate a new topical or systemic medication or supplement?
A
No
Yes
B
Did onset occur within minutes of sun exposure?
Did onset occur within minutes to hours of sun exposure?
No
E
Yes
D
No
C
Yes
Erythematous, minimally pruritic papules, vesicles, or plaques arising within hours of sun exposure with predilection for malar face, V of neck, outer arms, dorsal hands; pinhead papules in dark-skinned individuals; lesions last days to weeks; normal MED testing
Urticarial, pruritic lesions on sun-exposed sites (particularly the upper chest, outer arms) within 30 minutes; lesions resolve within 24 hours; urticaria induced within minutes of phototesting; normal MEDs
Onset of eczematous eruption 24+ hours after exposure; eruption often persists after medication withdrawal
Exaggerated sunburn-like reaction +/– bullae affecting sun-exposed skin only; may exhibit pigmentary changes
4
5
3
2
1
Consider Polymorphous Light Eruption
Consider Solar Urticaria
Consider Photoallergic Reaction
Consider Phototoxicity

80 Chronic Photodistributed Rash

Nayha Shetty and Henry W. Lim

Photodermatoses are characterized by the development of a cutaneous eruption after exposure to ultraviolet radiation (UVR), and less commonly, to visible light. They commonly present as a photodistributed eruption affecting the forehead, cheeks, neck, upper chest, upper back, and extensor arms with sparing of the nasolabial folds, upper eyelids, submental chin, and postauricular area. Chronic photodistributed dermatoses include photoaggravated dermatoses, hereditary photodermatoses, hydroa vacciniforme (HV), actinic prurigo (AP), porphyrias, and chronic actinic dermatitis (CAD). Management is centered around photoprotection and can include topical steroids, phototherapy, and systemic immunosuppressants.

A. The initial evaluation of patients with a chronic photodistributed rash should involve recording a detailed history and a thorough physical examination of the skin, nails, and mucosal surfaces while paying special attention to distribution and morphology. A detailed history should include timing of onset of rash after light exposure, whether flares occur after exposure to natural or artificial light, duration of eruption, history of underlying dermatoses, topical and systemic (both prescription and over-the-counter) medications, exposure to topical photosensitizing agents (e.g., foods, soaps, plants), occupation, diet (e.g., malnutrition), and family history. Laboratory evaluation may involve skin biopsy, serum studies for autoimmune antibodies, plasma porphyrins, phototesting, or photopatch testing.

B. **Photoaggravated dermatoses** are conditions in which the underlying condition is exacerbated, but not caused, by UVR. Diseases known to be exacerbated by UVR include cutaneous lupus erythematosus, dermatomyositis, atopic dermatitis, pellagra, rosacea, Darier disease, and less frequently acne, cutaneous T-cell lymphoma, and pemphigus. The severity of exacerbation with UVR exposure can vary between primary dermatoses. The eruption is typically limited to sites that are characteristically involved by the primary condition and, uncommonly, will involve all exposed skin. With the exception of lupus and atopic dermatitis, phototesting is typically normal. Management is centered around photoprotection and treatment of the underlying disease.

C. In patients exhibiting systemic signs or organ involvement (e.g., growth retardation, intellectual impairment, ophthalmologic findings), consider a **hereditary photodermatosis**. These conditions are caused by defects in DNA repair, chromosomal instability, or localized or systemic biochemical abnormalities. Conditions caused by nucleotide excision repair defects include xeroderma pigmentosum, trichothiodystrophy, Cockayne syndrome, cerebro-oculo-facio-skeletal syndrome, and UV-sensitive syndrome. Conditions caused by defects in double-strand break repair include Rothmund-Thomson syndrome and Bloom syndrome, and those caused by abnormal biochemical substances include Smith-Lemli-Opitz syndrome and Hartnup disease. In addition to cutaneous photosensitivity, many of these conditions exhibit specific extracutaneous abnormalities and a predisposition to malignancy. Early recognition, diagnosis, and initiation of photoprotection are essential to minimization of long-term complications.

D. If onset occurred in childhood, consider a diagnosis of **hydroa vacciniforme (HV)**, **actinic prurigo (AP)**, or **erythropoietic protoporphyria (EPP)**.

HV is characterized by deep-seated vesicles that heal with varioliform scars. Onset is in early childhood and typically subsides in late teens but may persist into adult life. Lesions recur in spring and summer. Conjunctivitis and cheilitis are uncommon. Lymphoproliferative disorders have been reported in severe cases, usually in adults.

AP mainly affects Native Americans and is characterized by persistent pruritic papulonodules with exacerbations in spring and summer. In contrast to HV, conjunctivitis and cheilitis (lower > upper lip) are very common in AP. AP typically manifests in childhood with a tendency for spontaneous remission in adulthood; however, adult-onset cases tend to exhibit a chronic course. Phototesting is abnormal in approximately 75% of patients.

EPP is a genetically determined deficiency in ferrochelatase and is characterized by burning and pain within minutes of UVR exposure. Cobblestone-like scars, particularly on the knuckles, may be seen. Uncommonly, patients may be at risk of liver disease.

E. In a patient with the onset of a chronic photodistributed eruption in adulthood, consider a diagnosis of **porphyria cutanea tarda (PCT)** or **chronic actinic dermatitis (CAD)**.

PCT, the most common cutaneous porphyria, is characterized by skin fragility and chronic vesiculobullous lesions that heal with milia, most often on the dorsal hands. Photosensitivity in this condition has a delayed onset. Additional findings may include periorbital hypertrichosis, and in severe cases, scarring alopecia, sclerodermoid changes, and onycholysis. PCT has been associated with alcohol use, hepatitis C and human immunodeficiency virus infections, and iron overload.

CAD is characterized by a chronic progressive pruritic eruption with lichenification and sharp cutoffs at clothing lines. It is a relatively common condition, more commonly seen in older males. Phototesting demonstrates a reduction of the minimal erythema dose to UVA, UVB, or visible light. Photoprotection alone is typically insufficient for disease control.

See Appendix 1 for Further Reading and Image References.

Patient presenting with a chronic photodistributed cutaneous eruption

↓

Does the patient show signs of or have a history of an underlying dermatosis (e.g., atopic dermatitis)? Ⓐ

- **Yes**
  - 1
  - 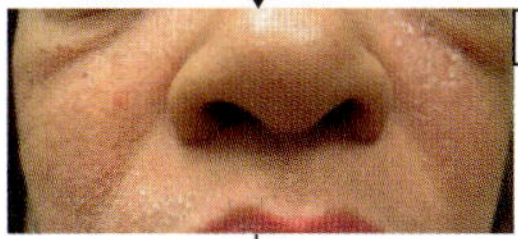
  - Patient with facial rash consistent with Acute Cutaneous Lupus Erythematosus
  - → Consider Photoaggravated dermatoses (e.g., atopic dermatitis, cutaneous lupus) Ⓑ
- **No**
  - Does the patient have systemic/organ involvement (e.g., growth retardation, intellectual impairment, ophthalmologic findings)?
    - **Yes**
      - 2
      - 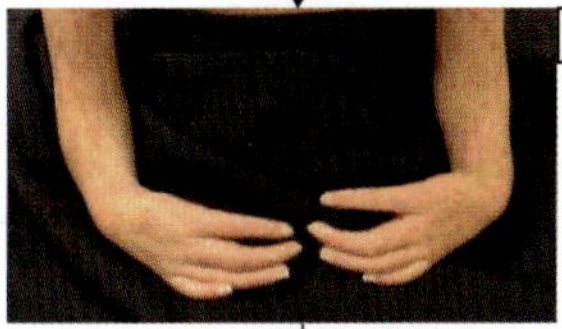
      - Skeletal abnormalities in a patient with Rothmund-Thomson Syndrome
      - → Consider Hereditary photodermatoses (e.g., XP, Cockayne syndrome, Bloom syndrome) Ⓒ
    - **No**
      - Did onset occur in childhood?
        - **No** Ⓔ
          - Older patient with persistent eczematous, lichenified eruption that worsens in summer and exhibits sharp cutoff at clothing lines; decreased MEDs to UVA, UVB, or visible light
            - 7
            - 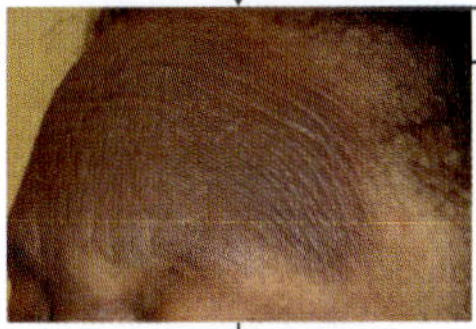
            - → Consider Chronic Actinic Dermatitis
          - Middle-aged patient with skin fragility, bullae, crusts, milia, scarring on sun-exposed areas +/−periorbital hypertrichosis, hyperpigmentation, sclerodermoid changes; associated with hepatitis C; phototesting normal
            - 6
            - 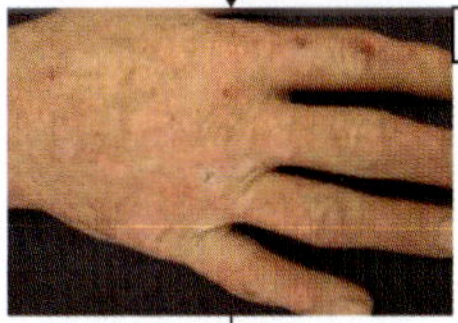
            - → Consider Porphyria Cutanea Tarda
        - **Yes** Ⓓ
          - Erythematous macules, papules, vesicles, crusts, and vacciniform scars on the face, dorsal hands that present within hours of sun exposure; rarely positive family history; severe cases in adults associated with lymphoproliferative disease
            - 3
            - 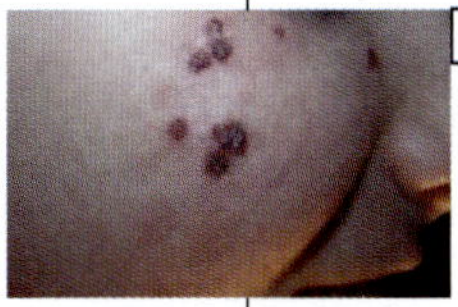
            - → Consider Hydroa Vacciniforme
          - Persistent pruritic papulonodules, crusts, excoriations, lichenification, cheilitis, conjunctivitis that occurs during summer but may be present year-round; up to 50% with positive family history; improves in adolescence, but may persist; adult onset may occur; more common in American Indians and mestizos
            - 4
            - 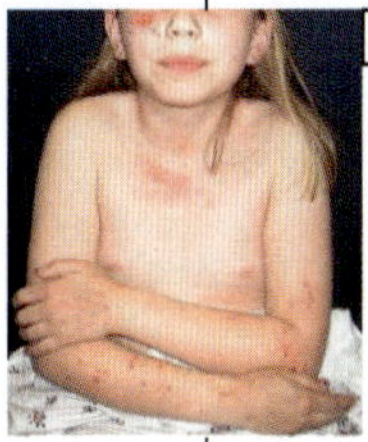
            - → Consider Actinic Prurigo
          - Early childhood onset of burning, pain, stinging > pruritus within minutes of sun exposure, improves in winter; characterized by erythema, edema, purpura, cobblestoning of knuckles; may have positive family history; may develop liver disease
            - 5
            - 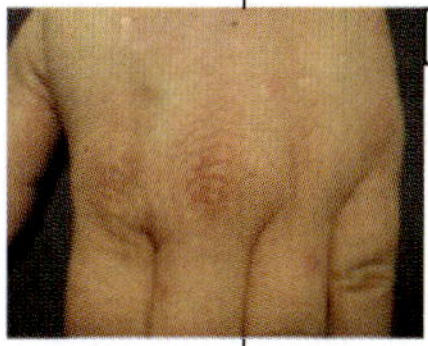
            - → Consider Erythropoietic Protoporphyria

PART XVII
Sweating Disorder

81 Hyperhidrosis

Isabella Inez Sanchez and Christina Nicole Kraus

Hyperhidrosis, or excessive sweating, results from overstimulation of cholinergic receptors on eccrine glands. This leads to an increase in sweat production, greater than that required for normal thermoregulation. The highest density of eccrine glands is on the palms, soles, axillae, and face, which is why these areas are most associated with hyperhidrosis.

Hyperhidrosis can be classified as primary or secondary and focal or generalized. Distinguishing these is important, as management differs between primary and secondary hyperhidrosis. The initial evaluation of a patient presenting with hyperhidrosis should involve a detailed history: medical and family history, current medications, timing and location of sweating, and triggers of sweating, including emotional and environmental. In some patients, excess sweat may be visible on physical examination. The iodine-starch test can be used to detect the presence of sweat. For this test, iodine solution is applied to the skin and allowed to dry, followed by a light application of cornstarch to the area. The appearance of a dark blue to purple stain indicates that sweat is present.

A. The first step in the diagnostic algorithm is to rule out secondary causes of hyperhidrosis. Secondary hyperhidrosis is less common, presents later in life, may be nonsymmetric, and persists during the night. It is associated with underlying medical conditions and medications. Key clinical history includes the age of onset, duration of symptoms, time of day when symptoms are exacerbated, triggers, body areas involved, family history, and extent of functional impairment. A complete past medical history, including an accurate medication history, and surgical history should be obtained. The physical examination should include a careful visual inspection of common areas involved, such as the face, axillae, palms, and soles. It should also be noted if the patient has flushing or changes in sensation at the site(s) of hyperhidrosis. Laterality and symmetry should also be assessed. Visible sweating may be present in some patients. Otherwise, the areas of excessive sweating can be outlined using the starch-iodine test.

B. Secondary hyperhidrosis can present in a focal or generalized pattern. Causes of focal secondary hyperhidrosis include **Frey syndrome** (auriculotemporal syndrome) occurring after parotidectomy, **Harlequin syndrome**, **peripheral neuropathy**, **anxiety disorder**, spinal cord injury, and **compensatory hyperhidrosis** (e.g., following botulinum toxin or sympathectomy). Nonfocal secondary hyperhidrosis can arise as a **medication side effect**. Offending medications include antidepressants (e.g., fluoxetine, amitriptyline), anticholinesterases (e.g., pyridostigmine), opioids (e.g., morphine), nonsteroidal anti-inflammatory drugs (e.g., aspirin), sialogogues (e.g., cevimeline), among others. Recreational drugs such as cocaine can also induce hyperhidrosis.

C. If medication-induced hyperhidrosis is ruled out, an underlying medical condition may be the cause. Medical conditions to consider include **infections** (e.g., tuberculosis), **neoplasms** (e.g., lymphoma), endocrine conditions (e.g., **menopause, hyperthyroidism, diabetes, pheochromocytoma, carcinoid syndrome**), pregnancy, and **Parkinson's disease**. Laboratory workup includes thyroid function tests, complete blood count, comprehensive metabolic panel, hemoglobin A1c, QuantiFERON gold (or purified protein derivative skin test), and any other symptom-guided evaluation. Therapies for secondary hyperhidrosis should be directed toward the underlying condition. For patients with secondary hyperhidrosis, the inciting agent (if medication-induced) should be discontinued if feasible, or the underlying medical condition should be treated.

D. **Primary hyperhidrosis** is idiopathic and the most common form of hyperhidrosis. It is typically focal, and the pathophysiology is not fully understood. In general, patients first notice symptoms during puberty and often have a family history of hyperhidrosis. Other distinguishing features include a duration of symptoms that exceeds 6 to 12 months and cessation of sweating during sleep. The axilla is the most frequently affected site, and bilateral, symmetric involvement is common.

In addition to behavioral modifications such as trigger avoidance, topical treatments are generally considered first-line. Topical therapies include aluminum chloride, topical glycopyrronium pads, and oxybutynin gel. Systemic medications are second-line therapies for treatment-resistant focal hyperhidrosis and generalized hyperhidrosis. These include anticholinergics such as glycopyrrolate, oxybutynin, clonidine; propranolol is another treatment option for performance anxiety–induced hyperhidrosis. Noninvasive and minimally invasive treatments include botulinum toxin injections, iontophoresis, and microwave thermolysis. Surgical therapies include local excision of eccrine glands or curettage or liposuction of sweat glands. Sympathectomy may be considered for severe, recalcitrant disease.

See Appendix 1 for Further Reading and Image References.

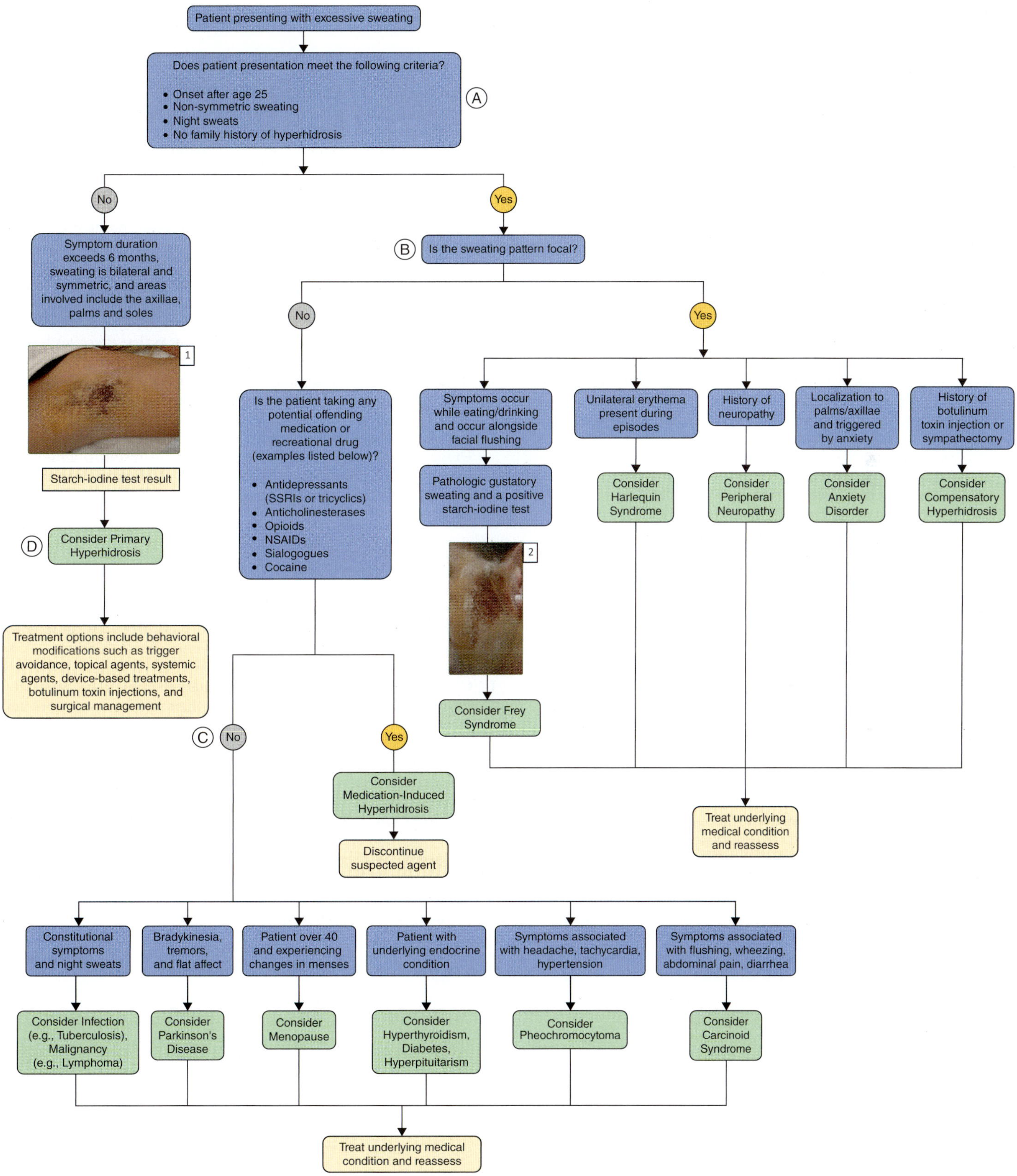
Patient presenting with excessive sweating
Does patient presentation meet the following criteria?
• Onset after age 25
• Non-symmetric sweating
• Night sweats
• No family history of hyperhidrosis
A
No
Yes
Symptom duration exceeds 6 months, sweating is bilateral and symmetric, and areas involved include the axillae, palms and soles
1
Starch-iodine test result
D
Consider Primary Hyperhidrosis
Treatment options include behavioral modifications such as trigger avoidance, topical agents, systemic agents, device-based treatments, botulinum toxin injections, and surgical management
B
Is the sweating pattern focal?
No
Yes
Is the patient taking any potential offending medication or recreational drug (examples listed below)?
• Antidepressants (SSRIs or tricyclics)
• Anticholinesterases
• Opioids
• NSAIDs
• Sialogogues
• Cocaine
C
No
Yes
Consider Medication-Induced Hyperhidrosis
Discontinue suspected agent
Symptoms occur while eating/drinking and occur alongside facial flushing
Pathologic gustatory sweating and a positive starch-iodine test
2
Consider Frey Syndrome
Unilateral erythema present during episodes
Consider Harlequin Syndrome
History of neuropathy
Consider Peripheral Neuropathy
Localization to palms/axillae and triggered by anxiety
Consider Anxiety Disorder
History of botulinum toxin injection or sympathectomy
Consider Compensatory Hyperhidrosis
Treat underlying medical condition and reassess
Constitutional symptoms and night sweats
Consider Infection (e.g., Tuberculosis), Malignancy (e.g., Lymphoma)
Bradykinesia, tremors, and flat affect
Consider Parkinson's Disease
Patient over 40 and experiencing changes in menses
Consider Menopause
Patient with underlying endocrine condition
Consider Hyperthyroidism, Diabetes, Hyperpituitarism
Symptoms associated with headache, tachycardia, hypertension
Consider Pheochromocytoma
Symptoms associated with flushing, wheezing, abdominal pain, diarrhea
Consider Carcinoid Syndrome
Treat underlying medical condition and reassess

82 Anhidrosis/Hypohidrosis

Isabella Inez Sanchez and Christina Nicole Kraus

Anhidrosis is the absence of sweating, and hypohidrosis is decreased sweating. Either can be focal or generalized. While hyperhidrosis affects about 5% of the population, hypohidrosis and anhidrosis are less common. Dysfunction at various points along the normal physiologic pathway of sweating, from neurologic changes to dysfunction of the sweat glands themselves, can result in anhidrosis/hypohidrosis. Furthermore, patients with focal anhidrosis/hypohidrosis may develop compensatory hyperhidrosis in other anatomical regions with a high density of eccrine glands.

A. Overall, treatment of anhidrosis is challenging and consists of identifying and managing the underlying disorder or, in cases of medication-induced anhidrosis, removing the inciting medication. Broad measures include behavioral modifications to prevent hyperthermia and cooling measures, such as frequent use of water spray bottles. If the mechanism of anhidrosis involves physical obstruction of the glands, gentle exfoliation may be helpful, in addition to other cooling modifications. Prompt recognition of anhidrosis/hypohidrosis is important to prevent heat injuries.

B. For any patient presenting with anhidrosis/hypohidrosis, a detailed medical history including a review of any offending medications and history of neurologic and cardiovascular disease is important. A comprehensive family history and physical examination with attention to the hair, nails, and teeth can help determine whether a genetic etiology should be considered.

C. The first step is to identify whether anhidrosis is associated with a known genetic condition. Genetic disorders can result in anhidrosis due to various mechanisms, including reduced or absent sweat glands or dysfunction of sweat glands. Patients with **X-linked hypohidrotic ectodermal dysplasia** can have almost complete absence of sweat glands (males) or reduced sweating (female carriers). Other ectodermal dysplasias associated with anhidrosis/hypohidrosis include **Rapp-Hodgkin syndrome** and **Naegeli-Franceschetti-Jadassohn syndrome**. Patients with **ectodermal dysplasias** have an abnormal development of hair and teeth in addition to eccrine glands. **Lamellar ichthyosis** causes obstruction of sweat glands due to the thickened stratum corneum. Incontinentia pigmenti (IP) can result in anhidrosis/hypohidrosis due to fibrosis of eccrine glands. In adolescents/adults, the vesicular and verrucous lesions in IP are no longer present; instead, hyperpigmentation or hypopigmentation along the lines of Blaschko are seen. Anhidrosis can be also seen in **Bazex-Dupré-Christol syndrome** and **congenital insensitivity to pain with anhidrosis. Fabry disease** can have a variety of autonomic abnormalities, including both hypohidrosis and hyperhidrosis. **Crisponi/cold-induced sweating syndrome 1 (CISS1)** can also present with anhidrosis in childhood that later progresses to cold-induced sweating in puberty.

D. **Medications** can cause anhidrosis through disruption of synaptic transmission in neural pathways between the hypothalamus and eccrine glands or through direct dysfunction of the eccrine glands. Nicotinic acetylcholine receptor antagonists (trimethaphan) and muscarinic acetylcholine receptor antagonists (glycopyrrolate) block neurotransmission leading to sweating. Antipsychotics, tricyclic antidepressants, and certain antihistamines can also have anticholinergic effects. Topiramate and 5-fluorouracil can interfere with synaptic transmission in the autonomic ganglia. Eccrine gland necrosis can be seen with the use of some medications, including chemotherapies (cytarabine, doxorubicin). Aldehydes and aluminum salts applied topically can cause eccrine gland dysfunction.

E. **Central or neuropathic causes** include factors that affect any level of innervation between the brain and the eccrine glands. Medications (discussed in Section D) may play a role in these pathways. Tumors, infarction, injuries, and other lesions of the hypothalamus, pons, or medulla can lead to anhidrosis. Spinal cord trauma and tumors as well as degenerative syndromes (multiple system atrophy or Shy-Drager syndrome) and multiple sclerosis can result in anhidrosis. Finally, peripheral neuropathies (diabetes, alcoholism, leprosy) can lead to anhidrosis through damage to the peripheral sympathetic nerves.

F. **Local destruction of the eccrine glands** can cause anhidrosis. Prior radiation, trauma, burns, and tumors can cause anhidrosis in the affected areas. Graft-versus-host disease can lead to eccrine gland destruction. Connective tissue diseases, including systemic sclerosis, morphea, and, less commonly, Sjögren syndrome, can cause anhidrosis through a similar mechanism of fibrosis and scarring.

G. **Obstruction of the eccrine glands** (also seen in some congenital causes of anhidrosis) can occur with inflammatory dermatoses and in the setting of heat and humidity (miliaria). Some inflammatory dermatoses leading to anhidrosis/hypohidrosis include psoriasis, atopic dermatitis, and other eczematous dermatoses, as well as bullous dermatoses.

H. **Acquired idiopathic generalized anhidrosis (AIGA)** is an uncommon variant of anhidrosis that is idiopathic. Unlike the prior causes discussed, it is responsive to oral or intravenous steroids. Some studies have shown improvement in AIGA with the use of other medications such as cyclosporine and intravenous immunoglobulin. AIGA has also been reported to spontaneously resolve.

See Appendix 1 for Further Reading and Image References.

(A) Patient presenting with decreased/absent sweating → Treatment broadly consists of behavioral approaches to prevent hyperthermia and cooling measures, including use of water spray bottles. If there is an underlying cause/medication, treating this or removing the medication is important. If sweat glands are blocked, gentle exfoliation is recommended. The idiopathic variant may respond to systemic steroid treatment.

(B) Detailed medical history, family history, and physical examination

Is it congenital or associated with a genetic syndrome?

- **No** → Is it associated with a medication?
  - (D) **Yes** → Potential Medications:
    - Anticholinergics
    - Tricyclic antidepressants
    - Antiepileptics
    - Antihistamines
    - Antiemetics
    - Opioids
    - Muscle relaxants

    → Consider Medication-Induced Anhidrosis (H)
  - **No** → Does the patient have a medical condition that could cause anhidrosis/hypohidrosis?
    - **No** → Consider Acquired Idiopathic Generalized Anhidrosis
    - **Yes** →
      - History of stroke, spinal cord injury or tumor, degenerative syndromes, autoimmune autonomic neuropathy / Diabetes, alcohol use disorder, leprosy, amyloidosis → Consider Central or Neuropathic Cause (Example: Horner syndrome causing changes in innervation of sweat glands) (E)
      - Tissue destruction from tumor, radiation, burn, morphea, graft-versus-host disease, systemic sclerosis, Sjögren syndrome → Consider Peripheral Cause: Destruction (Example: Burn scar causing destruction of sweat glands) (F)
      - Associated with psoriasis, miliaria, eczematous dermatoses, or bullous disease → Consider Peripheral Cause: Obstruction (Example: Psoriasis plaques causing sweat gland obstruction) (G)
- (C) **Yes** →
  - Painful acroparesthesias and angiokeratomas → Consider Fabry Disease
  - Insensitivity to pain → Consider Congenital Insensitivity to Pain With Anhidrosis
  - Patient presenting with camptodactyly → Consider Crisponi/CISS1 Syndrome
  - Presence of hair, teeth, and/or nail abnormalities →

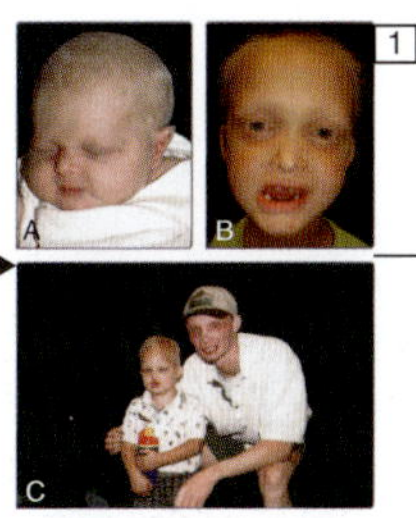

Features consistent with hypohidrotic ectodermal dysplasia

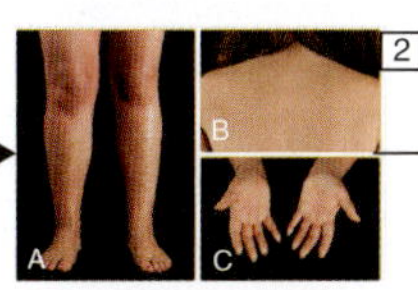

Autosomal recessive congenital ichthyosis (TGM1 mutations, classic lamellar ichthyosis, moderate)

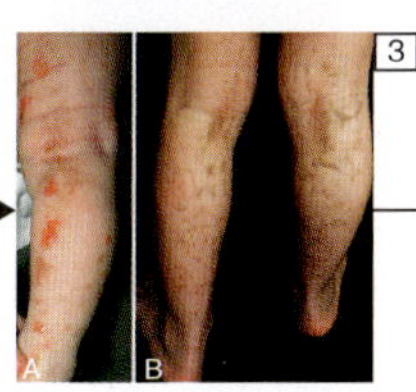

Skin manifestations of incontinentia pigmenti: (A) Vesiculobullous stage and (B) hyperpigmented stage

→ Consider genetic disorders such as:
- Ectodermal Dysplasias (Hypohidrotic Ectodermal Dysplasia, Rapp-Hodgkin Syndrome, Naegeli-Franceschetti-Jadassohn)
- Incontinentia Pigmenti
- Bazex-Dupré-Christol
- Lamellar Ichthyosis

PART XVIII
Pregnancy Rash

83 Pregnancy Dermatoses

Sarah E. Park and Jennifer L. Hsiao

Dermatoses of pregnancy are a group of inflammatory skin conditions that occur during pregnancy or immediately postpartum. They include **intrahepatic cholestasis of pregnancy (ICP), atopic eruption of pregnancy (AEP), pustular psoriasis of pregnancy (PPP), polymorphic eruption of pregnancy (PEP)**, and **pemphigoid gestationis (PG)**. Important considerations for each condition include fetal risk, maternal risk, and risk of recurrence with subsequent pregnancies.

A. Initial evaluation involves eliciting a detailed obstetric history (multiparity or primigravida, multiple gestation pregnancy, and history of skin conditions in prior pregnancies), history of underlying dermatosis, family history of dermatosis, and performing a thorough physical examination of the skin. The initial anatomic area of involvement and pattern of spread, morphology, distribution of lesions, and laboratory findings help guide diagnosis. A skin biopsy may be warranted to rule out specific dermatoses, such as PG and PPP.

B. If the patient presents with pruritus without primary skin lesions, the provider should evaluate for underlying causes of pruritus. If the patient has elevated total serum bile acids and extreme pruritus, **ICP** should be considered. ICP classically presents in the second or third trimester with severe generalized pruritus that often also affects the palms and soles and is worse at night. Secondary skin changes such as excoriations or prurigo nodule-like lesions may be seen. The incidence of ICP varies widely among geographic regions and ethnic groups; specifically, in the United States, the incidence ranges from 0.32% in predominantly White populations to 5.6% in predominantly Latina populations. Jaundice occurs in 10% to 15% of cases, typically within 4 weeks of the onset of pruritus. Pruritus often resolves within 2 to 3 weeks after delivery. Maternal risk includes bleeding, steatorrhea, cholelithiasis, cholesterol gallstones, and subsequent diagnosis of hepatobiliary disease. Fetal risk includes stillbirth, preterm delivery, intrapartum fetal distress, respiratory distress, and meconium staining.

If total serum bile acids are normal, laboratory workup for **other potential causes of pruritus** should be performed, including other hepatic disease or renal or thyroid disease. If laboratory workup is normal, consider a diagnosis of **pruritus gravidarum**, or maternal pruritus without a discernible cause.

C. In a patient with primary lesions who presents with an eczematous or papular pruritic eruption in the first or second trimester, consider **AEP**. AEP is the most common dermatosis of pregnancy, with a prevalence of 5% to 20%. There are two types: E-type (eczematous papules and plaques in classic atopic sites) and P-type (prurigo-like papules and nodules, typically on the extensor surfaces of limbs and trunk). Pruritic folliculitis of pregnancy is considered to be a form of P-type AEP, presenting with follicular papules and pustules on the trunk that may spread and become generalized. AEP is typically diagnosed clinically; however, laboratory tests may reveal an elevated serum IgE level. Histopathology is nonspecific. AEP is not associated with any maternal and fetal risk, and the risk of recurrence in subsequent pregnancies is variable.

D. If a patient presents with pustules late in pregnancy, **PPP**, a rare variant of generalized pustular psoriasis, should be considered. There is typically no personal or family history of psoriasis. Patients present with erythematous plaques studded with sterile pustules at the margins that begin in flexural regions and spread centrifugally. PPP may be associated with hypocalcemia and systemic symptoms such as fever and malaise. Histopathology shows spongiform pustules with neutrophils. The condition typically resolves quickly postpartum. Maternal risk includes complications of hypocalcemia, which can be avoided with prompt treatment. There is an increased risk of intrauterine fetal demise, stillbirth, fetal growth restriction, and neonatal death. PPP may recur in subsequent pregnancies with increased severity.

E. Late-onset pregnancy rashes that do not present with pustules include **PEP** and **PG**. Patients with PEP typically present with a history of an abrupt eruption of pruritic urticarial papules within abdominal striae in the third trimester or in the immediate postpartum period. Lesions spare the face, umbilicus, palms, and soles. The incidence of PEP is estimated to be 1 in 200 pregnancies. Primiparous females and females with multiple gestational pregnancies are more commonly affected. Other clinical presentations include eczematous lesions, polycyclic erythema, and targetoid lesions. Laboratory tests are normal. A skin biopsy is nonspecific, although it can help differentiate PEP from PG. PEP is typically self-limited to 4 to 6 weeks, resolving within 2 weeks postpartum. There is no associated maternal or fetal risk.

F. **PG** typically occurs during the second or third trimester but can also occur postpartum. The incidence of PG is more rare than PEP, estimated to be 1 in 50,000 to 60,000 pregnancies. PG presents with an abrupt onset of urticarial papules, plaques, vesicles, and bullae on the abdomen that spread across the trunk and extremities. The face, mucous membranes, palms, and soles are usually spared. Unlike PEP, PG classically involves the umbilicus. Anti-BP180 antibodies are elevated. Histology shows subepidermal vesicles with a perivascular lymphocytic and eosinophilic infiltrate, and direct immunofluorescence reveals a linear deposit of C3 at the basement membrane zone. Typically, there is spontaneous remission within weeks to months post delivery. Maternal risk includes persistent PG that becomes indistinguishable from bullous pemphigoid (rare) and a long-term increased risk of Graves' disease. Fetal risk includes preterm birth and small-for-gestational-age babies. PG typically recurs in all subsequent pregnancies and often with increased severity and an earlier presentation in gestation.

See Appendix 1 for Further Reading and Image References.

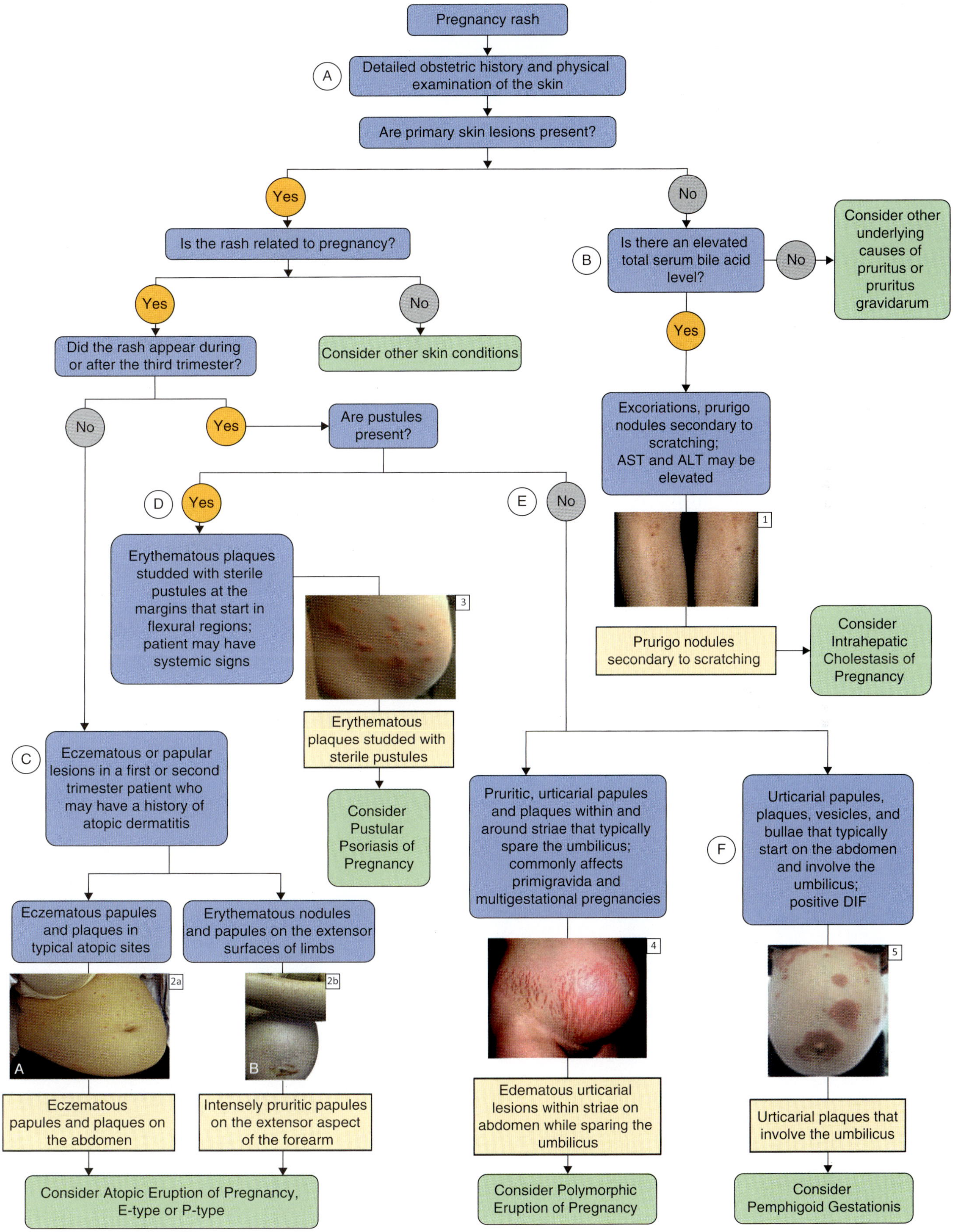
Pregnancy rash
A
Detailed obstetric history and physical examination of the skin
Are primary skin lesions present?
Yes
Is the rash related to pregnancy?
Yes
Did the rash appear during or after the third trimester?
No
Yes
Are pustules present?
D
Yes
Erythematous plaques studded with sterile pustules at the margins that start in flexural regions; patient may have systemic signs
3
Erythematous plaques studded with sterile pustules
Consider Pustular Psoriasis of Pregnancy
E
No
No
Consider other skin conditions
C
Eczematous or papular lesions in a first or second trimester patient who may have a history of atopic dermatitis
Eczematous papules and plaques in typical atopic sites
2a
A
Eczematous papules and plaques on the abdomen
Erythematous nodules and papules on the extensor surfaces of limbs
2b
B
Intensely pruritic papules on the extensor aspect of the forearm
Consider Atopic Eruption of Pregnancy, E-type or P-type
No
B
Is there an elevated total serum bile acid level?
No
Consider other underlying causes of pruritus or pruritus gravidarum
Yes
Excoriations, prurigo nodules secondary to scratching; AST and ALT may be elevated
1
Prurigo nodules secondary to scratching
Consider Intrahepatic Cholestasis of Pregnancy
Pruritic, urticarial papules and plaques within and around striae that typically spare the umbilicus; commonly affects primigravida and multigestational pregnancies
4
Edematous urticarial lesions within striae on abdomen while sparing the umbilicus
Consider Polymorphic Eruption of Pregnancy
F
Urticarial papules, plaques, vesicles, and bullae that typically start on the abdomen and involve the umbilicus; positive DIF
5
Urticarial plaques that involve the umbilicus
Consider Pemphigoid Gestationis

PART XIX
Lip Disorders

84 Facial Swelling

Maria C. Bell and Edita M. Newton

A diverse group of diseases may be responsible for patient concerns of facial swelling. Clinicians should consider the timing of symptoms, distribution, affected layers of the skin, and associated symptoms to determine the diagnosis.

A. **Wheals** are transient, pruritic subcutaneous papules and plaques due to superficial dermal edema. They are typically skin-colored to light pink with a flare of surrounding erythema. A variety of culprits must be considered for a patient with wheals, including an acute hypersensitivity reaction such as a food allergy or other systemic exposure or physical urticaria due to heat or friction, although many of these patients have no identifiable cause.

B. **Angioedema** is characterized by deep dermal and subcutaneous swelling without epidermal change. It may develop in patients who have wheals such as in allergic or spontaneous urticaria, although angioedema without wheals has a different differential and may be either hereditary or acquired. The face, especially the lips and eyelids, is the most commonly and obviously affected area of the skin, although the extremities may also be involved. Some patients develop gastrointestinal involvement or laryngeal edema. While uncommon during infancy, hereditary angioedema typically presents in the first or second decades of life with recurrent cutaneous edema, painful abdominal episodes, and upper airway edema, whereas acquired angioedema is more likely to present after age 40.

C. **Contact dermatitis** is a type IV hypersensitivity reaction that presents following exposure to an external allergen and can range in appearance from a bullous or edematous eruption in an acute form to an eczematous rash in a more subacute to chronic form. The reaction may be localized if the area of exposure is limited or may be more generalized as in airborne contact dermatitis, where patients may have profound edema of the eyelids and cheeks and pruritus of all exposed skin.

D. A localized, poorly defined area of redness, warmth, edema, and pain is suggestive of **cellulitis** or infection of the skin. Patients may also have an associated fever or leukocytosis, and in some cases, a history of trauma may be present. **Erysipelas** is a more superficial and well-demarcated form of infection that shares symptoms of tenderness, warmth, and edema. *Streptococcus A* is the most common culprit for erysipelas of the face. Trauma or nasopharyngeal infection may precipitate this disease.

E. **Drug reaction with eosinophilia and systemic symptoms (DRESS)**, also known as drug-induced hypersensitivity syndrome or drug-induced delayed multiorgan hypersensitivity syndrome, is a rare drug eruption characterized by a generalized morbilliform rash alongside eosinophilia, lymphadenopathy, and visceral organ involvement. Generalized facial swelling is another common manifestation. DRESS generally manifests about 2 to 6 weeks after initial exposure to the culprit medication, and patients are frequently hospitalized due to the severity of disease.

F. **Subcutaneous emphysema**, the presence of gas in the subcutaneous tissue of the skin, can lead to the sudden appearance of swelling of the face and neck. This is most likely to be caused by trauma, including procedural trauma such as dental surgery or intubation but can also occur due to infection. Gas migrates along the fascial planes from the point of injury to the surrounding tissue, and the presence of crepitus on examination is diagnostic.

G. **Orofacial granulomatosis** may cause chronic swelling of the lips due to granulomatous inflammation. This may affect only the lips or cause more extensive facial swelling. At first presentation, this may be episodic and last for only a few days at a time, but eventually it becomes more persistent and chronic. Melkersson-Rosenthal syndrome is a variant, which presents with a triad of lip swelling, unilateral facial paralysis, and fissuring of the tongue. Unlike angioedema, orofacial granulomatosis is generally painless, although patients may develop associated fissuring and scaling of the lips. A similar presentation may be seen with systemic granulomatous disease, such as sarcoidosis.

H. Another cause of chronic facial swelling is **Morbihan disease** or persistent edema of rosacea. This is an uncommon and severe form of rosacea that affects the forehead, glabella, eyelids, and cheeks with gradually worsening redness and swelling that becomes firmer and has been described as having a "woody" consistency.

I. **Superior vena cava syndrome** also causes insidious facial swelling. Obstruction of venous flow through the superior vena cava may lead to chronic redness and facial swelling, most commonly due to the mass effect from a thoracic tumor. Gradual onset of symptoms with concomitant cough, dyspnea, and hoarseness is suggestive of this diagnosis, as well as visible distention of the veins of the neck. Symptoms tend to worsen when the patient is in a supine position, and imaging can confirm the diagnosis.

J. **Leonine facies** describe a clinical presentation with exaggerated convexities and deepened creases of the face, which look like worsening facial swelling. A variety of underlying disorders have been implicated, including lepromatous leprosy, cutaneous T-cell lymphoma, granulomatous and depositional diseases, leishmaniasis, and contact dermatitis. Associated systemic symptoms and identification of the underlying disorder are important for diagnosis and management, and the chronic worsening nature argues against more acute pathologies.

See Appendix 1 for Further Reading and Image References.

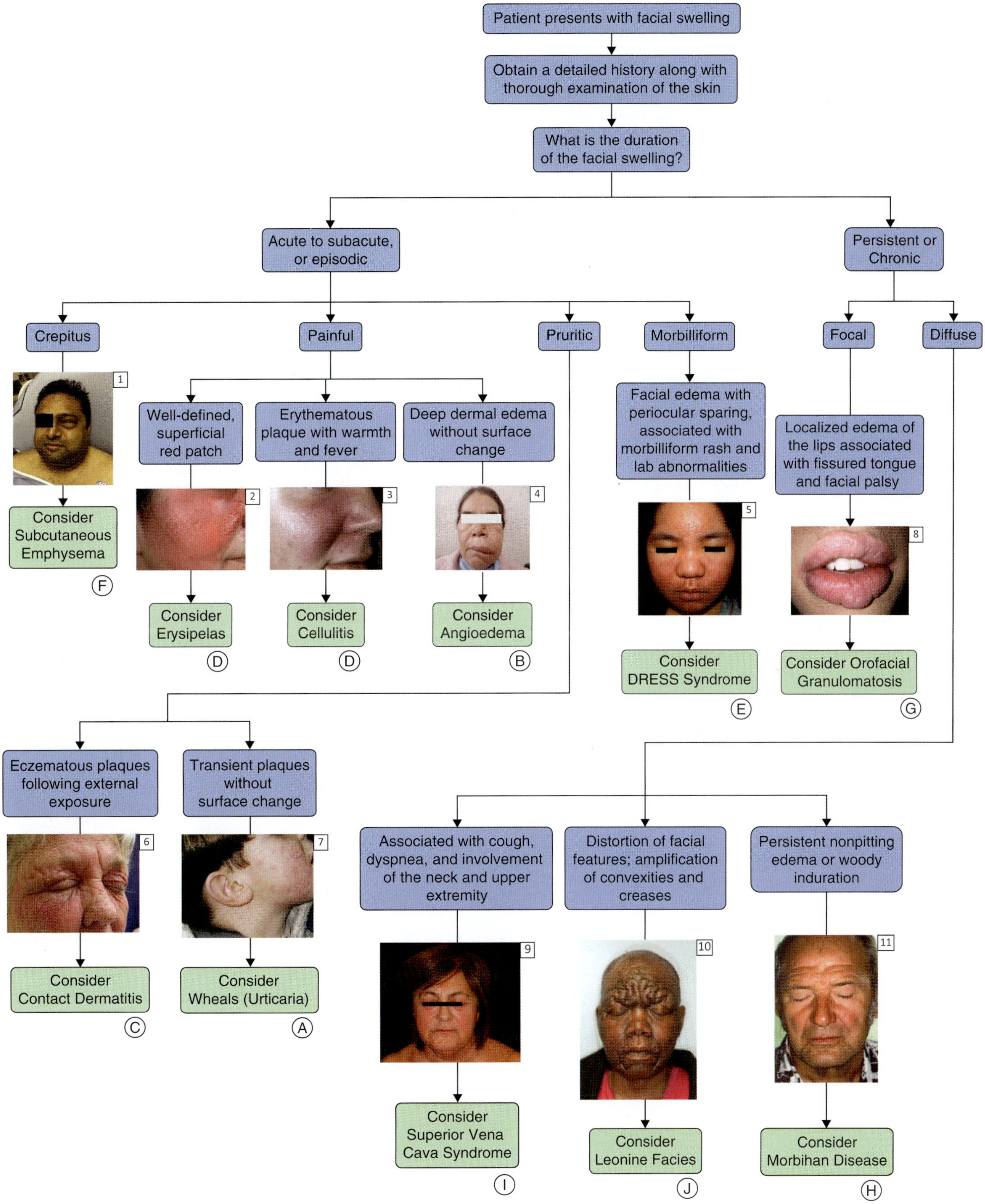
Patient presents with facial swelling
Obtain a detailed history along with thorough examination of the skin
What is the duration of the facial swelling?
Acute to subacute, or episodic
Persistent or Chronic
Crepitus
Painful
Pruritic
Morbilliform
Focal
Diffuse
1
Consider Subcutaneous Emphysema
F
Well-defined, superficial red patch
2
Consider Erysipelas
D
Erythematous plaque with warmth and fever
3
Consider Cellulitis
D
Deep dermal edema without surface change
4
Consider Angioedema
B
Facial edema with periocular sparing, associated with morbilliform rash and lab abnormalities
5
Consider DRESS Syndrome
E
Localized edema of the lips associated with fissured tongue and facial palsy
8
Consider Orofacial Granulomatosis
G
Eczematous plaques following external exposure
6
Consider Contact Dermatitis
C
Transient plaques without surface change
7
Consider Wheals (Urticaria)
A
Associated with cough, dyspnea, and involvement of the neck and upper extremity
9
Consider Superior Vena Cava Syndrome
I
Distortion of facial features; amplification of convexities and creases
10
Consider Leonine Facies
J
Persistent nonpitting edema or woody induration
11
Consider Morbihan Disease
H

85 Cheilitis

Suha Zawawi and Alison J. Bruce

Cheilitis, also known as inflammation of the lips, can be caused by multiple etiologies. Cheilitis may arise as a primary lip disorder but can also occur as a manifestation of a more widespread or systemic condition. Cheilitis may be reactive to a nearby source of inflammation. We discuss the following six important types:

A. **Cheilitis simplex**, also known to patients as chapped lips, is one of the most common forms of cheilitis. Lesions may present as dry, scaly, swollen lips with fissuring of the surface. Environmental factors often play a role in drying the vermilion and mucosal surfaces of the lips. Excessive licking may exacerbate the fissures of the lips. Chronically chapped lips may result in crusting of the surface and, oftentimes, bleeding. Diagnosis is clinical.

B. **Angular cheilitis (AC)** presents as erythematous, fissured patches of the commissures of the lips. Crusting is common. The lesions are typically bilateral and can cause burning and pain. AC is multifactorial in nature and includes infectious, nutritional, or immunological components. The infectious component includes *Candida* and *Staphylococci* as the most common etiologies. In the elderly, denture stomatitis is the most prevalent etiology. Poorly fitted dentures can impair the normal flow of saliva, leading to an overgrowth of *Candida*. The presence of excessive or lax skin around the commissures of the mouth can provide favorable conditions for *Candida* to thrive. Nutritional causes include, but are not limited to, deficiencies of vitamin B_{12}, folate, riboflavin, iron, zinc, and general malnutrition. AC may also be a sign of severe immunodeficiency and therefore should be investigated further in select cases. The diagnosis of AC is usually clinical.

C. **Cheilitis granulomatosa (CG)** is a rare inflammatory disorder characterized by recurrent or persistent swelling of one or both lips in the absence of systemic disease. The soft angioedematous swelling will evolve into an indurated firm swelling. Slowly progressive cosmetic deformity may develop. Biopsy will typically demonstrate granulomatous inflammation. The clinician must exclude Crohn's disease, sarcoidosis, tooth root abscesses, Melkersson-Rosenthal syndrome, solid facial edema, and allergic contact cheilitis.

D. **Exfoliative cheilitis (EC)** is a hyperkeratotic, desquamating cheilitis with thick, scaly, and crusting lesions. EC may be a result of infections, medications, chronically inflamed lips, or activities such as repetitive biting, licking, or picking of the lips following psychological stressors. The psychological variant of EC may be "factitious" or artifactual in nature. Patients with artifactual cheilitis present with intense distress about their condition and are usually unaware of their habits. A 2021 case series (Burns et al.) on artifactual pseudo-cheilitis reported that lesions commonly started during stressful periods, and diagnosis required a high level of clinical suspicion. Every potential cause must be excluded before giving the patient an opportunity to accept the diagnosis of a self-inflicted condition. Differential includes infectious, autoimmune, allergic forms of cheilitis, cheilitis glandularis, and cheilitis simplex.

E. **Contact cheilitis** is an eczematous or dry inflammatory lip reaction that may be irritant or allergic in nature. Patients may have a predisposition to atopic dermatitis. Allergic causes include but are not limited to lipsticks, lip balms, toothpaste, and citrus fruit peels. Irritant causes include, but are not limited to, dryness, humidity, sunlight, and maceration. Contact cheilitis may present as a dry, scaly, fissured cheilitis or an acute, eczematous, crusted papulovesicular cheilitis. Patch testing confirms the allergen(s) in allergic contact cheilitis.

Patch testing should be performed on patients with suspicious findings, and the offending agent must be removed. The tests that may be used to identify the causative agent for allergic contact stomatitis include elimination and provocation tests, patch tests, and immunotoxicologic tests. Differential diagnoses include cheilitis simplex, cheilitis glandularis, CG, oral lichen planus, and oral lichenoid reactions.

F. **Chronic actinic cheilitis (AC)**, also referred to as solar cheilitis, is a premalignant condition of the lips that usually presents in patients with a prolonged history of sun exposure. With AC, the epithelium thickens and may develop warty papules or atrophic plaques, which become eroded. The vermilion of the lower lip is typically involved. Diagnosis is usually clinical; however, a biopsy to exclude invasive squamous cell carcinoma may be indicated. Differential diagnoses such as lupus erythematosus and lichen planus must also be excluded. A 2021 systematic review evaluated treatment outcomes and concluded that surgical treatment is more effective compared to topical treatment options (Trager et al.).

See Appendix 1 for References.

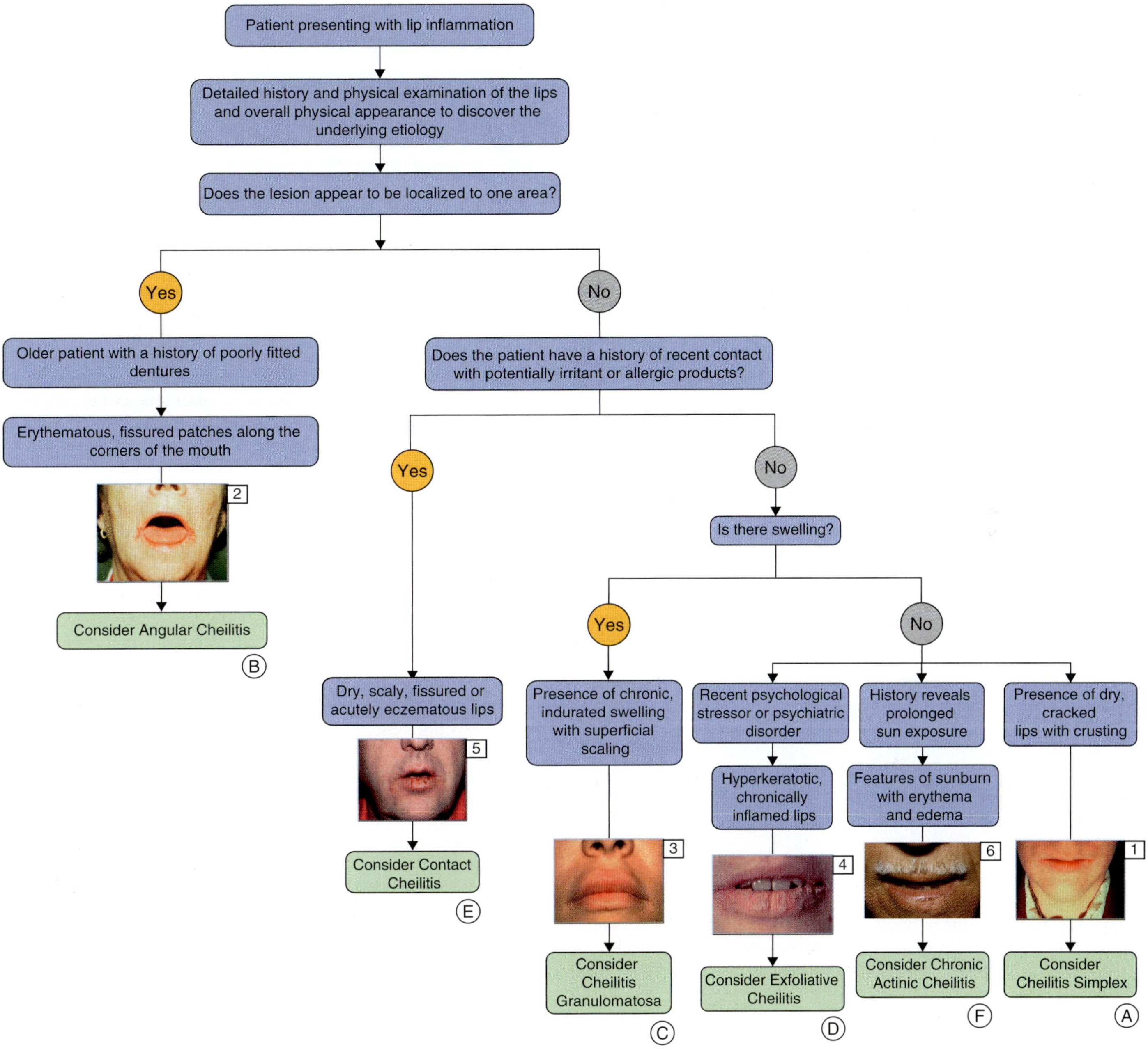

Patient presenting with lip inflammation
Detailed history and physical examination of the lips and overall physical appearance to discover the underlying etiology
Does the lesion appear to be localized to one area?
Yes
Older patient with a history of poorly fitted dentures
Erythematous, fissured patches along the corners of the mouth
2
Consider Angular Cheilitis
B
No
Does the patient have a history of recent contact with potentially irritant or allergic products?
Yes
Dry, scaly, fissured or acutely eczematous lips
5
Consider Contact Cheilitis
E
No
Is there swelling?
Yes
Presence of chronic, indurated swelling with superficial scaling
3
Consider Cheilitis Granulomatosa
C
No
Recent psychological stressor or psychiatric disorder
Hyperkeratotic, chronically inflamed lips
4
Consider Exfoliative Cheilitis
D
History reveals prolonged sun exposure
Features of sunburn with erythema and edema
6
Consider Chronic Actinic Cheilitis
F
Presence of dry, cracked lips with crusting
1
Consider Cheilitis Simplex
A

86 Lip Lesions

Suha Zawawi and Alison J. Bruce

Many benign and malignant lesions affect the lips. We discuss the common presenting signs and symptoms of vascular/nonvascular benign and premalignant/malignant lesions. Most of the lip lesions have overlapping symptoms, making it difficult to differentiate one from another. This chapter provides an algorithm to lead you to the most probable diagnosis.

A. **Venous lakes** are venous ectasias presenting as soft purple macules or papules of the lips. They can commonly be seen on the lower lip, ears, or face of older individuals with a history of increased sun exposure. There is a higher prevalence in males. The surrounding skin may reveal actinic damage. Lesions may be purple, red, or blue and are multilocular connections of venous spaces that can be emptied by sustained pressure. The diagnosis is largely clinical with a reddish-blue macule or papule that blanches on pressure due to compression of the dilated venule (diascopy). Dermoscopy shows an irregular pattern of globules with purple, red, or blue discoloration.

B. **Caliber-persistent labial artery (CPLA)** is a prominence of the inferior labial artery that appears as a soft elevation of the labial mucosa. It is more commonly found on the lower lip and is often bluish in color. Lesions are usually asymptomatic and can be detected by the appearance of pulsation upon inspection or palpation. However, pulsation may be absent in some cases, and a biopsy may become necessary to obtain a diagnosis. CPLA may become tender or ulcerated due to trauma or injury and therefore could be confused with carcinoma of the lips. Once a diagnosis of CPLA is made, no treatment is required. Differentials include mucocele, fibroma, and other soft tissue swellings of the lips.

C. **Warts,** also known as verruca vulgaris, may occur on the cutaneous or vermilion lip or intraorally. Warts are caused by the human papillomavirus and usually appear as solitary, hyperkeratotic raised papules. The diagnosis is clinical.

D. **Fordyce granules** are 1 to 3 mm ectopic sebaceous glands. These small macules are painless, and most commonly present on the buccal mucosa or the vermilion border of the lips. Fordyce granules may appear as a single lesion or multiple lesions clumped together. All age groups are affected, but lesions are more noticeable during adolescence/early adulthood. The diagnosis is clinical.

E. **Mucoceles** are smooth, painless, round, mucus-filled cysts 1 mm to 2 cm in size. Mucoceles are the result of traumatic obstruction and rupture of minor salivary glands or ducts. They are usually caused by trauma (lip biting) or chronic inflammation caused by smoking. The most common location of a mucocele is the lower lip lateral to midline. The diagnosis is clinical, and spontaneous remission is rare.

F. The **labial melanotic macule** is a solitary, well-defined pigmented macule of the lower lip. It usually occurs in adult females with a history of excessive sun exposure. The lesion clinically simulates an early malignant melanoma and can be differentiated based on clinical and histological findings. Dermoscopy shows patterns of lines and dots with gray and brown discoloration.

G. **Actinic keratoses (AKs)** are irregular scaly lesions caused by chronic sun damage. AKs have the potential to progress to squamous cell carcinoma. AKs occur in fair-skinned elderly individuals with excessive sun exposure. Lesions can be skin colored or erythematous and may exhibit ulceration/fissuring. A biopsy may be performed to distinguish between actinic keratosis and squamous cell carcinoma.

H. **Squamous cell carcinoma** is the most common malignancy of the lips. It presents as a thick, scaly papule, or a crusted ulceration of the lips. Lesions most commonly arise on the lower lip. Squamous cell carcinomas generally occur in individuals with long-term sun exposure. Fair-skinned individuals with a history of chronic exposure to sunlight are more susceptible. Other risk factors include tobacco smoking, poor dentition, infection with herpes simplex virus or papillomavirus, and immune suppression. The risk of metastasis is of concern. Squamous cell carcinoma may progress from an AK. The diagnosis of squamous cell carcinoma requires a biopsy.

I. **Basal cell carcinoma** is a malignant neoplasm that presents as a pearly, sometimes ulcerated, papule or nodule. Lesions are commonly present around the mouth. In contrast to squamous cell carcinoma, basal cell carcinoma occurs more commonly on the upper cutaneous lip. Lesions may be pigmented, resembling melanomas, and biopsy is required for confirmation.

J. **Kaposi sarcoma** is an acquired immunodeficiency syndrome (AIDS)–defining condition that commonly presents as an asymptomatic red, blue, or purple macule. Lesions most commonly occur on the face and may affect the lips. Lesions may progress to papules, nodules, or ulcers and may become painful. Diagnosis must be supported by biopsy.

See Appendix 1 for Further Reading and Image References.

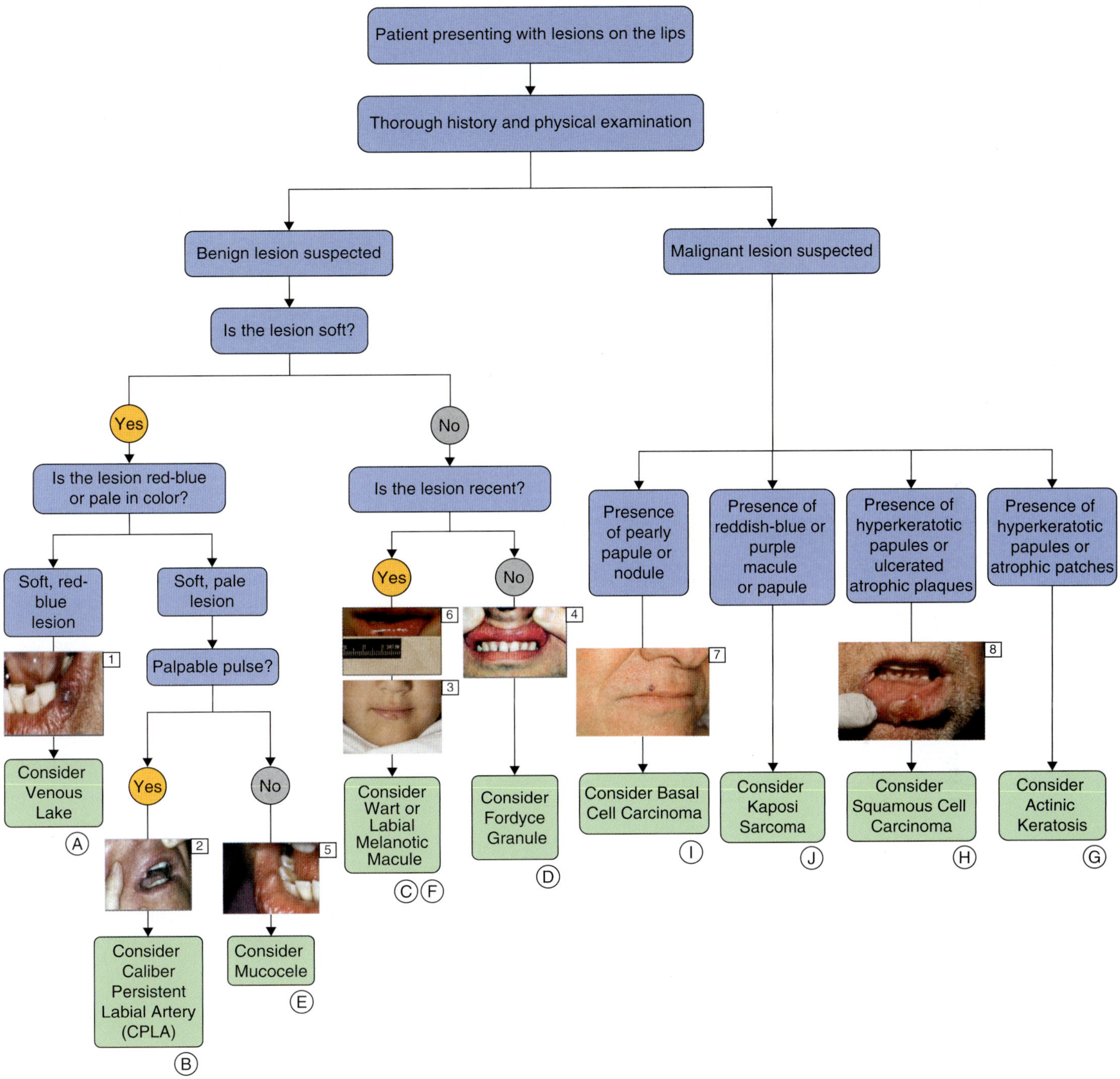
Patient presenting with lesions on the lips
Thorough history and physical examination
Benign lesion suspected
Malignant lesion suspected
Is the lesion soft?
Yes
No
Is the lesion red-blue or pale in color?
Is the lesion recent?
Soft, red-blue lesion
Soft, pale lesion
1
Palpable pulse?
Yes
No
2
5
Consider Venous Lake
A
Consider Caliber Persistent Labial Artery (CPLA)
B
Consider Mucocele
E
Yes
No
6
3
4
Consider Wart or Labial Melanotic Macule
C F
Consider Fordyce Granule
D
Presence of pearly papule or nodule
Presence of reddish-blue or purple macule or papule
Presence of hyperkeratotic papules or ulcerated atrophic plaques
Presence of hyperkeratotic papules or atrophic patches
7
8
Consider Basal Cell Carcinoma
I
Consider Kaposi Sarcoma
J
Consider Squamous Cell Carcinoma
H
Consider Actinic Keratosis
G

PART XX
Hair Disorders

87 Focal Alopecia

Amy McMichael and Hannah Y. Gantz

Focal alopecia describes hair loss of the scalp with various clinical presentations and etiologies. The two predominant subtypes of alopecia include cicatricial (scarring) alopecia and noncicatricial (nonscarring) alopecia. Cicatricial alopecia can be further divided into primary and secondary subtypes, with the latter often beginning as nonscarring with progression to scarring, if untreated. General evaluation includes clinical examination, pull test, and trichoscopy. Semi-invasive evaluation includes trichogram, although not often performed. Invasive evaluation includes biopsy, usually two 4 mm punch biopsies cut horizontally and vertically.

Noncicatricial focal alopecias include androgenetic alopecia (AGA), alopecia areata, and trichotillomania.

A. **Androgenetic alopecia (AGA)**, or patterned hair loss, is linked to genetic factors and serum androgens, presenting with a decline in production of terminal hairs with miniaturization on trichoscopy. In males, the average age of onset is 25 years and presents as regression in the vertex and frontotemporal scalp. In females, the average age of onset is 30 years, although any time after puberty is possible. Presentation in females includes a history of effluvium with widening of the central part, reduction in hair density in the vertex and frontoparietal scalp, and commonly a sparing of the frontal hairline.

B. **Alopecia areata** is a nonscarring, immune-mediated process that may be associated with other autoimmune diseases, such as rheumatoid arthritis or type I diabetes. This presents as circular patchy hair loss that may appear anywhere throughout the scalp and may resolve quickly. Nail findings may be associated. Trichoscopy will show exclamation mark hairs, yellow dots, and black dot hairs. Regrowth of nonpigmented hairs may indicate active disease. Biopsy will show patchy focal peribulbar lymphocytic infiltrate. Alopecia totalis is the loss of all scalp hair, while alopecia universalis is the loss of all body hair.

C. Classified by the Diagnostic and Statistical Manual of Mental Disorders, Fourth Edition (DSM-IV) as "hair pulling disorder," a subtype of "obsessive-compulsive and related disorders," **trichotillomania** presents as irregular hair loss that predominantly affects the crown of the scalp. Mechanical pulling of the scalp hair, eyebrows, or eyelashes will be observed, and trichoscopy will show broken hairs and perifollicular erythema, with decreased density of hair of varying lengths.

Several conditions are part of the category, primary focal cicatricial alopecia.

D. **Central centrifugal cicatricial alopecia** is a lymphocytic process seen primarily in females of African descent and may be attributed to genetic predisposition and long-term hair care practices. Clinically, this typically starts at the vertex and progresses to the parietal scalp. Itching or stinging may be associated, or the patient may be asymptomatic, with an enlarging area of hair loss over time. Trichoscopy will show peripilar gray/white halos, honeycomb patterning of the scalp, and loss of follicular openings due to fibrosis. Diffuse alopecia may occur.

E. **Lichen planopilaris (LPP)** is a lymphocytic process primarily affecting middle-aged females, although males can also be affected. Clinically, this can be symptomatic with burning, itching, and pain of the scalp. Patchy alopecia or diffuse thinning of hairs is present, and the nails or buccal membranes may have associated findings. Trichoscopy will show perifollicular erythema and scaling at the margins of alopecia (distinguishing factor from discoid lupus). Diffuse alopecia may occur.

F. **Frontal fibrosing alopecia** is variant-LPP, presenting as banded hair loss across the frontotemporal hairline that can progress to the temporal-parietal, and in severe cases, occipital scalp. Loss of eyebrows can occur.

   Pseudopelade of Brocq is variant-LPP presenting as irregularly merging patches of alopecia with atrophic indentations in the skin, often described as "footprints in the snow." This condition is usually asymptomatic, and trichoscopy often lacks the perifollicular scaling observed in LPP.

G. **Chronic cutaneous lupus erythematosus**, or **discoid lupus**, is a lymphocytic process more commonly affecting females than males. Clinically, round or annular scaling plaques of alopecia present with scalp tenderness, itching, or burning. Trichoscopy will show follicular plugging and dyspigmentation of the scalp. Erythema, scaling, and pigment changes often present at the center of the alopecia, whereas many other cicatricial alopecias present with these findings on the perimeter of the patch (see Section E on LPP). Diffuse alopecia may occur.

H. **Folliculitis decalvans** is a neutrophilic process affecting both males and females that presents with tender or painful erythematous patchy hair loss in any area of the scalp. Trichoscopy will demonstrate follicular pustules, compounded follicles at the margins of active alopecia, and loss of follicular openings. Diffuse alopecia may occur.

I. **Acne keloidalis nuchae** is a mixed lymphocytic-neutrophilic process that occurs mostly in males of African descent and others who have coarse and/or curly hair. Clinically, this begins as small pustules and papules at the lower margin of the occipital scalp with progression to larger plaques containing purulence and scars.

Secondary focal cicatricial alopecia can present as traction alopecia or tinea capitis.

J. **Traction alopecia** primarily affects females of African descent and is attributed to various forms of long-term traumatic hairstyling practices. This presents similarly to frontal fibrosing alopecia but preserves the "fringe sign" along the frontotemporal border with increased vellus hairs. Trichoscopy demonstrates decreased hair density, perifollicular hematoma or gray color, hair casts, and interfollicular black dots.

K. **Tinea capitis** is the most common superficial fungal infection in children, predominantly caused in the United States by *Trichophyton tonsurans*. Clinical presentation largely depends on the organism and host response, but commonly presents as patchy alopecia with superficial scaling and follicular pustules. Trichoscopy demonstrates comma and corkscrew hairs, and black dots within the follicular openings. Occipital and cervical adenopathy may be observed. Fungal culture is gold standard for diagnosis, and KOH staining may detect the presence of dermatophytes.

See Appendix 1 for Further Reading and Image References.

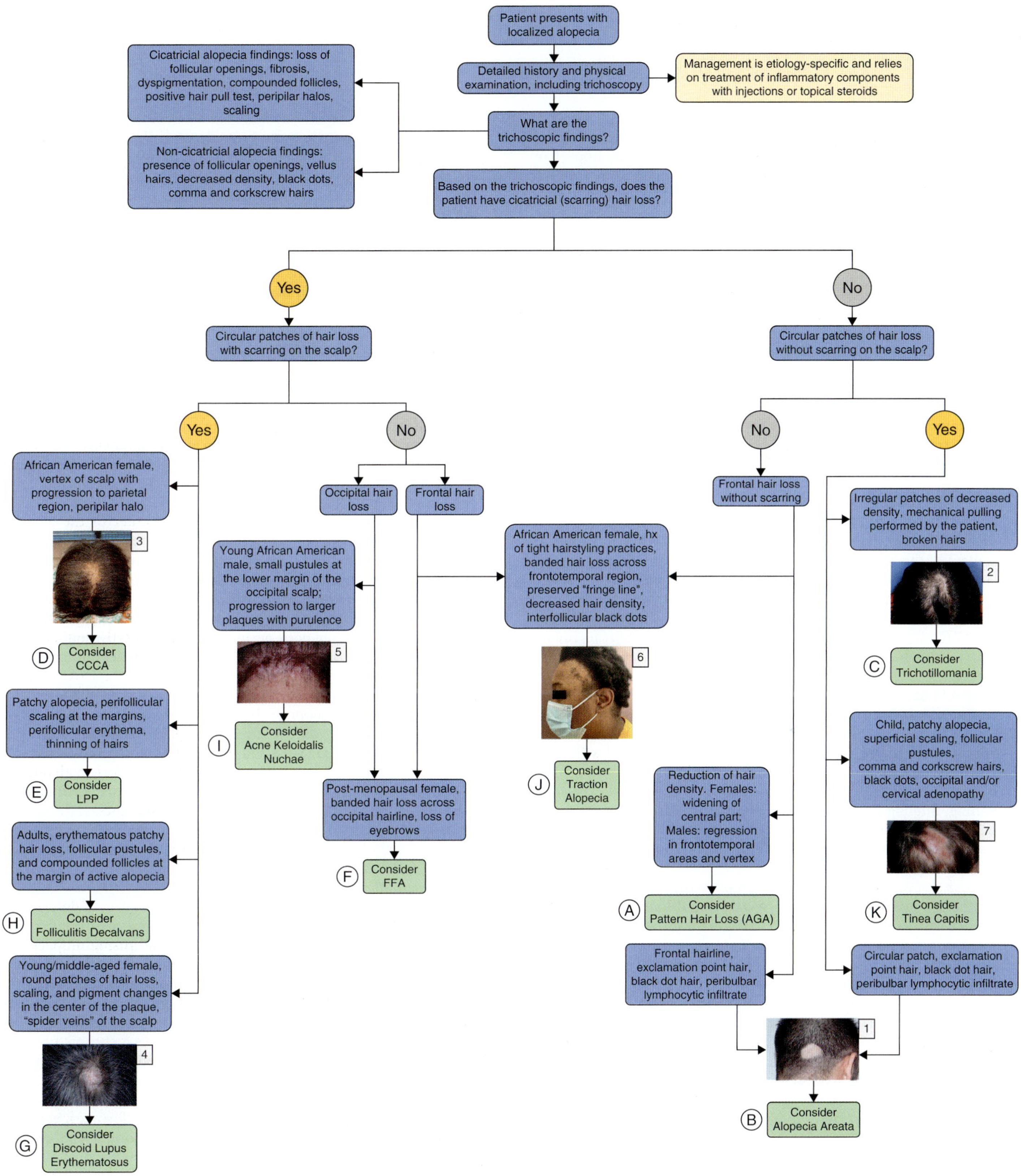
Patient presents with localized alopecia
Detailed history and physical examination, including trichoscopy
Management is etiology-specific and relies on treatment of inflammatory components with injections or topical steroids
What are the trichoscopic findings?
Cicatricial alopecia findings: loss of follicular openings, fibrosis, dyspigmentation, compounded follicles, positive hair pull test, peripilar halos, scaling
Non-cicatricial alopecia findings: presence of follicular openings, vellus hairs, decreased density, black dots, comma and corkscrew hairs
Based on the trichoscopic findings, does the patient have cicatricial (scarring) hair loss?
Yes
Circular patches of hair loss with scarring on the scalp?
Yes
African American female, vertex of scalp with progression to parietal region, peripilar halo
3
D Consider CCCA
Patchy alopecia, perifollicular scaling at the margins, perifollicular erythema, thinning of hairs
E Consider LPP
Adults, erythematous patchy hair loss, follicular pustules, and compounded follicles at the margin of active alopecia
H Consider Folliculitis Decalvans
Young/middle-aged female, round patches of hair loss, scaling, and pigment changes in the center of the plaque, "spider veins" of the scalp
4
G Consider Discoid Lupus Erythematosus
No
Occipital hair loss
Frontal hair loss
Young African American male, small pustules at the lower margin of the occipital scalp; progression to larger plaques with purulence
5
I Consider Acne Keloidalis Nuchae
Post-menopausal female, banded hair loss across occipital hairline, loss of eyebrows
F Consider FFA
African American female, hx of tight hairstyling practices, banded hair loss across frontotemporal region, preserved "fringe line", decreased hair density, interfollicular black dots
6
J Consider Traction Alopecia
No
Circular patches of hair loss without scarring on the scalp?
No
Frontal hair loss without scarring
Reduction of hair density. Females: widening of central part; Males: regression in frontotemporal areas and vertex
A Consider Pattern Hair Loss (AGA)
Frontal hairline, exclamation point hair, black dot hair, peribulbar lymphocytic infiltrate
1
B Consider Alopecia Areata
Yes
Irregular patches of decreased density, mechanical pulling performed by the patient, broken hairs
2
C Consider Trichotillomania
Child, patchy alopecia, superficial scaling, follicular pustules, comma and corkscrew hairs, black dots, occipital and/or cervical adenopathy
7
K Consider Tinea Capitis
Circular patch, exclamation point hair, black dot hair, peribulbar lymphocytic infiltrate

88 Diffuse Alopecia

Amy McMichael and Madison H. Read

Diffuse alopecia describes hair loss that affects close to the full or full scalp in a generalized manner. It often has a considerable impact on patients' lives. There is no miracle drug for treatment, but systemic immunosuppressive agents are usually best for inflammatory diffuse hair loss. However, each type of diffuse alopecia warrants its own treatment plan, unique to a patient and their goals, medical history, and other factors.

A. The first step in management should be taking a detailed history, including the location of hair loss, past medical history, styling practices, family history of hair loss, duration, hair loss progression, scalp symptoms, recent laboratory work, current medications, and prior treatments. Next, a thorough examination of the scalp and face should be performed. Trichoscopic evaluation will also provide important clues to the patient's diagnosis. A detailed history, physical examination (PE), and trichoscopic evaluation are often enough to determine the type of alopecia present. However, if there is still doubt, a biopsy should be taken to confirm the diagnosis.

B. If a patient presents with abrupt diffuse scalp shedding, consider **telogen effluvium (TE)**, which often presents after a triggering event such as surgery, pregnancy, illness, or other physiologic stress. In acute TE, the shedding begins 2 to 3 months after the insult and lasts for 6 to 9 months. However, chronic TE, which primarily affects females aged 30 to 60 years, involves shedding that lasts more than 6 to 9 months. PE findings that indicate active TE include a positive pull test, and common trichoscopic findings are short regrowing hairs, empty follicles, and a normal hair shaft diameter.

C. **Alopecia areata (AA)** can rarely present as diffuse hair loss. More commonly, it is circular patchy hair loss (see Chapter 87). It is a chronic, remitting, and relapsing, autoimmune form of hair loss that affects both genders, all ages, and races. AA is associated with atopy and other autoimmune diseases, so gathering a detailed past medical history is important. A small percentage of patients will experience itching, tingling, and formication of the scalp. On trichoscopic evaluation, yellow dots, black dots, exclamation point hairs, and short vellus hairs are often seen.

D. Diffuse alopecia can also be the result of medication, especially chemotherapy agents. **Chemotherapy-associated hair loss** presents as diffuse hair loss 2 to 4 weeks after treatment initiation due to cytotoxic agents attacking hair matrix cells. Certain drugs such as akylating agents, cytotoxics, antimicrotubule agents, and topoisomerase inhibitors cause the most severe hair loss. Lower-dose treatment hair loss is usually less compared with high-dose aggressive treatments. On trichoscopy, black dots, broken hairs, and short regrowing hairs can be seen.

E. **Androgenetic alopecia** occurs in both males and females and likely involves a genetic predisposition. Androgen-stimulated follicular miniaturization contributes to bitemporal recess and vertex balding in males and diffuse crown and frontal thinning and a widened part in females with varying degrees of severity (see Chapter 87). More males than females are affected. Men are most likely affected between the ages 20–30 and women after age 50. Trichoscopically, hair miniaturization is present.

F. Diffuse alopecia can also be associated with aging and hormonal changes. Specifically, **senescent alopecia** is a nonandrogen-dependent thinning in patients >60 years. Patients with senescent alopecia have a reduced number of hairs and a decreased quality of scalp hair. Interestingly, the hair loss does not always follow a perfectly regular course. Periods of worsening, stability, and slight regrowth might occur over time. Trichoscopically, a decrease in active hair follicles and follicular diameter can be seen diffusely rather than in just the vertex, frontal, and temporal scalp as seen in androgenetic alopecia. Senescent alopecia often occurs with androgenetic alopecia.

G. In contrast to nonscarring alopecia, scarring alopecia is more challenging to treat because inflammation causes the destruction of hair follicles. Early diagnosis and treatment initiation yield better results for patients. The scarring forms of alopecia are either a lymphocytic or neutrophilic process. One of the lymphocytic alopecias, **lichen planopilaris (LPP)**, presents as diffuse patches of hair thinning that become more confluent over time and affects primarily middle-aged females. Patches may be erythematous with perifollicular scaling and pili multigemini. It rarely involves the entire scalp, but loss of eyebrows can occur (see Chapter 87 for focal LPP). During trichoscopic evaluation, common findings include white dots (fibrosis), peripilar casts, hyperkeratotic perifollicular white scale, perifollicular erythema, dystrophic hairs, and blue-gray dots.

H. In an African-American female with hair loss at the vertex of the scalp, consider another lymphocytic form of hair loss, **central centrifugal cicatricial alopecia**. The hair loss usually expands outward in an oval or teardrop shape. It can be focal (see Chapter 87), or in severe cases, only posterior occipital hair may remain. Trichoscopically, white dots, peripilar halo around hair follicles, perifollicular erythema, hair shaft variability, and preservation of honeycomb pigmented network are common.

I. The last lymphocytic alopecia, **lupus-related hair loss,** can take several forms, including diffuse discoid lupus, TE, alopecia areata, or lupus-specific alopecia. Most common is discoid lupus, which presents as round or annular erythematous plaques often with scaling and dyspigmentation. It can be diffuse or focal (see Chapter 87). Lesions are often accompanied by scalp itching and tenderness. It is more common in females than in males. Distinct trichoscopic findings include arborizing telangiectasia, hyperkeratotic plugs, loss of follicles, white central plaque, blue-gray dots, and scalp dyspigmentation.

J. **Dissecting cellulitis** is a mixed lymphocytic and neutrophilic type of hair loss. It primarily affects young African-American males and can be associated with acne and hidradenitis suppurativa. The primary PE findings are subcutaneous boggy nodules that present with sterile pus forming interconnecting tracts on any area of the scalp. With trichoscopy, "3D" yellow dots, dystrophic hairs, white dots with white halo, and yellow dots can be observed. As a chronic progressive disease, it is important to find treatment options that minimize symptoms and control new lesions.

K. Lastly, **folliculitis decalvans** is a neutrophilic form of hair loss that affects both males and females from adulthood to middle age. Diagnostic findings include patchy hair loss with perifollicular scale and pustules involving any region of the scalp and trichoscopically with tufting, follicular scaling and inflammation, perifollicular pustules, peripilar white dots (fibrosis), and chrysalis structures. It can present as either focal (see Chapter 87) or diffuse hair loss.

See Appendix 1 for Further Reading and Image References.

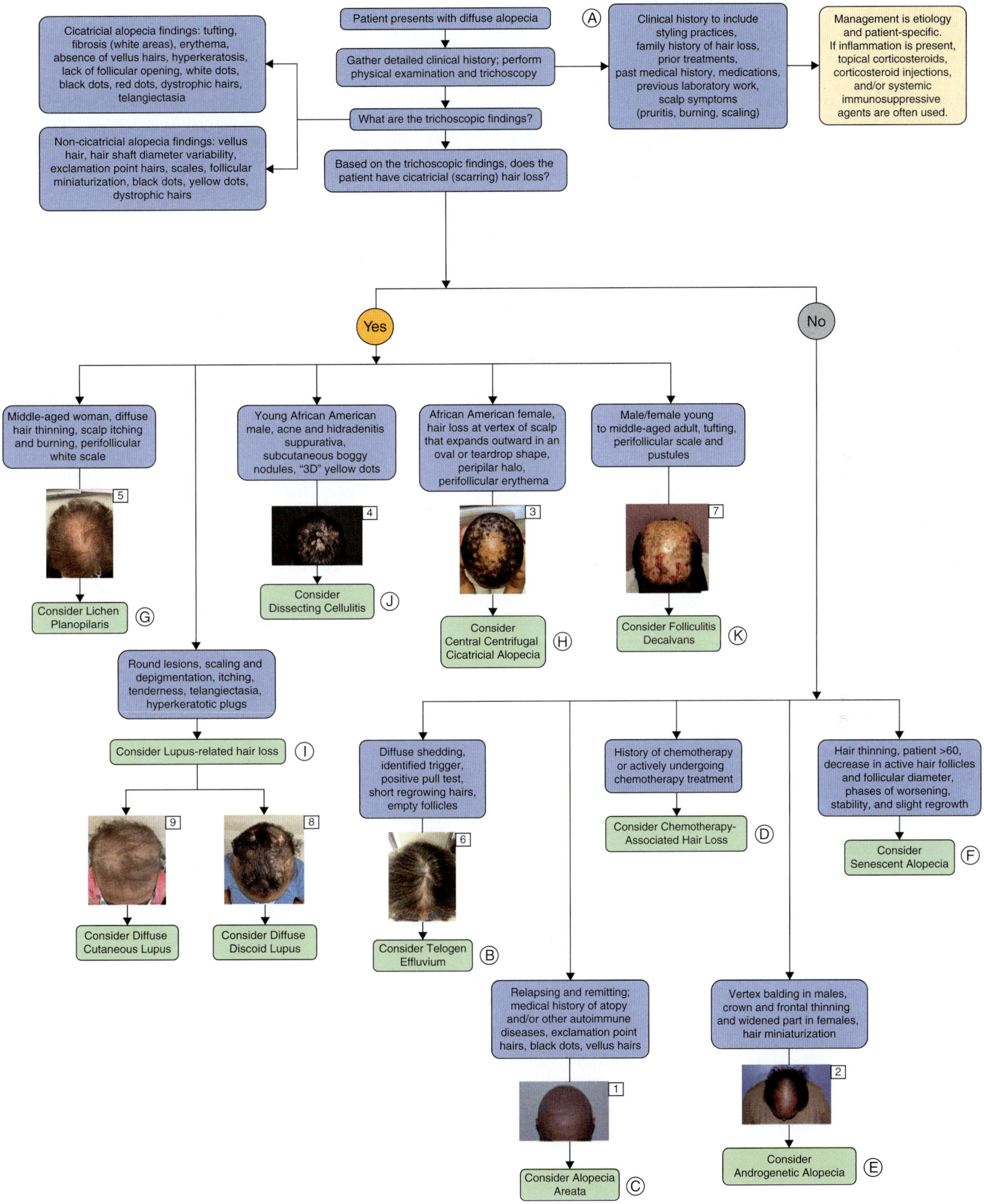
Patient presents with diffuse alopecia
Gather detailed clinical history; perform physical examination and trichoscopy
A
Clinical history to include styling practices, family history of hair loss, prior treatments, past medical history, medications, previous laboratory work, scalp symptoms (pruritis, burning, scaling)
Management is etiology and patient-specific. If inflammation is present, topical corticosteroids, corticosteroid injections, and/or systemic immunosuppressive agents are often used.
What are the trichoscopic findings?
Cicatricial alopecia findings: tufting, fibrosis (white areas), erythema, absence of vellus hairs, hyperkeratosis, lack of follicular opening, white dots, black dots, red dots, dystrophic hairs, telangiectasia
Non-cicatricial alopecia findings: vellus hair, hair shaft diameter variability, exclamation point hairs, scales, follicular miniaturization, black dots, yellow dots, dystrophic hairs
Based on the trichoscopic findings, does the patient have cicatricial (scarring) hair loss?
Yes
No
Middle-aged woman, diffuse hair thinning, scalp itching and burning, perifollicular white scale
5
Consider Lichen Planopilaris
G
Young African American male, acne and hidradenitis suppurativa, subcutaneous boggy nodules, "3D" yellow dots
4
Consider Dissecting Cellulitis
J
African American female, hair loss at vertex of scalp that expands outward in an oval or teardrop shape, peripilar halo, perifollicular erythema
3
Consider Central Centrifugal Cicatricial Alopecia
H
Male/female young to middle-aged adult, tufting, perifollicular scale and pustules
7
Consider Folliculitis Decalvans
K
Round lesions, scaling and depigmentation, itching, tenderness, telangiectasia, hyperkeratotic plugs
Consider Lupus-related hair loss
I
9
Consider Diffuse Cutaneous Lupus
8
Consider Diffuse Discoid Lupus
Diffuse shedding, identified trigger, positive pull test, short regrowing hairs, empty follicles
6
Consider Telogen Effluvium
B
History of chemotherapy or actively undergoing chemotherapy treatment
Consider Chemotherapy-Associated Hair Loss
D
Hair thinning, patient >60, decrease in active hair follicles and follicular diameter, phases of worsening, stability, and slight regrowth
Consider Senescent Alopecia
F
Relapsing and remitting; medical history of atopy and/or other autoimmune diseases, exclamation point hairs, black dots, vellus hairs
1
Consider Alopecia Areata
C
Vertex balding in males, crown and frontal thinning and widened part in females, hair miniaturization
2
Consider Androgenetic Alopecia
E

89 Hypertrichosis

Jonathan Rick

Hypertrichosis is an examination finding common in several different and unrelated clinical entities. Strictly defined, hypertrichosis is the presence of excessive hair growth. As such, the declaration of hypertrichosis can vary based on location, patient demographics, or the interpreting clinician—what is normal for one patient may be atypical for another. Hypertrichosis may be overgrowth of vellus, lanugo or terminal hair, and various hair colors may be appreciated.

The first major distinction is the distribution of hypertrichosis, which is either diffuse or localized.

A. Localized hypertrichosis is a common finding in some **melanocytic nevi** and is likely the most familiar etiology of hypertrichosis. However, hypertrichosis can be an important clue in the diagnosis of **Becker nevus**, **spinal dysraphism** (incomplete spinal fusion), and **aplasia cutis** (hair collar sign). Hypertrichosis is nonspecific for any of these entities, and lesion-specific workup/examination is needed to diagnose these lesions. Melanocytic nevi, Becker nevi, and **vascular tumors** may be found anywhere on the body and may not develop hair growth until later in life. The hair collar sign is found on the scalp around aplasia cutis and is typically present at birth. Similarly, hypertrichosis associated with spina bifida is usually present at birth and is found near the spine, where the underlying dysraphism is present.

B. Patterned hypertrichosis, however, may clue the physician to a specific diagnosis. Specific congenital genodermatoses such as **hypertrichosis of the palms and soles**, **hypertrichosis cubiti**, and **primary faun tail deformity** are named after their hypertrichosis findings. Hypertrichosis is found in several other genodermatoses, but it is not altogether diagnostic.

C. Acquired patterned hypertrichosis is more common than hypertrichosis caused by genodermatoses. **Hirsutism** and virilization from androgenizing tumor secretions may cause male-patterned hair growth. Porphyrias such as **porphyria cutanea tarda** and **hepatoerythropoietic porphyria** may cause hypertrichosis of the affected skin. Hypertrichosis has been identified in **systemic lupus erythematosus** and **frictional dermatitis** as well. For these latter syndromes, a history of rash or friction will assist in the diagnosis. Lastly, **topical minoxidil** and bimatoprost may cause localized hypertrichosis in the areas they are applied to, and oral minoxidil may cause a patterned hypertrichosis to responsive, hair-bearing areas.

D. Diffuse generalized hypertrichosis similarly has congenital and acquired causes. Congenital hypertrichosis is often striking and can present as diffuse vellus hairs (**hypertrichosis universalis congenita**, universal hypertrichosis) or diffuse lanugo hair (**congenital hypertrichosis lanuginosa**). Given the rarity of these conditions, multispecialty care for these patients is appropriate, as tooth deformities and deafness have been reported.

E. Acquired diffuse generalized hypertrichosis has several disparate etiologies that should be considered. Initially, several medications have been associated with new-onset diffuse hypertrichosis, and cessation of these agents should be considered if medically appropriate. However, hypertrichosis has also been associated with **human immunodeficiency virus infection**, **acromegaly**, and **dermatomyositis**. In appropriate contexts, further workup of these conditions should be considered. Lastly, **hypertrichosis lanuginosa acquisita** is a well-documented but rare paraneoplastic phenomenon. This syndrome is associated with lung, colorectal, and breast cancer.

Medications known to cause hypertrichosis include antibiotics, corticosteroids, nonsteroidal antiinflammatory medications, vasodilators (most notably minoxidil), diuretics, anticonvulsants, cyclosporine, mycophenolate, tacrolimus, penicillamine, interferon, and estimated glomerular filtration rate inhibitors.

See Appendix 1 for Image References.

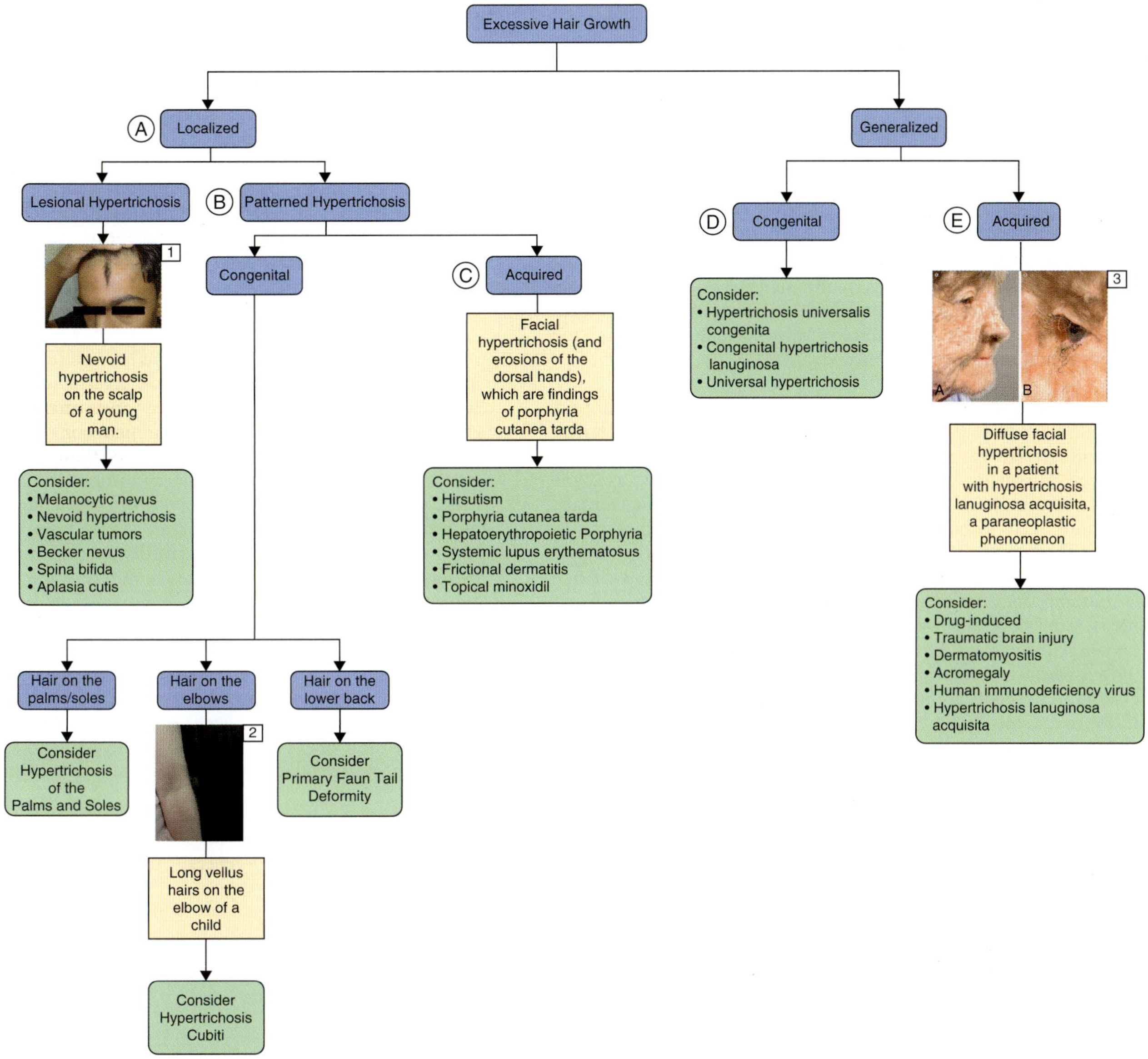
Excessive Hair Growth
A Localized
Generalized
Lesional Hypertrichosis
B Patterned Hypertrichosis
1
Nevoid hypertrichosis on the scalp of a young man.
Consider:
• Melanocytic nevus
• Nevoid hypertrichosis
• Vascular tumors
• Becker nevus
• Spina bifida
• Aplasia cutis
Congenital
C Acquired
Facial hypertrichosis (and erosions of the dorsal hands), which are findings of porphyria cutanea tarda
Consider:
• Hirsutism
• Porphyria cutanea tarda
• Hepatoerythropoietic Porphyria
• Systemic lupus erythematosus
• Frictional dermatitis
• Topical minoxidil
Hair on the palms/soles
Consider Hypertrichosis of the Palms and Soles
Hair on the elbows
2
Long vellus hairs on the elbow of a child
Consider Hypertrichosis Cubiti
Hair on the lower back
Consider Primary Faun Tail Deformity
D Congenital
Consider:
• Hypertrichosis universalis congenita
• Congenital hypertrichosis lanuginosa
• Universal hypertrichosis
E Acquired
3
A
B
Diffuse facial hypertrichosis in a patient with hypertrichosis lanuginosa acquisita, a paraneoplastic phenomenon
Consider:
• Drug-induced
• Traumatic brain injury
• Dermatomyositis
• Acromegaly
• Human immunodeficiency virus
• Hypertrichosis lanuginosa acquisita

90 Hirsutism

Jonathan Rick

Hirsutism is the development of excessive male-patterned terminal hair in females. These changes can be found on the lips, chin, jawline, chest, and back. However, in certain patients, excessive terminal hair growth may be noted on the arms/legs as well. These dark course hairs are often cosmetically distressing to patients. The most common cause of these changes is polycystic ovary syndrome (PCOS), and many cases are thought to be secondary to an increase in androgenizing hormones. However, many patients have serologically normal androgens, and other, less common, causes have been identified.

A. It must first be outlined that hirsutism changes may be a normal variant in certain patients. There is natural variation in terminal hair growth in male-specific patterns based on patient's race and age. Hirsutism becomes more common as patients age, and Mediterranean, Middle Eastern, European, and South Asian females are more likely to be affected. When no underlying cause is suspected, the hirsutism changes are often minimal and slowly progressive. The overall pattern (as outlined above) is identical, but the hair is thin and does not progress. These patients have age-appropriate menses and normal ovarian ultrasounds. Patients may endorse that female relatives have similar findings. In these patients, discontinuing medications that may worsen hirsutism is helpful (section C), even if these agents are not unilaterally causative. Additionally, cosmetic treatments may be pursued as well. In general, patients with slowly progressive and mild changes do not have underlying physiological abnormalities.

B. On the other end of the spectrum, patients may notice rapidly progressive and severe changes in terminal hair patterns. These findings are suggestive of a relatively acute elevation in androgenizing hormones, which can be caused by tumors secreting androgens. These cases warrant a prompt evaluation of serum androgens and likely imaging to determine the etiology. These tumors may arise in a myriad of locations, but ovaries and adrenals have well-documented origins. Hirsutism from androgen-secreting tumors may also be associated with genital changes and deepening of the voice, a phenomenon known as virilization. Surgical removal of these tumors is often curative.

C. A more nuanced evaluation is required for patients who do not lie on either extreme. Most patients will present with moderate hirsutism changes that are not rapidly progressive and are not entirely explained by natural variation. The most common driver for these changes is **PCOS**, which may be a clinical diagnosis if suspicion is strong. Evaluation for metabolic syndrome and androgen levels may support this diagnosis. Other, much less common, causes of hirsutism include hyperprolactinemia (likely from a pituitary **prolactinoma**), **acromegaly**, **hypothyroidism**, and **congenital adrenal hyperplasia**. The treatment of these conditions may be deferred to appropriate specialists.

In all situations, a thorough patient medication reconciliation is important to uncover any medications associated with hirsutism. Discontinuation of these may slow, and at times reverse, the progression of hair growth. Suspected medications include bimatoprost, androgens, progestins, estrogen antagonists, glucocorticosteroids, minoxidil (oral or topical), interferon, mycophenolate, tacrolimus, phenytoin, D-penicillamine, cyclosporine, and danazol.

See Appendix 1 for Image References.

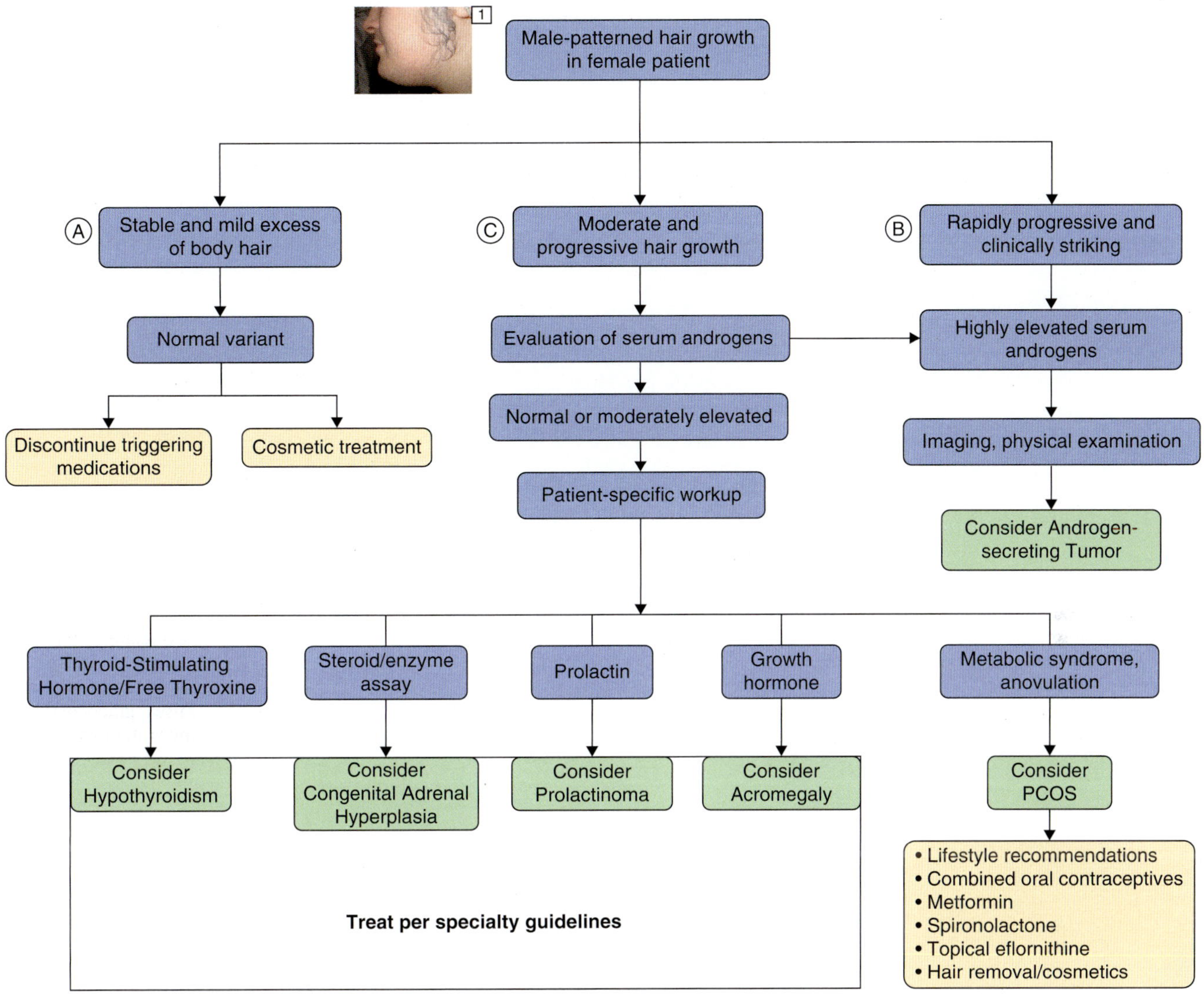
1
Male-patterned hair growth in female patient
Ⓐ Stable and mild excess of body hair
Normal variant
Discontinue triggering medications
Cosmetic treatment
Ⓒ Moderate and progressive hair growth
Evaluation of serum androgens
Normal or moderately elevated
Patient-specific workup
Ⓑ Rapidly progressive and clinically striking
Highly elevated serum androgens
Imaging, physical examination
Consider Androgen-secreting Tumor
Thyroid-Stimulating Hormone/Free Thyroxine
Consider Hypothyroidism
Steroid/enzyme assay
Consider Congenital Adrenal Hyperplasia
Prolactin
Consider Prolactinoma
Growth hormone
Consider Acromegaly
Treat per specialty guidelines
Metabolic syndrome, anovulation
Consider PCOS
• Lifestyle recommendations
• Combined oral contraceptives
• Metformin
• Spironolactone
• Topical eflornithine
• Hair removal/cosmetics

PART XXI

Nail Disorders

91 Nail Shape Changes

Jennifer Adams and Robert Borucki

Changes in nail shape are a challenging yet crucial component of the dermatologic examination, as they can be harbingers of underlying systemic diseases. These changes may be inherited or acquired and are often chronic and distressing to the patient. The first step to discerning etiology is based on examination to determine if the nail abnormality is a change in nail growth direction, nail curvature, or size.

The first step in determining the cause of a nail growth direction abnormality is to determine if onset was in childhood or later in life.

A. **Onychogryphosis** affects a single or a few toenails (typically the great toenail). The nail plate grows asymmetrically in a thickened "ram's horn" shape with a yellow-brown color. Onychogryphosis is almost exclusively seen in the elderly, resulting from neglected care of the nails. Mechanical debridement and offloading pressure on the affected nail can be helpful, but nail avulsion and matricectomy are the definitive treatments.

B. **Congenital malalignment of the great toenails** is a condition in which the nail plate of the great toes deviates laterally. It typically presents early in childhood due to an unknown cause. The nail plate is often thickened and curved, leading to a common cause of ingrown nails in children. Conservative treatment is recommended for minimally symptomatic cases, whereas procedural options exist for more complicated or painful cases.

C. When a patient's nail(s) are abnormally curved, important diagnostic considerations include first whether the nail is concave (koilonychia) and second if not concave, whether the nails are entirely involved. The nail plates are thinned and flattened in **koilonychia**, often with an upward curve at the outer edges of the nail plate, resembling a spoon. This can be a normal finding in children, which spontaneously resolves over time. In adults, koilonychia can be secondary to a range of conditions, including iron storage abnormalities, coronary artery disease, amyloidosis, or an underlying inflammatory dermatosis.

D. **Nail clubbing** can be attributed to a number of systemic causes, most commonly respiratory disease. The condition is a result of growth in the soft tissue of the distal fingers, leading to a round or bulbous distal phalanx. The nail plate is, in turn, enlarged and overly curved to cover the enlarged digit. The condition typically develops over the course of years; however, inherited forms of the condition have been reported.

E. Clubbing must be differentiated from a "**parrot beak**" deformity of the nail where there is excessive forward curvature of solely the free nail edge. Parrot beak nails can be an isolated feature in patients neglecting nail trimming or associated with systemic diseases, such as systemic sclerosis or skeletal abnormalities.

F. **Pincer nails**, or trumpet nails, have an increased transverse curvature in the nail plate. This condition typically affects the larger toes and can be hereditary or acquired. The acquired form is usually the result of wearing poorly fitting tight shoes over time, but patients should be evaluated to ensure that there is no corresponding subungual exostosis. Pincer nails are commonly associated with painful ingrown nails, which may be the presenting complaint.

When nails are of abnormal size, important diagnostic considerations include whether the increased size is the result of length alone or whether it is due to the overall surface area change.

G. **Brachyonychia**, or racquet nails, is a congenital malformation causing a shortened distal phalanx, which results in short widened nails. It is typically inherited as an isolated condition, although it has also been reported as acquired in the setting of hyperparathyroidism and psoriatic arthropathy. Brachyonychia more commonly affects the thumbs, although all digits can be affected. In contrast, **dolichonychia** is characterized by long narrow fingernails as seen in cases of Marfan syndrome.

H. **Macronychia** is the enlargement of the nails in comparison to the digits, which is often the result of local gigantism. **Micronychia** is proportionally smaller nails compared with the digits and can occur in the setting of plexiform neuromas.

See Appendix 1 for Further Reading and Image References.

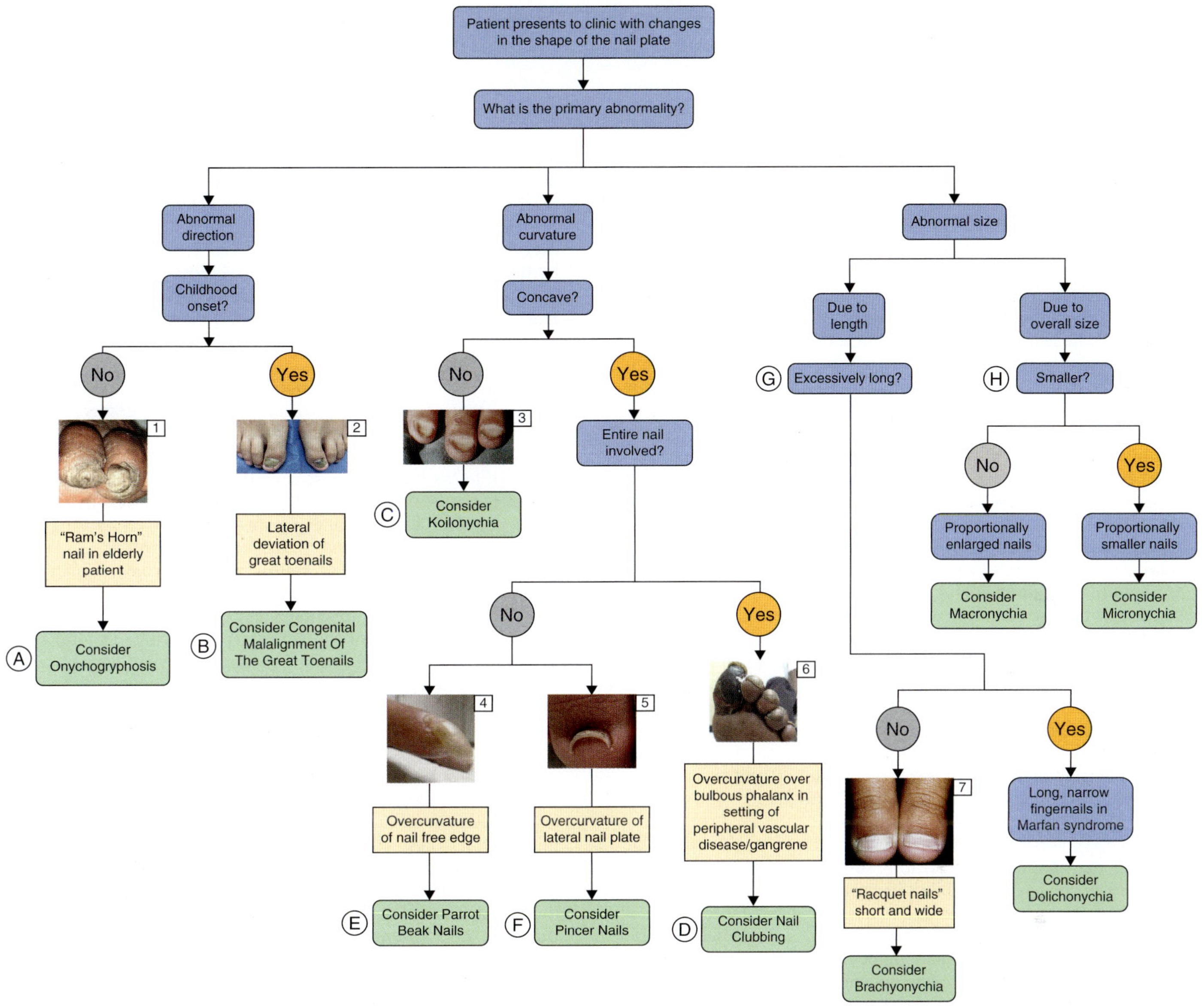
Patient presents to clinic with changes in the shape of the nail plate
What is the primary abnormality?
Abnormal direction
Childhood onset?
No
1
"Ram's Horn" nail in elderly patient
A
Consider Onychogryphosis
Yes
2
Lateral deviation of great toenails
B
Consider Congenital Malalignment Of The Great Toenails
Abnormal curvature
Concave?
No
3
C
Consider Koilonychia
Yes
Entire nail involved?
No
4
Overcurvature of nail free edge
E
Consider Parrot Beak Nails
5
Overcurvature of lateral nail plate
F
Consider Pincer Nails
Yes
6
Overcurvature over bulbous phalanx in setting of peripheral vascular disease/gangrene
D
Consider Nail Clubbing
Abnormal size
Due to length
G
Excessively long?
No
7
"Racquet nails" short and wide
Consider Brachyonychia
Yes
Long, narrow fingernails in Marfan syndrome
Consider Dolichonychia
Due to overall size
H
Smaller?
No
Proportionally enlarged nails
Consider Macronychia
Yes
Proportionally smaller nails
Consider Micronychia

92 Discolored Nails

Jennifer Adams and Robert Borucki

Colors on nails can give insight into external and internal influences, from nicotine pigment residue to underlying dermatologic or systemic diseases. Identifying the color and pattern is crucial but can often be more challenging due to the frequent use of nail polish or other finishes, which obscure pathologic findings.

A. Pigment following the shape of the proximal nail fold (concave pattern) indicates an **external etiology,** and a detailed examination and history can be helpful to elicit the source. Color affecting all fingernail plates may indicate work with dyes, whereas yellowing preferentially of the dominant index fingernail over other nails can be a clue to cigarette smoking.

B. A white discoloration of the nail is referred to as leukonychia, which must be sorted into true and apparent leukonychia. **True leukonychia** does not resolve with pressure on the nail plate. It is more common in a punctate or striate pattern and secondary to trauma to the distal nail matrix, whereas diffuse true leukonychia (leukonychia totalis) is rarer and results from an underlying genetic disorder.

Apparent leukonychia is a white discoloration due to edema of the nail bed that resolves with pressure on the nail plate. **Muehrcke lines, half-and-half nails**, and **Terry nails** are all patterns of apparent leukonychia and are signs of underlying systemic diseases. Muehrcke nails are transverse white lines seen in hypoalbuminemia or in chemotherapy patients. Half-and-half nails have white discoloration of the proximal half of the nails and are frequently associated with chronic renal disease history and hemodialysis. Terry nails are a common sign of liver cirrhosis; leukonychia is found over the majority of the nail but spares the distal 1 to 2 mm.

C. Pink or red coloration (erythronychia) affecting a single nail can be due to a hematoma or neoplasm. A **subungual hematoma** can be deep red, purple, or almost black in appearance (often with splinter hemorrhages at the periphery). Dermoscopy is helpful to differentiate blood from melanonychia. Pink or red of a single nail can also point to a **neoplasm**—this may be benign (i.e., onychopapilloma, verruca, or glomus tumor) or malignant (i.e., Bowen disease, melanoma). Longitudinal erythronychia with splinter hemorrhage and corresponding hyponychial papule is typical of onychopapilloma. Verrucae present as keratotic papules with pinpoint hemorrhages and must be differentiated from squamous cell carcinoma with biopsy, if necessary. A glomus tumor often has extreme sensitivity and pain, especially with cold.

Pink or red spots (erythronychia) affecting multiple nails can be due to systemic disease (i.e., amyloidosis, hemiplegia, graft-versus-host disease, or epidermolysis bullosa) or to a primary dermatologic disease (i.e., lichen planus, Darier disease, or psoriasis). A detailed history and examination should be able to distinguish these diagnoses. Nail psoriasis often has pink salmon patches which may border onycholysis and can be seen in conjunction with irregular pits or oil drop spots. The involvement of nail disease in psoriasis can also be a harbinger for psoriatic arthritis, thus involvement of the nails should lead to a thorough review of systems and physical examination. **Darier disease** manifests on the nails as longitudinal erythronychia with distal "V-shaped nicking".

D. **Green nail syndrome** is a discoloration of the nail plate due to *Pseudomonas aeruginosa*. This discoloration can range from a yellow-green to green-black and is due to pyocyanin and pyoverdin produced by the bacteria. The discoloration is subungual and often localized to the central nail, sparing the lateral nail. Green nail syndrome is more common in patients with occupations that require frequent and prolonged nail exposure to water.

E. Yellow nails can be due to **yellow nail syndrome**, which is an uncommon syndrome with yellow discoloration of slow-growing nails associated with lymphedema and chronic respiratory diseases. There is a typical loss of the cuticle as well, which can aid in the diagnosis of yellow nail syndrome. Careful review of medications can identify **drug-induced yellowing of the nails**, and a review of history may elicit a **systemic cause (jaundice or carotenemia)**. Hyperkeratosis with yellowing can be another feature of **nail psoriasis** or **onychomycosis**.

F. A blue-gray discoloration affecting multiple nails is likely secondary to medications, including silver, chemotherapy, antimalarials, or minocycline. These discolorations are due to pigment deposition in the nail bed or dermis and are frequently permanent despite discontinuation of the offending medication. History can be helpful with the blue discoloration of a single nail in the evaluation for a **glomus tumor** or other **vascular malformation.**

G. Black or brown pigment of a single nail is often due to **melanocytic hyperplasia** (i.e., lentigo, nevus, or melanoma). Features such as asymmetry, width >3 mm, new onset in an older patient, or rapid growth should direct the clinician toward biopsy. Darkening of multiple nails is more consistent with **melanocytic activation** due to physiologic, medication, endocrine, or systemic disease etiologies.

See Appendix 1 for Further Reading and Image References.

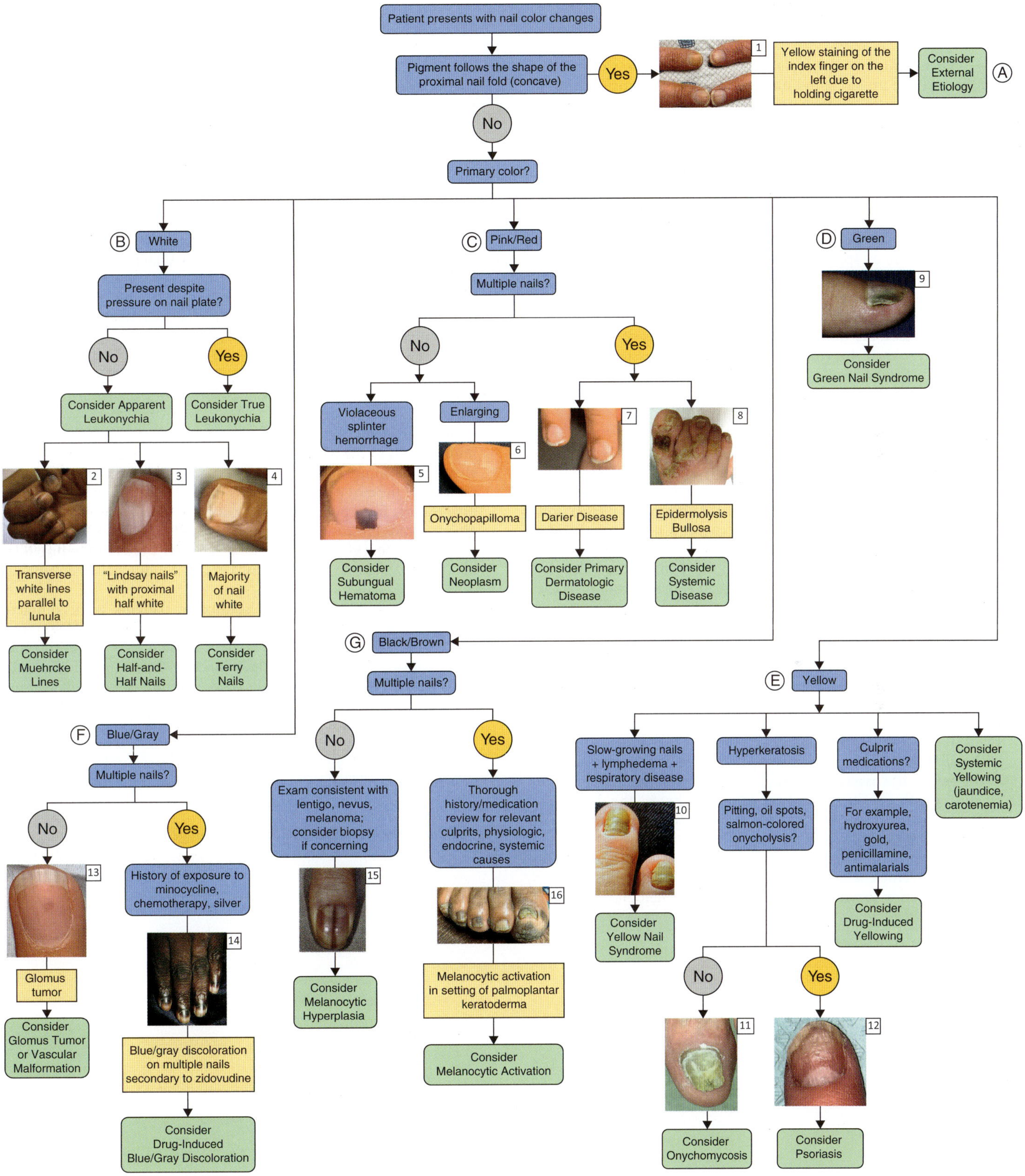
Patient presents with nail color changes
Pigment follows the shape of the proximal nail fold (concave)
Yes
1
Yellow staining of the index finger on the left due to holding cigarette
Consider External Etiology
A
No
Primary color?
B
White
Present despite pressure on nail plate?
No
Yes
Consider Apparent Leukonychia
Consider True Leukonychia
2
3
4
Transverse white lines parallel to lunula
"Lindsay nails" with proximal half white
Majority of nail white
Consider Muehrcke Lines
Consider Half-and-Half Nails
Consider Terry Nails
C
Pink/Red
Multiple nails?
No
Yes
Violaceous splinter hemorrhage
5
Consider Subungual Hematoma
Enlarging
6
Onychopapilloma
Consider Neoplasm
7
Darier Disease
Consider Primary Dermatologic Disease
8
Epidermolysis Bullosa
Consider Systemic Disease
D
Green
9
Consider Green Nail Syndrome
G
Black/Brown
Multiple nails?
No
Yes
Exam consistent with lentigo, nevus, melanoma; consider biopsy if concerning
15
Consider Melanocytic Hyperplasia
Thorough history/medication review for relevant culprits, physiologic, endocrine, systemic causes
16
Melanocytic activation in setting of palmoplantar keratoderma
Consider Melanocytic Activation
F
Blue/Gray
Multiple nails?
No
Yes
13
Glomus tumor
Consider Glomus Tumor or Vascular Malformation
History of exposure to minocycline, chemotherapy, silver
14
Blue/gray discoloration on multiple nails secondary to zidovudine
Consider Drug-Induced Blue/Gray Discoloration
E
Yellow
Slow-growing nails + lymphedema + respiratory disease
10
Consider Yellow Nail Syndrome
Hyperkeratosis
Pitting, oil spots, salmon-colored onycholysis?
No
Yes
11
Consider Onychomycosis
12
Consider Psoriasis
Culprit medications?
For example, hydroxyurea, gold, penicillamine, antimalarials
Consider Drug-Induced Yellowing
Consider Systemic Yellowing (jaundice, carotenemia)

93 Transverse/Longitudinal Nail Changes

Jana S. Guenther and Scott D. Worswick

Insults to the nail matrix or nail plate can result in a variety of nail disorders that present in a longitudinal (spanning the long orientation of the nail) or transverse manner. Distinguishing between them can be important, as they may provide clues to underlying pathologies requiring further investigation. Physical examination of all 20 nails is thus important for all patients.

A. After determining the orientation of the nail changes, the next important distinguishing factor to consider is if there is discoloration. White nail discoloration is called leukonychia and can be classified as true or apparent, depending on the origin of the color change. True transverse leukonychia (**Mees lines**) results from abnormal keratinization of the nail matrix and is thus unaffected by the application of pressure to the nail. On the contrary, apparent leukonychia (**Muehrcke lines**) results from anomalies of the nail bed vasculature, so the color change disappears with pressure. Muehrcke and Mees lines tend to affect all nails since both are due to systemic causes (arsenic classically in the case of Mees lines, and low albumin in the case of Muehrcke lines).

B. Larger areas of apparent leukonychia may represent **Terry nails, Lindsay nails,** or **onycholysis**. Terry and Lindsay nails are distinguished by the amount of nail involvement. Terry nails (often found in patients with cirrhosis, congestive heart failure, or diabetes) present as leukonychia of the entire nail except for a 1- to 2 mm band at the distal free edge. On the contrary, Lindsay nails (found in patients on hemodialysis) are also called half-and-half nails, as they affect the proximal 40% to 80% of the nail, creating an appearance of nails that are half-white.

While the prior abnormalities affect the proximal nail, onycholysis causes apparent leukonychia of the distal nail. It results from the separation of the nail plate from the nail bed and progresses proximally from the distal or lateral free margins.

C. Multiple transverse nail abnormalities present without discoloration. **Beau lines** are transverse grooves in the nail that progress distally with nail growth. They are caused by decreased keratinocyte activity in the nail matrix as a result of a stressor. The width of the depression correlates with the duration of the stressor, whereas the depth correlates with the degree of damage to the nail matrix. **Onychomadesis** is a full-thickness depression, in which the insult is severe enough to cause complete separation and eventual shedding of the nail plate. In contrast, **onychoschizia** is limited to the distal nail plate. It results from impaired intercellular adhesion within the nail plate and presents as fine, peeling, horizontal layers at the nails' distal free edge.

D. There are many nail changes that present with longitudinal color change. **Melanonychia** (brown or black discoloration) and **erythronychia** (red discoloration) are discussed in more detail in Chapter 92.

Splinter hemorrhages evolve from erythronychia to melanonychia over days. They are 1- to 3 mm linear subungual hemorrhages, typically on the distal third of the nail; their name derives from their resemblance to wood splinters. They can be a sign of endocarditis, but they are also found in other patients, including those with psoriasis.

E. Structural longitudinal nail disorders may affect the entirety of the involved nail(s) or only part of the nail(s). In general, **longitudinal nail splitting** can occur at the distal edge, the proximal nail fold, or evenly dividing the entire nail plate into two. It develops due to injury to the nail plate itself or to the nail matrix.

A **longitudinal groove** originates from the proximal nail fold and typically affects only one nail. These grooves are most often the result of damage to the nail matrix from a small tumor such as a fibroma or myxoid cyst in the nail fold.

Median canaliform dystrophy of Heller presents as a single midline split in the nail plate with oblique furrows along both sides, giving it the appearance of a fir tree. It can affect one nail (most commonly the thumb) or multiple. It is often due to self-induced repetitive trauma from pushing on the cuticle and proximal nail fold, but oral retinoids are another common cause.

Dorsal pterygium occurs due to scarring between the proximal nail fold and matrix and is most commonly due to lichen planus.

F. The two main nail changes described in patients with complete nail involvement are trachyonychia and onychorrhexis. Most commonly due to lichen planus, **trachyonychia** affects the entire nail plate, causing longitudinal ridges throughout a thinned, dull nail plate with a roughened sandpaper-like texture. It can involve one nail but often causes "twenty nail dystrophy." **Onychorrhexis** also presents with longitudinal ridging as well as thinning and splitting, although it does not have the rough texture of trachyonychia. It is most often caused by handwashing and dermatitis. The term "brittle nails" typically refers to onychorrhexis and onychoschizia.

See Appendix 1 for Further Reading and Image References.

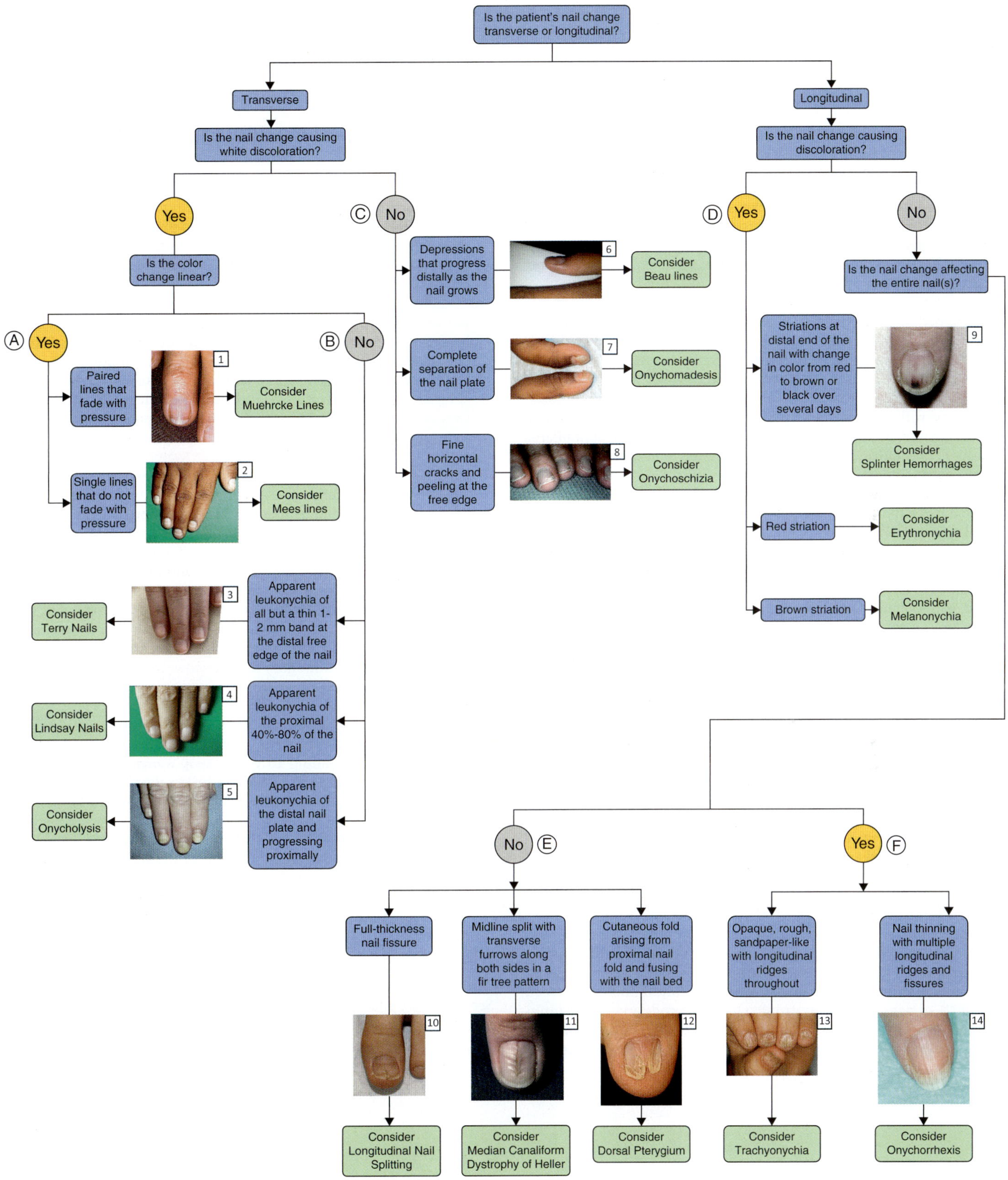
Is the patient's nail change transverse or longitudinal?
Transverse
Is the nail change causing white discoloration?
Yes
Is the color change linear?
A Yes
Paired lines that fade with pressure
1
Consider Muehrcke Lines
Single lines that do not fade with pressure
2
Consider Mees lines
B No
Apparent leukonychia of all but a thin 1-2 mm band at the distal free edge of the nail
3
Consider Terry Nails
Apparent leukonychia of the proximal 40%-80% of the nail
4
Consider Lindsay Nails
Apparent leukonychia of the distal nail plate and progressing proximally
5
Consider Onycholysis
C No
Depressions that progress distally as the nail grows
6
Consider Beau lines
Complete separation of the nail plate
7
Consider Onychomadesis
Fine horizontal cracks and peeling at the free edge
8
Consider Onychoschizia
Longitudinal
Is the nail change causing discoloration?
D Yes
Striations at distal end of the nail with change in color from red to brown or black over several days
9
Consider Splinter Hemorrhages
Red striation
Consider Erythronychia
Brown striation
Consider Melanonychia
No
Is the nail change affecting the entire nail(s)?
No E
Full-thickness nail fissure
10
Consider Longitudinal Nail Splitting
Midline split with transverse furrows along both sides in a fir tree pattern
11
Consider Median Canaliform Dystrophy of Heller
Cutaneous fold arising from proximal nail fold and fusing with the nail bed
12
Consider Dorsal Pterygium
Yes F
Opaque, rough, sandpaper-like with longitudinal ridges throughout
13
Consider Trachyonychia
Nail thinning with multiple longitudinal ridges and fissures
14
Consider Onychorrhexis

94 Thickened Nails

Karen M. Ly and Natalie M. Fragoso

Nail thickening is a common type of nail dystrophy. It can be an isolated finding or occur alongside other nail and skin findings, which may provide a clue to the underlying diagnosis.

A. A detailed history and physical examination of the skin, nails, and hair should be performed. The history should include the age of onset of nail thickening, history of dermatologic disease, relevant family history, a review of patient footwear and exposures, and any pertinent systemic symptoms.

B. Thickened nails can be broadly categorized as nail thickening due to subungual hyperkeratosis, with the accumulation of subungual scaling from the increased proliferation of keratinocytes, or thickening of the nail plate itself, also called onychauxis.

C. Patients with subungual hyperkeratosis may have an associated inflammatory skin disease, such as psoriasis, pityriasis rubra pilaris, or hand dermatitis. **Nail psoriasis** occurs due to inflammation of the nail matrix and nail bed and is seen in 7% to 56% of patients with psoriasis. Fingernails are affected more often than toenails. Other associated nail findings include multiple coarse pits, salmon patches, and splinter hemorrhages. Patients with **pityriasis rubra pilaris** may have nails that are thickened with yellow-brown discoloration and subungual debris. Skin examination will likely reveal perifollicular keratotic papules, salmon-colored plaques with islands of sparing, and palmoplantar keratoderma. **Chronic hand dermatitis**, which can be due to atopic dermatitis or contact dermatitis, can present with subungual hyperkeratosis, onycholysis, and fissuring of the nail plate. There may be edema and inflammation of the nail fold and dermatitis of the digits and hands, which suggests the underlying cause.

D. **Onychomycosis (tinea unguium)** is a fungal infection of the nail that is caused by dermatophytes, yeasts, or nondermatophyte molds. It is a common condition that represents 50% of all nail diseases; it presents with a combination of white or yellow nail discoloration, onycholysis, subungual hyperkeratosis, and nail thickening. Concurrent tinea pedis may be seen with toenail involvement.

Nail plate thickening, or onychauxis, is caused by hypertrophy of the nail plate. The nail is hyperkeratotic and discolored, with a loss of translucency.

E. Presentation of onychauxis at birth in conjunction with other dermatologic findings is suggestive of a genetic disorder. **Pachyonychia congenita** is a group of autosomal dominant genodermatoses caused by mutations in keratin proteins. Three key clinical findings are seen in 90% of patients: nail dystrophy, focal keratoderma, and palmoplantar pain. Toes, thumbs, and index fingers are most commonly affected, but all digits may be involved. Nails are very thickened, and hyperkeratosis of the nail bed produces increased transverse curvature of the nail plate.

Epidermolysis bullosa (EB) is a group of genetic disorders characterized by mechanically fragile skin that blisters after minor trauma. Nail abnormalities can be seen in all types of EB, including nail thickening, which presents with a yellow, thick, and short nail plate due to scarring of the nail bed. Onychogryphosis, granulation tissue of the nail bed, nail atrophy, and anonychia from frequent blistering can also be seen.

Ectodermal dysplasias are a group of inherited disorders involving abnormalities in at least two ectodermally derived structures: hair, nail, skin, and sweat glands. Nails may be normal or a defining characteristic of the disease. In hidrotic ectodermal dysplasia, infants have milky white nails that gradually thicken during childhood. Hair is brittle, pale, and wiry, which distinguishes it from pachyonychia congenita. Thickened nails may also be seen in ankyloblepharon-ectodermal dysplasia-clefting syndrome.

F. Patients with laterally deviated great toenails present since birth or childhood without any other findings of the skin, hair, or nails may have **congenital malalignment of the great toenails**. The nail plates of the great toes are laterally deviated from their longitudinal axes and may be markedly thickened.

G. A patient with systemic symptoms and onset of nail abnormalities in adulthood may have **yellow nail syndrome**. The nails are strikingly yellow and thickened, with increased curvature. Typically, all 20 nails are involved. It is characterized by a triad of yellow nails, lymphedema, and pulmonary disease; however, nail changes may be an isolated finding.

H. Nail thickening can also occur due to chronic **trauma**. Abnormalities in foot or digit anatomy or poorly fitting shoes can predispose to repeated trauma, leading to onychauxis. **Onychogryphosis** is an exaggerated thickening and lateral enlargement of the nail plate most commonly seen in the elderly, giving the nail the appearance of a rams horn.

I. **Onychomatricoma** is a benign tumor of the nail matrix suspected to be due to abnormal nail matrix differentiation. Clinical findings include a localized or diffuse thickening of the nail plate, transverse and longitudinal curvature, multiple splinter hemorrhages, and swelling of the proximal nail fold. When the nail is avulsed, a tumor with fingerlike projections is seen near the proximal nail fold.

See Appendix 1 for Further Reading and Image References.

- Patient presenting with thickened nails
- (A) Detailed history and physical examination of the skin, nails, and hair
- (B) Does the examination reveal subungual hyperkeratosis or thickened nail plate?
  - **Subungual hyperkeratosis**
    - Is there an associated inflammatory skin condition?
      - (C) **Yes**
        - Nail pitting, salmon patches, psoriatic plaques on the extensors, inflammatory arthritis
          - 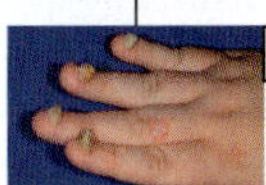
          - 1
          - Subungual hyperkeratosis in a patient with an adjacent cutaneous psoriatic plaque on the third finger
          - Consider Psoriasis
        - Perifollicular papules, salmon-colored plaques with islands of sparing, palmoplantar keratoderma
          - Consider Pityriasis Rubra Pilaris
        - Erythematous scaly plaques of the hands, +/– fissuring, +/– lichenification
          - Consider Chronic Hand Dermatitis
      - (D) **No**
        - Onycholysis, yellow discoloration, subungual debris +/– tinea pedis
          - Consider Onychomycosis
  - **Thickened nail plate**
    - Were the nail changes present at birth or early in life?
      - **Yes**
        - Are there also other skin, hair, or nail findings?
          - (E) **Yes**
            - Severely thickened nails with increased curvature, painful keratoderma
              - 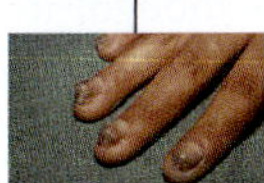
              - 2
              - Markedly thickened, discolored fingernails with an upward projection at the free edge
              - Consider Pachyonychia Congenita
            - Mechanically fragile skin that blisters with trauma, thickened nail plates
              - 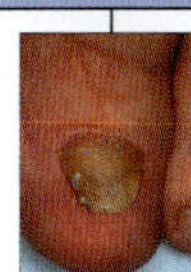
              - 3
              - Thickened, yellowed, and shortening of the great toe
              - Consider Epidermolysis Bullosa
            - Thickened nails, +/– hair abnormalities (brittle, wiry hair), +/– skin or sweat gland abnormalities
              - Consider Ectodermal Dysplasias
          - (F) **No**
            - Lateral deviation of the great toenails
              - Consider Congenital Malalignment of the Great Toes
      - **No**
        - Are there associated systemic symptoms?
          - **Yes** (G)
            - Yellow, thickened nails involving all 20 nails, +/– lymphedema, +/– pulmonary disease
              - 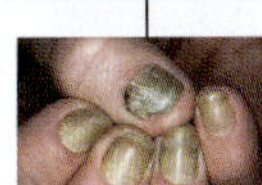
              - 4
              - Pale yellow discoloration and thickening of the nail plates with an increased transverse curvature
              - Consider Yellow Nail Syndrome
          - **No** (H) (I)
            - Evidence of bony deformities of the digits or ill-fitting shoes
              - Consider Trauma
            - Marked lateral enlargement of the nail plates
              - 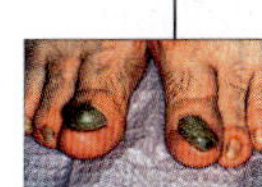
              - 5
              - Thickened and elongated yellow-green toenails resembling a Ram's horn
              - Consider Onychogryphosis
            - Thickening of the nail plate, increased curvature, +/– swelling of the proximal nail fold
              - 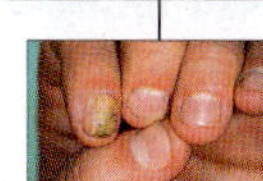
              - 6
              - Longitudinal yellow and thickened band of the index finger
              - Consider Onychomatricoma

95 Other Textural Nail Changes

Gabrielle E. Duprat and Natalie M. Fragoso

Textural nail changes can occur as an isolated finding or may be a clue to identifying underlying systemic disorders. A careful history and physical examination can help elucidate the etiology of the underlying textural nail changes.

A. The character of the textural change should be assessed; do the nails have pitting, is there general roughness on the external surface of the nail plate, or is there detachment from the nail bed?

B. Nail pitting refers to punctate depressions on the nail plate surface caused by abnormal keratinization. The number and quality of pits can help determine the diagnosis.

If the patient presents with pits that are small, geometrically distributed, and less numerous, then **alopecia areata (AA)** should be considered.

If the pits are large, deep, and irregularly spaced, then **psoriasis** should be considered. Other clues to indicate psoriasis include the presence of more than 20 pits, whereas the presence of 60 pits confirms psoriasis. Nail psoriasis can also present with crumbling, oil spots, onychomadesis, and onycholysis.

C. Patients with nail roughness should be assessed for a history of distal nail splitting. **Brittle nail syndrome (onychoschizia)** presents with roughness of the nail plate, splitting (onychoschizia), ridging, and onycholysis. It typically affects elderly females. Exposure to certain chemicals causes damage to adhesion between corneocytes and is thought to play a role in pathogenesis.

D. General roughness of the nail plate in the setting of self-induced trauma suggests onychotillomania, including **nail biting, habit-tic deformity**, and **median canaliform dystrophy**. If only the thumb is involved, then this suggests either median canaliform dystrophy or habit-tic deformity.

Median canaliform dystrophy presents with a longitudinal split in the middle of the nail, which gives a fir-tree appearance. This typically presents symmetrically on the bilateral thumbnails. The etiology is unknown but is thought to be secondary to trauma or from isotretinoin.

E. **Habit-tic deformity** is secondary to repeatedly rubbing the nail fold. This typically presents on the thumb as multiple midline Beau lines. Instruments may also be used to destroy the nails, and patients may lack insight into the condition. This is associated with a variety of psychiatric disorders, including obsessive-compulsive disorder, depression, and body dysmorphia. First-line therapy includes occluding the nail from trauma (adhesive bandages or occlusive dressings).

F. **Nail biting (onychophagia)** typically affects the nail plate or the proximal nail fold. This can lead to nail surface irregularities, splinter hemorrhages, and longitudinal melanonychia.

G. The presence of roughness over the entire nail plate without a history of self-induced trauma suggests **trachyonychia**. Trachyonychia is due to diffuse damage to the proximal nail matrix, often from underlying inflammatory conditions, and can affect 1 to 20 nails. It is most common in children, where it typically affects all 20 nails and is usually idiopathic. In adults, trachyonychia is most commonly due to AA. Patients with more severe AA are more likely to have nail changes, including pitting, trachyonychia, onycholysis, and ridging. Trachyonychia represents 12% of nail changes associated with AA in children and 3% in adults. Other associations include lichen planus, atopic dermatitis, and psoriasis.

H. If there is detachment from the nail plate, it may be proximal, lateral, or distal. If the nail is detached from the distal or lateral edge, it is called **onycholysis**. Onycholysis can frequently be caused by environmental insults (trauma and exposure to irritants), especially in patients with hand dermatitis. In such instances, fingernails are more commonly involved than toenails. Onycholysis can also be secondary to metabolic disorders, including hyperthyroidism. Patients will typically present with multiple nails involved and additional cutaneous findings consistent with hyperthyroidism. Infections such as candidiasis and human papillomavirus may also cause onycholysis; patients may present with nail color changes (yellow or green) and nail thickening. Patients with psoriasis can develop onycholysis but will also often have other nail changes, including oil drops and pits. Tetracycline antibiotics are among the most common drug causes of onycholysis in the fingernails, especially after sun exposure. If only one nail is involved, this is a clue to indicate that the change may be due to an underlying tumor, such as squamous cell carcinoma, melanoma, or fibroma.

I. **Onychomadesis** refers to the detachment of the nail plate from the proximal nail fold. This is thought to be a severe form of a Beau line. A detailed history can help elucidate the cause. Trauma is a common cause of onychomadesis. Major medical illnesses such as Stevens-Johnson syndrome, major depression, pneumonia, and Guillan-Barré syndrome have been associated with onychomadesis. Medications have also been implicated, including chemotherapeutics (capecitabine, doxorubicin, and etoposide) and antiepileptics (carbamazepine and valproic acid). This cause should be suspected if all nails are affected at the same level and a drug was taken 2 to 3 weeks prior to the onset of nail changes. Hand-foot-and-mouth disease is the most common cause of onychomadesis in children.

See Appendix 1 for Further Reading and Image References.

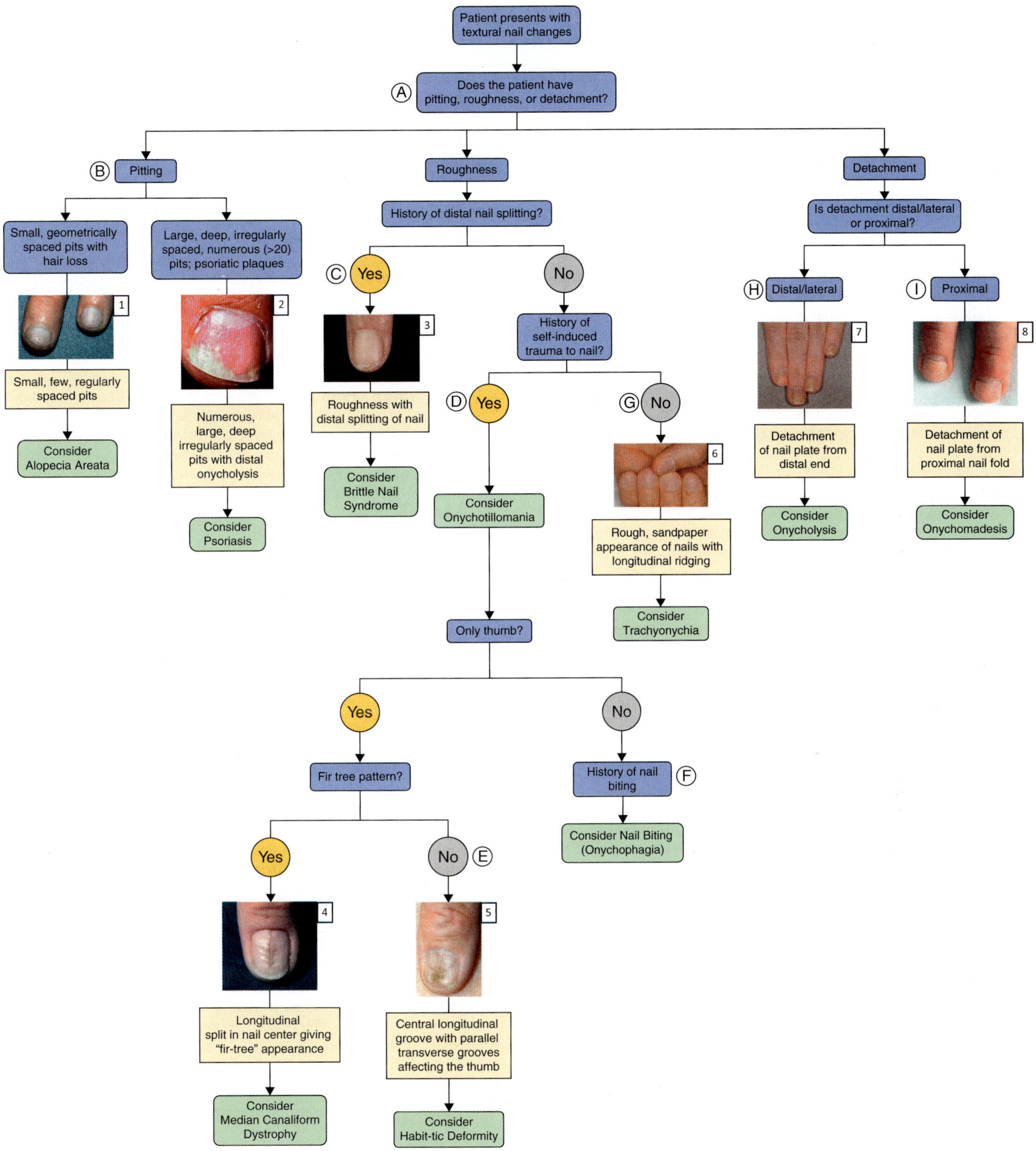
Patient presents with textural nail changes
A
Does the patient have pitting, roughness, or detachment?
B
Pitting
Roughness
Detachment
Small, geometrically spaced pits with hair loss
Large, deep, irregularly spaced, numerous (>20) pits; psoriatic plaques
1
Small, few, regularly spaced pits
Consider Alopecia Areata
2
Numerous, large, deep irregularly spaced pits with distal onycholysis
Consider Psoriasis
History of distal nail splitting?
C
Yes
No
3
Roughness with distal splitting of nail
Consider Brittle Nail Syndrome
History of self-induced trauma to nail?
D
Yes
G
No
Consider Onychotillomania
6
Rough, sandpaper appearance of nails with longitudinal ridging
Consider Trachyonychia
Only thumb?
Yes
No
Fir tree pattern?
History of nail biting
F
Consider Nail Biting (Onychophagia)
Yes
No
E
4
Longitudinal split in nail center giving “fir-tree” appearance
Consider Median Canaliform Dystrophy
5
Central longitudinal groove with parallel transverse grooves affecting the thumb
Consider Habit-tic Deformity
Is detachment distal/lateral or proximal?
H
Distal/lateral
I
Proximal
7
Detachment of nail plate from distal end
Consider Onycholysis
8
Detachment of nail plate from proximal nail fold
Consider Onychomadesis

96 Isolated Nail Growths

Katrina H. Lee and Marcia Hogeling

Neoplasms of the nail often have unique findings that may aid clinicians in diagnosis and further management. It is important for clinicians to identify growths concerning for malignancy so that prompt referral for biopsy and appropriate treatment may be initiated. Management is specific to each condition but may include reassurance, monitoring, destruction, or surgical intervention.

A. The initial evaluation of isolated nail growths should involve obtaining a detailed history, especially regarding duration, progression of the lesion, and any associated symptoms. A thorough examination of both the affected and all unaffected finger and toenail units is essential. The nail plate, nail bed, lunula, eponychium, hyponychium, nail folds, and surrounding skin should be closely assessed. Palpation of the neoplasm will reveal the lesion's contour and consistency and may elicit tenderness in cases of malignancy or glomus tumors. Dermoscopy and radiographic imaging may be useful diagnostic tools.

B. Determining whether the isolated nail growth is melanocytic or nonmelanocytic will greatly narrow the differential diagnosis. Clinical features that may indicate a benign neoplasm include young age of onset, a band even in width and homogeneous in color, involvement of multiple nails, or pigmentation at other mucocutaneous sites (suggestive of genodermatoses such as Peutz-Jeghers or Laugier-Hunziker). In an adult with new-onset or changing melanonychia, consider the diagnosis of **subungual melanoma**. Features suggestive of melanoma include 50 years or older at onset, rapid change in appearance, irregular pigmentation, uneven width of band (particularly increased width at the base of the nail), nail dystrophy, and extension of pigment onto the proximal nail fold (Hutchinson sign). If there is any clinical concern for subungual melanoma, the patient should be promptly referred for biopsy. See Chapter 92 for a more detailed differential.

C. In a patient presenting with a thin longitudinal growth isolated to the nail plate with associated longitudinal erythronychia, consider the diagnosis of **onychopapilloma**. The keratotic tumor can be visualized on the underside of the plate when looking at the nail en face. Additional features include distal V-nicking, thinning of the nail plate directly over the tumor, and distal splinter hemorrhages.

D. **Onychomatricomas** present with localized thickening of the nail plate, leading to overcurvature of the nail with yellow-hued streaking. At the distal end, multiple holes and cavities are present. Occasionally, associated splinter hemorrhages or melanonychia may be present. Onychomatricomas are benign and typically painless.

E. Tender blue or red subungual macules should raise suspicion for **glomus tumors**. Palpation of the lesion on physical examination should elicit highly localized pain, known as the Love sign. The patient may also describe increased sensitivity to the cold. A magnetic resonance imaging with contrast may be obtained to aid in diagnosis. Characteristic glomus cells should be identified on the histology of excisional specimens.

F. **Squamous cell carcinoma (SCC)** is the most common malignancy of the nail unit. Up to three-fourths of periungual SCCs are caused by the human papillomavirus. Thus any wart that is progressive despite treatment should raise suspicion for malignancy. Helpful clues include pain, oozing, crusting, and disruption of nail architecture. **Keratoacanthomas (KA)** are typically painful and grow rapidly over weeks. **Verrucous carcinoma (VC)** is a low-grade variant of SCC that rarely metastasizes but can be locally destructive.

G. If there is a history of rapidly growing and bleeding periungual or subungual growth with a friable exophytic papulonodule on examination, the diagnosis of **pyogenic granuloma (PG)** should be considered. There is often a history of preceding trauma in the affected area. PGs may also be drug induced. Common culprits include oral contraceptives, retinoids, and epidermal growth factor receptor (EGFR) inhibitors.

H. In a patient with a known history of tuberous sclerosis (TS), the diagnosis of **periungual fibroma (Koenen tumor)** should be considered for any periungual growths. They present as firm, skin-colored papulonodules over the proximal nail folds. The tip of the lesion is often keratotic. Patients with TS begin to form periungual fibromas during adolescence and often have lesions involving multiple digits as they reach adulthood. In the general population, these neoplasms typically involve a single nail.

I. History of preceding trauma resulting in a firm bony growth under the nail should prompt the diagnosis of **subungual exostosis**. This benign nail tumor commonly affects the great toe. Diagnosis may be confirmed by a radiograph.

J. **Digital myxoid cysts** present as soft, compressible translucent papulonodules over the proximal nail fold or distal interphalangeal joint. Longitudinal nail grooves or dystrophy is appreciated when the pseudocyst compresses the nail matrix. Jellylike contents are expressed from the lesion when aspirated with an 18-gauge needle. Relapse of the myxoid cysts is common despite various treatment modalities. Excision offers the highest cure rate.

K. The diagnosis of **warts** relies heavily on clinical findings. Verrucous papules may be peri- or subungual. Dermoscopy reveals characteristic thrombosed capillary loops. Fingernails are more commonly affected than toenails.

See Appendix 1 for Further Reading and Image References.

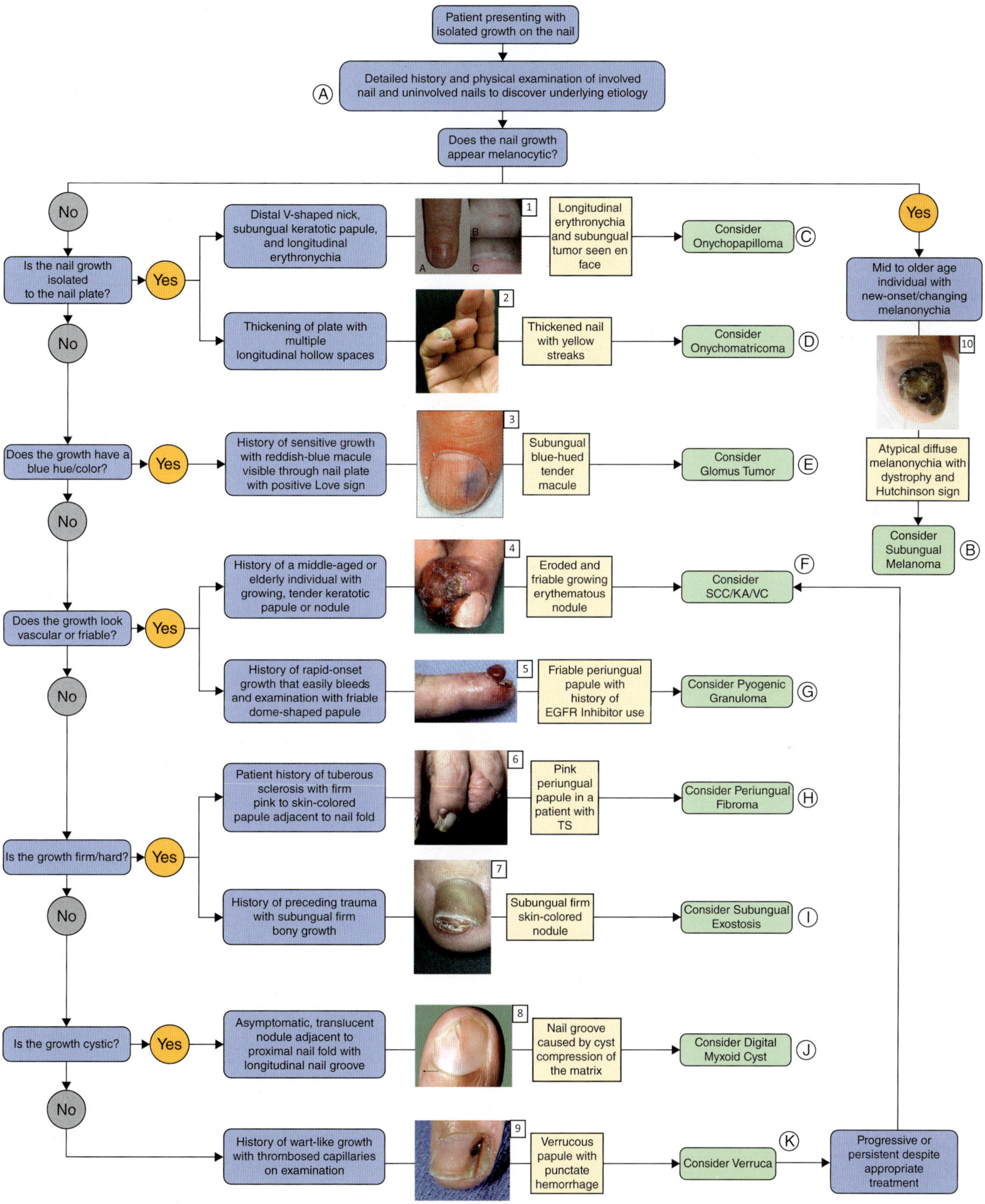
Patient presenting with isolated growth on the nail
A
Detailed history and physical examination of involved nail and uninvolved nails to discover underlying etiology
Does the nail growth appear melanocytic?
No
Is the nail growth isolated to the nail plate?
Yes
Distal V-shaped nick, subungual keratotic papule, and longitudinal erythronychia
1
A
B
C
Longitudinal erythronychia and subungual tumor seen en face
Consider Onychopapilloma
C
Thickening of plate with multiple longitudinal hollow spaces
2
Thickened nail with yellow streaks
Consider Onychomatricoma
D
No
Does the growth have a blue hue/color?
Yes
History of sensitive growth with reddish-blue macule visible through nail plate with positive Love sign
3
Subungual blue-hued tender macule
Consider Glomus Tumor
E
No
Does the growth look vascular or friable?
Yes
History of a middle-aged or elderly individual with growing, tender keratotic papule or nodule
4
Eroded and friable growing erythematous nodule
F
Consider SCC/KA/VC
History of rapid-onset growth that easily bleeds and examination with friable dome-shaped papule
5
Friable periungual papule with history of EGFR Inhibitor use
Consider Pyogenic Granuloma
G
No
Is the growth firm/hard?
Yes
Patient history of tuberous sclerosis with firm pink to skin-colored papule adjacent to nail fold
6
Pink periungual papule in a patient with TS
Consider Periungual Fibroma
H
History of preceding trauma with subungual firm bony growth
7
Subungual firm skin-colored nodule
Consider Subungual Exostosis
I
No
Is the growth cystic?
Yes
Asymptomatic, translucent nodule adjacent to proximal nail fold with longitudinal nail groove
8
Nail groove caused by cyst compression of the matrix
Consider Digital Myxoid Cyst
J
No
History of wart-like growth with thrombosed capillaries on examination
9
Verrucous papule with punctate hemorrhage
K
Consider Verruca
Progressive or persistent despite appropriate treatment
Yes
Mid to older age individual with new-onset/changing melanonychia
10
Atypical diffuse melanonychia with dystrophy and Hutchinson sign
Consider Subungual Melanoma
B

APPENDIX 1
Additional Materials

Further Reading and Image References

Chapter 1

FURTHER READING

Callen J. Approach to the patient with facial erythema. *UpToDate*. 2021. Available from: https://www.uptodate.com/contents/approach-to-the-patient-with-facial-erythema?search=facial%20erythema&source=search_result&selectedTitle=1~150&usage_type=default&display_rank=1#H1132364904.

Cobos GA, Femia A, Vleugels RA. Dermatomyositis: an update on diagnosis and treatment. *Am J Clin Dermatol.* 2020;1(3):339–353. https://doi.org/10.1007/s40257-020-00502-6.

Drucker AM, Rosen CF. Drug-induced photosensitivity: culprit drugs, management and prevention. *Drug Saf.* 2011;34(10):821–837. https://doi.org/10.2165/11592780-000000000-00000.

Marks J, Miller J. *Lookingbill and Marks' Principles of Dermatology*. 6th ed. Elsevier; 2019.

Okon LG, Werth VP. Cutaneous lupus erythematosus: diagnosis and treatment. *Best Pract Res Clin Rheumatol.* 2013;27(3):391–404. https://doi.org/10.1016/j.berh.2013.07.008.

IMAGE REFERENCES

1. From https://www.jaad.org/article/S0190-9622(20)30127-4/fulltext
2. From https://www.jaad.org/article/S0190-9622(17)32603-8/fulltext
3. From https://www.jaad.org/article/S0190-9622(05)00929-1/fulltext
4. From https://www.jaadcasereports.org/article/S2352-5126(22)00182-5/fulltext
5. Plant Dermatitis. Available from: https://www.sciencedirect.com/science/article/abs/pii/S0733862724000415.
6. Type I hypersensitivity in photoallergic contact dermatitis. Available from: https://www.jaadcasereports.org/article/S2352-5126(23)00458-7/fulltext.
7. *Dermatology: An Illustrated Colour Text*. Chapter 65, 142–143.
8. Phototoxic drug eruption induced by vandetanib used for the treatment of metastatic medullary thyroid cancer. Available from: https://www.sciencedirect.com/science/article/pii/S0365059622001337?via%3Dihub.
9. From https://phil.cdc.gov/details.aspx?pid=2874 (public domain)
10. Non-tuberculous Mycobacterium facial cellulitis in an immunocompromised rheumatoid arthritis patient--Skin biopsy can help. Available from: https://www.sciencedirect.com/science/article/pii/S2214250923001932?via%3Dihub.
11. From Marks JG, Miller JJ, Lookingbill DP. *Lookingbill and Marks' Principles of Dermatology* (6th ed.). Elsevier; 2019.
12. From https://www.jaadcasereports.org/article/S2352-5126(19)30416-3/fulltext
13. From https://www.sciencedirect.com/science/article/pii/S0738081X06001076#fig1
14. Reprinted with permission from Momen SE, Diaz-Cano S, Walsh S, Creamer D. Discriminating minor and major forms of drug reaction with eosinophilia and systemic symptoms: Facial edema aligns to the severe phenotype. *J Am Acad Dermatol.* 2021;84(5):1157–1158.

Chapter 2

FURTHER READING

Kang S, Amagai M, Bruckner AL, McMichael AJ, Orringer JS, et al. *Fitzpatrick's Dermatology*. 9th ed. McGraw Hill; 2019. https://accessmedicine.mhmedical.com/content.aspx?bookid=2570&sectionid=210413309.

Bolognia JL, Schaffer JV, Cerroni L. *Dermatology*. 4th ed. Elsevier; 2017. https://www.elsevier.com/books/dermatology-2-volume-set/bolognia/978-0-7020-6275-9.

Mauskar MM, Marathe K, Venkatesan A, Schlosser BJ, Edwards L. Vulvar diseases: approach to the patient. *J Am Acad Dermatol.* 2020;82(6):1277–1284. PubMed ID: 31712174.

Bayers S, Shulman ST, Paller AS. Kawasaki disease: part I. Diagnosis, clinical features, and pathogenesis. *J Am Acad Dermatol.* 2013;69(4): 501.e1-11; quiz 511-2. PubMed ID: 24034379.

Sheth KR, Keays M, Grimsby GM, et al. Diagnosing testicular torsion before urological consultation and imaging: validation of the TWIST score. *J Urol.* 2016;195(6):1870–1876. PubMed ID: 26835833.

IMAGE REFERENCES

2. Dinulos JGH. Infestations and bites. In: *Habif's Clinical Dermatology: A Color Guide to Diagnosis and Therapy*. 7th ed. Elsevier; 2019:571–630. https://www.elsevier.com/books/habifs-clinical-dermatology/dinulos/978-0-323-61269-2
3. Dinulos JGH. Candida balanitis. In: *Habif's Clinical Dermatology: A Color Guide to Diagnosis and Therapy*. 7th ed. Elsevier; 2019:483–524. https://www.elsevier.com/books/habifs-clinical-dermatology/dinulos/978-0-323-61269-2
4. Dinulos JGH. Psoriasis and other papulosquamous diseases. In: *Habif's Clinical Dermatology: A Color Guide to Diagnosis and Therapy*. 7th ed. Elsevier; 2019: 483–524. https://www.elsevier.com/books/habifs-clinical-dermatology/dinulos/978-0-323-61269-2
5. Dinulos JGH. Psoriasis and other papulosquamous diseases. In: *Habif's Clinical Dermatology: A Color Guide to Diagnosis and Therapy*. 7th ed. Elsevier; 2019: 483–524. https://www.elsevier.com/books/habifs-clinical-dermatology/dinulos/978-0-323-61269-2
6. Bolognia JL, Schaffer JV, Cerroni L. *Dermatology*. 4th ed. Elsevier; 2018. Courtesy Robert Hartman, MD.
7. JA de Hullu and AGJ van der Zee. "Surgery and radiotherapy in vulvar cancer" in Critical Reviews in Oncology/Hematology 2006 October; 60(1):38-58.
8. Partin AW, Dmochowski RR, Kavoussi LR, et al. Management of abnormalities of the external genitalia in boys. In: *Campbell Walsh Wein Urology*. 12th ed. Elsevier; 2022:871–904. https://www.us.elsevierhealth.com/campbell-walsh-wein-urology-9780323546423.html
9. Courtesy Anne W. Lucky, MD
10. Robert G. Micheletti, William D. James, Dirk M. Elston, Patrick J. McMahon. Andrews' Diseases of the Skin Clinical Atlas, 2nd ed. Elsevier; 2023.
11. Dinulos JGH. Eczema and hand dermatitis. In: *Habif's Clinical Dermatology: A Color Guide to Diagnosis and Therapy*. 7th ed. Elsevier; 2019:483–524. https://www.elsevier.com/books/habifs-clinical-dermatology/dinulos/978-0-323-61269-2
12. Dinulos JGH. Eczema and hand dermatistis. In: *Habif's Clinical Dermatology: A Color Guide to Diagnosis and Therapy*. 7th ed. Elsevier; 2019:483–524. https://www.elsevier.com/books/habifs-clinical-dermatology/dinulos/978-0-323-61269-2
13. Dinulos JGH. Psoriasis and other papulosquamous diseases. In: *Habif's Clinical Dermatology: A Color Guide to Diagnosis and Therapy*. 7th ed. Elsevier; 2019: 483–524. https://www.elsevier.com/books/habifs-clinical-dermatology/dinulos/978-0-323-61269-2
14. Courtesy Scott D. Worswick.
15. Abbas, et al. Red scrotum syndrome: an update on clinicopathologic features, pathogenesis, diagnosis, and management. *J Am Acad Dermatol.* 2022; 87(3).
16. Reproduced with permission from Reid A. Waldman, Jane M. Grant-Kels Dermatology for the Primary Care Provider, 1e:119-133 Elsevier; 2022.
17. Dinulos JGH. Warts, herpes simplex, and other viral infections. In: *Habif's Clinical Dermatology: A Color Guide to Diagnosis and Therapy*. 7th ed. Elsevier; 2019:483–524. https://www.elsevier.com/books/habifs-clinical-dermatology/dinulos/978-0-323-61269-2
18. Marks JG Jr, Miller JJ. Eczematous rashes. In: *Lookingbill and Mark's Principles of Dermatology*. 6th ed. Elsevier; 2006:95–112. https://www.sciencedirect.com/book/9781416031857/lookingbill-and-marks-principles-of-dermatology
19. Dinulos JGH. Hypersensitivity syndromes and vasculitis. In: *Habif's Clinical Dermatology: A Color Guide to Diagnosis and Therapy*. 7th ed. Elsevier; 2019: 713–747. https://www.elsevier.com/books/habifs-clinical-dermatology/dinulos/978-0-323-61269-2
20. From the Fitzsimons Army Medical Center Collection, Aurora, Colorado.
21. Pride H. Crohn's disease: erythema, swelling, and a dusky cyanotic discoloration in early cutaneous disease. *Pediatric Dermatol.* 2009.

Chapter 3

FURTHER READING

Bolognia J, Jorizzo JL, Schaffer JV. *Dermatology*. 4th ed. Elsevier Saunders; 2017.

Bolognia J, Schaffer JV, Duncan KO, Ko CJ. *Dermatology Essentials*. 2nd ed. Elsevier; 2021.

Dinulos JG. *Habif's Clinical Dermatology*. 7th ed. Elsevier; 2021.

James WD, Elston D, Treat JR, Rosenbach MA. *Andrews' Diseases of the Skin: Clinical Dermatology*. 13th ed. Elsevier; 2019.

Paller AS, Mancini AJ. *Hurwitz Clinical Pediatric Dermatology*. 6th ed. Elsevier; 2022.

IMAGE REFERENCES

1. Bolognia JL, Schaffer JV, Cerroni L. *Dermatology*. 4th ed. Elsevier; 2018. (A) Courtesy Robert Hartman, MD; (B) Courtesy Mary Stone, MD; (C,D) Courtesy Julie V. Schaffer, MD.
2. Li AW, Yin ES, Stahl M, et al. The skin as a window to the blood: cutaneous manifestations of myeloid malignancies. *Blood Rev.* 2017;31(6):370–388.

3. Cleminson K, Cunningham N. Acute generalized exanthematous pustulosis. *CMAJ*. 2020;192(42):E1268.
4. High WA, Prok LD. Dermatology Secrets. 6th ed. Elsevier; 2021.
5. Courtesy of Karolyn Wanat, Medical College of Wisconsin.
6. Krooks J, Minkov M, Weatherall AG. Langerhans cell histiocytosis in children: history, classification, pathobiology, clinical manifestations, and prognosis. *J Am Acad Dermatol*. 2018;78(6):1035–1044.
7. Courtesy of Karolyn Wanat, Medical College of Wisconsin.
8. Bolognia JL, Schaffer JV, Cerroni L. *Dermatology*. 4th ed. Elsevier; 2018. Courtesy Kalman Watsky, MD.
9. Bolognia JL, Schaffer JV, Cerroni L. *Dermatology*. 4th ed. Elsevier; 2018. A, Courtesy Lorenzo Cerroni, MD; B, Courtesy Mary Stone, MD; C, D, Courtesy Julie V. Schaffer, MD.
10. Sheila S. Galbraith, MD.
11. Courtesy of Karolyn Wanat, Medical College of Wisconsin.
12. Courtesy of Karolyn Wanat, Medical College of Wisconsin.
13. Courtesy of Karolyn Wanat, Medical College of Wisconsin.

Chapter 4

FURTHER READING

Bolognia J, Schaffer J, Duncan K, Ko C. *Dermatology Essentials*. 2nd ed. Elsevier; 2022.

Nelson C, Stephen S, Ashchyan H, James W, Micheletti R, Rosenbach M. Neutrophilic dermatoses: pathogenesis, Sweet syndrome, neutrophilic eccrine hidradenitis, and Behçet disease. *J Am Acad Dermatol*. 2018;79(6):987–1006. https://doi.org/10.1016/j.jaad.2017.11.064.

Nyssen A, Benhadou F, Magnée M, André J, Koopmansch C, Wautrecht JC. Chilblains. *J Vasc Dis*. 2020;49(2):133–140. https://doi.org/10.1024/0301-1526/a000838.

Raieli V, Compagno A, D'Amelio M. Red ear syndrome. *Curr Pain Headache Rep*. 2016;20(3):19. https://doi.org/10.1007/s11916-016-0547-y.

Serrao R, Zirwas M, English J. Palmar erythema. *Am J Clin Dermatol*. 2007;8(6):347–356. https://doi.org/10.2165/00128071-200708060-00004.

IMAGE REFERENCES

1. Reprinted with permission from Hustchison RL: Frostbite of the hand. *J Hand Surg Am*. 39:183, 2014.

2A. Dinulos J. *Habif's Clinical Dermatology: A Color Guide to Diagnosis and Therapy*. 7th ed. Elsevier; 2021.

2B. Dinulos J. *Habif's Clinical Dermatology: A Color Guide to Diagnosis and Therapy*. 7th ed. Elsevier; 2021.

3. James W, Elston D, Treat J, Rosenbach M, Neuhaus I. *Andrew's Diseases of the Skin*. 13th ed. Elsevier; 2020.
4. Courtesy Kalman Watsky, MD.
5. Courtesy Christopher Baker, MD, and Robert Kelly, MD.

6A. Hochberg M, Gravallese E, Silman A, Smolen J, Wienblatt M, Weisman M. *Rheumatology*. 7th ed. Elsevier; 2019.

6B. Hochberg M, Gravallese E, Silman A, Smolen J, Wienblatt M, Weisman M. *Rheumatology*. 7th ed. Elsevier; 2019.

7. From Moitri MO, Banglawala SM, Archibald J. Red ear syndrome: literature review and a pediatric case report. *Int J Pediatr Otorhinolaryngol*. 2015;79(3):281–285; Fig. 1.
8. From Yu Y, Cheng AS, Wang L, et al. Hot tub folliculitis or hot hand-foot syndrome caused by Pseudomonas aeruginosa. *J Am Acad Dermatol*. 2007;57:596–600.
9. Courtesy Jeffrey P. Callen, MD.
10. James W, Elston D, Treat J, Rosenbach M, Neuhaus I. *Andrew's Diseases of the Skin*. 13th ed. Elsevier; 2020.

11A. James W, Elston D, Treat J, Rosenbach M, Neuhaus I. *Andrew's Diseases of the Skin*. 13th ed. Elsevier; 2020.

11B. From Miller KK, Gorcey L, McLellan BN. Chemotherapy-induced hand-foot syndrome and nail changes: a review of clinical presentation, etiology, pathogenesis, and management. *J Am Acad Dermatol*. 2014;71(4):787–794.

11C. James W, Elston D, Treat J, Rosenbach M, Neuhaus I. *Andrew's Diseases of the Skin*. 13th ed. Elsevier; 2020.

Chapter 5

FURTHER READING

Bolognia JL, Schaffer JV, Duncan KO, Ko CJ. *Dermatology Essentials*. 2nd ed. Elsevier; 2022.

Marchionne EM, McCalmont TH, Pincus LB, LeBoit PE, Fox LP. Acute inflammatory edema: a mimicker of cellulitis in critically ill patients. *J Am Acad Dermatol*. 2019;81(4):931–936. https://doi.org/10.1016/j.jaad.2019.05.083.

Nadelman RB. Erythema migrans. *Infect Dis Clin North Am*. 2015;29(2):211–239. https://doi.org/10.1016/j.idc.2015.02.001.

Luis Rodríguez-Peralto J, Carrillo R, Rosales B, Rodríguez-Gil Y. Superficial thrombophlebitis. *Semin Cutan Med Surg*. 2007;26(2):71–76. https://doi.org/10.1016/j.sder.2007.02.002.

Bolognia J, Schaffer JV, Cerroni L. *Dermatology*. 4th ed. Elsevier; 2018.

IMAGE REFERENCES

1. Dinulos JG. *Habif's Clinical Dermatology*. 7th ed. Elsevier; 2019.
2. Reprinted with permission from Dermatology Essentials, 2nd ed. Ko CJ. Bolognia JL. Schaffer JV. Duncan KO. Elsevier; 2022. Courtesy, NYUDSC
3. Whitley, Richard J. *Mandell, Douglas, and Bennett's Principles and Practice of Infectious Diseases*. 2019. 1849–1856.e2.
4. James WD, Elston D, Treat JR, Rosenbach MA. *Andrews' Diseases of the Skin*. 13th ed. Elsevier; 2020.
5. Robert G. Micheletti, William D. James, Dirk M. Elston, Patrick J. McMahon. *Andrews' Diseases of the Skin Clinical Atlas*. 2nd ed. Elsevier; 2023.
6. Micheletti RG, James WD, Elston DM, McMahon PJ. *Andrews' Diseases of the Skin Clinical Atlas*. 2nd ed. Elsevier; 2021.

Chapter 6

FURTHER READING

Betrains A, Staels F, Schrijvers R, et al. Systemic autoinflammatory disease in adults. *Autoimmun Rev*. 2021;20(4):1–12. https://doi.org/10.1016/j.autrev.2021.102774.

Drago F, Ciccarese G, Gasparini G, et al. Contemporary infectious exanthems: an update. *Future Microbiol*. 2017;12:171–193. https://doi.org/10.2217/fmb-2016-0147.

Hughey L. Fever and erythema in the emergency room. *Semin Cutan Med Surg*. 2007;26(3):133–138. https://doi.org/10.1016/j.sder.2007.09.007.

Hannah-Shmouni F, Stratakis C, Koch C. Flushing in (neuro)endocrinology. *Rev Endocr Metab Disord*. 2016;17(3):373–380. https://doi.org/10.1007/s11154-016-9394-8.

Roccuzzo G, Giordano S, Avallone G, et al. Sézary syndrome: different erythroderma morphological features with proposal for a clinical score system. *Cells*. 2022;11(3):1–8. https://doi.org/10.3390/cells11030333.

IMAGE REFERENCES

1. Courtesy Scott D. Worswick, MD.
2. Courtesy Scott D. Worswick, MD.
3. Cohen B. *Pediatric Dermatology*. 5th ed. Elsevier; 2022.
4. James W. *Andrew's Diseases of the Skin*. 13th ed. Elsevier; 2020.
5. From Kliegman, R. M., Stanton, B. F., St. Geme, J. W., et al. [Eds.]. [2011]. *Nelson textbook of pediatrics* [19th ed.]. Saunders.

Chapter 7

FURTHER READING

Bolognia J, Schaffer JV, Cerroni L, España A. *Figurate erythemas. Dermatology*. Elsevier; 2008:277–285 [essay].

James WD, Berger TG, Elston DM. Erythema and urticaria. In: James WD, Berger TG, Elston DM, eds. *Andrews' Diseases of The Skin: Clinical Dermatology*. 12th ed. Elsevier; 2016:139–140 [essay].

Boehner A, Neuhauser R, Zink A, Ring J. Figurate erythemas—update and diagnostic approach. *J Dtsch Dermatol Ges*. 2021;19(7):963–972. https://doi.org/10.1111/ddg.14450.

McDaniel B, Cook C. *Erythema annulare centrifugum. StatPearls*. StatPearls Publishing; 2022.

Katayama I, Kotobuki Y, Kiyohara E, Murota H. Annular erythema associated with Sjögren's syndrome: review of the literature on the management and clinical analysis of skin lesions. *Mod Rheumatol*. 2010;20(2):123–129. https://doi.org/10.1007/s10165-009-0257-y.

IMAGE REFERENCES

1. Courtesy Donald Lookingbill, MD.
2. Micheletti RG, et al. *Andrews' Diseases of the Skin Clinical Atlas*. 2nd ed. Elsevier; 2023.

3. Courtesy of Karolyn Wanat, Medical College of Wisconsin.
4. Eichenfield LF, et al. *Neonatal Dermatology*. 2nd ed. Elsevier; 2008.
5. Courtesy of Karolyn Wanat, Medical College of Wisconsin.
6. Courtesy Scott D. Worswick, MD.

Chapter 8

FURTHER READING

Bhushan P, Manjul P, Baliyan V. Flagellate dermatoses. *Indian J Dermatol Venereol Leprol*. 2014;80(2):149–152. https://doi.org/10.4103/0378-6323.129397.

Constantinou A, Kotecha D, Laouris P, de Paula B. A closer look at chemotherapy-induced flagellate dermatitis. *Skin Health Dis*. 2022;2(1):e92. https://doi.org/10.1002/ski2.92.

Homayounfar G, Zimarowski MJ, Burgin S. A woman with night sweats, arthritis, and two distinct eruptions. Adult-onset Still's disease (AOSD). *Int J Dermatol*. 2015;54(8):865–867. https://doi.org/10.1111/ijd.12742.

Wang AS, Barr KL, Jagdeo J. Shiitake mushroom-induced flagellate erythema: a striking case and review of the literature. *Dermatol Online J*. 2013;19(4):5.

Yamamoto T, Nishioka K. Flagellate erythema. *Int J Dermatol*. 2006;45(5):627–631. https://doi.org/10.1111/j.1365-4632.2005.02647.x.

IMAGE REFERENCES

1. Courtesy Brandon Adler, MD.
2. Hochberg MCC, ed. *Rheumatology*. 7th ed. Elsevier; 2019.
3. Micheletti RG, James WD, Elston DM, McMahon PJ. *Andrews' Diseases of the Skin Clinical Atlas*. 2nd ed. Elsevier; 2021.
4. Mancini AJ, Paller AS. *Paller and Mancini—Hurwitz Clinical Pediatric Dermatology: A Textbook of Skin Disorders of Childhood and Adolescence*. 6th ed. Elsevier; 2022.
5. Ibrahimi OA, Anderson RR. Images in clinical medicine. Bleomycin-induced flagellate hyperpigmentation. *N Engl J Med*. 2010;363(24):e36. https://doi.org/10.1056/NEJMicm1002334.
6. Jaheersha Pakran, Amani Abdulla AlFalasi, Anwar H.A. Al Hammadi. Flagellate erythema as manifestation of food hypersensitivity. *Journal of Dermatology & Dermatologic Surgery*. 2017;21(2):95-97.
7. Vinay K, Saikia UN, Dogra S. Image gallery: flagellate bullous exanthem in chikungunya. *Br J Dermatol*. 2017;177(4):e162. https://doi.org/10.1111/bjd.15872.
8. Courtesy Steven Binnick, MD.

Chapter 9

FURTHER READING

Bolognia J, Schaffer J, Cerroni L, Callen J. *Systemic sclerosis and related disorders. Dermatology*. 4th ed. Elsevier; 2018.

Bolognia J, Schaffer J, Cerroni L, Callen J. *Morphea and lichen sclerosus. Dermatology*. 4th ed. Elsevier; 2018.

Shah SS, Chhabra M. *Parry Romberg syndrome. StatPearls [Internet]*. StatPearls Publishing; 2021.

Myers KL, Mir A, Schaffer JV, Meehan SA, Orlow SJ, Brinster NK. Segmental stiff skin syndrome (SSS): a distinct clinical entity. *J Am Acad Dermatol*. 2016;75(1):163–168.

Volksbeck SI, Nashan D, Bruckner-Tuderman L, Braun-Falco M. Localized sclerosis of the scalp (alopecia porphyrinica) as predominant presentation of porphyria cutanea tarda. *J Eur Acad Dermatol Venereol*. 2007;21(8):1125–1127.

IMAGE REFERENCES

4. Kaidar-Person O, Oldenborg S, Poortmans P. Re-irradiation and hyperthermia in breast cancer. *Clin Oncol*. 2018;30(2):73–84. Courtesy Elsevier.

Chapter 10

FURTHER READING

Bolognia J, Schaffer J, Cerroni L, Callen J. *Systemic sclerosis and related disorders. Dermatology*. 4th ed. Elsevier; 2018.

Goldman N, Han J, LaChance A. Diagnosis and management of cutaneous manifestations of autoimmune connective tissue diseases. *Clin Cosmet Investig Dermatol*. 2022;15:2285–2312.

High WA, Ayers RA, Chandler J, et al. Gadolinium is detectable within the tissue of patients with nephrogenic systemic fibrosis. *J Am Acad Dermatol*. 2007;56:21–26.

Shulman LE. Diffuse fasciitis with eosinophilia: a new syndrome? *Trans Assoc Am Physicians*. 1975;88:70–86.

Peñas PF, Jones-Caballero M, Aragüés M, Fernández-Herrera J, Fraga J, García-Díez A. Sclerodermatous graft-vs-host disease: clinical and pathological study of 17 patients. *Arch Dermatol*. 2002;138(7):924–934.

Chapter 11

FURTHER READING

Canavan TN, Mathes EF, Frieden I, Shinkai K. Mycoplasma pneumoniae-induced rash and mucositis as a syndrome distinct from Stevens-Johnson syndrome and erythema multiforme: a systematic review. *J Am Acad Dermatol*. 2015;72(2):239–245. https://doi.org/10.1016/j.jaad.2014.06.026. PMID: 25592340.

Lu A, Endicott A, Tan SY, et al. Toxic epidermal necrolysis-like toxic erythema of chemotherapy: 2 illustrative cases. *JAAD Case Rep*. 2021;15:56–59. https://doi.org/10.1016/j.jdcr.2021.07.010. PMID: 34401432; PMCID: PMC8358280.

Bolognia JL, et al. *Dermatology*. Elsevier; 2018.

Cooper CL, Wiseman M, Brunham R. Bullous cellulitis caused by Serratia marcescens. *Int J Infect Dis*. 1998;3(1):36–38. https://doi.org/10.1016/s1201-9712(98)90093-5. PMID: 9831674.

IMAGE REFERENCES

1. Dinulos JG, Habif TP. *Habif's Clinical Dermatology: A Color Guide to Diagnosis and Therapy*. 7th ed. Elsevier; 2021.
2. Canavan TN, Mathes EF, Frieden I, Shinkai K. Mycoplasma pneumoniae-induced rash and mucositis as a syndrome distinct from Stevens-Johnson syndrome and erythema multiforme: a systematic review. *J Am Acad Dermatol*. 2015;72(2):239–245.
3. Courtesy Scott D. Worswick, MD.
4. Dinulos JG, Habif TP. *Habif's Clinical Dermatology: A Color Guide to Diagnosis and Therapy*. 7th ed. Elsevier; 2021.
5. Nix DP, Bryant RA. *Acute and Chronic Wounds: Intraprofessionals From Novice to Expert*. 6th ed. Elsevier; 2024.
6. Allen CM, et al. *Oral and Maxillofacial Pathology*. 5th ed. Elsevier; 2024.
7. Allen CM, et al. *Oral and Maxillofacial Pathology*. 5th ed. Elsevier; 2024.
8. Bolick BN, et al. *Pediatric Acute Care: A Guide for Interprofessional Practice*. 2nd ed. Elsevier; 2021.
9. From Cohen BA, ed. *Pediatric Dermatology*. 5th ed. Elsevier; 2022.
10. Humphrey, Stephen R.; *Cutaneous Fungal Infections in Nelson Textbook of Pediatrics*, Twenty Second Edition. Elsevier.
11. Dinulos JG, Habif TP. *Habif's Clinical Dermatology: A Color Guide to Diagnosis and Therapy*. 7th ed. Elsevier; 2021.
12. Photo courtesy of Eric Meinhardt, MD.
13. Paller AS, Mancini AJ. *Hurwitz Clinical Pediatric Dermatology*. Elsevier; 2021.
14. Dinulos JG, Habif TP. *Habif's Clinical Dermatology: A Color Guide to Diagnosis and Therapy*. 7th ed. Elsevier; 2021.
15. Courtesy Scott D. Worswick, MD.
16. Courtesy of Timmie Sharma.
17. Courtesy University of Southern California Dermatology Residents' Slide Collection.
18. Courtesy Edward W. Cowen, MD.
19. Sens MA, Hughes R. Diagnostic Pathology: Forensic Autopsy. "Cutaneous Burn: Superficial thermal injuries commonly have an erythematous appearance with associated skin slip." 2021.
20. Thomas Romanelli _Smith's Anesthesia for Infants and Children, 41, 1113-1131.e5. Copyright © 2022 by Elsevier Inc; Figure 41.1 B.

Chapter 12

FURTHER READING

Duong TA, Valeyrie-Allanore L, Wolkenstein P, Chosidow O. Severe cutaneous adverse reactions to drugs. *Lancet*. 2017;390(10106):1996–2011. https://doi.org/10.1016/S0140-6736(16)30378-6. Epub 2017 May 2. Erratum in: *Lancet*. 2017;390(10106):1948. PMID: 28476287.

Canavan TN, Mathes EF, Frieden I, Shinkai K. Mycoplasma pneumoniae-induced rash and mucositis as a syndrome distinct from Stevens-Johnson syndrome and erythema multiforme: a systematic review. *J Am Acad Dermatol*. 2015;72(2):239–245. https://doi.org/10.1016/j.jaad.2014.06.026. PMID: 25592340.

Handler MZ, Schwartz RA. Staphylococcal scalded skin syndrome: diagnosis and management in children and adults. *J Eur Acad Dermatol Venereol*. 2014;28(11):1418–1423. https://doi.org/10.1111/jdv.12541. Epub 2014 May 20. PMID: 24841497.

Bolognia JL, et al. *Dermatology*. Elsevier; 2018.
Miller SJ. Nutritional deficiency and the skin. *J Am Acad Dermatol*. 1989;21(1): 1–30. https://doi.org/10.1016/s0190-9622(89)70144-4. PMID: 2663932.

IMAGE REFERENCES

1. Courtesy Scott D. Worswick.
2. Courtesy Scott D. Worswick.
3. Courtesy Scott D. Worswick.
4. Nowicki J, et al. *Textbook of Natural Medicine*. 5th ed. Elsevier; 2020.
5. Cho YT, Lin JW, Chen YC, et al. Generalized bullous fixed drug eruption is distinct from Stevens-Johnson syndrome/toxic epidermal necrolysis by immunohistopathological features. *J Am Acad Dermatol*. 2014;70(3):539–548. https://doi.org/10.1016/j.jaad.2013.11.015. Epub 2014 Jan 2. PMID: 24388722.
6. Courtesy Scott D. Worswick.
7. Hung YT, Chen YW, Huang Y, Lin YJ, Chen CB, Chung WH. Acute graft-versus-host disease presenting as Stevens-Johnson syndrome and toxic epidermal necrolysis: a retrospective cohort study. *J Am Acad Dermatol*. 2022: S0190–9622(22)02961-9. https://doi.org/10.1016/j.jaad.2022.10.035. Epub ahead of print. PMID: 36280000.
8. Dinulos JG, Habif TP. *Habif's Clinical Dermatology: A Color Guide to Diagnosis and Therapy*. 7th ed. Elsevier; 2021.
9. Dinulos JG, Habif TP. *Habif's Clinical Dermatology: A Color Guide to Diagnosis and Therapy*. 7th ed. Elsevier; 2021.
10. Khanna N. *Illustrated Synopsis of Dermatology & Sexually Transmitted Diseases*. 7th ed. Elsevier; 2024.
11. Courtesy Campbell Stewart, MD.
12. de Oliveira Alves A, Bortolato T, Bernardes Filho F. Pellagra. *J Emerg Med*. 2018;54(2):238–240. Copyright © 2017 Elsevier Inc.

Chapter 13

FURTHER READING

Wang C, Pusic I, Anadkat M. Association of leukemia cutis with survival in acute myeloid leukemia. *JAMA Dermatol*. 2019;155(7):826–832. https://doi.org/10.1001/jamadermatol.2019.0052.
Pulitzer M. Cutaneous T-cell lymphoma. *Clin Lab Med*. 2017;37(3):527–546. https://doi.org/10.1016/j.cll.2017.06.006.
Schneiderman P, Grossman M. *The Clinician's Guide to Dermatologic Differential Diagnosis*. 2nd ed. Elsevier; 2022.
James W, Elston D, Treat J, Rosenbach M, Neuhaus I, Andrews G. *Andrews' Diseases of the Skin: Clinical Dermatology*. 13th ed. Elsevier; 2020.

IMAGE REFERENCES

1. James W, Elston D, Treat J, Rosenbach M, Neuhaus I, Andrews G. *Andrews' Diseases of the Skin: Clinical Dermatology*. 13th ed. Elsevier; 2020. Courtesy Chris Miller, MD.
2. James W, Elston D, Treat J, Rosenbach M, Neuhaus I, Andrews G. *Andrews' Diseases of the Skin: Clinical Dermatology*. 13th ed. Elsevier; 2020.
3. James W, Elston D, Treat J, Rosenbach M, Neuhaus I, Andrews G. *Andrews' Diseases of the Skin: Clinical Dermatology*. 13th ed. Elsevier; 2020.
4. James W, Elston D, Treat J, Rosenbach M, Neuhaus I, Andrews G. *Andrews' Diseases of the Skin: Clinical Dermatology*. 13th ed. Elsevier; 2020.
5. Bolognia JL, Schaffer JV, Cerroni L, *Dermatology*. 4th ed. Elsevier; 2018. Courtesy Lorenzo Cerroni, MD.

Chapter 14

FURTHER READING

Wong CYB, Helm MA, Helm TN, Zeitouni N. Patterns of skin metastases: a review of 25 years' experience at a single cancer center. *Int J Dermatol*. 2014;53(1):56–60. https://doi.org/10.1111/j.1365-4632.2012.05635.x.
Goldstein AO. Overview of benign lesions of the skin. In: Post TW, ed. *UpToDate*; 2023 Available from: https://www.uptodate.com/contents/overview-of-benign-lesions-of-the-skin.
Gandhi SA, Kampp J. Skin cancer epidemiology, detection, and management. *Med Clin North Am*. 2015;99(6):1323–1335. https://doi.org/10.1016/j.mcna.2015.06.002.
Suárez AL, Pulitzer M, Horwitz S, Moskowitz A, Querfeld C, Myskowski PL. Primary cutaneous B-cell lymphomas: part I. Clinical features, diagnosis, and classification. *J Am Acad Dermatol*. 2013;69(3):329.e1–329.e13. https://doi.org/10.1016/j.jaad.2013.06.012.

Chapter 15

FURTHER READING

Bolognia JL, Jorizzo JL, Rapini RP. *Dermatology*. Elsevier; 2012.
James WD, Elston DM, Berger TG, Andrews GC. *Andrews' Diseases of The Skin: Clinical Dermatology*. Elsevier; 2011.
Calonje E, Brenn T, Lazar A, Billings SD. *McKee's Pathology of the Skin: With Clinical Correlations*. 5th ed. Elsevier; 2020.
Callen JP. *Dermatological Signs of Systemic Disease*. 5th ed. Elsevier; 2017.
H DJG, Habif TP. *Habif's Clinical Dermatology: A Color Guide to Diagnosis and Therapy*. 7th ed. Elsevier; 2021.

Chapter 16

FURTHER READING

Bolognia JL, Jorizzo JL, Schaffer JV. *Dermatology E-Book*. Elsevier Health Sciences; 2012.
Borroni G, Torti S, D'ospina RM, Pezzini C. Drug-induced panniculitides. *G Ital Dermatol Venereol*. 2014;149(2):263–270.
Guhl G, García-Díez A. Subcutaneous sweet syndrome. *Dermatol Clin*. 2008; 26(4):541–551.
Morita TCAB, Trés GFS, García MSC, Halpern I, Criado PR, Carvalho JFD. Panniculitides of particular interest to the rheumatologist. *Adv Rheumatol*. 2019:59.
Wick M.R. Panniculitis: a summary. In *Seminars in Diagnostic Pathology*. Vol. 34, No. 3. WB Saunders; 2017:261–272.

IMAGE REFERENCES

3. Courtesy Ian Odell, MD, PhD.
4. Bolognia JL, Schaffer JV, Cerroni L. *Dermatology*. 4th ed. Elsevier; 2018. Courtesy Kenneth E. Greer, MD.

Chapter 17

FURTHER READING

Legat F, Weisshaar E, Fleischer Jr. AB Bernhard JD, Cropley TG. Pruritus and dysesthesia. In: Bolognia JL, Schaffer JV, Cerroni L, eds. *Dermatology*. 4th ed. Elsevier; 2018. https://www.clinicalkey.com/#!/content/book/3-s2.0-B9780702062759000064?scrollTo=%23top.
Kwon CD, Khanna R, Williams KA, Kwatra MM, Kwatra SG. Diagnostic workup and evaluation of patients with prurigo nodularis. *Medicines (Basel)*. 2019;6(4):97. https://doi.org/10.3390/medicines6040097.
Montag A. Diseases caused by arthropods. In: Plewig G, French L, Ruzicka T, Kaufmann R, Hertl M, eds. *Braun-Falco's Dermatology*. Springer; 2022. https://doi.org/10.1007/978-3-662-63709-8-23.
Vornicescu C, Şenilă SC, Cosgarea R, Candrea E, Pop AD, Ungureanu L. Pemphigoid nodularis—rare presentation of bullous pemphigoid: a case report and literature review. *Exp Ther Med*. 2019;17(2):1132–1138. https://doi.org/10.3892/etm.2018.7057.

IMAGE REFERENCES

2. Bolognia, JL, Schaffer JV, Cerroni L. *Dermatology*. 4th ed. Elsevier; 2018. Courtesy Lorenzo Cerroni, MD.
3. Bolognia, JL, Schaffer JV, Cerroni L. *Dermatology*. 4th ed. Elsevier; 2018.
4. Bolognia, JL, Schaffer JV, Cerroni L. *Dermatology*. 4th ed. Elsevier; 2018. Courtesy of Yale Residents' Slide Collection.

Chapter 18

FURTHER READING

Bogdanov I, Darlenski R, Hristakieva E, Manuelyan K. The rash that presents as a vesiculobullous eruption. *Clin Dermatol*. 2020;38(1):19–34. https://doi.org/10.1016/j.clindermatol.2019.10.012.
Chan CX, Zug KA. Diagnosis and management of dermatitis, including atopic, contact, and hand eczemas. *Med Clin North Am*. 2021;105(4):611–626. https://doi.org/10.1016/j.mcna.2021.04.003.
Ständer S, Kasperkiewicz M, Thaçi D, et al. Prevalence and presumptive triggers of localized bullous pemphigoid. *J Dermatol*. 2021;48(8):1257–1261. https://doi.org/10.1111/1346-8138.15912.

Davis MDP, Moschella SL. Neutrophilic dermatoses. In: Bolognia J, Schaffer J, Cerroni L, Callen J, eds. *Dermatology*. 4th ed. Elsevier; 2018:453–471.e2.

Weiss EH, Ko CJ, Leung TH, et al. Neutrophilic dermatoses: a clinical update. *Curr Dermatol Rep*. 2022;11(2):89–102. https://doi.org/10.1007/s13671-022-00355-8.

IMAGE REFERENCES

1. Micheletti RG, James WD, Elston DM, McMahon PJ. *Andrews' Diseases of the Skin Clinical Atlas*. 2nd ed. Elsevier; 2021.
2. Dinulos JGH, Habif TP. *Habif's Clinical Dermatology*. 7th ed. Elsevier; 2021.
3. Kliegman RM, St Geme JW, Blum NJ, Shah SS, Tasker RC, Wilson KM. *Nelson Textbook of Pediatrics*. 21st ed. Elsevier; 2019.
4. Zitelli BJ, McIntire SC, Nowalk AJ, Garrison J. *Zitelli and Davis' Atlas of Pediatric Physical Diagnosis*. 8th ed. Elsevier; 2021.
5. James WD, Elston DM, Treat JR, Rosenbach MA, Neuhaus IM. *Andrews' Diseases of the Skin*. 13th ed. Elsevier; 2019.
6. Dinulos JGH, Habif TP. *Habif's Clinical Dermatology*. 7th ed. Elsevier; 2021.
7. Dinulos JGH, Habif TP. *Habif's Clinical Dermatology*. 7th ed. Elsevier; 2021.
8. Callen JP, Jorizzo JL, Zone JJ, Piette W, Rosenbach MA, Vleugels RA. *Dermatological Signs of Systemic Disease*. 5th ed. Elsevier; 2017.

Chapter 19

FURTHER READING

Bolognia J, Schaffer J, Cerroni L, Callen J. *Dermatology*. 4th ed. Elsevier; 2018.

Dinulos JGH, Habif TP. *Habif's Clinical Dermatology: A Color Guide to Diagnosis and Therapy*. 7th ed. Elsevier; 2020.

James W, Elston D, Treat J, et al. *Andrews' Diseases of the Skin*. 13th ed. Elsevier; 2019.

Kang S, Amagai M, Bruckner A, et al. *Fitzpatrick's Dermatology*. 9th ed. McGraw Hill; 2019.

Saavedra A, Roh E, Mikailov A. *Fitzpatrick's Color Atlas and Synopsis of Clinical Dermatology*. 9th ed. McGraw Hill; 2023.

IMAGE REFERENCES

1. Carneiro-Leão L, Cernadas J. *J Allergy Clin Immunol Pract*. 2019;7(5).
2. Nelson CA, Tomayko MM. Targeting the FcRn: A novel approach to the treatment of pemphigus. *J Invest Dermatol*. 2021;141-2:2777–2780.
3. James W, Elston D, Treat J, et al. *Andrews' Diseases of the Skin*. 13th ed. Elsevier; 2019.
4. Callen J, Jorizzo J, Zone J, et al. *Dermatological Signs of Systemic Disease*. 5th ed. Elsevier; 2017.
5. Courtesy Dr. Lawrence Lieblich, Northwell Health.
6. James W, Elston D, Treat J, et al. *Andrews' Diseases of the Skin*. 13th ed. Elsevier; 2019.
7. Lee H. *J Am Acad Dermatol*. 2018;79(4).
8. Buonavoglia A, Leone P, Dammacco R, et al. *Autoimmunity Rev*. 2019;18(4).
9. From Antaya RJ, Robinson DM. Blisters and pustules in the newborn. *Pediatr Ann*. 2010;39:635-645.
10. Dinulos JG. *Habif's Clinical Dermatology: A Color Guide to Diagnosis and Therapy*. 7th ed. Elsevier; 2020.
11. Paller A, Mancini A. *Hurwitz Clinical Pediatric Dermatology: A Textbook of Skin Disorders of Childhood and Adolescence*. 5th ed. Elsevier; 2016.
12. González-Gay M, Pina T. *Dermatological Signs of Systemic Disease*. 5th ed. Elsevier; 2017.
13. Basam K. *Dermatopathology: Foundations in Diagnostic Pathology*. 2nd ed. Elsevier; 2016.
14. Abel M, Suresh R, Raffi J, et al. *JAAD Case Rep*. 2019;5(12).
15. Lukács J, Schliemann S, Elsner P. *Clin Dermatol*. 2015;33(5).
16. Sparks J, Sheriff S, Burruss J. *JAAD Case Rep*. 2023;35.
17. Murrell DT. *Autoimmune Blistering Diseases, Part II - Diagnosis and Management, An Issue of Dermatologic Clinics*. Vol. 29-4; 1st ed. Elsevier; 2011.
18. Photograph courtesy of Dirk Elston, MD.
19. Courtesy Daniela Kroshinsky, MD MPH.
20. Reprinted with permission from Mandell, Douglas, and Bennett's Principles and Practices of Infectious Diseases. 9th ed. © 2020 by Elsevier, Inc. All rights reserved.
21. Ryder C, Pedersen E, Mancuso J. *JAAD Case Rep*. 2021;18.
22. Harrell J, Rubio X, Nielson, et al. *Clin Dermatol*. 2019;37(6).

Chapter 20

FURTHER READING

Lodi G, Varoni E, Robledo-Sierra J, Villa A, Jontell M. Oral ulcerative lesions. In: Farah C, Balasubramaniam R, McCullough M, eds. *Contemporary Oral Medicine*. Springer; 2017. https://doi.org/10.1007/978-3-319-28100-1-12-1.

Amagai M, et al. Pemphigus. In: Bolognia JL, ed. *Dermatology*. Elsevier; 2018:494–509.

Bolognia J, Jorizzo JL, Rapini RP, Allen C, Camisa C, McNamara K. *Oral disease. Dermatology*. Mosby/Elsevier; 2008. [essay].

Bolognia JL, Schaffer JV, Cerroni L, et al. *Dermatology*. Elsevier; 2018. [essay].

IMAGE REFERENCES

1. Kohanim S, et al. Stevens-Johnson syndrome/toxic epidermal necrolysis—a comprehensive review and guide to therapy. I. Systemic disease. *Ocul Surf*. 2016;14(1):2–19. https://doi.org/10.1016/j.jtos.2015.10.002.
2. Özkaya E. Oral mucosal fixed drug eruption: characteristics and differential diagnosis. *J Am Acad Dermatol*. 2013;69(2):e51–e58. https://doi.org/10.1016/j.jaad.2012.08.019.
3. Aw M, Gresham L, Spurr A, Gavigan G. Reactive infectious mucocutaneous eruption following COVID-19 infection in vaccinated patients. *JAAD Case Rep*. 2023;31:35–41. https://doi.org/10.1016/j.jdcr.2022.10.018.
4. Seibt CE, Munerato MC. Secondary syphilis in the oral cavity and the role of the dental surgeon in STD prevention, diagnosis and treatment: a case series study. *Braz J Infect Dis*. 2016;20(4):393–398. https://doi.org/10.1016/j.bjid.2016.03.008.
5. Cui RZ, et al. Recurrent aphthous stomatitis. *Clin Dermatol*. 2016;34(4):475–481. https://doi.org/10.1016/j.clindermatol.2016.02.020.
6. Crovetto-Martinez R, et al. Mucocutaneous leishmaniasis must be included in the differential diagnosis of midline destructive disease: two case reports. *Oral Surg Oral Med Oral Pathol Oral Radiol*. 2015;119(1):e20–e26. https://doi.org/10.1016/j.oooo.2014.09.008.
7. Bagan J, Sarrion G, Jimenez Y. Oral cancer: clinical features. *Oral Oncol*. 2010;46(6):414–417. https://doi.org/10.1016/j.oraloncology. 2010.03.009.
8. Warnakulasuriya S. Clinical features and presentation of oral potentially malignant disorders. *Oral Surg Oral Med Oral Pathol Oral Radiol*. 2018;125(6):582–590. https://doi.org/10.1016/j.oooo.2018.03.011.
9. Ventarola D, Bordone L, Silverber N. Update on hand-foot-and-mouth disease. *Clin Dermatol*. 2015;33(3):340–346. https://doi.org/10.1016/j.clindermatol.2014.12.011.
10. Reprinted with permission from Samaranayake L. Essential Microbiology for Dentistry, 6th ed. ISBN-978-0-443-11721-3; Fig. 21.8.
11. Siegel M. Diagnosis and management of recurrent herpes simplex infections. *J Am Dent Assoc*. 2002;133(9):1245–1249. https://doi.org/10.14219/jada.archive.2002.0366.
12. Buonavoglia A, et al. Pemphigus and mucous membrane pemphigoid: an update from diagnosis to therapy. *Autoimmun Rev*. 2019;18(4):349–358. https://doi.org/10.1016/j.autrev.2019.02.005.
13. Buonavoglia A, et al. Pemphigus and mucous membrane pemphigoid: an update from diagnosis to therapy. *Autoimmun Rev*. 2019;18(4):349–358. https://doi.org/10.1016/j.autrev.2019.02.005.

Chapter 21

FURTHER READING

Bandow GD. Diagnosis and management of vulvar ulcers. *Dermatol Clin*. 2010;28(4):753–763. https://doi.org/10.1016/j.det.2010.08.008.

Roett MA, Mayor MT, Uduhiri KA. Diagnosis and management of genital ulcers. *Am Fam Physician*. 2012;85(3):254–262. PMID: 22335265.

Sehgal VN, et al. Nonspecific genital ulcers. *Clin Dermatol*. 2014;32(2):259–274. https://doi.org/10.1016/j.clindermatol.2013.08.024.

Bolognia JL, Schaffer JV, Cerroni L, Cooper S, Wojnarowska F. *Anogenital (non-venereal) disease. Dermatology*. Elsevier; 2018.

IMAGE REFERENCES

1. Bunker CB. Skin conditions of the male genitalia. *Medicine*. 2010;38(6): 294–299. Elsevier BV. https://doi.org/10.1016/j.mpmed. 2010.03.006.
2. Pipkin C. Erosive disease of the vulva. *Dermatol Clin*. 2010;28:737–751. https://doi.org/10.1016/j.det.2010.08.005.
3. Lotery HE, Galask RP. Erosive lichen planus of the vulva and vagina. *Obstet Gynecol*. 2003;101(5):1121–1125. https://doi.org/10.1016/S0029-7844(02)02383-9.

4. Fistarol SK, Itin PH. Diagnosis and treatment of lichen sclerosus: an update. *Am J Clin Derm.* 2013;14(1):27–47. Springer Science and Business Media LLC. https://doi.org/10.1007/s40257-012-0006-4.
5. Matthews N, et al. Genital diseases in the mature woman. *Clin Dermatol.* 2018;36(2):208–221. https://doi.org/10.1016/j.clindermatol. 2017.10.012.
6. Nakai N, Katoh N. A case of fixed drug eruption caused by loxoprofen sodium hydrate. *Allergol Int.* 2015;64(4):377–378. Elsevier BV. https://doi.org/10.1016/j.alit.2015.04.007.
7. Kleine C, Stich A. 53—Lymphogranuloma venereum. *Hunter's Tropical Medicine and Emerging Infectious Diseases (Tenth Edition).* 2020:521–523. https://doi.org/10.1016/B978-0-323-55512-8.00053-3.
8. de Vries HJC. Skin as an indicator for sexually transmitted infections. *Clin Dermatol.* 2014;32(2):196–208. https://doi.org/10.1016/j.clindermatol.2013.08.003.
9. Sukthankar A. Syphilis. *Medicine.* 2010;38(5):263–266. Elsevier BV. https://doi.org/10.1016/j.mpmed.2010.01.016.
10. Reprinted with permission from Velho PE, Souza EM, Belda Junior W. Donovanosis. *Braz J Infect Dis.* 2008;12(6):523. Figure 1.
11. Pipkin C. Erosive disease of the vulva. *Dermatol Clin.* 2010;28:737–751. https://doi.org/10.1016/j.det.2010.08.005.
12. Photo courtesy of Connie Celum, Walter Stamm; Seattle STD/HIV Prevention Training Center, University of Washington.
13. Reprinted with permission from Sharma R, Dronen SC. Herpes simplex in emergency medicine. Medscape Reference. http://emedicine.medscape.com/article/783113-overview.
14. Dessinioti C, Katsambas A, Antoniou C. Hidradenitis suppurrativa (acne inversa) as a systemic disease. *Clin Dermatol.* 2014;32(3):397–408. https://doi.org/10.1016/j.clindermatol.2013.11.006.
15. Lehman J, et al. Reactive nonsexually related acute genital ulcers: review of cases evaluated at Mayo Clinic. *J Am Acad Dermatol.* 2010;63(1):44–51. https://doi.org/10.1016/j.jaad.2009.08.038.
16. Hagen J, Swoger J, Grandinetti L. Cutaneous manifestations of Chron disease. *Dermatol Clin.* 2015;33(3):417–431. https://doi.org/10.1016/j.det.2015.03.007.
17. Georgala S, Georgala C, Nicolaidou E. Pyoderma gangrenosum of the penis: a potentially dramatic skin disease. *Urology.* 2008;72(5):1185.e9–1185.e10. https://doi.org/10.1016/j.urology.2008.01.034.

Chapter 22

FURTHER READING

Fife CE, Carter MJ, Walker D. Why is it so hard to do the right thing in wound care? *Wound Repair Regen.* 2009;18:154–158.
Hammer P, Latour E, Bohnett MC, et al. The utility and challenges of histopathologic evaluation in the diagnosis of nonmalignant skin ulcers. *Wound Repair Regen.* 2020;28(2):219–223.
Haynes D, Hammer P, Malachowski SJ, et al. Characterisation and diagnosis of ulcers in inpatient dermatology consultation services: a multi-centre study. *Int Wound J.* 2019;16(6):1440–1444.
Isoherranen K, O'Brien JJ, Barker J, et al. Atypical wounds. Best clinical practice and challenges. *J Wound Care.* 2019;28(suppl 6):S1–S92.

Chapter 23

FURTHER READING

Bolognia J, Schaffer J, Cerroni L, Callen J. *Dermatology.* 4th ed. Elsevier; 2018.
Bolognia J, Schaffer JV, Duncan KO, Ko CJ. *Dermatology Essentials.* 1st ed. Elsevier; 2022.
Marks JG, Miller JJ, Lookingbill DP. *Lookingbill and Marks' Principles of Dermatology.* 6th ed. Elsevier; 2019.
Panda S, Khanna S, Singh SK, Gupta SK. Squamous cell carcinoma developing in a diabetic foot ulcer. *Int J Low Extrem Wounds.* 2011;10(2):101–103. https://doi.org/10.1177/1534734611412001.
Karagounis T, Belmont HM, Caplan AS. A woman with painful digital ulcers. *JAMA.* 2022;327(16):1608. https://doi.org/10.1001/jama.2022.3667.

IMAGE REFERENCES

1. James WD, Elston DM, Mcmahon PJ, Andrews GC. *Andrews' Diseases of the Skin Clinical Atlas.* Elsevier; 2018.
2. Marks JG, Miller JJ, Lookingbill DP. *Lookingbill and Marks' Principles of Dermatology.* 6th ed. Elsevier; 2019.
3. James WD, Elston DM, Mcmahon PJ, Andrews GC. *Andrews' Diseases of the Skin Clinical Atlas.* Elsevier; 2018.
4. Panda S, Khanna S, Singh SK, Gupta SK. Squamous cell carcinoma developing in a diabetic foot ulcer. *Int J Low Extrem Wounds.* 2011;10(2):101–103.
5. Marks JG, Miller JJ, Lookingbill DP. *Lookingbill and Marks' Principles of Dermatology.* 6th ed. Elsevier; 2019.
6. Courtesy Brandon Adler, MD.
7. James WD, Elston DM, Mcmahon PJ, Andrews GC. *Andrews' Diseases of the Skin Clinical Atlas.* Elsevier; 2018.
8. James WD, Elston DM, Mcmahon PJ, Andrews GC. *Andrews' Diseases of the Skin Clinical Atlas.* Elsevier; 2018.
9. Courtesy Curt Samlaska, MD.
10. James WD, Elston DM, Mcmahon PJ, Andrews GC. *Andrews' Diseases of the Skin Clinical Atlas.* Elsevier; 2018.
11. Jeong HS, Dominguez AR. Calciphylaxis: controversies in pathogenesis, diagnosis and treatment.*Am J Med Sci.*2016;351(2):217–227.
12. James WD, Elston DM, Treat JR, Rosenbach MA, Neuhaus I. *Andrews' Diseases of the Skin Clinical Dermatology.* Elsevier; 2020.
13. Marks JG, Miller JJ, Lookingbill DP. *Lookingbill and Marks' Principles of Dermatology.* 6th ed. Elsevier; 2019.
14. Hughes M, Bruni C, Ruaro B, Confalonieri M, Matucci-Cerinic M, Bellando-Randone S. Digital ulcers in systemic sclerosis. *La Presse Médicale.*2021;50(1):104064.

Chapter 24

FURTHER READING

James WD, Elston DM, Treat JR, Rosenbach MA, Neuhaus IM. *Andrews' Diseases of the Skin: Clinical Dermatology.* 13th ed. Elsevier; 2020.
Edgar NR, Saleh D, Miller RA. Recurrent aphthous stomatitis: a review. *J Clin Aesthet Dermatol.* 2017;10(3):26–36.
Ikeda T, Gion Y, Yoshino T, Sato Y. A review of EBV-positive mucocutaneous ulcers focusing on clinical and pathological aspects. *J Clin Exp Hematop.* 2019;59(2):64–71. https://doi.org/10.3960/jslrt.18039.
Aoyama Y, Sugiyama S, Yamamoto T. Anti-cytomegalovirus therapy: whether and when to initiate, those are the questions. *Pharmaceuticals (Basel).* 2022;15(7):797. https://doi.org/10.3390/ph15070797.
Ramien ML, Bahubeshi A, Lara-Corrales I, et al. Blistering severe cutaneous adverse reactions in children: proposal for paediatric-focused clinical criteria. *Br J Dermatol.* 2021;185(2):447–449.

IMAGE REFERENCES

2. Paller A, Mancini S. *Hurwitz Clinical Pediatric Dermatology.* 6th ed. Elsevier; 2020.
5. James WD, Elston DM, Treat JR, Rosenbach MA, Neuhaus IM. *Andrews' Diseases of the Skin: Clinical Dermatology.* 13th ed. Elsevier; 2020.
6. Courtesy Dr. Aimee Smidt.
7. Courtesy Steven Binnick, MD.
8. James WD, Elston DM, Treat JR, Rosenbach MA, Neuhaus IM. *Andrews' Diseases of the Skin: Clinical Dermatology.* 13th ed. Elsevier; 2020.
9. Paller A, Mancini S. *Hurwitz Clinical Pediatric Dermatology.* 6th ed. Elsevier; 2020.
11. Cheng SX, Chapman MS, Margesson LJ, Birenbaum D. Genital ulcers caused by Epstein-Barr virus. *JAAD.* 2004;51(5):824–826.
12. Curtiss P, Cobos G, Hoffmann R, Seminara N, Liebman T, Brinster N, Lo Sicco K. Genital ulcers in an immunocompromised man. *JAAD Case Rep.* 2018;14;4(7):619–621.
13. Callen JP, Jorizzo JL, Zone JJ, Piette WW, Rosenbach MA, Vleugels RA. *Dermatological Signs of Systemic Disease.* 5th ed. Elsevier; 2017.
14. Paller A, Mancini S. *Hurwitz Clinical Pediatric Dermatology.* 6th ed. Elsevier; 2020.
15. James WD, Elston DM, Treat JR, Rosenbach MA, Neuhaus IM. *Andrews' Diseases of the Skin: Clinical Dermatology.* 13th ed. Elsevier; 2020.
16. James WD, Elston DM, Treat JR, Rosenbach MA, Neuhaus IM. *Andrews' Diseases of the Skin: Clinical Dermatology.* 13th ed. Elsevier; 2020.
17. Paller A, Mancini S. *Hurwitz Clinical Pediatric Dermatology.* 6th ed. Elsevier; 2020.
18. James WD, Elston DM, Treat JR, Rosenbach MA, Neuhaus IM. *Andrews' Diseases of the Skin: Clinical Dermatology.* 13th ed. Elsevier; 2020.
19. Callen JP, Jorizzo JL, Zone JJ, Piette WW, Rosenbach MA, Vleugels RA. (2017). *Dermatological Signs of Systemic Disease.* 5th ed. Elsevier; 2017.
20. Paller A, Mancini S, *Hurwitz Clinical Pediatric Dermatology.* 6th ed. Elsevier; 2020.

Chapter 25

FURTHER READING

Welsh JP, Skvarka CB, Allen HB. A novel visual clue for the diagnosis of hypertrophic lichen planus. *Arch Dermatol.* 2006;142(7):954. https://doi.org/10.1001/archderm.142.7.954. PMID: 16847230.

Sussman ME, Pousti BT, Grossman SK, Lee JB, Hsu S. Verrucous sarcoidosis: a rare clinical presentation of sarcoidosis. *Cureus.* 2021;13(5):e15175. https://doi.org/10.7759/cureus.15175. PMID: 34178497; PMCID: PMC8216646.

Noparstak M, McDaniel B, King J, et al. Verrucous sarcoidosis associated with human papillomavirus infection: a case report. *JAAD Case Rep.* 2015;1(5):247–250. https://doi.org/10.1016/j.jdcr.2015.05.006. PMID: 27051743; PMCID: PMC4809230.

Chee SN, Ge L, Agar N, Lowe P. Spiny keratoderma: case series and review. *Int J Dermatol.* 2017;56(9):915–919. https://doi.org/10.1111/ijd.13680. Epub 2017 Jul 5. PMID: 28681429.

Caldito EG, Antia C, Petronic-Rosic V. Cutaneous *blastomycosis. JAMA Dermatol.* 2022;158(9):1064. https://doi.org/10.1001/jamadermatol.2022.3151. PMID: 35947397.

IMAGE REFERENCES

1. James WD, Elston DM, Treat JR, Rosenbach MA, Nuehaus IM. *Andrews' Diseases of the Skin.* 2019:587–635.e7.
2. James WD, Elston DM, Treat JR, Rosenbach MA, Nuehaus IM. *Andrews' Diseases of the Skin.* 2019:205–214.e2.
3. J. Tuberculosis verrucosa cutis. James WD, Elston DM, Treat JR, Rosenbach MA, Nuehaus IM. *Andrews' Diseases of the Skin.* 2019:324–335.e2.
4. Giulia P, Ilaria M, Enrico R, Mario C. *J Pediatr.* 2013;63(3):920–920.e1.
5. Hagan CE, Offiah M, Brodell RT, Jackson JD. Chronic verrucous sarcoidosis associated with human papillomavirus infection: improvement with adalimumab. *JAAD Case Reports.* 2018;4(9):866.
6. Ferreira CP, Miranda A, Nery JA. Kaposi's sarcoma simulating verrucous syndrome. *Braz J Infect Dis.* 2015;19:444–445.
9. Elliott H. Campbell, Charlie Becknell. Spiny keratoderma exposes underlying renal cell carcinoma. *JAAD Case Reports.* 2018;4(4):382–383.
11. Courtesy Debabrata Bandyopadhyay, MD.

Chapter 26

FURTHER READING

Mevorah B, Gat A, Golan H, Brenner S. Unilateral spiny hyperkeratosis. *Dermatology.* 2008;217(2):181–186. https://doi.org/10.1159/000140678.

Chee SN, Ge L, Agar N, Lowe P. Spiny keratoderma: case series and review. *Int J Dermatol.* 2017;56(9):915–919. https://doi.org/10.1111/ijd.13680.

Caccetta TP, Dessauvagie B, McCallum D, Kumarasinghe SP. Multiple minute digitate hyperkeratosis: a proposed algorithm for the digitate keratoses. *J Am Acad Dermatol.* 2012;67(1):e49–e55. https://doi.org/10.1016/j.jaad.2010.07.023.

Miller A, Aires D, Fraga G. Multiple minute digitate hyperkeratoses: a case report. *Dermatol Online J.* 2011;17(5):1.

Leerunyakul K, Chirasuthat P, Suchonwanit P. A case report of idiopathic follicular hyperkeratotic spicules and literature review. *Case Rep Dermatol.* 2019;11(3):278–285. https://doi.org/10.1159/000503272.

IMAGE REFERENCES

1. Marks JG, Miller JJ. Inflammatory papules. In: *Lookingbill and Marks' Principles of Dermatology.* Elsevier; 2019:151–165. https://www.doi.org.10.1016/B978-0-323-43040-1.00011-7.
2. Chun Wong JL, Wilson N. Prurigo nodularis. In: *Treatment of Skin Disease.* Elsevier; 2018:672–675. https://www.doi.org.10.1016/B978-0-7020-6912-3.00203-2.
3. Weingarten M, Silverberg N. Follicular eczema and accentuation: a survey of published data. *J Am Acad Dermatol.* 2022;87(4):860–862. https://www.doi.org.10.1016/j.jaad.2021.11.008.
4. Hinojosa JA, Williams CL, Vandergriff T, Le LQ. Arsenical keratosis secondary to Fowler solution. *JAAD Case Rep.* 2018;4(1):72–74. https://www.doi.org.10.1016/j.jdcr.2017.11.008.
5. Frigerio A, Toptan T, Chang Y, Abbott J, Cipriano SD, Bowen AR. Widespread keratosis pilaris-like eruption in an immunocompromised child. *JAAD Case Rep.* 2019;5(4):352–354. https://www.doi.org.10.1016/j.jdcr.2019.02.001.
6. Jack A, Mauro MJ, Ehst BD. Pityriasis rubra pilaris-like eruption associated with the multikinase inhibitor ponatinib. *J Am Acad Dermatol.* 2013;69(5):e249–e250. https://www.doi.org.10.1016/j.jaad.2013.04.061.
7. Gaufin G, Guo EL, Cardis MA. Hyperkeratotic spicules in a woman with breast cancer. *Int J Women's Dermatol.* 2021;7(5):803–804. https://www.doi.org.10.1016/j.ijwd.2021.06.006.
8. Paller AS, Mancini AJ. Disorders of hair and nails. In: *Hurwitz Clinical Pediatric Dermatology.* Elsevier; 2011:130–166. https://www.doi.org.10.1016/B978-1-4377-0412-9.00007-1.
9. Marks JG, Miller JJ. Inflammatory papules. In: *Lookingbill and Marks' Principles of Dermatology.* Elsevier; 2019:151–165. https://www.doi.org.10.1016/B978-0-323-43040-1.00011-7.
10. De Cerqueira AMM, De Souza Cardoso F. Nutritional diseases. In: *Tropical Dermatology.* Elsevier; 2017:407–426. https://www.doi.org.10.1016/B978-0-323-29634-2.00033-X.
11. Tobin AM, Kirby B, Lebwohl M. Pityriasis rubra pilaris. In: *Treatment of Skin Disease.* Elsevier; 2018:629–631. https://www.doi.org.10.1016/B978-0-7020-6912-3.00191-9.
12. Micheletti RG, Elston DM, James WD, McMahon PJ. *Andrews' Diseases of the Skin Clinical Atlas.* 2nd ed. Elsevier; 2023.
13. Maouni S, El Anzi O, Sqalli A, Znati K, Meziane M, Hassam B. Erythromelanosis follicularis faciei et colli: dermoscopy and dermatopathology correlates. *JAAD Case Rep.* 2019;5(6):535–536. https://www.doi.org.10.1016/j.jdcr.2019.04.011.
14. Muniesa C, Estrach T, Pujol RM, et al. Folliculotropic mycosis fungoides: clinicopathological features and outcome in a series of 20 cases. *J Am Acad Dermatol.* 2010;62(3):418–426. https://www.doi.org.10.1016/j.jaad.2009.03.014.
15. Paul C, Fermand JP, Flageul B, et al. Hyperkeratotic spicules and monoclonal gammopathy. *J Am Acad Dermatol.* 1995;33(2):346–351. https://www.doi.org.10.1016/0190-9622(95)91431-5.
16. Stonesifer CJ, Husain SA, Niedt GW, Gallitano SM. Dermatoscopy case of the month: trichodysplasia spinulosa. *JAAD Case Rep.* 2021;17:116–118. https://www.doi.org.10.1016/j.jdcr.2021.09.018.
17. Courtesy of Dr. Kenneth E. Greer, MD.
18. Díez-Madueño K, Buendía Castaño D, Alonso-García S, de la Cueva Dobao P. Perforating folliculitis. *Med Clin.* 2022;159(9):456. https://www.doi.org.10.1016/j.medcle.2022.07.013 [in English].
19. Lonergan CL, Cropley TG. Renal disease and the skin. In: *Dermatological Signs of Internal Disease.* Elsevier; 2009:305–309. https://www.doi.org.10.1016/B978-1-4160-6111-3.00038-0.
20. Russo T, Piccolo V, Mascolo M, Staibano S, Alfano R, Argenziano G. Dermoscopy of Kyrle disease. *Am Acad Dermatol.* 2016;75(3).
21. Dinulos JGH. *Habif's Clinical Dermatology: A Color Guide to Diagnosis and Therapy.* 7th ed. Elsevier; 2021.
22. Linares-Gonzalez L, Ródenas-Herranz T, Ruiz-Villaverde R. Spiny keratoderma as a paraneoplastic condition in clear cell renal cell carcinoma. *Actas Dermosifiliogr.* 2022; 113(5):T514–T515. https://doi.org/10.1016/j.ad.2021.08.015.
23. Caccetta TP, Dessauvagie B, McCallum D, Kumarasinghe SP. Multiple minute digitate hyperkeratosis: a proposed algorithm for the digitate keratoses. *J Am Acad Dermatol.* 2012;67(1):e49–e55. https://www.doi.org.10.1016/j.jaad.2010.07.023.

Chapter 27

FURTHER READING

Weinkle A, Pettit C, Jani A, et al. Distinguishing Stevens-Johnson syndrome/toxic epidermal necrolysis from clinical mimickers during inpatient dermatologic consultation—a retrospective chart review. *J Am Acad Dermatol.* 2019;81(3):749–757.

Melnick L, Samimi S, Elder D, et al. Targetoid lesions in the emergency department. Bed bug bites (Cimex lectularius) with targetoid lesions on initial presentation. *JAMA Dermatol.* 2013;149(6):751–756.

Bolognia JL, Jorizzo JJ, Schaffer JV, et al. *Dermatology.* 3rd ed. Elsevier; 2012.

IMAGE REFERENCES

4. Courtesy Teri Greiling, MD, PhD.

Chapter 28

FURTHER READING

Wang JF, Orlow SJ. Keratosis pilaris and its subtypes: associations, new molecular and pharmacologic etiologies, and therapeutic options. *Am J Clin Dermatol.* 2018;19(5):733–757.

Stibich AS, Schwartz RA. Papular urticaria. *Cutis.* 2001;68(2):89–91.

Liu YS, Cheng YP, Liu CI, Yang CY, Yang CY. Presenile diffuse familial sebaceous hyperplasia successfully treated with low-dose isotretinoin: a report of two cases and review of the published work. *J Dermatol.* 2016;43(10):1205–1208.

Husar K, Skerlev M. Molluscum contagiosum from infancy to maturity. *Clin Dermatol.* 2002;20(2):170–172. https://doi.org/10.1016/s0738-081x(02)00209-2. PMID: 11973052.

Berk DR, Bayliss SJ. Milia: a review and classification. *J Am Acad Dermatol.* 2008;59(6):1050–1063.

IMAGE REFERENCES

3. Vishwanath T, et al. Immersion cryoanasthesia: a low-cost, easy-to-do technique to reduce pain during injections into digits. *J Am Acad Dermatol.* 2019;81(4):e91–e92.
4. Schadler ED, Mehlis SL, Cibull TL, Ortel B. Two cases of treatment with aromatase inhibitors and development of miliary osteoma cutis—is there an association? *JAAD Case Rep.* 2018;4(7):648–650.
5. Behera B, Mathews I, Vinupriya S, Chandrashekar L, Thappa DM, Srinivas BH. Milia: a dermoscopic pitfall. *J Am Acad Dermatol.* 2017;77(2):e29–e31.
6. Hengge UR, Ruzicka T, Schwartz RA, Cork MJ. Adverse effects of topical glucocorticosteroids. *J Am Acad Dermatol.* 2006;54(1):1–15; quiz 16–18.
7. Nedorost ST. Medical Pearl: the evaluation of perioral dermatitis: use of an extended patch test series. *J Am Acad Dermatol.* 2007;56(5 Suppl):S100–S102.
8. Quiñonez RL, Agbai ON, Burgess CM, Taylor SC. An update on cosmetic procedures in people of color. Part 1: scientific background, assessment, preprocedure preparation. *J Am Acad Dermatol.* 2022;86(4):715–725.
11. Wofford J, Fenves AZ, Jackson JM, Kimball AB, Menter A. The spectrum of nephrocutaneous diseases and associations: genetic causes of nephrocutaneous disease. *J Am Acad Dermatol.* 2016;74(2):231–244; quiz 245–246.
12. Free R, Pflederer RT, Fraga GR, Rajpara A. Flesh-colored papules and nodules on the face. *JAAD Case Rep.* 2018;4(6):512–514.
14. Smith DR, Mathias CG, Mutasim DF. Multiple eccrine hidrocystomas treated with glycopyrrolate. *J Am Acad Dermatol.* 2008;59(5 Suppl):S122–S123.
15. Yanagi T, Sawamura D, Nishie W, Abe M, Shibaki A, Shimizu H. Multiple apocrine hidrocystoma showing plane pigmented macules. *J Am Acad Dermatol.* 2006;54(2 Suppl):S53–S54.
18. Yoshiya H, Okuyama R, Uhara H. Effectiveness of topical maxacalcitol for acquired perforating disorder. *J Am Acad Dermatol.* 2013;68(6):e181–e182.
19. Valdebran M, Terrero D, Xue R. Dermoscopic findings in hyperkeratosis lenticularis perstans. *J Am Acad Dermatol.* 2016;75(6):e211–e213.
20. Pruitt LG, Hsia LL, Burke WA. Disseminated superficial porokeratosis involving the groin and genitalia in a 72-year-old immunocompetent man. *JAAD Case Rep.* 2015;1(5):277–279.
21. Berry CT, Berry KG, Abbott J, et al. Resolution of acquired palmoplantar keratoderma and scurvy after treatment of multivitamin deficiencies. *JAAD Case Rep.* 2022;22:27–30.
22. Bleasel NR, Stapleton KM, Lee MS, Sullivan J. Vitamin A deficiency phrynoderma: due to malabsorption and inadequate diet. *J Am Acad Dermatol.* 1999;41(2 Pt 2):322–324.
23. Habif TP. *Clinical Dermatology: A Color Guide to Diagnosis and Therapy.* 6th ed. Elsevier; 2016.
26. Hongcharu W, Baldassano M, Gonzalez E. Generalized lichen amyloidosis associated with chronic lichen planus. *J Am Acad Dermatol.* 2000;43(2 Pt 2):346–348.
27. Wenzel FG, Horn TD. Nonneoplastic disorders of the eccrine glands. *J Am Acad Dermatol.* 1998;38(1):1–17; quiz 18–20.
28. Prindaville B, Belazarian L, Levin NA, Wiss K. Pityrosporum folliculitis: a retrospective review of 110 cases. *J Am Acad Dermatol.* 2018;78(3):511–514.
29. de Abreu L, Guimarães Cordeiro NG, Buçard AM, Quintella DC, Argenziano G. Dermoscopy of Grover disease. *J Am Acad Dermatol.* 2017;76(2 Suppl 1):S60–S63.
30. Haddad V Jr, Cardoso JL, Lupi O, Tyring SK. Tropical dermatology: venomous arthropods and human skin: part I. Insecta. *J Am Acad Dermatol.* 2012;67(3):331.e1–331.e14; Figure 23.

Chapter 29

FURTHER READING

Meza-Romero R, Navarrete-Dechent C, Downey C. Molluscum contagiosum: an update and review of new perspectives in etiology, diagnosis, and treatment. *Clin Cosmet Investig Dermatol.* 2019;12:373.

Badri T, Gandhi GR. *Molluscum contagiosum. StatPearls.* StatPearls Publishing; 2022.

Bauer JH, Miller OF, Peckham SJ. Medical Pearl: confirming the diagnosis of molluscum contagiosum using 10% potassium hydroxide. *J Am Acad Dermatol.* 2007;56(5 Suppl).

Bolognia J, Schaffer JV, Cerroni L. In: Bolognia J, Schaffer JV, Cerroni L, eds. *Dermatology.* 4th ed. Elsevier; 2018.

Thornhill JP, Barkati S, Walmsley S, et al. Monkeypox virus infection in humans across 16 countries—April-June 2022. *N Engl J Med.* 2022;387(8):679–691.

Bubna A. Umbilicated lesions in dermatology. *Clin Dermatol Rev.* 2019;3(1):99.

Centers for Disease Control and Prevention. Monkeypox. Updated September 28, 2022. https://www.cdc.gov/poxvirus/monkeypox/vaccines/vaccine-basics.html

Dogra S, Mehta H, Gupta S, Suri V. Monkeypox: a new global health emergency with predominant dermatological manifestations. *Int J Dermatol.* 2022 Published online.

Ayoade F, Kumar S. *Varicella zoster. StatPearls.* StatPearls Publishing; 2022.

Wollina U. Variations in herpes zoster manifestation. *Indian J Med Res.* 2017;145(3):294.

Karray M, Kwan E, Souissi A. *Kaposi varicelliform eruption. StatPearls.* StatPearls Publishing; 2022.

Reddy KA, Satyanarayana MA, Aryasomayajula S, Krishna BAR. Basal cell carcinoma developing from trichoepithelioma: review of three cases. *J Clin Diagn Res.* 2016;10(3): PD17.

Guidelines for the prevention and treatment of opportunistic infections in adults and adolescents with HIV. Clinical Info HIV.gov. Updated September 28, 2022. https://clinicalinfo.hiv.gov/en/guidelines.

IMAGE REFERENCES

2. Courtesy Karl Saardi, MD.
5. Eleryan M, Friedman A. *The Full Spectrum of Dermatology: A Diverse and Inclusive Atlas.* 1st ed. SanovaWorks and Educational Testing & Assessment Systems; 2021.

Chapter 30

FURTHER READING

Dessinioti C, Antoniou C, Katsambas A. Acneiform eruptions. *Clin Dermatol.* 2014;32:24–34.

Du-Thanh A, Kluger N, Bensalleh H, Guillot B. Drug-induced acneiform eruption. *Am J Clin Dermatol.* 2011;12:233–245.

McFarland S, Polcari I. Morphology-based diagnosis of acneiform eruptions. *Pediatr Ann.* 2015;44:e188–e193.

Cheung M, Taher M, Lauzon G. Acneiform facial eruptions: a problem for young women. *Can Fam Physician.* 2005;51:527–533.

Momin S, Peterson A, Del Rosso J. A status report on drug-associated acne and acneiform eruptions. *J Drugs Dermatol.* 2010;9:627–636.

Bolognia J, Schaffer JV, Cerroni L. In: Bolognia J, Schaffer JV, Cerroni L, eds. *Dermatology.* 4th ed. Elsevier; 2018.

Nair P, Salazar F. *Acneiform eruptions. StatPearls.* StatPearls Publishing; 2022.

McDermott MF, Aksentijevich I. The autoinflammatory syndromes. *Curr Opin Allergy Clin Immunol.* 2002;2(6):511–516.

Dierselhuis MP, Frenkel J, Wulffraat NM, Boelens JJ. Anakinra for flares of pyogenic arthritis in PAPA syndrome. *Rheumatology (Oxford).* 2005 Epub ahead of print.

Braun-Falco M, Kovnerystyy O, Lohse P, Ruzicka T. Pyoderma gangrenosum, acne, and suppurative hidradenitis (PASH)—a new autoinflammatory syndrome distinct from PAPA syndrome. *J Am Acad Dermatol.* 2012;66(3):409–415.

IMAGE REFERENCES

1. Friedman A. George Washington University Medical Faculty Associates, Department of Dermatology, George Washington University School of Medicine and Health Sciences, Washington, DC.
2. Friedman A. George Washington University Medical Faculty Associates, Department of Dermatology, George Washington University School of Medicine and Health Sciences, Washington, DC.
3. Friedman A. George Washington University Medical Faculty Associates, Department of Dermatology, George Washington University School of Medicine and Health Sciences, Washington, DC.
4. Friedman A. George Washington University Medical Faculty Associates, Department of Dermatology, George Washington University School of Medicine and Health Sciences, Washington, DC.
5. Friedman A. George Washington University Medical Faculty Associates, Department of Dermatology, George Washington University School of Medicine and Health Sciences, Washington, DC.
6. Friedman A. George Washington University Medical Faculty Associates, Department of Dermatology, George Washington University School of Medicine and Health Sciences, Washington, DC.

Chapter 31

FURTHER READING

Calonje E, Brenn T, Lazar AJ, Billings SD. Granulomatous, necrobiotic and perforating dermatoses. In: Calonje E, Brenn T, Lazar AJ, Billings SD, eds. *McKee's Pathology of the Skin*. 5th ed. Elsevier; 2020:306–350.

Harbaoui S, Litaiem N. *Acquired perforating dermatosis. StatPearls*. StatPearls Publishing; 2022.

Rapini RP. Perforating diseases. In: Bolognia J, Schaeffer J, Cerroni L, Callen J, eds. *Dermatology*. 4th ed. Elsevier; 2018:1690–1696.

IMAGE REFERENCES

1. Gontijo JRV, Júnior FF, Pereira LB, Pedrosa MS. Trauma-induced acquired reactive perforating collagenosis. *An Bras Dermatol*. 2021;96(3):392–393. https://doi.org/10.1016/j.abd.2020.06.022. Epub 2021 Mar 20. PMID: 33840572; PMCID: PMC8178551.
2. From James WD et al. *Andrews' diseases of the skin*. 12th ed. Elsevier; 2016.
3. Lal NR, Bandyopadhyay D, Verma R, Shukla AK. Perforating calcific elastosis: revisiting a rare entity. *Indian J Dermatol*. 2018;63(2):186–188. https://doi.org/10.4103/ijd.IJD_111_17. PMID: 29692466; PMCID: PMC5903054.
4. Courtesy Dr. Blake St. Clair, MD.
5. Reprinted with permission from Dusek P, Litwin T, Czlonkowska A. Wilson disease and other neurodegenerations with metal accumulations. *Neurol Clin*. 2015;33-1:175–204.
9. Lucas C, Aranha J, da Rocha I, Sousa D. Case report: pseudoxanthoma elasticum. *F1000Res*. 2020;9:9. https://doi.org/10.12688/f1000research.21431.1. PMID: 32742638; PMCID: PMC7372526.

Chapter 32

FURTHER READING

Brandt O, Abeck D, Gianotti R, Burgdorf W. Gianotti-Crosti syndrome. *J Am Acad Dermatol*. 2006;54(1):136–145. https://doi.org/10.1016/j.jaad.2005.09.033. Epub 2005 Dec 2. PMID: 16384769.

Antia C, Baquerizo K, Korman A, Bernstein JA, Alikhan A. Urticaria: a comprehensive review: epidemiology, diagnosis, and work-up. *J Am Acad Dermatol*. 2018;79(4):599–614. https://doi.org/10.1016/j.jaad.2018.01.020. PMID: 30241623.

Cohen PR, Kurzrock R. Sweet's syndrome revisited: a review of disease concepts. *Int J Dermatol*. 2003;42:761–778. https://doi.org/10.1046/j.1365-4362.2003.01891.x.

Wisnieski JJ. Urticarial vasculitis. *Curr Opin Rheumatol*. 2000;12(1):24–31. https://doi.org/10.1097/00002281-200001000-00005. PMID: 10647951.

Critchlow WA, Chang D. Cheilitis granulomatosa: a review. *Head Neck Pathol*. 2014;8(2):209–213. https://doi.org/10.1007/s12105-013-0488-2.

Chapter 33

IMAGE REFERENCES

1. Antia C, Baquerizo K, Korman A, Bernstein JA, Alikhan A. Urticaria: a comprehensive review: epidemiology, diagnosis, and work-up. *J Am Acad Dermatol*. 2018;79(4):599–614. https://doi.org/10.1016/j.jaad.2018.01.020.
2. Saleh D, Crane JS. Tumid lupus erythematosus. In: *StatPearls* [Internet]. StatPearls Publishing; 2019. https://www.ncbi.nlm.nih.gov/books/NBK482515/
3. Hsu S, Le EH, Khoshevis MR. Differential diagnosis of annular lesions. *Am Fam Physician*. 2001;64(2):289–296.
4. Reich HL, Nguyen JT, James WD. Annular lichen planus: a case series of 20 patients. *J Am Acad Dermatol*. 2004;50(4):595–599. https://doi.org/10.1016/j.jaad.2003.08.011.

Chapter 34

FURTHER READING

Bolognia JL, Jorizzo JJ, Schaffer JV, et al. In: Callen JP, Cerroni L, Heymann WR, McGrath J, Patterson JW, Schwarz T, eds. *Dermatology*. 3rd ed. Elsevier; 2012.

IMAGE REFERENCES

6. From VisualDx. 2018. Available at: https://www.visualdx.com/visualdx/diagnosis/?moduleId=17&diagnosisId=52126
7. From VisualDx. 2021. Available at: https://www.visualdx.com/visualdx/diagnosis/?moduleId=101&diagnosisId=52339
8. From VisualDx. 2023. Available at: https://www.visualdx.com/visualdx/diagnosis/?moduleId=101&diagnosisId=1424
9. From VisualDx. 2021. Available at: https://www.visualdx.com/visualdx/diagnosis/?moduleId=101&diagnosisId=51858

Chapter 35

FURTHER READING

Bolognia J, Schaffer JV, Cerroni L, eds. *Dermatology*. 4th ed. Elsevier; 2018.

Calonje E, Brenn T, Lazar AJ, MacKee PH, Billings SD, eds. *McKee's Pathology of the Skin: With Clinical Correlations*. 5th ed. Elsevier; 2020.

Dinulos JGH. *Habif's Clinical Dermatology: A Color Guide to Diagnosis and Therapy*. 7th ed. Elsevier; 2021.

James WD, Elston DM, Treat JR, et al. *Epidermal nevi, neoplasms, and cysts. Andrews' Diseases of the Skin*. 13th ed. Elsevier Inc; 2020:636–685.e7.

Patterson JW, Weedon D. *Weedon's Skin Pathology*. 5th ed. Elsevier; 2021.

IMAGE REFERENCES

1. From Calonje E, Brenn T, Lazar AJ, Billings SD. Granulomatous, necrobiotic and perforating dermatoses. *McKee's Pathology of the Skin*, 306–350.e15 [Chapter 9].
2. From James WD, Elston DM, Treat JR, Rosenbach MA, Neuhaus IM. Syphilis, yaws, bejel, and pinta. *Andrews' Diseases of the Skin*, 18, 347–361.e3.
3. From James WD, Elston DM, Treat JR, Rosenbach MA, Neuhaus IM. Cutaneous lymphoid hyperplasia, cutaneous T-cell lymphoma, other malignant lymphomas, and allied diseases. *Andrews' Diseases of the Skin*, 32, 731–749.e4.
4. From James WD, Elston DM, Treat JR, Rosenbach MA, Neuhaus IM. Connective tissue diseases. *Andrews' Diseases of the Skin*, 8, 157–183.e8.
5. From Rosenbach M, English JC. Reactive granulomatous dermatitis in dermatologic clinics. *Dermatol Clin*. 2015;33(3):373–387. Copyright © 2015 Elsevier Inc.
6. From Rosenbach M, English JC. *Dermatol Clin*. 2015;33(3):373–387. Copyright © 2015 Elsevier Inc.
7. From James GH, Dinulos MD. Cutaneous manifestations of internal disease. *Habif's Clinical Dermatology*, 990–1012.e1 [Chapter 26].
8. From Ibbotson SH. Dermatology. *Davidson's Principles and Practice of Medicine*, 27, 1063–1117.

9A. From James WD, Elston DM, Treat JR, Rosenbach MA, Neuhaus IM. Macrophage/monocyte disorders. *Andrews' Diseases of the Skin*, 31, 704–730.e2.

9B. From James WD, Elston DM, Treat JR, Rosenbach MA, Neuhaus IM. Macrophage/monocyte disorders. *Andrews' Diseases of the Skin*, 31, 704–730.e2.

10. Courtesy Dr. Debabrata Bandyopadhyay.

11A. Islam MP, Roach ES, Handbook of Clinical Neurology. vol. 132 Elsevier B.V; 2015. All rights reserved.

11B. Islam MP, Roach ES, Handbook of Clinical Neurology. vol. 132 Elsevier B.V; 2015. All rights reserved.

12. From Dinulos JGH. Urticaria, angioedema, and pruritus. *Habif's Clinical Dermatology*, 176–214.e1 [Chapter 6].
13. From James WD, Elston DM, Treat JR, Rosenbach MA, Neuhaus IM. Errors in metabolism. *Andrews' Diseases of the Skin*, 26, 515–546.e3.
14. From James WD, Elston DM, Treat JR, Rosenbach MA, Neuhaus IM. Cutaneous vascular diseases. *Andrews' Diseases of the Skin*, 35, 813–861.e5.
15. From James WD, Elston DM, Treat JR, Rosenbach MA, Neuhaus IM. Erythema and urticaria. *Andrews' Diseases of the Skin*, 7, 140–156.e3.
16. From James WD, Elston DM, Treat JR, Rosenbach MA, Neuhaus IM. Cutaneous lymphoid hyperplasia, cutaneous T-cell lymphoma, other malignant lymphomas, and allied diseases. *Andrews' Diseases of the Skin*, 32, 731–749.e4.
17. From James WD, Elston DM, Treat JR, Rosenbach MA, Neuhaus IM. Cutaneous lymphoid hyperplasia, cutaneous T-cell lymphoma, other malignant lymphomas, and allied diseases. *Andrews' Diseases of the Skin*, 32, 731–749.e4.

18A. From Dinulos JGH. Premalignant and malignant nonmelanoma skin tumors. *Habif's Clinical Dermatology*, 815–862.e1 [Chapter 21].

18B. From Dinulos JGH. Premalignant and malignant nonmelanoma skin tumors. *Habif's Clinical Dermatology*, 815–862.e1 [Chapter 21].

19. From James WD, Elston DM, Treat JR, Rosenbach MA, Neuhaus IM. Cutaneous lymphoid hyperplasia, cutaneous T-cell lymphoma, other malignant lymphomas, and allied diseases. *Andrews' Diseases of the Skin*, 32, 731–749.e4.
20. From James WD, Elston DM, Treat JR, Rosenbach MA, Neuhaus IM. Mucinoses. *Andrews' Diseases of the Skin*, 9, 184–190.e2.
21. From James WD, Elston DM, Treat JR, Rosenbach MA, Neuhaus IM. Connective tissue diseases. *Andrews' Diseases of the Skin*, 8, 157–183.e8.

22. Langlois S, Brochot P, Reguiai Z. et al. Necrobiotic xanthogranuloma with multiple myeloma. *Case Reports and pathogenic hypotheses, Joint Bone Spine*, 2006;73(1):120–122.
23. From James WD, Elston DM, Treat JR, Rosenbach MA, Neuhaus IM. Macrophage/monocyte disorders. *Andrews' Diseases of the Skin*, 31, 704–730.e2.
24A. From Dinulos JGH. Cutaneous manifestations of internal disease. *Habif's Clinical Dermatology*, 990–1012.e1 [Chapter 26].
24B. From Dinulos JGH. Cutaneous manifestations of internal disease. *Habif's Clinical Dermatology*, 990–1012.e1 [Chapter 26].
25. From James WD, Elston DM, Treat JR, Rosenbach MA, Neuhaus IM. Errors in metabolism. *Andrews' Diseases of the Skin*, 26, 515–546.e3.
26. From Dinulos JGH. Cutaneous manifestations of internal disease. *Habif's Clinical Dermatology*, 990–1012.e1 [Chapter 26].
27. From Micheletti RG, James WD, Elston DM, McMahon PJ. Errors in metabolism. *Andrews' Diseases of the Skin Clinical Atlas*. 26, 361–378.
28. Courtesy Dr. Debabrata Bandyopadhyay.

Chapter 36

FURTHER READING

Forton FMN, De Maertelaer V. Papulopustular rosacea and rosacea-like demodicosis: two phenotypes of the same disease? *J Eur Acad Dermatol Venereol.* 2018;32(6):1011–1016. https://doi.org/10.1111/jdv.14885. Epub 2018 Mar 23. PMID: 29478301; PMCID: PMC6001808.

Curman P, Näsman A, Brauner H. Trichodysplasia spinulosa: a comprehensive review of the disease and its treatment. *J Eur Acad Dermatol Venereol.* 2021;35(5):1067–1076. https://doi.org/10.1111/jdv.17081. Epub 2021 Jan 6. PMID: 33559344; PMCID: PMC8247895.

Panchaprateep R, Tanus A, Tosti A. Clinical, dermoscopic, and histopathologic features of body hair disorders. *J Am Acad Dermatol.* 2015;72(5):890–900. https://doi.org/10.1016/j.jaad.2015.01.024. Epub 2015 Mar 5. PMID: 25748313.

Ma BC, Sahni VN, Sahni DR, Secrest AM. Disseminate and recurrent infundibulofolliculitis: an under-recognized yet treatable entity. *J Drugs Dermatol.* 2021;20(12):1353–1354. https://doi.org/10.36849/jdd.6173. PMID: 34898159.

Martorell A, Jfri A, Koster SBL, et al. Defining hidradenitis suppurativa phenotypes based on the elementary lesion pattern: results of a prospective study. *J Eur Acad Dermatol Venereol.* 2020;34(6):1309–1318. https://doi.org/10.1111/jdv.16183. Epub 2020 Feb 16. PMID: 31919904.

IMAGE REFERENCES

12. James WD, Elston DM, Treat JR, Rosenbach MA, Nuehaus IM. *Andrews' Diseases of the Skin*. 2019:475–484.e2.
13. James WD, Elston DM, Treat JR, Rosenbach MA, Nuehaus IM. *Andrews' Diseases of the Skin*. 2019:92–139.e3.
14. Gawkrodger DJ, Ardern-Jones MR. *Dermatology: An Illustrated Colour Text.* 2021:110–111.

Chapter 37

FURTHER READING

Bolognia J, Schaffer JV, Cerroni L. *Dermatology*. Elsevier; 2018.

Drago F, Ciccarese G, Parodi A. Pityriasis rosea and pityriasis rosea-like eruptions: how to distinguish them? *JAAD Case Rep.* 2018;4(8):800–801.

James WD, Elston DM, Treat JR, Rosenbach MA, Neuhaus I. *Andrews' Diseases of the Skin Clinical Dermatology*. 13th ed. Elsevier; 2020.

Ko CJ. *Dermatology: Visual Recognition and Case Reviews*. Elsevier; 2022.

IMAGE REFERENCES

1. Dinulos JG, Habif TP. *Habif's Clinical Dermatology: A Color Guide to Diagnosis and Therapy*. Elsevier; 2021.
2. Zabel M, Hile GA, Shefler A, Harms PW, Chan MP, Mancuso JB. Dupilumab-induced pityriasis rosea. *JAAD Case Rep.* 2023;33:27–29. https://www.doi.org/10.1016/j.jdcr.2023.01.001.
3. Dinulos JG, Habif TP. *Habif's Clinical Dermatology: A Color Guide to Diagnosis and Therapy*. Elsevier; 2021.
4. Dinulos JG, Habif TP. *Habif's Clinical Dermatology: A Color Guide to Diagnosis and Therapy*. Elsevier; 2021.
5. Dinulos JG, Habif TP. *Habif's Clinical Dermatology: A Color Guide to Diagnosis and Therapy*. Elsevier; 2021.
6. Dinulos JG, Habif TP. *Habif's Clinical Dermatology: A Color Guide to Diagnosis and Therapy*. Elsevier; 2021.
9. Courtesy Fitzsimons Army Medical teaching files.
10. Dinulos JG, *Habif TP. Habif's Clinical Dermatology: A Color Guide to Diagnosis and Therapy*. Elsevier; 2021.
11. Dinulos JG, Habif TP. *Habif's Clinical Dermatology: A Color Guide to Diagnosis and Therapy*. Elsevier; 2021.

Chapter 38

FURTHER READING

Daoud MS, Pittelkow MR. Chapter 26. Lichen planus. In: Goldsmith LA, Katz SI, Gilchrest BA, Paller AS, Leffell DJ, Wolff K, eds. *Fitzpatrick's Dermatology in General Medicine*. 8th ed. McGraw Hill; 2012. https://accessmedicine.mhmedical.com/content.aspx?bookid=392&sectionid=41138721.

Kumarasinghe SPW, Pandya A, Chandran V, et al. A global consensus statement on ashy dermatosis, erythema dyschromicum perstans, lichen planus pigmentosus, idiopathic eruptive macular pigmentation, and Riehl's melanosis. *Int J Dermatol.* 2019;58(3):263–272.

Moffarah AS, Al Mohajer M, Hurwitz BL, Armstrong DG. Skin and soft tissue infections. *Microbiol Spectr.* 2016;4(4). https://doi.org/10.1128/microbiolspec.DMIH2-0014-2015.

Vyas A. Genital lichen sclerosus and its mimics. *Obstet Gynecol Clin North Am.* 2017;44(3):389–406.

Lotti T, Buggiani G, Prignano F. Prurigo nodularis and lichen simplex chronicus. *Dermatol Ther.* 2008;21(1):42–46.

IMAGE REFERENCES

1. Klaisiri, Iamaroon A, Neff A, Pitak-Arnnop P. Oral lichenoid lesion related to dental amalgam: A case report. *J Stomatol Oral Maxillofac Surg*, 2019;120(6):591–594.
2. Chirravur P, Sroussi H, Treister N, et al. Hydroxychloroquine for the management of recalcitrant oral lichen planus. *Oral Surg Oral Med Oral Pathol Oral Radiol.* 2024;137(4):355–361.
3. James WD, Berger TG, Elston DM, Neuhaus IM. *Andrews' Diseases of the Skin: Clinical Dermatology*. 12th ed. Elsevier; 2016.
4. *Courtesy of Debabrata Bandyopadhyay, MD.*
5. James WD, Berger TG, Elston DM, Neuhaus IM. *Andrews' Diseases of the Skin: Clinical Dermatology*. 12th ed. Elsevier; 2016.
6. James WD, Berger TG, Elston DM, Neuhaus IM. *Andrews' Diseases of the Skin: Clinical Dermatology*. 12th ed. Elsevier; 2016.
7. James WD, Berger TG, Elston DM, Neuhaus IM. *Andrews' Diseases of the Skin: Clinical Dermatology*. 12th ed. Elsevier; 2016.
8. Leung N, Oliveira M, Selim MA, McKinley-Grant L, Lesesky E. Erythema dyschromicum perstans: A case report and systematic review of histologic presentation and treatment. *Int J Womens Dermatol.* 2018;4(4):216–222.
9. James WD, Berger TG, Elston DM, Neuhaus IM. *Andrews' Diseases of the Skin: Clinical Dermatology*. 12th ed. Elsevier; 2016.
10. Dinulos JG. *Habif's Clinical Dermatology: A Color Guide to Diagnosis and Therapy*. 7th ed. Elsevier; 2020.
11. James WD, Berger TG, Elston DM, Neuhaus IM. *Andrews' Diseases of the Skin: Clinical Dermatology*. 12th ed. Elsevier; 2016.
12. James WD, Berger TG, Elston DM, Neuhaus IM. *Andrews' Diseases of the Skin: Clinical Dermatology*. 12th ed. Elsevier; 2016.
13. James WD, Berger TG, Elston DM, Neuhaus IM. *Andrews' Diseases of the Skin: Clinical Dermatology*. 12th ed. Elsevier; 2016.
14. James WD, Berger TG, Elston DM, Neuhaus IM. *Andrews' Diseases of the Skin: Clinical Dermatology*. 12th ed. Elsevier; 2016.

Chapter 39

FURTHER READING

Blum AE, Burgin S. Eczematous drug eruptions. *Am J Clin Dermatol.* 2021;22(3):349–366.

Ilkit M, Durdu M, Karakaş M. Cutaneous id reactions: a comprehensive review of clinical manifestations, epidemiology, etiology, and management. *Crit Rev Microbiol.* 2012;38(3):191–202.

James WD, Elston DM, Treat JR, et al., eds. Contact dermatitis and drug eruptions. *Andrews' Diseases of the Skin.* 13th ed. Elsevier Health Sciences; 2020: 92–139.e3.

James WD, Elston DM, Treat JR, et al., eds. Eczema, atopic dermatitis, and noninfectious immunodeficiency disorders. *Andrews' Diseases of the Skin.* 13th ed. Elsevier Health Sciences; 2020:63–91.e2.

Ständer S. Atopic dermatitis. *N Engl J Med.* 2021;384(12):1136–1143.

Chapter 40

FURTHER READING

Bologna JL, Jorizzo JJ, Schaffer JV, et al. *Dermatology*. 3rd ed. Elsevier; 2012. Edited by Callen JP, Cerroni L, Heymann WR, et al.

Chapter 41

FURTHER READING

Stern RS. Exanthematous drug eruptions. *N Engl J Med*. 2012;366(26):2492–2501.

Isaacs M, Cardones AR, Rahnama-Moghadam S. DRESS syndrome: clinical myths and pearls. *Cutis*. 2018;102(5):322–326.

Kardaun SH, Sekula P, Valeyrie-Allanore L, Liss Y, Chu CY, Creamer D, RegiSCAR Study Group Drug reaction with eosinophilia and systemic symptoms (DRESS): an original multisystem adverse drug reaction. Results from the prospective Regi SCAR study. *Br J Dermatol*. 2013;169(5):1071–1080.

Korman AM, Alikhan A, Kaffenberger BH. Viral exanthems: an update on laboratory testing of the adult patient. *J Am Acad Dermatol*. 2017;76(3):538–550.

Burns JC, Glodé MP. Kawasaki syndrome. *Lancet*. 2004;364(9433):533–544.

IMAGE REFERENCES

1. Lew BL, Haw CR, Lee MH. Cutaneous drug eruption from cetirizine and hydroxyzine. *J Am Acad Dermatol*. 2004;50(6):953–956.
2. Saberi SA, Kumar AM, Davis D, Nambudiri VE. Florid cutaneous morbilliform eruption in the setting of primary Epstein-Barr virus infection. *JAAD Case Reports*. 2024;45:102–105.
3. Fatima S, Veenstra J, Antonyan AS, Kohen L. Severe recalcitrant morbilliform eruption from dual immune checkpoint blockade. *JAAD Case Reports*. 2018;4(6):593–595.
4. Letko E, Papaliodis DN, Papaliodis GN, Daoud YJ, Ahmed AR, Foster CS. Stevens-Johnson syndrome and toxic epidermal necrolysis: a review of the literature. *Ann Allergy Asthma Immunol*. 2005;94(4):419–436.
5. Lowndes S, Darby A, Mead G, Lister A. Stevens–Johnson syndrome after treatment with rituximab. *Ann Oncol*. 2002;13(12):1948–1950.
6. Momen SE, Diaz-Cano S, Walsh S, Creamer D. Discriminating minor and major forms of drug reaction with eosinophilia and systemic symptoms: facial edema aligns to the severe phenotype. *J Am Acad Dermatol*. 2021;85(3):645–652.
7. Photograph courtesy of M. Hartwell.
8. Reprinted with permission from Elsevier. *The Lancet*. 364(9433), 533–544.
9. Pincus LB, Grossman ME, Fox LP. The exanthem of dengue fever: clinical features of two US tourists traveling abroad. *J Am Acad Dermatol*. 2008;58(2):308–316.
10. Paller AS, Mancini AJ. *Paller and Mancini-Hurwitz Clinical Pediatric Dermatology E-Book: A textbook of skin disorders of childhood and adolescence*. Elsevier Health Sciences; 2020. Figure 16.10.
11. Fukuda M, Harada T, Shimizu T, Hiroshige J. Forchheimer spots in rubella. *Intern Med*. 2020;59(13):1673.
12. Paller AS, Mancini AJ. *Paller and Mancini-Hurwitz Clinical Pediatric Dermatology E-Book: A textbook of skin disorders of childhood and adolescence*. Elsevier Health Sciences; 2020. Figure 16.7.

Chapter 42

FURTHER READING

César A, Cruz M, Mota A, Azevedo F. Erythroderma. A clinical and etiological study of 103 patients. *J Dermatol Case Rep*. 2016;10(1):1–9. https://doi.org/10.3315/jdcr.2016.1222.

Khaled A, Sellami A, Fazaa B, Kharfi M, Zeglaoui F, Kamoun MR. Acquired erythroderma in adults: a clinical and prognostic study. *J Eur Acad Dermatol Venereol*. 2010;24(7):781–788. https://doi.org/10.1111/j.1468-3083.2009.03526.x.

Mistry N, Gupta A, Alavi A, Sibbald RG. A review of the diagnosis and management of erythroderma (generalized red skin). *Adv Skin Wound Care*. 2015;28(5):228–236. https://doi.org/10.1097/01.ASW.0000463573.40637.73. quiz 237–238.

Miyashiro D, Sanches JA. Erythroderma: a prospective study of 309 patients followed for 12 years in a tertiary center. *Sci Rep*. 2020;10(1):9774. https://doi.org/10.1038/s41598-020-66040-7.

Navrotski BRde F, Nihi FM, Camilleri MJ, Cerci FB. Wet wrap dressings as a rescue therapy option for erythrodermic psoriasis. *An Bras Dermatol*. 2018;93(4):598–600. https://doi.org/10.1590/abd1806-4841.20186414.

IMAGE REFERENCES

1. van der Velden HMJ, et al. Fingernail psoriasis reconsidered: A case-control study. *JAAD*. 2013;69(2):245–252.
2. From Hurwitz Clinical Pediatric Dermatology: A Textbook of Skin Disorders of Childhood and Adolescence. 5th ed. 2015.
3. From James WD, et al. *Andrews' diseases of the skin*. 12th ed. Elsevier; 2016.
5. Copyright Richard P. Usatine, MD.
6. Courtesy Hsui CK, MD, and Lee JYY, MD, National Cheng Kung University Hospital, Tainan, Taiwan.
7. From Callen JP, Jorizzo JL, Zone JJ, Piette W, Rosenbach MA, Vleugels RA. *Dermatological Signs of Systemic Disease*. 5th ed. Elsevier; 2017.

Chapter 43

FURTHER READING

Bolognia J, Schaffer J, Cerroni L, Callen J. *Dermatology*. 4th ed. Elsevier; 2018.

Itin PH, Fistarol SK. Palmoplantar keratodermas. *Clin Dermatol*. 2005;23(1): 15–22.

Rosenstein NE, Perkins BA, Stephens DS, Popovic T, Hughes JM. Meningococcal disease. *N Engl J Med*. 2001;344(18):1378–1388.

Deleuran M, Vestergaard C. Clinical heterogeneity and differential diagnosis of atopic dermatitis. *Br J Dermatol*. 2014;170(suppl 1):2–6.

Shih S, Khachemoune A. Acquired digital fibrokeratoma: review of its clinical and dermoscopic features and differential diagnosis. *Int J Dermatol*. 2019;58(2):151–158.

IMAGE REFERENCES

1. Karatas E, Nazim A, Patel P, et al. Erythema multiforme reactions after Pfizer/BioNTech (BNT162b2) and Moderna (mRNA-1273) COVID-19 vaccination: a case series. *JAAD Case Rep*. 2023;32:55–58.
2. Beaulieu A, Rehman HU. Janeway lesions. *CMAJ*. 2010;182(10):1075.
3. Landy J, Djogovic D, Sligl W. Gonococcal septic shock, acute respiratory distress syndrome, and multisystem organ failure: a case report. *Int J Infect Dis*. 2010;14:e239–e241.
4. Pace D. Paediatric Infectious Diseases Clinic, Mater Dei Hospital, Malta.
5. Dourmishev LA, Dourmishev AL. Syphilis: uncommon presentations in adults. *Clin Dermatol*. 2005;23(6):555–564.
6. Han B, Hur K, Ohn J, Lim SS, Mun JH. Acral lentiginous melanoma in situ: dermoscopic features and management strategy. *Sci Rep*. 2020;10(1):20503.
7. Wada M, Lee S, Curnow P, Simpson I, Mar A. A case of pityriasis rubra pilaris following AstraZeneca COVID-19 vaccine. *JAAD Case Rep*. 2022;24:74–77.
8. Lebowitz E, Kim JS, Magro C. Reactive arthritis following COVID-19 vaccination with BNT162b2. *JAAD Case Rep*. 2022;24:108–111.
9. McLean WI, Hansen CD, Eliason MJ, Smith FJ. The phenotypic and molecular genetic features of pachyonychia congenita. *J Invest Dermatol*. 2022;131(5):1015–1017.

Chapter 44

FURTHER READING

Tolaymat L, Hall MR. *Perioral Dermatitis*. StatPearls Publishing; 2022. https://www.ncbi.nlm.nih.gov/books/NBK525968/.

Dessinioti C, Antoniou C, Katsambas A. Acneiform eruptions. *Clin Dermatol*. 2014;32:24–34.

Maarouf M, Saberian C, Lio PA, Shi VY. Head-and-neck dermatitis: diagnostic difficulties and management pearls. *Pediatr Dermatol*. 2018;35:748–753.

Al-Qassabi A, Al-Busaidi K, Al Baccouche K, Al Ismaili A. Granulomatous periorificial dermatitis in an adult: a case report with review of literature. *Sultan Qaboos Univ Med J*. 2020;20(1):e101–103.

Leung AKC, Barankin B. Herpes labialis: an update. *Recent Pat Inflamm Allergy Drug Discov*. 2017;11(2):107–113.

IMAGE REFERENCES

7. James WD, Berger TG, Elston DM. *Andrews' Disease of the Skin Clinical Dermatology*. 11th ed. Elsevier; 2011.

Chapter 45

FURTHER READING

Bolognia J, Schaffer JV, Cerroni L. *Dermatology*. Elsevier; 2018.

James WD, Elston DM, Treat JR, Rosenbach MA, Neuhaus I. *Andrews' Diseases of the Skin Clinical Dermatology*. 13th ed. Elsevier; 2020.

Ko CJ. *Dermatology: Visual Recognition and Case Reviews*. Elsevier; 2022.
Rosen T. Update on genital lesions. *JAMA*. 2003;290(8):1001–1005. https://doi.org/10.1001/jama.290.8.1001. PMID: 12941660.
Matthews N, Wong V, Brooks J, Kroumpouzos G. Genital diseases in the mature woman. *Clin Dermatol*. 2018;36(2):208–221. https://doi.org/10.1016/j.clindermatol.2017.10.012. Epub 2017 Oct 3. PMID: 29566925.

IMAGE REFERENCES

1. Dinulos JG, Habif TP. *Habif's Clinical Dermatology: A Color Guide to Diagnosis and Therapy*. Elsevier; 2021.
2. From Wu IB, Schwartz RA. Reiter's syndrome: the classic triad and more. *J Am Acad Dermatol*. 2008;59(1):117; with permission.
3. Dinulos JG, Habif TP. *Habif's Clinical Dermatology: A Color Guide to Diagnosis and Therapy*. Elsevier; 2021.
4. Dinulos JG, Habif TP. *Habif's Clinical Dermatology: A Color Guide to Diagnosis and Therapy*. Elsevier; 2021.
5. Hinten F, Meeuwis KAP, van Rossum MM, de Hullu JA. HPV-related (pre) malignancies of the female anogenital tract in renal transplant recipients. *Crit Rev Oncol Hematol*. 2012;84(2):161–180. https://www.doi.org.10.1016/j.critrevonc.2012.02.008.
6. Dinulos JG, Habif TP. *Habif's Clinical Dermatology: A Color Guide to Diagnosis and Therapy*. Elsevier; 2021.
7. Dinulos JG, Habif TP. *Habif's Clinical Dermatology: A Color Guide to Diagnosis and Therapy*. Elsevier; 2021.
8. Photo is courtesy of Tiffany Mayo, MD.
10. Waldman RA, Grant-Kels JM. *Dermatology for the Primary Care Provider*. Elsevier; 2022.

Chapter 46

FURTHER READING

Dinulos JGH, Habif TP. *Habif's Clinical Dermatology: A Color Guide to Diagnosis and Therapy*. 7th ed. Elsevier; 2021.
Bolognia JL, Schaffer JV, Cerroni L, et al. *Dermatology*. Vol. 2. 4th ed. Elsevier; 2017.
Urso B, Lu KB, Khachemoune A. Axillary manifestations of dermatologic diseases: a focused review. *Acta Dermatovenerol Alp Pannonica Adriat*. 2018;27(4):185–191.
Marks JG, Miller JJ. *Scaling papules, plaques, and patches. Lookingbill and Marks' Principles of Dermatology*. 6th ed. Elsevier Masson; 2019.
Ashton R, Leppard B. *Differential Diagnosis in Dermatology*. 5th ed. Radcliffe; 2005.

IMAGE REFERENCES

1. Courtesy of Richard Antaya, MD.
2. Gawkrodger D, Ardern-Jones MR. *Dermatology: An Illustrated Color Text*. 7th ed. Elsevier.
3. Bolognia JL, Schaffer JV, Cerroni L. *Dermatology*. 4th ed. Elsevier; 2018. Courtesy Lorenzo Cerroni, MD.
4. Stewart RW. Skin, hair, and nails. In: *Seidels Guide to Physical Examination*. Elsevier Health Sciences Division; 2014.
5. Fitzsimons Army Medical Center Collection.
6. From the Fitzsimons Army Medical Center Collection, Aurora, CO.
7. Higgins E. Psoriasis. *Medicine*. 2021;49(6). https://www.doi.org.10.1016/j.mpmed.2021.03.005.
8. Gawkrodger DJ, DSc MD FRCP FRCPE; Ardern-Jones MR, BSc MBBS DPhil FRCP. *Dermatology: An Illustrated Colour Text*. Published December 31, 2020. Pages 110–111. © 2021.
9. Bolognia JL, Schaffer JV, Cerroni L. *Dermatology*. 4th ed. Elsevier; 2018. Courtesy Kalman Watsky, MD.
10. Calonje E, Brenn T, Lazar A, Billings SD. *McKee's Pathology of the Skin: With Clinical Correlations*. 5th ed. Elsevier; 2020.
11. Drago F, Broccolo F, Rebora A. Pityriasis rosea: an update with a critical appraisal of its possible herpesviral etiology. *J Am Acad Dermatol*. 2009;61(2):303–318. https://www.doi.org.10.1016/j.jaad.2008.07.045.
12. Busam KJ. *Dermatopathology*. 2nd ed. Elsevier; 2014.
13. Yang C-C, Shih I-H, Lin W-L, et al. Juvenile pityriasis rubra pilaris: report of 28 cases in Taiwan. *J Am Acad Dermatol*. 2008;59(6):943–948. https://www.doi.org.10.1016/j.jaad.2008.07.054.
14. Reprinted with permission from Drago F, Broccolo F, Rebora A. Pityriasis rosea: An update with a critical appraisal of its possible herpesviral etiology. *JAAD*. 2009;61(2):303–318.
15. Reprinted with permission from Busam KJ. *Dermatopathology*. 2nd ed. Elsevier; 2016.

Chapter 47

FURTHER READING

Montagnon CM, Tolkachjov SN, Murrell DF, Camilleri MJ, Lehman JS. Intraepithelial autoimmune blistering dermatoses: clinical features and diagnosis. *J Am Acad Dermatol*. 2021;84(6):1507–1519. https://doi.org/10.1016/j.jaad.2020.11.075.
Luelmo-Aguilar J, Santandreu MS. Folliculitis: recognition and management. *Am J Clin Dermatol*. 2004;5(5):301–310. https://doi.org/10.2165/00128071-200405050-00003.
Ross EK, Tan E, Shapiro J. Update on primary cicatricial alopecias. *J Am Acad Dermatol*. 2005;53(1):1–40. https://doi.org/10.1016/j.jaad.2004.06.015.
Bolduc C, Sperling LC, Shapiro J. Primary cicatricial alopecia: other lymphocytic primary cicatricial alopecias and neutrophilic and mixed primary cicatricial alopecias. *J Am Acad Dermatol*. 2016;75(6):1101–1117. https://doi.org/10.1016/j.jaad.2015.01.056.

IMAGE REFERENCES

3. Image used with permission from VisualDx (www.visualdx.com).
4. Image used with permission from VisualDx (www.visualdx.com).
9. Image used with permission from VisualDx (www.visualdx.com).
10. Image used with permission from VisualDx (www.visualdx.com).

Chapter 48

FURTHER READING

Veraldi S, Schianchi R, Nazzaro G, et al. Seven cases of blistering dactylitis. *Acta Derm Venereol*. 2020;100:adv00196.
Choi E, Huang J, Chew KL, Jaffar H, Tan C. Pustular tinea manuum from *Trichophyton erinacei* infection. *JAAD Case Rep*. 2018;4(6):518–520. https://doi.org/10.1016/j.jdcr.2018.01.019.
Toussirot É, Aubin F. Paradoxical reactions under TNF-α blocking agents and other biological agents given for chronic immune-mediated diseases: an analytical and comprehensive overview. *RMD Open*. 2016;2(2):e000239.
Croitoru DO, Brooks SG, Nathanielsz N. et al. Predictors of severity in paradoxical psoriasis from biologic therapies: a systematic review. *J Am Acad Dermatol*. 2022:S0190-9622(22)01010-6. https://www.doi.org.10.1016/j.jaad.2022.06.019. Epub ahead of print. PMID: 35718193.
Räßler F, Goetze S, Elsner P. Acrokeratosis paraneoplastica (Bazex syndrome)—a systematic review on risk factors, diagnosis, prognosis and management. *J Eur Acad Dermatol Venereol*. 2017;31(7):1119–1136.

Chapter 49

FURTHER READING

Bolognia J, Schaffer J, Cerroni L, Callen J. *Dermatology*. 4th ed.2018.
Hoegler KM, John AM, Handler MZ, Schwartz RA. Generalized pustular psoriasis: a review and update on treatment. *J Eur Acad Dermatol Venereol*. 2018;32(10):1645–1651.
Kurtzman DJ, Jones T, Lian F, Peng LS. Metastatic Crohn's disease: a review and approach to therapy. *J Am Acad Dermatol*. 2014;71(4):804–813.
Nelson CA, Stephen S, Ashchyan HJ, James WD, Micheletti RG, Rosenbach M. Neutrophilic dermatoses: pathogenesis, Sweet syndrome, neutrophilic eccrine hidradenitis, and Behçet disease. *J Am Acad Dermatol*. 2018;79(6):987–1006.

IMAGE REFERENCES

1. Image C and G. Courtesy Charles Phillips, MD.
2. Image D. Adapted from Ashchyan HJ, Nelson CA, Stephen S, James WD, Micheletti RG, Rosenbach M. Neutrophilic dermatoses. *J Am Acad Dermatol*. 2018;79(6):1009–1022.
3. Image E. Adapted from Wu IB, Schwartz RA. Reiter's syndrome: the classic triad and more. *J Am Acad Dermatol*. 2008;59(1):113–121.
4. Image F. Adapted from Earle M, Nelson D. A teen with a rash and arthralgia; a reminder to keep gonococcal disease on the differential. *Vis J Emerg Med*. 2021;22:100914.

Chapter 50

FURTHER READING

Bolognia J, Schaffer J, Cerroni L, Callen J. *Dermatology*. 4th ed. Elsevier; 2018.

Mengesha YM, Bennett ML. Pustular skin disorders: diagnosis and treatment. *Am J Clin Dermatol.* 2002;3(6):389–400. https://doi.org/10.2165/00128071-200203060-00003.

Patterson JW. *Skin pathology. Dermatopathology.* 4th ed. Elsevier; 2015.

IMAGE REFERENCES

3. Lebowitz E, Kim J, Magro C. Reactive arthritis following COVID-19 vaccination with BNT162b2. *JAAD Case Rep.* 2022;24:108–111. https://doi.org/10.1016/j.jdcr.2022.04.026.

Chapter 51

FURTHER READING

Schieving JH, Schoenaker M, Weemaes CM, et al. Telangiectasias: small lesions referring to serious disorders. *Eur J Paediatr Neurol.* 2017;21(6):807–815. https://doi.org/10.1016/j.ejpn.2017.07.016.

Gupta R, Gautam RK, Bhardwaj M, Chauhan A. A clinical approach to diagnose patients with localized telangiectasia. *Int J Dermatol.* 2015;54(8):e294–e301. https://doi.org/10.1111/ijd.12629.

Requena L, Sangueza OP. Cutaneous vascular anomalies. Part I. Hamartomas, malformations, and dilation of preexisting vessels. *J Am Acad Dermatol.* 1997;37(4):523–552. https://doi.org/10.1016/s0190-9622(97)70169-5.

Valdivielso-Ramos M, Martin-Santiago A, Azaña JM, et al. Capillary malformation-arteriovenous malformation syndrome: a multicentre study. *Clin Exp Dermatol.* 2021;46(2):300–305. https://doi.org/10.1111/ced.14428.

Wiznia LE, Steuer AB, Penn LA, Meehan SA, Femia AN. Generalized essential telangiectasia. *Dermatol Online J.* 2018;24(12): 13030/qt2926z3f5.

IMAGE REFERENCES

3. Diociaiuti A, Cutrone M, Rotunno R, et al. Angioma serpiginosum: a case report and review of the literature. *Ital J Pediatr.* 2019;45(1):53.
4. Gallo RL, Granstein RD, Kang S, et al. Standard classification and pathophysiology of rosacea: the 2017 update by the National Rosacea Society Expert Committee. *J Am Acad Dermatol.* 2018;78(1):148–155.
5. James W, Berger T, Elston D. *Andrews' Diseases of the Skin: Clinical Dermatology.* 11th ed. Elsevier; 2011.
6. Sachs DL, Varani J, Chubb H, et al. Atrophic and hypertrophic photoaging: clinical, histologic, and molecular features of 2 distinct phenotypes of photoaged skin. *J Am Acad Dermatol.* 2019;81(2):480–488.
7. Perez A, Wain ME, Robson A, Groves RW, Stefanato CM. Cutaneous collagenous vasculopathy with generalized telangiectasia in two female patients. *J Am Acad Dermatol.* 2010;63(5):882–885.
8. Thrash B, Patel M, Shah KR, Boland CR, Menter A. Cutaneous manifestations of gastrointestinal disease: part II. *J Am Acad Dermatol.* 2013;68(2):211.e1–246.
9. Valdivielso-Ramos M, Martin-Santiago A, Azaña JM, et al. Capillary malformation-arteriovenous malformation syndrome: a multicentre study. *Clin Exp Dermatol.* 2021;46(2):300–305.
10. Greenberger S, Berkun Y, Ben-Zeev B, Levi YB, Barziliai A, Nissenkorn A. Dermatologic manifestations of ataxia-telangiectasia syndrome. *J Am Acad Dermatol.* 2013;68(6):932–936.
11. Ciatti S, Varga J, Greenbaum SS. The 585 nm flashlamp-pumped pulsed dye laser for the treatment of telangiectases in patients with scleroderma. *J Am Acad Dermatol.* 1996;35(3 Pt 1):487–488.
12. Huang A, Desai A, Brinster N, Marmon S. Telangiectasia macularis eruptiva perstans in the presence of liver cirrhosis. *JAAD Case Rep.* 2020;6(5):438–440.

Chapter 52

FURTHER READING

Diociaiuti A, Paolantonio G, Zama M, et al. Vascular birthmarks as a clue for complex and syndromic vascular anomalies. *Front Pediatr.* 2021;9:730393. https://doi.org/10.3389/fped.2021.730393.

Maria C, et al. Vascular malformations: part I. *J Am Acad Dermatol.* 2007;56(3): 353–370. quiz 371-374. https://doi.org/10.1016/j.jaad.2006.05.069.

Garzon MC, Huang JT, Enjolras O, Frieden IJ. Vascular malformations. Part II: associated syndromes. *J Am Acad Dermatol.* 2007;56(4):541–564. https://doi.org/10.1016/j.jaad.2006.05.066.

Mahajan P, Bergstrom KL, Phung TL, Metry DW. The genetics of vascular birthmarks. *Clin Dermatol.* 2022;40(4):313–321. https://doi.org/10.1016/j.clindermatol.2022.02.006.

Wassef M, Blei F, Adams D, et al. Vascular anomalies classification: recommendations from the International Society for the Study of Vascular Anomalies. *Pediatrics.* 2015;136(1):e203–e214. https://doi.org/10.1542/peds.2014-3673.

IMAGE REFERENCES

1. Iga, N, Endo, Y, Fujisawa, A, et al. Possible association between cutaneous angiosarcoma of the scalp and nuchal salmon patch. *J Dermatol.* 2013;40(12):1049–1050.
2. Boos MD, Bozarth XL, Sidbury R, et al. Forehead location and large segmental pattern of facial port-wine stains predict risk of Sturge-Weber syndrome. *J Am Acad Dermatol.* 2020;83(4), 1110–1117. https://doi.org/10.1016/j.jaad.2020.05.017.
5. Alluhaibi R, Alkhayat LN, Aqeeli W. Capillary malformation-arteriovenous malformation syndrome. *Cureus.* 2021;13(1):e12562.
6. Patel, R., Durant, E. J., & Freed, R. (2021). Parkes-Weber syndrome in the emergency department. *BMJ Case Rep.* 14(9), e241649. Figure 1 & Figure 3.
7. Yang X, Su L, Wang D, Shen Y. Interventional therapy of Cobb syndrome (spinal arteriovenous metameric syndrome). *Ann Neurol.* 2023. https://doi.org/10.1002/ana.26810. Advance online publication.

Chapter 53

FURTHER READING

Angelo C, Provini A, Ferranti G, Palermi G, Paradisi M. Eruptive pseudoangiomatosis. *Pediatr Dermatol.* 2002;19:243–245. https://doi.org/10.1046/j.1525-1470.2002.00072.x.

Hoeger P, Colmenero I. Vascular tumours in infants. Part I: benign vascular tumours other than infantile haemangioma. *Br J Dermatol.* 2014;171:466–473. https://doi.org/10.1111/bjd.12650.

Requena L, Sangueza OP. Cutaneous vascular proliferation. Part II. Hyperplasias and benign neoplasms. *J Am Acad Dermatol.* 1997;37(6):887–919. https://doi.org/10.1016/s0190-9622(97)70065-3. quiz 920-2.

Udondo González del Tánago B, Aguirre Meñica M, Zaldumbide Dueñas L, Martínez Expósito Ó, González-Hermosa MR. Hundreds of vasculoproliferative skin lesions in a paediatric renal transplant recipient. *Clin Exp Dermatol.* 2022;47:1748–1751. https://doi.org/10.1111/ced.15234.

Xu X, Xu C, Chen H, et al. Eruptive microvenular hemangiomas in 4 Chinese patients: clinicopathologic correlation and review of the literature. *Am J Dermatopathol.* 2010;32(8):837–840. https://doi.org/10.1097/DAD.0b013e3181d74290.

IMAGE REFERENCES

3. Shinozaki-Ushiku A, Higashihara T, Ikemura M, et al. Glomeruloid hemangioma associated with TAFRO syndrome. Hum Pathol. 2018;82:172–176.
4. Linos K, Csaposs J Carlson JA. Microvenular hemangioma presenting with numerous bilateral macules, patches, and plaques: a case report and review of the literature. *Am J Dermatopathol.* 2013;35(1):98–101.
5. Zaballos P, Llambrich A, Del Pozo LJ, et al. Dermoscopy of targetoid hemosiderotic hemangioma: a morphological study of 35 cases. *Dermatology.* 2015;231(4):339–344.
6. Requena L, Sangueza OP. Cutaneous vascular anomalies. Part I. Hamartomas, malformations, and dilation of preexisting vessels. *J Am Acad Dermatol.* 1997;37(4):523–552.
9. Wambier CG, Cappel MA, Danilau Ostroski TK, et al. Familial outbreak of eruptive pseudoangiomatosis with dermoscopic and histopathologic correlation. *J Am Acad Dermatol.* 2017;76(2 suppl 1):S12–S15.
10. Jiang HZ, Jin XH, Huang XY, et al. Three cases report of idiopathic angiosarcoma of the head and neck and literature review. *Ann Palliat Med.* 2020;9(4):2333–2340.

Chapter 54

FURTHER READING

Thomas AE, Baird SF, Anderson J. Purpuric and petechial rashes in adults and children: initial assessment. *BMJ.* 2016;352:i1285. https://doi.org/10.1136/bmj.i1285. Published 2016 Mar 22.

Dabiri G, Damstetter E, Chang Y, Baiyee Ebot E, Powers JG, Phillips T. Coagulation disorders and their cutaneous presentations: diagnostic work-up and treatment. *J Am Acad Dermatol.* 2016;74(5):795–806. https://doi.org/10.1016/j.jaad.2015.08.071.

McGrath A, Barrett MJ. *Petechiae. StatPearls.* StatPearls Publishing; 2022.

Bolognia JL, Schaffer JV, Cerroni L. *Purpura: mechanisms and differential diagnosis. Dermatology.* 4th ed. Elsevier; 2018:376–389.e1.

Marks J, Miller J. *Purpura. Lookingbill and Marks' Principles of Dermatology*. 6th ed. Elsevier; 2017:234–245.

IMAGE REFERENCES

2. Marks J, Miller J. Purpura. *Lookingbill and Marks' Principles of Dermatology*. 6th ed. Elsevier; 2017:234–245.
3. Bolognia JL, Schaffer JV, Cerroni L. *Dermatology*. 4th ed. Elsevier; 2018. Courtesy of Yale Residents' Slide Collection.
4. Photo courtesy of Bryan E. Anderson, MD.

Chapter 55

FURTHER READING

Arakaki R, Fox L. Updates in the approach to the patient with purpura. *Curr Derm Rep*. 2017;6:55–62. https://doi.org/10.1007/s13671-017-0184-7.

Weiser J, Scully B, Bulman W, Husain S, Grossman M. Periumbilical parasitic thumbprint purpura: strongyloides hyperinfection syndrome acquired from a cadaveric renal transplant. *Transpl Infect Dis*. 2011;13(1):58–62. https://doi.org/10.1111/j.1399-3062.2010.00516.x.

Schneiderman P, Grossman M. *The Clinician's Guide to Dermatologic Differential Diagnosis*. 2nd ed. Elsevier; 2022.

James W, Elston D, Treat J, Rosenbach M, Neuhaus I, Andrews G. *Andrews' Diseases of the Skin: Clinical Dermatology*. 13th ed. Elsevier; 2020.

IMAGE REFERENCES

1. Palmer M, Brodell RT, Mostow EN. Elder abuse: dermatologic clues and critical solutions. *J Am Acad Dermatol*. 2013;68(2):e37–42.
2. Marks JG, Miller JJ, Hollins LC. Lookingbill and Marks' Principles of Dermatology. 7th ed. Elsevier; 2025:242–254.

Chapter 56

FURTHER READING

Cutaneous vascular diseasesJames WD, Elston D, Treat JR, Rosenbach MA, Neuhaus I, eds. *Andrews' Diseases of the Skin: Clinical Dermatology*. 13th ed. Elsevier; 2019.

Wick MR, Patterson JW. Cutaneous paraneoplastic syndromes. *Semin Diagn Pathol*. 2019;36(4):211–228. https://doi.org/10.1053/j.semdp.2019.01.001. Epub 2019 Jan 31. PMID: 30736994.

Marquez J, Aguirre L, Muñoz C, Echeverri A, Restrepo M, Pinto LF. Cocaine-levamisole-induced vasculitis/vasculopathy syndrome. *Curr Rheumatol Rep*. 2017;19(6):36. https://doi.org/10.1007/s11926-017-0653-9. PMID: 28612332.

Johnson EF, Wetter DA, Lehman JS, Hand JL, Davis DM, Tollefson MM. Leukocytoclastic vasculitis in children: clinical characteristics, subtypes, causes and direct immunofluorescence findings of 56 biopsy-confirmed cases. *J Eur Acad Dermatol Venereol*. 2017;31(3):544–549. https://doi.org/10.1111/jdv.13952. Epub 2016 Sep 19. PMID: 27580419.

IMAGE REFERENCES

1. Monjazeb S, Philips RC, Wilkerson M. A case of leukocytoclastic vasculitis following influenza vaccination. *JAAD Case Rep*. 2016;2(4):340–342. https://doi.org/10.1016/j.jdcr.2016.06.007. PMID: 27570819; PMCID: PMC4992000.
2. Archambault LJ, Chen JY, Obeid RA, Hill HE, DiCaudo DJ, Renszel K. Concurrent pulmonary coccidioidomycosis and immunoglobulin A vasculitis with hemorrhagic bullae. *JAAD Case Rep*. 2020;7:50–53. https://doi.org/10.1016/j.jdcr.2020.11.001. PMID: 33319005; PMCID: PMC7727300.
3. Kwon HJ, Park KD, Yoon JH. Leukocytoclastic vasculitis as a cutaneous paraneoplastic syndrome in malignant mesothelioma. *JAAD Case Rep*. 2022;26:20–22. https://doi.org/10.1016/j.jdcr.2022.06.006. PMID: 35865729; PMCID: PMC9294479.

Chapter 57

FURTHER READING

Georgesen C, Fox LP, Harp J. Retiform purpura: a diagnostic approach. *J Am Acad Dermatol*. 2020;82(4):783–796. https://doi.org/10.1016/j.jaad.2019.07.112. Epub 2019 Aug 31. PMID: 31479689.

Karimi K, Odhav A, Kollipara R, Fike J, Stanford C, Hall JC. Acute cutaneous necrosis: a guide to early diagnosis and treatment. *J Cutan Med Surg*. 2017;21(5):425–437. https://doi.org/10.1177/1203475417708164. Epub 2017 May 4. PMID: 28470091.

Klein GF, Kofler H, Wolf H, Fritsch PO. Eczema-like, erythematous, infiltrated plaques: a common side effect of subcutaneous heparin therapy. *J Am Acad Dermatol*. 1989;21(4 Pt 1):703–707.

Lee KC, Ladizinski B, Nutan FN. Systemic complications of levamisole toxicity. *J Am Acad Dermatol*. 2012;67(4):791–792. PubMed ID: 22980252.

IMAGE REFERENCES

1. Ward KM, Celebi JT, Gmyrek R, Grossman ME. Acute infectious purpura fulminans associated with asplenism or hyposplenism. *J Am Acad Dermatol*. 2002;47(4):493–496. https://doi.org/10.1067/mjd.2002.124701. PMID: 12271289.
2. Shields BE, Rosenbach M, Brown-Joel Z, Berger AP, Ford BA, Wanat KA. Angioinvasive fungal infections impacting the skin: background, epidemiology, and clinical presentation. *J Am Acad Dermatol*. 2019;80(4):869–880.e5. https://doi.org/10.1016/j.jaad.2018.04.059. Epub 2018 Aug 10. PMID: 30102951.
3. Georgesen C, Fox LP, Harp J. Retiform purpura: a diagnostic approach. *J Am Acad Dermatol*. 2020;82(4):783–796. https://doi.org/10.1016/j.jaad.2019.07.112. Epub 2019 Aug 31. PMID: 31479689.
4. Photograph courtesy of Christine Ahn, MD.
5. Bryan J, Skopis PK, Saikaly SK, Nguyen K, Motaparthi K. Comparing cases of type I cryoglobulinemia with histopathologic findings of vasculitis. *JAAD Case Rep*. 2022;23:160–161. https://doi.org/10.1016/j.jdcr.2022.02.014. PMID: 35519798; PMCID: PMC9062339.
7. Horváth B, Demeter J, Eros N, et al. Intravascular large B-cell lymphoma: remission after rituximab-cyclophosphamide, doxorubicin, vincristine, and prednisolone chemotherapy. *J Am Acad Dermatol*. 2009;61(5):885–888. https://doi.org/10.1016/j.jaad.2008.12.045. Epub 2009 Jul 25. PMID: 19632742.

Chapter 58

FURTHER READING

Bolognia JL, Schaffer JV, Cerroni L. *Dermatology: 2-Volume Set*. 4th ed. Elsevier Health Sciences; 2017.

Antia C, Baquerizo K, Korman A, Bernstein JA, Alikhan A. Urticaria: a comprehensive review: epidemiology, diagnosis, and work-up. *J Am Acad Dermatol*. 2018;79(4):599–614. https://doi.org/10.1016/j.jaad.2018.01.020. PMID: 30241623.

Antia C, Baquerizo K, Korman A, Alikhan A, Bernstein JA. Urticaria: a comprehensive review: treatment of chronic urticaria, special populations, and disease outcomes. *J Am Acad Dermatol*. 2018;79(4):617–633. https://doi.org/10.1016/j.jaad.2018.01.023. PMID: 30241624.

IMAGE REFERENCES

1. Paller AS, Mancini AJ. *Paller and Mancini—Hurwitz Clinical Pediatric Dermatology: A Textbook of Skin Disorders of Childhood & Adolescence*. 6th ed. Elsevier-Health Sciences Division; 2021.
2. Paller AS, Mancini AJ. *Paller and Mancini—Hurwitz Clinical Pediatric Dermatology: A Textbook of Skin Disorders of Childhood & Adolescence*. 6th ed. Elsevier-Health Sciences Division; 2021.
3. James WD, Elston D, Treat JR, Rosenbach MA. *Andrews' Diseases of the Skin: Clinical Dermatology*. 13th ed. Elsevier-Health Sciences Division; 2019.
4. Paller AS, Mancini AJ. *Paller and Mancini—Hurwitz Clinical Pediatric Dermatology: A Textbook of Skin Disorders of Childhood & Adolescence*. 6th ed. Elsevier-Health Sciences Division; 2021.
5. James WD, Elston D, Treat JR, Rosenbach MA. *Andrews' Diseases of the Skin: Clinical Dermatology*. 13th ed. Elsevier-Health Sciences Division; 2019.

Chapter 59

FURTHER READING

Antia C, Baquerizo K, Korman A, Bernstein JA, Alikhan A. Urticaria: a comprehensive review: epidemiology, diagnosis, and work-up. *J Am Acad Dermatol*. 2018;79(4):599–614. https://doi.org/10.1016/j.jaad.2018.01.020. PMID: 30241623.

Hogan SR, Mandrell J, Eilers D. Adrenergic urticaria: review of the literature and proposed mechanism. *J Am Acad Dermatol*. 2014;70(4):763–766. https://doi.org/10.1016/j.jaad.2013.10.062. Epub 2013 Dec 25. PMID: 24373776.

Saini S. Chronic spontaneous urticaria: clinical manifestations, diagnosis, pathogenesis, and natural history. In: Post TW, ed. UpToDate; 2023.

IMAGE REFERENCES

1. Bolognia JL, Schaffer JV, Cerroni L. *Dermatology*. 4th ed. Elsevier; 2018. Courtesy Jeffrey P. Callen, MD.
2. James WD, Elston D, Treat JR, Rosenbach MA. *Andrews' Diseases of the Skin: Clinical Dermatology*. 13th ed. Elsevier—Health Sciences Division; 2019.
3. James WD, Elston D, Treat JR, Rosenbach MA. *Andrews' Diseases of the Skin: Clinical Dermatology*. 13th ed. Elsevier—Health Sciences Division; 2019.
4. James WD, Elston D, Treat JR, Rosenbach MA. *Andrews' Diseases of the Skin: Clinical Dermatology*. 13th ed. Elsevier—Health Sciences Division; 2019.
5. Bolognia JL, Schaffer JV, Cerroni L. *Dermatology*. 4th ed. Elsevier; 2018.

Chapter 60

FURTHER READING

Antia C, Baquerizo K, Korman A, Bernstein JA, Alikhan A. Urticaria: a comprehensive review: epidemiology, diagnosis, and work-up. *J Am Acad Dermatol.* 2018;79(4):599–614. https://doi.org/10.1016/j.jaad.2018.01.020.

Davis M, van der Hilst J. Mimickers of urticaria: urticarial vasculitis and autoinflammatory diseases. *J Allergy Clin Immunol Pract.* 2018;6(4):1162–1170. https://doi.org/10.1016/j.jaip.2018.05.006.

Schocket AL. Chronic urticaria: pathophysiology and etiology, or the what and why. *Allergy Asthma Proc.* 2006;27(2):90–95.

Morris AE, Hall AG, Marshall Jr GD. Not all that itches is urticaria. *Ann Allergy Asthma Immunol.* 2012;109(1):10–13. https://doi.org/10.1016/j.anai.2012.05.012.

Marzano AV, Genovese G. Eosinophilic dermatoses: recognition and management. *Am J Clin Dermatol.* 2020;21(4):525–539. https://doi.org/10.1007/s40257-020-00520-4.

IMAGE REFERENCES

1. Davis M, van der Hilst J. Mimickers of urticaria: urticarial vasculitis and autoinflammatory diseases. *J Allergy Clin Immunol Pract.* 2018;6(4):1162–1170. https://doi.org/10.1016/j.jaip.2018.05.006.
2. Courtesy Dr. D. L. Kastner, National Institutes of Health, Bethesda, Md.
4. Blake, S. C., & Daniel, B. S. (2019). Cutaneous lupus erythematosus: A review of the literature. *International journal of women's dermatology*, 5(5): 320–329. https://doi.org/10.1016/j.ijwd.2019.07.004.
6. Hochbery M, et al. *Rheumatoid Arthritis*. Elsevier; 2009 [Chapter 5 A].
7. Krecak I, Karaman I, Jakelic S. Darier's sign. *Eur J Int Med.* 2022;97.
8. ISSN-0738-081X: Annular urticarial lesions. 2022. Image Identifier: pii:S0738081X21002686/gr12, Elsevier.

Chapter 61

FURTHER READING

Cunniff C, Bassetti JA, Ellis NA. Bloom's syndrome: clinical spectrum, molecular pathogenesis, and cancer predisposition. *Mol Syndromol.* 2017;8(1):4–23.

Giordano CN, Yew YW, Spivak G, Lim HW. Understanding photodermatoses associated with defective DNA repair: syndromes with cancer predisposition. *J Am Acad Dermatol.* 2016;75(5):855–870.

Lehmann AR, Fassihi H. Molecular analysis directs the prognosis, management and treatment of patients with xeroderma pigmentosum. *DNA Repair (Amst).* 2020;93 102907.

Nahhas AF, Oberlin DM, Braunberger TL, Lim HW. Recent developments in the diagnosis and management of photosensitive disorders. *Am J Clin Dermatol.* 2018;19(5):707–731.

Rayinda T, van Steensel M, Danarti R. Inherited skin disorders presenting with poikiloderma. *Int J Dermatol.* 2021;60(11):1343–1353.

IMAGE REFERENCES

1. Thomas ER, Shanley S, Walker L, Eeles R. Surveillance and treatment of malignancy in Bloom syndrome. *Clin Oncol (R Coll Radiol).* 2008;20(5):375–379.
2. In: Paller AS, Mancini AJ, eds. *Hurwitz Clinical Pediatric Dermatology*. 6th ed. Elsevier Saunders; 2022:520–540. Courtesy Sarah Chamlin, MD.
3. Concolino D, Sestito S, Falvo F, et al. Assessment of intrafamilial clinical variability of poikiloderma with neutropenia by a 10-year follow-up of three affected siblings. *Eur J Med Genet.* 2019;62(1):73–76.
4. Lai-Cheong JE, McGrath JA. Kindler syndrome. *Dermatol Clin.* 2010;28(1): 119–124.
5. Plante J, Strat N, Snyder A, Santa Lucia G, Winterfield L, Wine Lee L. Xeroderma pigmentosum presenting as a diffuse midline glioma in a patient with skin of color. *JAAD Case Rep.* 2021;13:141–143.
6. DeMaria D, Mejia-Lopez E, Kelting SM, Soukoulis V. A case of familial calcific aortic and mitral stenosis in association with hereditary sclerosing poikiloderma. *Cardiovasc Pathol.* 2016;25(3):195–199.
7. Savage SA, Alter BP. Dyskeratosis congenita. *Hematol Oncol Clin North Am.* 2009;23(2):215–231.

Chapter 62

FURTHER READING

Lin YL, Chu GY. Successful treatment of poikiloderma-like cutaneous amyloidosis: a case report and literature review. *Indian J Dermatol.* 2021;66(4): 434–437.

Nofal A, Salah E. Acquired poikiloderma: proposed classification and diagnostic approach. *J Am Acad Dermatol.* 2013;69(3):e129–e140.

Seghers AC, Lee JS, Tan CS, et al. Atopic dirty neck or acquired atopic hyperpigmentation? An epidemiological and clinical study from the National Skin Centre in Singapore. *Dermatology.* 2014;229(3):174–182.

Semkova K, Carr R, Grainger M, et al. Poikilodermatous plaque-like hemangioma: case series of a newly defined entity. *J Am Acad Dermatol.* 2019;81(6): 1257–1270.

Vasconcelos Berg R, Valente NYS, Fanelli C, et al. Poikilodermatous mycosis fungoides: comparative study of clinical, histopathological and immunohistochemical features. *Dermatology.* 2020;236(2):117–122.

IMAGE REFERENCES

1. Bilic M, Adams BB. Erythema ab igne induced by a laptop computer. *J Am Acad Dermatol.* 2004;50(6):973–974.
2. Kehe K, Thiermann H, Balszuweit F, Eyer F, Steinritz D, Zilker T. Acute effects of sulfur mustard injury—Munich experiences. *Toxicology.* 2009;263(1):3–8.
3. Hira K, Suga Y, Monma T, Mitsuishi K, Ogawa H. Tacrolimus ointment in the treatment of dirty neck lesions in atopic dermatitis. *J Am Acad Dermatol.* 2005;52(4):720–722.
4. Courtesy of Alexander C. Katoulis, MD, Athens, Greece.
5. Semkova K, Carr R, Grainger M, et al. Poikilodermatous plaque-like hemangioma: case series of a newly defined entity. *J Am Acad Dermatol.* 2019;81(6):1257–1270.
6. Nofal A, Salah E. Acquired poikiloderma: proposed classification and diagnostic approach. *J Am Acad Dermatol.* 2013;69(3):e129–e140.
7. Pramatarov K, Vassileva S, Miteva L. Subacute cutaneous lupus erythematosus presenting with generalized poikiloderma. *J Am Acad Dermatol.* 2000;42(2 Pt 1):286–288.
9. Chen TM. A much-delayed complication. *Am J Med.* 2005;118(8):833–835.
10. Ballester-Sánchez R, Navarro-Mira M, Sanz-Caballer J, Botella-Estrada R. Review of cutaneous graft-vs-host disease. *Actas Dermosifiliogr.* 2016;107(3):183–193.
12. Reprinted with permission from Elsevier (Lancet Infect Dis. 2011;11(10): 800).

Chapter 63

FURTHER READING

Cardenas-de la Garza JA, Cuellar-Barboza A, Arvizu-Rivera RI, et al. Acrodermatitis chronica atrophicans by Borrelia afzelii in an unusual geographical zone. *Rheumatology (Oxford).* 2020;59(12):3995–3996. https://doi.org/10.1093/rheumatology/keaa275.

Magro CM, Poe JC, Kim C, et al. Degos disease: a C5b-9/interferon-α–mediated endotheliopathy syndrome. *Am J Clin Pathol.* 2011;135(4):599–610. https://doi.org/10.1309/AJCP66QIMFARLZKI.

Chapter 64

FURTHER READING

Shen LY, Edmonson MB, Williams GP, Gottam CC, Hinshaw MA, Teng JM. Lipoatrophic panniculitis: case report and review of the literature. *Arch Dermatol.* 2010;146(8):877–881. https://doi.org/10.1001/archdermatol.2010.180.

Cao H, Hegele RA. LMNA is mutated in Hutchinson-Gilford progeria (MIM 176670) but not in Wiedemann-Rautenstrauch progeroid syndrome (MIM 264090). *J Hum Genet.* 2003;48:271–274. https://doi.org/10.1007/s10038-003-0025-3.

Tan SK, Tay YK. Linear atrophoderma of Moulin. *JAAD Case Rep.* 2016;2(1):10–12. https://doi.org/10.1016/j.jdcr.2015.10.005. PMID: 27051814; PMCID: PMC4809442.

Chapter 65

FURTHER READING

Vashi NA, Wirya SA, Inyang M, Kundu RV. Facial hyperpigmentation in skin of color: special considerations and treatment. *Am J Clin Dermatol.* 2017;18(2):215–230. https://doi.org/10.1007/s40257-016-0239-8.

Wang RF, Ko D, Friedman BJ, Lim HW, Mohammad TF. Disorders of hyperpigmentation. Part I. Pathogenesis and clinical features of common pigmentary disorders. *J Am Acad Dermatol.* 2023;88(2):271–288. https://doi.org/10.1016/j.jaad.2022.01.051.

Nicolaidou E, Antoniou C, Katsambas AD. Origin, clinical presentation, and diagnosis of facial hypermelanoses. *Dermatol Clin.* 2007;25(3):321–326. https://doi.org/10.1016/j.det.2007.05.002. viii.

Chang MW. Disorders of hyperpigmentation. *Dermatology.* 2012;2:939–964.

Kutlubay Z, Cesur SK, Aşkın Ö, Tüzün Y. The color of skin: brown diseases of the skin, nails, and mucosa. *Clin Dermatol.* 2019;37(5):487–506. https://doi.org/10.1016/j.clindermatol.2019.07.007.

Nahhas AF, Braunberger TL, Hamzavi IH. An update on drug-induced pigmentation. *Am J Clin Dermatol.* 2019;20(1):75–96. https://doi.org/10.1007/s40257-018-0393-2.

IMAGE REFERENCES

1. Reprinted with permission from Sqalli A, Meziane M, El Anzi O, Znati K, Hassam B, Maouni S. Erythromelanosis follicularis faciei et colli: dermoscopy and dermatopathology correlates. *J Dermatol Case Rep.* 2019;5(6).
2. Mancini AJ, Paller AS. Erythema dyschromicum perstans. Oval slate-gray macules, all oriented along the same axis, on the trunk of this otherwise healthy girl. 2022. Reprinted with permission from Paller A, Mancini A. *Paller and Mancini—Hurwitz Clinical Pediatric Dermatology: A Textbook of Skin Disorders of Childhood and Adolescence.* 6th ed. Elsevier; 2022.

3A. Reprinted with permission from Alikhan A, Hocker T. *Review of Dermatology.* Elsevier; 2017. Reprinted with permission from Molinar VE, et al. What's new in objective assessment and treatment of facial hyperpigmentation? *Dermatol Clin.* 2014;32(2):123–135.

3B. Friedman BJ, Wang RF, Ko D, Mohammad TF, Lim HW, 2023. Lichen planus pigmentosus in a Black female. 88(2). Reprinted with permission from Disorders of hyperpigmentation. Part I. Pathogenesis and clinical features of common pigmentary disorders. 2023.

4. Reprinted from Callen JP, Greer KE, Paller AS, Swinyer LJ. *Color Atlas of Dermatology.* 2nd ed. Saunders; 2000.
5. James WD, McMahon PJ, Elston DM. Reprinted with permission from James WD, Elston DM, Micheletti RM, McMahon PJ. *Andrews' Diseases of the Skin Clinical Atlas.* Elsevier; 2018.
6. Reprinted with permission from Micheletti R, James W, Elston D. et al. *Andrews' Diseases of the Skin Clinical Atlas.* 2nd ed. Elsevier; 2023.
7. Cobbett SL, Terman J, Lewis's Medical-Surgical Nursing in Canada: Assessment and Management of Clinical Problems. Fifth Edition. Elsevier, 2023.
8. Bolognia JL, Schaffer JV, Cerroni L. *Dermatology.* 4th ed. Elsevier; 2018. Courtesy, Henry Lim, MD.
9. Courtesy Henry Lim, MD. Reprinted with permission from Bolognia JL, Jorizzo JL, Schaffer JV. *Dermatology.* 3rd ed. Saunders; 2012.
10. Reprinted with permission from Savory SA, Agim NG, Mao R, et al. Reliability assessment and validation of the postacne hyperpigmentation index (PAHPI), a new instrument to measure postinflammatory hyperpigmentation from acne vulgaris. *J Am Acad Dermatol.* 2014;70(1):108–114.
11. Reprinted with permission from Ko CJ, Bolognia JL, Schaffer JV, Duncan KO. *Dermatology Essentials.* 2nd ed. Elsevier; 2022. Courtesy, Regional Dermatology Training Centre, Moshi, Tanzania.
12. Reprinted with permission from Ko CJ, Bolognia JL, Schaffer JV, Duncan KO. *Dermatology Essentials.* 2nd ed. Elsevier; 2022. Courtesy, YDRSC.
13. Reprinted with permission from Ko CJ, Bolognia JL, Schaffer JV, Duncan KO. *Dermatology Essentials.* 2nd ed. Elsevier; 2022. Courtesy YDRSC.

Chapter 66

FURTHER READING

Plensdorf S, Livieratos M, Dada N. Pigmentation disorders: diagnosis and management. *Am Fam Physician.* 2017;96(12):797–804.

Thawabteh AM, Jibreen A, Karaman D, Thawabteh A, Karaman R. Skin pigmentation types, causes and treatment—a review. *Molecules.* 2023;28(12):4839. https://doi.org/10.3390/molecules28124839.

Stulberg DL, Clark N, Tovey D. Common hyperpigmentation disorders in adults: part I. Diagnostic approach, café au lait macules, diffuse hyperpigmentation, sun exposure, and phototoxic reactions. *Am Fam Physician.* 2003;68(10):1955–1961.

Hassan S, Zhou XA. *Drug-induced pigmentation. StatPearls.* StatPearls Publishing; 2023. http://www.ncbi.nlm.nih.gov/books/NBK542253/.

García RMG, Molina SC. Drug-induced hyperpigmentation: review and case series. *J Am Board Fam Med.* 2019;32(4):628–638. https://doi.org/10.3122/jabfm.2019.04.180212.

Davis EC, Callender VD. Postinflammatory hyperpigmentation: a review of the epidemiology, clinical features, and treatment options in skin of color. *J Clin Aesthetic Dermatol.* 2010;3(7):20–31.

GARD Rare Disease Information. *Primary cutaneous amyloidosis.* National Organization for Rare Disorders; 2022https://rarediseases.org/gard-rare-disease/primary-cutaneous-amyloidosis/

Guillet C, Steinmann S, Maul JT, Kolm I. Primary localized cutaneous amyloidosis: a retrospective study of an uncommon skin disease in the largest tertiary care center in Switzerland. *Dermatology.* 2021;238(3):579–586. https://doi.org/10.1159/000518948.

Patel NU, Roach C, Alinia H, Huang WW, Feldman SR. Current treatment options for acanthosis nigricans. *Clin Cosmet Investig Dermatol.* 2018;11:407–413. https://doi.org/10.2147/CCID.S137527.

Brady MF, Rawla P. *Acanthosis nigricans. StatPearls.* StatPearls Publishing; 2023. http://www.ncbi.nlm.nih.gov/books/NBK431057/.

Le C, Bedocs PM. *Confluent and reticulated papillomatosis. StatPearls.* StatPearls Publishing; 2023. http://www.ncbi.nlm.nih.gov/books/NBK459130/.

Vachiramon V. Approach to reticulate hyperpigmentation. *Clin Exp Dermatol.* 2011;36(5):459–466. https://doi.org/10.1111/j.1365-2230.2011.04100.x.

Kettelhut EA, Traylor J, Sathe NC, Roach JP. *Erythema ab igne. StatPearls.* StatPearls Publishing; 2023. http://www.ncbi.nlm.nih.gov/books/NBK538250/.

Daroach M, Vinay K, Bishnoi A, Parsad D, Kumaran MS. Extrafacial melasma: a scenario less explored. *Indian Dermatol Online J.* 2022;13(4):484–486. https://doi.org/10.4103/idoj.idoj_463_21.

Xiao A, Kopelman H, Shitabata P, Nami N. Ketogenic diet-induced prurigo pigmentosa (the "Keto Rash"): a case report and literature review. *J Clin Aesthetic Dermatol.* 2021;14(12 suppl 1):S29–S32.

Alkhowailed MS, Otayf M, Albasseet A, Almousa A, Alajlan Z, Altalhab S. Clinical approach to linear hyperpigmentation: a review article. *Clin Cosmet Investig Dermatol.* 2021;14:23–35. https://doi.org/10.2147/CCID.S280819.

Cho E, Lim JH, Kim HS, Park YM, Lee JY, Kim HO. Type B pigmentary demarcation lines of pregnancy involving the anterior thighs and knees. *Ann Dermatol.* 2012;24(3):348–350. https://doi.org/10.5021/ad.2012.24.3.348.

Primary Care Dermatology Society. *Pigmentary demarcation lines* (syn. Futcher's lines; Voigt's lines)https://www.pcds.org.uk/clinical-guidance/futchers-lines-syn-voigts-lines

Jamalpur I, Mogili HR, Koratala A. Serpentine supravenous hyperpigmentation. *Clin Case Rep.* 2017;5(9):1546–1547. https://doi.org/10.1002/ccr3.1102.

Somasekharan D, Narayanan B. Serpentine supravenous hyperpigmentation—a rare cutaneous manifestation in non-neoplastic conditions. *J Skin Sex Transm Dis.* 2019;1(2):97–100. https://doi.org/10.25259/JSSTD_28_2019.

Vora RV, Gupta R, Mehta MJ, Chaudhari AH, Pilani AP, Patel N. Pregnancy and skin. *J Fam Med Prim Care.* 2014;3(4):318–324. https://doi.org/10.4103/2249-4863.148099.

George AO, Shittu OB, Enwerem E, Wachtel M, Kuti O. The incidence of lower mid-trunk hyperpigmentation (linea nigra) is affected by sex hormone levels. *J Natl Med Assoc.* 2005;97(5):685–688.

Harshman J, Quan Y, Hsiang D. Phytophotodermatitis. *Can Fam Physician.* 2017;63(12):938–940.

Abugroun A, Gaznabi S, Natarajan A, Daoud H. Lime-induced phytophotodermatitis. *Oxf Med Case Rep.* 2019;2019(11):470–472. https://doi.org/10.1093/omcr/omz113.

National Foundation for Ectodermal Dysplasias. I*ncontinentia pigmenti—symptoms and diagnosis.* https://www.nfed.org/learn/types/incontinentia-pigmenti/

Poziomczyk CS, Recuero JK, Bringhenti L, et al. Incontinentia pigmenti. *An Bras Dermatol.* 2014;89(1):26–36. https://doi.org/10.1590/abd1806-4841.20142584.

Chen YB, Rahemtullah A, Breeden E, Hochberg EP. Bleomycin-induced flagellate erythema. *J Clin Oncol.* 2007;25(7):898–900. https://doi.org/10.1200/JCO.2006.09.7691.

de Mendonça CN, Silva PMCE, Avelleira JCR, Nishimori FS, Cassia FdF. Shiitake dermatitis. *An Bras Dermatol.* 2015;90(2):276–278. https://doi.org/10.1590/abd1806-4841.20153396.

Shenoi SD, Rao R. Pigmented contact dermatitis. *Indian J Dermatol Venereol Leprol.* 2007;73:285. https://doi.org/10.4103/0378-6323.35728.

Daadaa N, Ben Tanfous A. *Riehl melanosis. StatPearls.* StatPearls Publishing; 2023. http://www.ncbi.nlm.nih.gov/books/NBK557437/.

Praetorius C, Sturm RA, Steingrimsson E. Sun-induced freckling: ephelides and solar lentigines. *Pigment Cell Melanoma Res.* 2014;27(3):339–350. https://doi.org/10.1111/pcmr.12232.

Rieder E, Kaplan J, Kamino H, Sanchez M, Pomeranz MK. Lichen planus pigmentosus. *Dermatol Online J.* 2013;19(12). https://doi.org/10.5070/D31912020713.

Ghosh A, Coondoo A. Lichen planus pigmentosus: the controversial consensus. *Indian J Dermatol.* 2016;61(5):482–486. https://doi.org/10.4103/0019-5154.190108.

IMAGE REFERENCES

1. Sinha S, Schwartz RA. Juvenile acanthosis nigricans. *J Am Acad Dermatol.* 2007;57(3):502–508. https://doi.org/10.1016/j.jaad.2006.08.016.
2. Silpa-Archa N, Kohli I, Chaowattanapanit S, Lim HW, Hamzavi I. Postinflammatory hyperpigmentation: a comprehensive overview: epidemiology, pathogenesis, clinical presentation, and noninvasive assessment technique. *J Am Acad Dermatol.* 2017;77(4):591–605. https://doi.org/10.1016/j.jaad.2017.01.035.
3. Wang RF, Ko D, Friedman BJ, Lim HW, Mohammad TF. Disorders of hyperpigmentation. Part I. Pathogenesis and clinical features of common pigmentary disorders. *J Am Acad Dermatol.* 2023;88(2):271–288. https://doi.org/10.1016/j.jaad.2022.01.051.
4. Love WE, Miedler JD, Smith MK, Mostow EN, Cooper KD, Gilliam AC. The spectrum of primary cutaneous nodular amyloidosis: two illustrative cases. *J Am Acad Dermatol.* 2008;58(2 suppl):S33–S35. https://doi.org/10.1016/j.jaad.2007.10.488.
5. Kwong HL, Lim SPR. Pigmented contact dermatitis in the axillae caused by hydroperoxides of limonene. *JAAD Case Rep.* 2020;6(6):476–478. https://doi.org/10.1016/j.jdcr.2020.04.00.
6. Wang RF, Ko D, Friedman BJ, Lim HW, Mohammad TF. Disorders of hyperpigmentation. Part I. Pathogenesis and clinical features of common pigmentary disorders. *J Am Acad Dermatol.* 2023;88(2):271–288. https://doi.org/10.1016/j.jaad.2022.01.051.
7. Wang RF, Ko D, Friedman BJ, Lim HW, Mohammad TF. Disorders of hyperpigmentation. Part I. Pathogenesis and clinical features of common pigmentary disorders. *J Am Acad Dermatol.* 2023;88(2):271–288. https://doi.org/10.1016/j.jaad.2022.01.051.
8. Bilic M, Adams BB. Erythema ab igne induced by a laptop computer. *J Am Acad Dermatol.* 2004;50(6):973–974.
9. Abrahams C, Chavez A. Hyperpigmented rashes: melasma. In: Waldman RA, Grant-Kels JM, eds. *Dermatology for the Primary Care Provider.* Elsevier; 2022: 165–175 [chapter 7].
10. Shevchenko A, Valdes-Rodriguez R, Hsu S, Motaparthi K. Prurigo pigmentosa: case series and differentiation from confluent and reticulated papillomatosis. *JAAD Case Rep.* 2017;4(1):77–80. https://doi.org/10.1016/j.jdcr.2017.07.027.
11. Pacheco TR, Levy M, Collyer JC, et al. Incontinentia pigmenti in male patients. *J Am Acad Dermatol.* 2006;55(2):251–255. https://doi.org/10.1016/j.jaad.2005.12.015.
12. Panicker VV, Riyaz N, Balachandran PK. A clinical study of cutaneous changes in pregnancy. J Epidemiol Glob Health. 2017;7(1):63–70. https://doi.org/10.1016/j.jegh.2016.10.002.
13. Carlsen K, Weismann K. Phytophotodermatitis in 19 children admitted to hospital and their differential diagnoses: child abuse and herpes simplex virus infection. *J Am Acad Dermatol.* 2007;57(5 suppl):S88–S91. https://doi.org/10.1016/j.jaad.2006.08.034.
14. Wang RF, Ko D, Friedman BJ, Lim HW, Mohammad TF. Disorders of hyperpigmentation. Part I. Pathogenesis and clinical features of common pigmentary disorders. *J Am Acad Dermatol.* 2023;88(2):271–288. https://doi.org/10.1016/j.jaad.2022.01.051.
15. Narang T, Dogra S, Sakia UN. Persistent serpentine supravenous hyperpigmented eruption in lepromatous leprosy after minocycline. *Leprosy Rev.* 2015;86(2):191–194. https://doi.org/10.1016/j.jaad.2011.09.001.
16. Adler MJ, Larsen WG. Clinical variability of shiitake dermatitis. *J Am Acad Dermatol.* 2012;67(4):e140–e141. https://doi.org/10.1016/j.jaad.2011.11.926.
17. Adler MJ, Larsen WG. Clinical variability of shiitake dermatitis. *J Am Acad Dermatol.* 2012;67(4):e140–e141. https://doi.org/10.1016/j.jaad.2011.11.926.

Chapter 67

FURTHER READING

Stulberg DL, Clark N, Tovey D. Common hyperpigmentation disorders in adults: part I. Diagnostic approach, café au lait macules, diffuse hyperpigmentation, sun exposure, and phototoxic reactions. *Am Fam Physician.* 2003;68(10):1955–1960.

Bolognia J, Schaffer JV, Cerroni L. *Dermatology.* 4th ed. Elsevier; 2018:286–1988.

Lipsker D, Lenormand C. [Hyperpigmentation]. *Ann Dermatol Venereol.* 2019;146(10):666–682. https://doi.org/10.1016/j.annder.2019.05.005. Hyperpigmentations.

IMAGE REFERENCES

1. Rosenbach MA, Treat JR, Neuhaus IM, Elston DM, James WD. *Andrews' Diseases of the Skin: Clinical Dermatology.* 13th ed. 2020. Reprinted with permission from *Andrews' Diseases of the Skin Clinical Atlas.* 2nd ed. Courtesy Steven Binnick, MD, 2023.
2. Reprinted with permission from *Ferri's Clinical Advisor* 2023; From Feldman M, et al. *Sleisenger and Fordtran's Gastrointestinal and Liver Disease.* 10th ed. Saunders; 2016.
3. Reprinted with permission from *Andrews' Diseases of the Skin Clinical Atlas.* 2nd ed. Courtesy Steven Binnick, MD, 2023.

Chapter 68

FURTHER READING

Kelly AP, Heidelberg KA. Nuances in skin of color. In: Taylor S, Kelly AP, Lim H, Serrano AM, eds. *Taylor and Kelly's Dermatology for Skin of Color.* 2nd ed. McGraw-Hill Education; 2016:123–129.

Passeron T, Ortonne JP. Vitiligo and other disorders of hypopigmentation. In: Bolognia JL, Schaffer JV, Cerroni L, eds. *Dermatology.* 4th ed. Elsevier; 2017.

Rodney IJ, Park J, Hexsel D, Halder RM. Disorders of hypopigmentation. In: Taylor S, Kelly AP, Lim H, Serrano AM, eds. *Taylor and Kelly's Dermatology for Skin of Color.* 2nd ed. McGraw-Hill Education; 2016.

Saleem MD, Oussedik E, Picardo M, Schoch JJ. Acquired disorders with hypopigmentation: a clinical approach to diagnosis and treatment. *J Am Acad Dermatol.* 2019;80(5):1233–1250. e10. PubMed ID: 30236514.

van Geel N, Speeckaert M, Chevolet I, De Schepper S, Lapeere H, Boone B, Speeckaert R. Hypomelanoses in children. *J Cutan Aesthet Surg.* 2013;6(2):65–72. https://doi.org/10.4103/0974-2077.112665. PMID: 24023426; PMCID: PMC3764650.

IMAGE REFERENCES

1. Manga P, Kromberg J, Turner A, Jenkins T, Ramsay M. In Southern Africa, brown oculocutaneous albinism (BOCA) maps to the OCA2 locus on chromosome 15q: P-gene mutations identified. *Am J Hum Genet.* 2001;68(3):782–787. https://doi.org/10.1086/318800. Epub 2001 Feb 9. PMID: 11179026; PMCID: PMC1274491.
2. Power B, Ferreira CR, Chen D, et al. Hermansky-Pudlak syndrome and oculocutaneous albinism in Chinese children with pigmentation defects and easy bruising. *Orphanet J Rare Dis.* 2019;14(1):52. https://doi.org/10.1186/s13023-019-1023-7. PMID: 30791930; PMCID: PMC6385472.
3. Malhotra AK, Bhaskar G, Nanda M, Kabra M, Singh MK, Ramam M. Griscelli syndrome. *J Am Acad Dermatol.* 2006;55(2):337–340. https://doi.org/10.1016/j.jaad.2005.11.1056. PMID: 16844525.
4. Ghosh SK, Bandyopadhyay D, Chatterjee G, Ghosh A, Sarkar S, Sarkar S. Mucocutaneous changes in tuberous sclerosis complex: a clinical profile of 27 Indian patients. *Indian J Dermatol.* 2009;54(3):255–257. https://doi.org/10.4103/0019-5154.55636. PMID: 20161858; PMCID: PMC2810693.
5. van Geel N, Speeckaert M, Chevolet I, et al. Hypomelanoses in children. *J Cutan Aesthet Surg.* 2013;6(2):65–72. https://doi.org/10.4103/0974-2077.112665. PMID: 24023426; PMCID: PMC3764650.
6. Gupta LK, Srivastava A, Khare AK, Mittal A, Balai M, Mehta S. Type B pigmentary demarcation lines. *Indian Dermatol Online J.* 2016;7(3):224–225. https://doi.org/10.4103/2229-5178.182366. PMID: 27294071; PMCID: PMC4886608.
7. Lopez AT, Rotemberg V, Husain S, Schneiderman P, Geskin L. Nevus anemicus: an island of sparing in the setting of drug-induced hypersensitivity. *JAAD Case Rep.* 2018;4(6):615–617. https://doi.org/10.1016/j.jdcr.2018.03.012. PMID: 30003132; PMCID: PMC6039754.
8. From Perine PL, Hopkins DR, Niemel PLA, et al. Handbook of endemic treponematoses?: yaws, endemic syphilis and pinta, 1984 GenevaWorld Health Organization http://apps.who.int/iris/handle/10665/37178?locale=en [accessed 2 May 2013].
9. From Perine PL, Hopkins DR, Niemel PLA, et al. Handbook of endemic treponematoses?: yaws, endemic syphilis and pinta, 1984 GenevaWorld Health Organization http://apps.who.int/iris/handle/10665/37178?locale=en [accessed 2 May 2013].
10. Zijlstra EE, Musa AM, Khalil EA, el-Hassan IM, el-Hassan AM. Post-kala-azar dermal leishmaniasis. *Lancet Infect Dis.* 2003;3(2):87–98. https://doi.org/10.1016/s1473-3099(03)00517-6. PMID: 12560194.
11. Uprety S, Vinay K, De D, Handa S, Saikia UN. Hypopigmented patches on a young man. *Clin Exp Dermatol.* 2016;41(1):100–102. https://doi.org/10.1111/ced.12678. Epub 2015 May 25. PMID: 26011253.

12. Silva VP, Fonseca HH, Sens MM, Bender AT. Indeterminate leprosy and lepromatous index case: four cases in the same family. *An Bras Dermatol.* 2013 Nov-Dec;88(6 Suppl 1):105-8. https://doi.org/10.1590/abd1806-4841.20132050. PMID: 24346893; PMCID: PMC3875986.
13. Katz KA, Mahlberg MJ, Honig PJ, Yan AC. Rice nightmare: Kwashiorkor in 2 Philadelphia-area infants fed Rice Dream beverage. *J Am Acad Dermatol.* 2005;52(5 suppl 1):S69–S72. https://doi.org/10.1016/j.jaad.2004.07.056. Erratum in: *J Am Acad Dermatol.* 2005;53(3):496. Mahlberg, Matthew H [corrected to Mahlberg, Matthew J]. PMID: 15858513.
14. Fan YM, Yang YP, Li W, Li SF. Bier spots: six case reports. *J Am Acad Dermatol.* 2009;61(3):e11–e12. https://doi.org/10.1016/j.jaad.2009.03.009. PMID: 19700009.
15. Ankad BS, Beergouder SL. Dermoscopic evaluation of idiopathic guttate hypomelanosis: a preliminary observation. *Indian Dermatol Online J.* 2015;6(3):164–167. https://doi.org/10.4103/2229-5178.156383. PMID: 26009709; PMCID: PMC4439743.
16. Noiles K, Vender R. Are all seborrheic keratoses benign? Review of the typical lesion and its variants. *J Cutan Med Surg.* 2008;12(5):203–210. https://doi.org/10.2310/7750.2008.07096. PMID: 18845088.
17. Siegfried EC, Hebert AA. Diagnosis of atopic dermatitis: mimics, overlaps, and complications. *J Clin Med.* 2015;4(5):884–917. https://doi.org/10.3390/jcm4050884. PMID: 26239454; PMCID: PMC4470205.
18. Alam HS, Ward JM, Davis LS. Generalized tinea versicolor following initiation of ixekizumab therapy. *JAAD Case Rep.* 2021;18:54–56. https://doi.org/10.1016/j.jdcr.2021.10.008. PMID: 34815994; PMCID: PMC8593516.
19. Lopez I, Ahmed A, Pandya AG. Topical PUVA for post-inflammatory hypopigmentation. *J Eur Acad Dermatol Venereol.* 2011;25(6):742–743. https://doi.org/10.1111/j.1468-3083.2010.03762.x. Epub 2010 Jun 21. PMID: 20569295.
20. Rodney IJ, Kindred C, Angra K, Qutub ON, Villanueva AR, Halder RM. Hypopigmented mycosis fungoides: a retrospective clinicohistopathologic study. *J Eur Acad Dermatol Venereol.* 2017;31(5):808–814. https://doi.org/10.1111/jdv.13843. Epub 2016 Aug 12. PMID: 27515575.

Chapter 69

FURTHER READING

Marçon CR, Maia M. Albinism: epidemiology, genetics, cutaneous characterization, psychosocial factors. *An Bras Dermatol.* 2019;94(5):503–520. https://doi.org/10.1016/j.abd.2019.09.023. Epub 2019 Sep 30. PMID: 31777350; PMCID: PMC6857599.

Passeron T, Ortonne JP. Vitiligo and other disorders of hypopigmentation. In: Bolognia JL, Schaffer JV, Cerroni L, eds. *Dermatology.* 4th ed. Elsevier; 2017.

Plensdorf S, Livieratos M, Dada N. Pigmentation disorders: diagnosis and management. *Am Fam Physician.* 2017;96(12):797–804. PMID: 29431372.

Rapini R.P. Practical Dermatopathology. 3rd ed. Elsevier; 2021:97803234178841–44 10.1016/B978-0-323-41788-4.00011-3. 139–150, 161–168, 241–255.

Takafuji M, Tanemura A, Hanaoka Y, et al. Non-invasive evaluation and differential diagnosis for pediatric leukoderma in a single institute. *J Cosmet Dermatol Sci Appl.* 2019;9:313–320. https://doi.org/10.4236/jcdsa.2019.94028.

IMAGE REFERENCES

1. Wang Y, Wang Z, Chen M, et al. Mutational analysis of the TYR and OCA2 genes in four Chinese families with oculocutaneous albinism. *PLoS One.* 2015;10(4):e0125651. https://doi.org/10.1371/journal.pone.0125651. PMID: 25919014; PMCID: PMC4412409.
2. Yang S, Dai P, Liu X, et al. Genetic and phenotypic heterogeneity in Chinese patients with Waardenburg syndrome type II. *PLoS One.* 2013;8(10):e77149. https://doi.org/10.1371/journal.pone.0077149. PMID: 24194866; PMCID: PMC3806753.
3. Agarwal S, Ojha A. Piebaldism: a brief report and review of the literature. *Indian Dermatol Online J.* 2012;3(2):144–147. https://doi.org/10.4103/2229-5178.96722. PMID: 23130293; PMCID: PMC3481873.
4. Lopez AT, Rotemberg V, Husain S, Schneiderman P, Geskin L. Nevus anemicus: an island of sparing in the setting of drug-induced hypersensitivity. *JAAD Case Rep.* 2018;4(6):615–617. https://doi.org/10.1016/j.jdcr.2018.03.012. PMID: 30003132; PMCID: PMC6039754.
5. Bari A, Rahman SB. Onchocerciasis: a review of a filarial disease of significant importance for dermatologists and ophthalmologists. *J Pak Asso Dermatol.* 2007;17:32–45.
6. Gupta D, Thappa DM. Dermatoses due to Indian cultural practices. *Indian J Dermatol.* 2015;60(1):3–12. https://doi.org/10.4103/0019-5154.147778. PMID: 25657390; PMCID: PMC4318059.
7. Tang H, Wang C, Fu L, Xu AE. Successful repigmentation of vitiligo after allogeneic bone marrow transplantation for Hodgkin's lymphoma by autologous noncultured melanocyte-keratinocyte transplantation. *Indian J Dermatol.* 2015;60(5):470–472. https://doi.org/10.4103/0019-5154.164364. PMID: 26538694; PMCID: PMC4601414.
8. Higashimori T, Kono T, Sakurai H, Nakazawa H, Groff WF. Treatment of mesh skin grafted scars using a plasma skin regeneration system. *Plast Surg Int.* 2010;2010:874348. https://doi.org/10.1155/2010/874348. Epub 2010 Jul 1. PMID: 22567232; PMCID: PMC3335560.
9. Bhagwat PV, Kudligi C, Shashikumar BM, Thirunavukkarasu A, Shendre ME. Extensive discoid lupus erythematosus in a HIV patient responding to hydroxychloroquine monotherapy. *Indian J Dermatol.* 2012;57(4):326–327. https://doi.org/10.4103/0019-5154.97687. PMID: 22837579; PMCID: PMC3401860.
10. Noiles K, Vender R. Are all seborrheic keratoses benign? Review of the typical lesion and its variants. *J Cutan Med Surg.* 2008;12(5):203–210.
11. Oliver B, Boehm M, Rosing DR, et al. Diffuse atrophic papules and plaques, intermittent abdominal pain, paresthesias, and cardiac abnormalities in a 55-year-old woman. *J Am Acad Dermatol.* 2016;75(6):1274–1277.

Chapter 70

FURTHER READING

Burr S. The assessment, history taking and differential diagnosis of pigmented skin lesions. *Dermatol Nurs.* 2015;14(4):18–22.

Mansur AT, Yildiz S. A diagnostic challenge: inflamed and pigmented seborrheic keratosis. Clinical, dermoscopic, and histopathological correlation. *Dermatol Online J.* 2019;25(3): 13030/qt0w56m5hq. PMID: 30982311.

Phadke PA, Zembowicz A. Blue nevi and related tumors. *Clin Lab Med.* 2011;31(2):345–358. https://doi.org/10.1016/j.cll.2011.03.011. PMID: 21549247.

Lao M, Weissler A, Siegfried E. Talon noir. *J Pediatr.* 2013;163(3):919. https://doi.org/10.1016/j.jpeds.2013.03.079.

Nazarian RS, Amin B, Papalezova K, Ohri N, McLellan BN. Radiation tattoos mimicking melanoma: a clinical observation. *Acta Oncol.* 2019;58(9):1283–1285. https://doi.org/10.1080/0284186X.2019.1632478.

Gunter Burg HK. *Atlas of Dermatopathology: Tumors, Nevi, and Cysts.* Wiley; 2018.

IMAGE REFERENCES

1. Dinulos JGH. *Habif's Clinical Dermatology.* 7th ed. Elsevier; 2021.
2. Dinulos JGH. *Habif's Clinical Dermatology.* 7th ed. Elsevier; 2021.
3. From the Fitzsimons Army Medical Center Collection, Aurora, CO.
11. Longo C, Scope A, Lallas A, et al. Blue lesions. *Dermatol Clin.* Elsevier; 2013.
12. James WD, Elston DM, Treat JR, Rosenbach MA, Neuhaus IM. *Andrews' Diseases of the Skin.* 13th ed. Elsevier; 2020.
13. H. Peter Soyer, Giuseppe Argenziano, Rainer Hofmann-Wellen, *Dermoscopy: The Essentials*, 1st ed. Elsevier; 2004.

Chapter 71

FURTHER READING

Longo C, Scope A, Lallas A, et al. Blue lesions. *Dermatol Clin.* 2013;31(4):637–647. ix. https://doi.org/10.1016/j.det.2013.07.001. Epub 2013 Aug 23. PMID: 24075551.

Borgenvik TL, Karlsvik TM, Ray S, Fawzy M, James N. Blue nevus-like and blue nevus-associated melanoma: a comprehensive review of the literature. *ANZ J Surg.* 2017;7:345–349. https://doi.org/10.1111/ans.13946.

Cohen PR. The color of skin: blue diseases of the skin, nails, and mucosa. *Clin Dermatol.* 2019;37(5):468–486. https://doi.org/10.1016/j.clindermatol.2019.07.006. Epub 2019 Jul 18. PMID: 31896403.

Franceschini D, Dinulos JG. Dermal melanocytosis and associated disorders. *Curr Opin Pediatr.* 2015;27(4):480–485. https://doi.org/10.1097/MOP.0000000000000247. PMID: 26087431.

Glazer AM, Rigel DS, Winkelmann RR, Farberg AS. Clinical diagnosis of skin cancer: enhancing inspection and early recognition. *Dermatol Clin.* 2017;35(4):409–416. https://doi.org/10.1016/j.det.2017.06.001. Epub 2017 Aug 7. PMID: 28886797.

IMAGE REFERENCES

1. James WD, et al. Chapter 28: Dermal and subcutaneous tumors. *Andrews' Diseases of the Skin: Clinical Atlas.* Elsevier; 2018.
2. Johar FM, Sulaiman WAW, Saad AZM, Basiron N, Sahid NA. Blue rubber bleb nevus syndrome in a Malay girl: a case report and literature review. *Int J Surg Case Rep.* 2020;72:202–206.
3. Elston DM, et al. Chapter 23: Clinical image atlas. *Dermatopathology.* 3rd ed. Elsevier; 2019.

4. James WD, et al. Chapter 30: Melanocytic nevi and neoplasms. *Andrews' Diseases of the Skin: Clinical Atlas.* Elsevier; 2018.
5. James WD, et al. Chapter 34: Disease of mucous membranes. *Andrews' Diseases of the Skin: Clinical Atlas.* Elsevier; 2018.
6. Courtesy Steven Binnick, MD.
7. Wise SR, Capra G, Martin P, Wallace D, Miller C. Malignant melanoma transformation within a nevus of Ito. *J Am Acad Dermatol.* 2010;62(5):869–874.
8. Manuskiatti W, Sivayathorn A, Leelaudomlipi P, Fitzpatrick RE. Treatment of acquired bilateral nevus of Ota-like macules (Hori's nevus) using a combination of scanned carbon dioxide laser followed by Q-switched ruby laser. *J Am Acad Dermatol.* 2003;48(4):584–591. ISSN 0190-9622. https://doi.org/10.1067/mjd.2003.193.
9. Elston DM, et al. Chapter 23: Clinical image atlas. *Dermatopathology.* 3rd ed. Elsevier; 2019.
10. Elston DM, et al. Chapter 6: Clinical image atlas. *Dermatopathology.* 3rd ed. Elsevier; 2019.
11. James WD, et al. Chapter 29: Epidermal nevi, neoplasms, and cysts. *Andrews' Diseases of the Skin: Clinical Atlas.* Elsevier; 2018.
12. James WD, et al. Chapter 29: Epidermal nevi, neoplasms, and cysts. *Andrews' Diseases of the Skin: Clinical Atlas.* Elsevier; 2018.
13. James WD, et al. Chapter 30: Melanocytic nevi and neoplasms. *Andrews' Diseases of the Skin: Clinical Atlas.* Elsevier; 2018.
14. Courtesy Steven Binnick, MD.
15. Micheletti RG, et al. *Andrews' Diseases of the Skin Clinical Atlas.* 2nd ed. Elsevier; 2023.

Chapter 72

FURTHER READING

Burr S. The assessment, history taking and differential diagnosis of pigmented skin lesions. *Dermatol Nurs.* 2015;14(4):18–22.

Mansur AT, Yildiz S. A diagnostic challenge: inflamed and pigmented seborrheic keratosis. Clinical, dermoscopic, and histopathological correlation. *Dermatol Online J.* 2019;25(3): 13030/qt0w56m5hq. PMID: 30982311.

Bolognia J, Schaffer JV, Cerroni L. In: Bolognia J, Schaffer JV, Cerroni L, eds. *Dermatology.* 4th ed. Elsevier; 2018.

IMAGE REFERENCES

1. Dinulos JGH. *Habif's Clinical Dermatology.* 7th ed. Elsevier; 2021.
9. Dinulos JGH. *Habif's Clinical Dermatology.* 7th ed. Elsevier; 2021.
12. Bonifaz A, Gómez-Daza F, Paredes V, Ponce RM. Tinea versicolor, tinea nigra, white piedra, and black piedra. *Clin Dermatol.* 2010;28(2).
13. Dinulos JGH. *Habif's Clinical Dermatology.* 7th ed. Elsevier; 2021.

Chapter 73

FURTHER READING

Al Hawsawi K, Alharazi A, Ashary A, Siddique A. Syringocystadenoma papilliferum: a case report and review of the literature. *Case Rep Dermatol.* 2019;11:36–39. https://doi.org/10.1159/000497054.

Bolognia JL, Schaffer JV, Cerroni L. *Dermatology.* Elsevier; 2018.

Chalfant V, Schriber T, Sabri A, et al. Primary cutaneous leiomyosarcoma of the lower extremity: a case report and literature review. *Cureus.* 2021;13(4): https://doi.org/10.7759/cureus.14282.

Gordon S, Fischer C, Martin A, Rosman IS, Council ML. Microcystic adnexal carcinoma: a review of the literature. *Dermatol Surg.* 2017;43(8):1012–1016. https://doi.org/10.1097/DSS.0000000000001142. PMID: 28654578.

Patterson JW, Hosler GA, Prenshaw KL. *Weedon's Skin Pathology.* 5th ed. Elsevier; 2021.

IMAGE REFERENCES

3. Laur WE, Posey RE, Waller JD. Lichen planus-like keratosis. A clinicohistopathologic correlation. *J Am Acad Dermatol.* 1981;4(3):329–336. https://www.doi.org.10.1016/S0190-9622(81)70034-3.
10. Winchester DS, Hocker TL, Roenigk RK. Skin metastases of leiomyosarcoma (LMS): a retrospective review of 21 cases. *J Am Acad Dermatol.* 2015;72(5): 910–912. https://doi.org/10.1016/j.jaad.2015.01.033. PMID: 25890461.
12. Huang HT, Ling Q. Is an accessory nipple associated with an intrapancreatic accessory spleen? *Hepatobiliary Pancreat Dis Int.* 2019;18(6):596–597. https://www.doi.org.10.1016/j.hbpd.2019.09.010.
17. Karaarslan I, Acar A, Yaman B, Ozdemir F. Reflectance confocal microscopic findings of a tiny syringocystadenoma papilliferum. *JAAD Case Rep.* 2019;5(4):323–325. https://doi.org/10.1016/j.jdcr.2019.02.023.
18. Guimerá Martín-Neda F, García Bustínduy M, Noda Cabrera A, Sánchez González R, García Montelongo R. A rapidly growing eccrine poroma in a pregnant woman. *J Am Acad Dermatol.* 2004;50(1):124–126. https://doi.org/10.1016/s0190-9622(03)00032-x. PMID: 14699381.
19. Casale F, Elwood HR, Tchanque-Fossuo CN. Exophytic growth on nasal ala. *JAAD Case Rep.* 2021;19:48–50. https://doi.org/10.1016/j.jdcr.2021.10.035.
20. Beatty CJ, Yousaf A, Al-Bouri A, Thompson AD, Kiavash K, Kolodney MS. Case report of syndromic multiple spiradenomas due to biallelic functional loss of *CYLD. JAAD Case Rep.* 2022;21:106–108. https://doi.org/10.1016/j.jdcr.2022.01.002.
21. Tiodorovic-Zivkovic D, Lallas A, Longo C, Moscarella E, Zalaudek I, Argenziano G. Dermoscopy of clear cell acanthoma. *J Am Acad Dermatol.* 2014;72(1):S47–S49. https://www.doi.org.10.1016/j.jaad.2014.06.039.
22. de Cambourg G, Cribier B. Fibrous papules of the face: a retrospective anatomoclinical study of 283 cases. *Ann Dermatol Venereol.* 2013;140(12): 763–770. https://www.doi.org.10.1016/j.annder.2013.09.163.

Chapter 74

FURTHER READING

Eisen DB, Michael DJ. Sebaceous lesions and their associatd syndromes: part I. *J Am Acad Dermatol.* 2009;61(4):549–560. https://doi.org/10.1016/j.jaad.2009.04.058.

Berk DR, Bayliss SJ. Milia: a review and classification. *J Am Acad Dermatol.* 2008;59(6):1050–1063. https://doi.org/10.1016/j.jaad.2008.07.034.

Reid SD, et al. Update on necrobiosis lipoidica: a review of etiology, diagnosis, and treatment options. *J Am Acad Dermatol.* 2013;69(5):783–791. https://doi.org/10.1016/j.jaad.2013.05.034.

Nair PA, Singhal R. Xanthelasma palpebrarum—a brief review. *Clin Cosmet Investig Dermatol.* 2018;11:1–5. https://doi.org/10.2147/CCID.S130116.

Ilias G, et al. Pseudoxanthoma elasticum, ocular manifestations, complications and treatment. *Clin Exp Optom.* 2011;94(2):169–180. https://doi.org/10.1111/j.1444-0938.2010.00559.x.

IMAGE REFERENCES

1. Martínez Pallás I, Conejero del Mazo R, Lezcano Biosca V. Pigmented purpuric dermatosis: a review of the literature. *Actas Dermosifiliogr (Engl Ed).* 2020;111(3):196–204. ISSN 1578-2190. https://www.doi.org.10.1016/j.jaad.2008.07.03410.1016/j.adengl.2020.03.007.
2. Baroni A. Long-wave plasma radiofrequency ablation for treatment of xanthelasma palpebrarum. *J Cosmet Dermatol.* 2019;18:121–123. https://www.doi.org.10.1016/j.jaad.2008.07.03410.1111/jocd.12509.
3. Ghanadan A, Khosravi M. Cutaneous syringoma: a clinicopathologic study of 34 new cases and review of the literature. *Indian J Dermatol.* 2013;58:326. https://www.doi.org.10.1016/j.jaad.2008.07.03410.4103/0019-5154.113956.
4. Jacobi H, Schreiber G. Pseudoxanthoma elasticum. Skin lesions as a signal to a systemic disease. Hautveränderungen als Wegweiser einer Systemerkrankung. *Hautarzt.* 1997;48:191–194. https://www.doi.org.10.1016/j.jaad.2008.07.03410.1007/s001050050569.
5. Castro Zayas PM, Aboukheir Aboukheir A, Martínez Bernal A, Ortíz Justiniano V. Nevus lipomatosus cutaneous superficialis. *J Pediatr Surg Case Rep.* 2021;74:102036. ISSN 2213-5766, https://www.doi.org.10.1016/j.jaad.2008.07.03410.1016/j.epsc.2021.102036.
6. Raymond J, Choi J. Nodular cutaneous amyloidosis effectively treated with intralesional methotrexate. *JAAD Case Rep.* 2016;2(5):373–376. ISSN 2352-5126, https://www.doi.org.10.1016/j.jaad.2008.07.03410.1016/j.jdcr.2016.04.006.
7. Zamora AB, Simón MP, Sánchez AT, Ponce Olivera RM. Adult colloid milium. An underdiagnosed and difficult to treat entity. *Rev Med Hosp Gen (Mex).* 2016;79(1):21–25. ISSN 0185-1063, https://www.doi.org.10.1016/j.jaad.2008.07.03410.1016/j.hgmx.2015.10.002.
8. Stark M, Stuart J. Eruptive xanthoma in the setting of hypertriglyceridemia and pancreatitis. *Am J Emerg Med.* 2018;36(8):1524.e5–1524.e7. ISSN 0735-6757, https://www.doi.org.10.1016/j.jaad.2008.07.03410.1016/j.ajem.2018.04.056.
9. Reid SD, Ladizinski B, Lee K, Baibergenova A, Alavi A. Update on necrobiosis lipoidica: a review of etiology, diagnosis, and treatment options. *J Am Acad Dermatol.* 2013;69(5):783–791. ISSN 0190-9622, https://www.doi.org.10.1016/j.jaad.2008.07.03410.1016/j.jaad.2013.05.034.
10. Poulopoulos AK, Epivatianos A, Zaraboukas T, Antoniades D. Verruciform xanthoma coexisting with oral discoid lupus erythematosus. *Br J Oral Maxillofac Surg.* 2007;45(2):159–160. ISSN 0266-4356, https://www.doi.org.10.1016/j.jaad.2008.07.03410.1016/j.bjoms.2005.06.020.
11. Truchuelo MT, et al. Pulsed dye laser treatment for multiple sebaceous hyperplasia secondary to ciclosporin. *Actas Dermosifiliogr.* 2011;102:470–471.

12. Zaballos P, Gómez-Martín I, Martin JM, Bañuls J. Dermoscopy of adnexal tumors. *Dermatol Clin.* 2018;36(4):397–412. https://doi.org/10.1016/j.det.2018.05.007. Epub 2018 Aug 16. PMID: 30201149.
13. Neto MPDS, de Assis BR, Andrade GR. Sebaceous nevus of Jadassohn: review and clinical-surgical approach. *An Bras Dermatol.* 2022;97(5):628–636. ISSN 0365-0596, https://www.doi.org.10.1016/j.jaad.2008.07.03410.1016/j.abd.2021.11.001.
14. Berk DR, Bayliss SJ. Milia: a review and classification. *J Am Acad Dermatol.* 2008;59(6):1050–1063. ISSN 0190-9622, https://www.doi.org.10.1016/j.jaad.2008.07.034.

Chapter 75

FURTHER READING

Bin Saif GA, Ericson ME, Yosipovitch G. The itchy scalp—scratching for an explanation. *Exp Dermatol.* 2011;20(12):959–968. https://doi.org/10.1111/j.1600-0625.2011.01389.x.

Shapiro J, Otberg N. *Hair Loss and Restoration.* CRC Press; 2015.

Vázquez-Herrera NE, Sharma D, Aleid NM, Tosti A. Scalp itch: a systematic review. *Skin Appendage Disord.* 2018;4(3):187–199. https://doi.org/10.1159/000484354.

Ju T, Vander Does A, Yosipovitch G. Scalp dysesthesia: a neuropathic phenomenon. *J Eur Acad Dermatol Venereol.* 2022;36(6):790–796. https://doi.org/10.1111/jdv.17985.

Hashimoto T, Yosipovitch G. Itching as a systemic disease. *J Allergy Clin Immunol.* 2019;144(2):375–380. https://doi.org/10.1016/j.jaci.2019.04.005.

IMAGE REFERENCES

1. Diniz Borges Figueira de Mello C, Fernandes Eloy da Costa França A, Magalhães RF. Entodermoscopy of *Pediculosis capitis*. *JAAD Case Rep.* 2022;22:70–71. https://doi.org/10.1016/j.jdcr.2022.02.011. PMID: 35330983; PMCID: PMC8938624.
2. Elewski BE. Clinical diagnosis of common scalp disorders. *J Investig Dermatol Symp Proc.* 2005;10(3):190–193. https://doi.org/10.1111/j.1087-0024.2005.10103.x. PMID: 16382661.
3. Berth-Jones J. Psoriasis. *Medicine.* 2009;37(5):235–241. https://doi.org/10.1016/j.mpmed.2009.02.005
4. Vázquez-Herrera NE, Sharma D, Aleid NM, Tosti A. Scalp itch: a systematic review. *Skin Appendage Disord.* 2018;4(3):187–199. https://doi.org/10.1159/000484354. Epub 2017 Nov 29. PMID: 30197900; PMCID: PMC6120392.
5. Silverberg NB, Weinberg JM, DeLeo VA. Tinea capitis: focus on African American women. *J Am Acad Dermatol.* 2002;46(2 Suppl Understanding):S120–124. https://doi.org/10.1067/mjd.2002.120793. PMID: 11807474.
6. Image courtesy of David Fiorentino, Stanford University.
7. Chiang C, Sah D, Cho BK, Ochoa BE, Price VH. Hydroxychloroquine and lichen planopilaris: efficacy and introduction of Lichen Planopilaris Activity Index scoring system. *J Am Acad Dermatol.* 2010;62(3):387–392. https://doi.org/10.1016/j.jaad.2009.08.054. Epub 2010 Jan 12. PMID: 20061052.
8. Fruhauf J, Schaider H, Massone C, Kerl H, Mullegger RR. Carbamazepine as the only effective treatment in a 52-year-old man with trigeminal trophic syndrome. *Mayo Clin Proc.* 2008;83(4):502–504. https://doi.org/10.4065/83.4.502. PMID: 18380997.

Chapter 76

FURTHER READING

Ansari P. Pruritus ani. *Clin Colon Rectal Surg.* 2016;29(1):38–42. https://doi.org/10.1055/s-0035-157039.

Khurana A, Tandon S, Marfatia YS, Madnani N. Genital lichen planus: an underrecognized entity. *Indian J Sex Transm Dis AIDS.* 2019;40(2):105–112. https://doi.org/10.4103/ijstd.IJSTD_45_19.

Meeuwis KA, de Hullu JA, Massuger LF, van de Kerkhof PC, van Rossum MM. Genital psoriasis: a systematic literature review on this hidden skin disease. *Acta Derm Venereol.* 2011;91(1):5–11. https://doi.org/10.2340/00015555-0988.

Savas JA, Pichardo RO. Female genital itch. *Dermatol Clin.* 2018;36(3):225–243. https://doi.org/10.1016/j.det.2018.02.006.

Swamiappan M. Anogenital pruritus—an overview. *J Clin Diagn Res.* 2016;10(4):WE01–WE03. https://doi.org/10.7860/JCDR/2016/18440.7703.

IMAGE REFERENCES

1. Maródi L. Mucocutaneous candidiasis. In: *Stiehm's Immune Deficiencies.* Vol 1. Academic Press; 2014:775–802.
2. Garland SM, Steben M. Genital herpes. *Best Pract Res Clin Obstet Gynaecol.* 2014;28(7):1098–1110. https://doi.org/10.1016/j.bpobgyn. 2014.07.015.
3. Reproduced from Dauendorffer JN, Renaud-Vilmer C, Cavelier-Balloy B. Le psoriasis génital chez l'homme [Male genital psoriasis]. *Ann Dermatol Venereol.* 2014;141(6–7):466–473. © 2014. Published by Elsevier Masson SAS. All rights reserved.
4. Nabavizadeh R, Vashi KB, Nabavizadeh B, Narayan VM, Master VA. Extramammary Paget's disease: updates in the workup and management. *Asian J Urol.* 2022;9(4):451–459. https://doi.org/10.1016/j.ajur.2022.08.001.
5. Savas JA, Pichardo RO. Female genital itch. *Dermatol Clin.* 2018;36(3):225–243. https://doi.org/10.1016/j.det.2018.02.006.

Chapter 77

FURTHER READING

Shumway NK, Cole E, Fernandez KH. Neurocutaneous disease: neurocutaneous dysesthesias. *J Am Acad Dermatol.* 2016;74(2):215–228. quiz 229-230.

Elmariah SB. Diagnostic work-up of the itchy patient. *Dermatol Clin.* 2018;36(3):179–188.

Chan CX, Zug KA. Diagnosis and management of dermatitis, including atopic, contact, and hand eczemas. *Med Clin North Am.* 2021;105(4):611–626.

Hamie L, Haddad I, Nasser N, Kurban M, Abbas O. Primary localized cutaneous amyloidosis of keratinocyte origin: an update with emphasis on atypical clinical variants. *Am J Clin Dermatol.* 2021;22(5):667–680.

Yosipovitch G, Mills KC, Nattkemper LA, et al. Association of pain and itch with depth of invasion and inflammatory cell constitution in skin cancer: results of a large clinicopathologic study. *JAMA Dermatol.* 2014;150(11):1160–1166. https://doi.org/10.1001/jamadermatol.2014.895. Erratum in: JAMA Dermatol. 2014;150(10):1122. PMID: 25055194; PMCID: PMC4229457.

IMAGE REFERENCES

1. Richey PM, Stone MS. Resolution of pseudoainhum with acitretin therapy in a patient with palmoplantar keratoderma and congenital alopecia. *JAAD Case Rep.* 2019;5(3):219–221.
2. Jung HM, Eun SH, Lee JH, Kim GM, Bae JM. Less painful and effective intralesional injection method for lichen simplex chronicus. *J Am Acad Dermatol.* 2018;79(6):e105–e106.
3. Abdullah F, Udelsman R. Cutaneous lichen amyloidosis in a family with familial medullary thyroid cancer. *Surgery.* 2004;135(5): 563–564.
4. Kazemi S, Murphrey M, Hawkes JE. Rapid resolution of widespread cutaneous lichen planus and generalized pruritus in an elderly patient following treatment with dupilumab. *JAAD Case Rep.* 2022;30:108–110.
5. Seuve É, Eyraud A, Desmoulière A. Physiopathologie du psoriasis. *Actual Pharm.* 2022;61(617):39–44.
6. Larocca CA, LeBoeuf NR. Overview of cutaneous T-cell lymphomas. *Hematol Oncol Clin North Am.* 2019;33(4):669–686.
7. Tully J, Woodruff CM. Allergic contact dermatitis from Grevillea masquerading as toxicodendron dermatitis. *JAAD Case Rep.* 2022;23:168–170.
8. Youssef S, Gallitano S, Bordone LA. Two cases of bullous pemphigoid successfully treated with oral tofacitinib. *JAAD Case Rep.* 2022;32:77–80.
9. Jackson Cullison SR, Jedrych JJ, James AJ. Porphyria cutanea tarda unmasked by supratherapeutic estrogen during gender-affirming hormone therapy. *JAAD Case Rep.* 2020;6(7):675–678.
10. Lago ADN, Fortes ABC, Furtado GS, Menezes CFS, Gonçalves LM. Association of antimicrobial photodynamic therapy and photobiomodulation for herpes simplex labialis resolution: case series. *Photodiagnosis Photodyn Ther.* 2020;32:102070.
11. Livshits D, Sokup B, Nguyen R. A typical case of herpes-zoster rash presenting as back pain. *Vis J Emerg Med.* 2022;26:101211.
12. Shah A, Goel K, Uchin J, Patibandla SK, Min Z, Bhanot N. Fever and rash in an adult: varicella re-infection in conjunction with newly diagnosed chronic lymphocytic leukemia. *Am J Med.* 2019;132(6):701–703.
13. From White G, Cox N. *Diseases of the Skin.* 2nd ed. St Louis, Mosby; 2006.
14. Kamler J, Piehl M, Chenevert L, Truong J. Adult presentation of hand, foot, and mouth disease. *Vis J Emerg Med.* 2022;29:101437.
15. Chan CX, Zug KA. Diagnosis and management of dermatitis, including atopic, contact, and hand eczemas. *Med Clin North Am.* 2021;105(4):611–626.
16. Pope E, Kowalski E, Tausk F. Topical ruxolitinib in the treatment of refractory facial seborrheic dermatitis. *JAAD Case Rep.* 2022;24:59–60.
17. Krzywanski J, Kuchar E, Mierzynski R. Cutaneous larva migrans in a beach volleyball player. *IDCases.* 2021;24:e01084.
18. Courtesy of Nicholas Compton, MD.
19. Walker HS, Hardwicke J. Non-melanoma skin cancer. *Surgery (Oxf).* 2022;40(1):39–45.
20. Cunha IM, Valadão I, Gomes E, Marinho A. Dupilumab: a safe and successful treatment in refractory prurigo nodularis. *J Allergy Clin Immunol Pract.* 2022;10(5):1365–1366.

21. Bautista Hernandez Y, Villavicencio Queijero MA, Quezada Bautista AA, Vazquez Tinajero A. Surface brachytherapy in the treatment of keloid scars in Mexico. *Rep Pract Oncol Radiother*. 2020;25(1): 133–138.
22. Kwatra SG, Stander S, Bernhard JD, Weisshaar E, Yosipovitch G. Brachioradial pruritus: a trigger for generalization of itch. *J Am Acad Dermatol.* 2013;68(5):870–873.
23. Ozen S, Cosar SN, Sozay S. Exercise, manipulative therapy, and physical modalities in the treatment of notalgia paresthetica: a case report. *J Chiropr Med*. 2021;20(4):224–228.
24. Shumway NK, Cole E, Fernandez KH. Neurocutaneous disease: neurocutaneous dysesthesias. *J Am Acad Dermatol.* 2016;74(2): 215–228.
25. Biz C, Ruggieri P. Distal metatarsal osteotomies for chronic plantar diabetic foot ulcers. *Foot Ankle Clin*. 2022;27(3):545–566.
26. Gandhi R, Vilke GM, Castillo EM. Intermittent transient flaring rash post herpes zoster. *J Emerg Med*. 2022;63(1):e37–e39.

Chapter 78

FURTHER READING

Berger TG, Shive M, Harper GM. Pruritus in the older patient: a clinical review. *JAMA*. 2013;310:2443–2450.

Matterne U, et al. Prevalence, correlates and characteristics of chronic pruritus: a population-based cross-sectional study. *Acta Derm Venereol.* 2011;91:674–679.

Etter L, Myers SA. Pruritus in systemic disease: mechanisms and management. *Dermatol Clin*. 2002;20:459–472.

Pitukweerakul S, Pilla S. Clinical images Terry's nails and Lindsay's nails: two nail abnormalities in chronic systemic diseases. *J Gen Intern Med.* 2016;31:970.

Millington GWM, et al. British Association of Dermatologists' guidelines for the investigation and management of generalized pruritus in adults without an underlying dermatosis, 2018. *Br J Dermatol.* 2018;178:34–60.

IMAGE REFERENCES

1. Yu ASL, Chertow GM, Luyckx VA, Marsden PA, Skorecki K, Taal MW, eds. *Brenner & Rector's the Kidney*. 11th ed. Elsevier; 2019.
2. Lebwohl M, Heymann WR, Coulson I, Murrell DF, eds. *Treatment of Skin Disease : Comprehensive Therapeutic Strategies*. 6th ed. Elsevier; 2021.
3. From Forbes CD, Jackson WF. *Color Atlas and Text of Clinical Medicine*. 3rd ed. Mosby; 2002. Reproduced by kind permission.
4. Kuo CC, Hung JB, Tsai CW, Chen YM. Uremic frost. *CMAJ*. 2010;182(17): E800–E800. https://www.doi.org.10.1503/cmaj.091779.
5. Bhandari A, Mahajan R. Skin changes in cirrhosis. *J Clin Exp Hepatol.* 2022;12(4):1215–1224. https://www.doi.org.10.1016/j.jceh.2021.12.013.
6. Ignacio-Cconchoy FL, Benites-Zapata VA, Yanac-Avila RL, Vela-Velàsquez CT. Myeloid sarcoma of the tongue as a first manifestation of acute promyelocytic leukemia: a case report. *Rep Pract Oncol Radiother*. 2020;25(2):174–177. https://www.doi.org.10.1016/j.rpor.2019.12.026.
7. Slater TA, Waduud MA, Ahmed N. *Pocketbook of Differential Diagnosis*. 5th ed. Elsevier; 2022.
8. Goldman L, Schafer AI, eds. *Goldman-Cecil Medicine*. 26th ed. Elsevier; 2020.

Chapter 79

FURTHER READING

Guan LL, Lim HW, Mohammad TF. Recognizing photoallergy, phototoxicitv and immune-mediated photodermatoses. *J Allergy Clin Immunol.* 2022;149(4):1206–1209. https://doi.org/10.1016/j.jaci.2022.02.013.

Lim HW, Epstein J. Photosensitivity diseases. *J Am Acad Dermatol.* 1997;36(1):84–90. https://doi.org/10.1016/s0190-9622(97)70330-x.

Gould JW, Mercurio MG, Elmets CA. Cutaneous photosensitivity diseases induced by exogenous agents. *J Am Acad Dermatol.* 1995;33(4):551–573. https://doi.org/10.1016/0190-9622(95)91271-1.

IMAGE REFERENCES

2. Amar L, Khalil M, Shulman K, Sami N. Dronedarone-induced photoallergic reaction. *JAAD Case Rep*. 2020;6(12):1208–1210. https://doi.org/10.1016/j.jdcr.2020.10.003.

Chapter 80

FURTHER READING

O'Gorman SM, Murphy GM. Photoaggravated disorders. *Dermatol Clin.* 2014;32(3):385. https://doi.org/10.1016/j.det.2014.03.008. ix.

Chantorn R, Lim HW, Shwayder TA. Photosensitivity disorders in children: part II. *J Am Acad Dermatol.* 2012;67(6):1113.e1. https://doi.org/10.1016/j.jaad.2012.07.032. 1127.

Gambichler T, Al-Muhammadi R, Boms S. Immunologically mediated photodermatoses: diagnosis and treatment. *Am Journal Clin Dermatol.* 2009;10(3):169–180. https://doi.org/10.2165/00128071-200910030-00003.

Bissell DM, Anderson KE, Bonkovsky HL. Porphyria. *N Engl J Med.* 2017;377(9):862–872. https://doi.org/10.1056/NEJMra1608634.

Rutter KJ, Farrar MD, Marjanovic EJ, Rhodes LE. Clinicophotobiological characterization of photoaggravated atopic dermatitis. *JAMA Dermatol.* 2022;158(9):1022–1030. https://doi.org/10.1001/jamadermatol.2022.2823.

IMAGE REFERENCES

2. Courtesy Tor Shwayder, MD (Henry Ford Health, Detroit).
4. Courtesy Tor Shwayder, MD (Henry Ford Health, Detroit).

Chapter 81

FURTHER READING

Henning MAS, Bouazzi D, Jemec GBE. Treatment of hyperhidrosis: an update. *Am J Clin Dermatol.* 2022;23(5):635–646.

Nawrocki S, Cha J. The etiology, diagnosis, and management of hyperhidrosis: a comprehensive review: therapeutic options. *J Am Acad Dermatol.* 2019;81(3):669–680.

Miller JL. Diseases of the eccrine and apocrine sweat glands. In: Bolognia JL, Schaffer JV, Cerroni L, eds. *Dermatology*. 4th ed. Elsevier; 2017.

Haider A, Solish N. Focal hyperhidrosis: diagnosis and management. *CMAJ*. 2005;172(1):69–75.

IMAGE REFERENCES

1. Kang S, Amagai M, Bruckner AL, et al. *Fitzpatrick's Dermatology*. 9th ed. McGraw Hill; 2019.
2. Kang S, Amagai M, Bruckner AL, et al. *Fitzpatrick's Dermatology*. 9th ed. McGraw Hill; 2019.

Chapter 82

FURTHER READING

Miller JL. Diseases of the eccrine and apocrine sweat glands. In: Bolognia JL, Schaffer JV, Cerroni L, eds. *Dermatology*. 4th ed. Elsevier; 2017.

Diseases of the skin appendages. In: James WD, Elston DM, Treat, JR, Rosenbach MA, Neuhaus IM, eds. *Andrews' Diseases of the Skin*. 13th ed. Elsevier; 2020.

Yilmaz Gulec E, Turgut GT, Gezdirici A, et al. Clinical and molecular genetic findings of Crisponi/cold-induced sweating syndrome (Cs/ciss) spectrum in patients from Turkey. *Clin Genet*. 2022;102(3):201–217.

Satoh T. Clinical analysis and management of acquired idiopathic generalized anhidrosis. *Curr Probl Dermatol.* 2016;51:75–79.

Mok ZR, Tey HL. Acquired idiopathic generalized anhidriosis: successful treatment with cyclosporine in two cases. *Dermatol Ther*. 2018;31(2): e12579.

IMAGE REFERENCES

1. Kang S, Amagai M, Bruckner AL, et al. *Fitzpatrick's Dermatology*. 9th ed. McGraw Hill; 2019.
2. Kang S, Amagai M, Bruckner AL, et al. *Fitzpatrick's Dermatology*. 9th ed. McGraw Hill; 2019.
3. Wataya-Kaneda M. Genetic disorders with dyshidrosis: ectodermal dysplasia, incontinentia pigmenti, Fabry disease, and congenital insensitivity to pain with anhidrosis. *Curr Probl Dermatol.* 51:42–49.

Chapter 83

FURTHER READING

Smith DD, Rood KM. Intrahepatic cholestasis of pregnancy. *Clin Obstet Gynecol.* 2020;63(1):134–151. https://doi.org/10.1097/GRF.0000000000000495.

Lehrhoff S, Pomeranz MK. Specific dermatoses of pregnancy and their treatment. *Dermatol Ther*. 2013;26(4):274–284. https://doi.org/10.1111/dth.12078.

Himeles JR, Pomeranz MK. Recognizing, diagnosing, and managing pregnancy dermatoses. *Obstet Gynecol.* 2022;140(4):679–695. https://doi.org/10.1097/AOG.0000000000004938.

Ambros-Rudolph CM, Müllegger RR, Vaughan-Jones SA, Kerl H, Black MM. The specific dermatoses of pregnancy revisited and reclassified: results of a retrospective two-center study on 505 pregnant patients. *J Am Acad Dermatol.* 2006;54(3):395–404. https://doi.org/10.1016/j.jaad.2005.12.012.

Sävervall C, Sand FL, Thomsen SF. Dermatological diseases associated with pregnancy: pemphigoid gestationis, polymorphic eruption of pregnancy, intrahepatic cholestasis of pregnancy, and atopic eruption of pregnancy. *Dermatol Res Pract.* 2015;2015: 979635. https://doi.org/10.1155/2015/979635.

IMAGE REFERENCES

1. Ambros-Rudolph CM, Müllegger RR, Vaughan-Jones SA, Kerl H, Black MM. The specific dermatoses of pregnancy revisited and reclassified: results of a retrospective two-center study on 505 pregnant patients. *J Am Acad Dermatol.* 2006;54(3):395–404. https://doi.org/10.1016/j.jaad.2005.12.012.
2. Roth MM, Cristodor P, Kroumpouzos G. Prurigo, pruritic folliculitis, and atopic eruption of pregnancy: facts and controversies. *Clin Dermatol.* 2016;34(3):392–400. https://doi.org/10.1016/j.clindermatol.2016.02.012.
3. Courtesy of Jennifer Hsiao, MD, Los Angeles, CA.
4. Dinulos JGH. Figure 6.27. In: Habif 's Clinical Dermatology: A Color Guide to Diagnosis and Therapy. 7th ed. Elsevier; 2021.
5. Bechtel MA. Pruritus in pregnancy and its management. *Dermatol Clin.* 2018;36(3):259–265. https://doi.org/10.1016/j.det.2018.02.012.

Chapter 84

FURTHER READING

Bolognia JL, Schaffer JV, Cerroni L. *Dermatology*. Elsevier; 2017.

Maurer M, Magerl M, Betschel S, et al. The international WAO/EAACI guideline for the management of hereditary angioedema—the 2021 revision and update. *Allergy*. 2022;77(7):1961–1990. PMID: 35006617.

Andersen MF, Longhurst HJ, Rasmussen ER, Bygum A. How not to be misled by disorders mimicking angioedema: a review of pseudoangioedema. *Int Arch Allergy Immunol.* 2016;169(3):163–170.

Al-Hamad A, Porter S, Fedele S. Orofacial granulomatosis. *Dermatol Clin.* 2015;33(3):433–446.

Brown DN, Wieser I, Wang C, Dabaja BS, Duvic M. Leonine facies (LF) and mycosis fungoides (MF): a single-center study and systematic review of the literature. *J Am Acad Dermatol.* 2015;73(6):976–986.

IMAGE REFERENCES

1. Rad MV, Chan EKY, Ahmed IH. Cervicofacial subcutaneous emphysema and pneumomediastinum secondary to dental treatment in a young man. *Respir Med Case Rep.* 2019;28:100918. https://doi:10.1016/j.rmcr.2019.100918.
4. Velasco-Medina AA, Cortés-Morales G, Barreto-Sosa A, Velázquez-Sámano G. Fisiopatología y avances en el tratamiento del Angioedema Hereditario [Pathophysiology and advances in the treatment of hereditary angioedema]. *Rev Alerg Mex.* 2011;58(2):112–119.
5. Cho YT, Yang CW, Chu CY. Drug reaction with eosinophilia and systemic symptoms (DRESS): an interplay among drugs, viruses, and immune system. *Int J Mol Sci.* 2017;18(6):1243. https://doi.org/10.3390/ijms18061243. PMID: 28598363; PMCID: PMC5486066.
6. Schloemer JA, Zirwas MJ, Burkhart CG. Airborne contact dermatitis: common causes in the USA. *Int J Dermatol.* 2015;54(3):271–274. https://doi.org/10.1111/ijd.12692. Epub 2014 Jul 1. PMID: 24981079.
7. Ventilacion L, Leech S. Recurrent urticaria. *Paediatr Child Health.* 2016;26(7): 292–297.
8. Bruett CT, Trump BR, Adams DR, Halpern LR. Orofacial granulomatosis: a case treated with azithromycin pulse therapy, review of the literature and an algorithm for diagnosis. *IDCases.* 2020;21. https://doi.org/10.1016/j.idcr.2020.e00924.
9. Tomás-Velázqez A, Quan López PL, Calvo Imirizaldu M, España Alonso A. Superior vena cava syndrome. *Actas Dermo-Sifiliográficas.* 2021;112(5):471–473. https://doi:10.1016./j.adengl.2021.02.012.
10. Brown DN, Wieser I, Wang C, Dabaja BS, Duvic M. Leonine facies (LF) and mycosis fungoides (MF): a single-center study and systematic review of the literature. *J Am Acad Dermatol.* 2015;73(6):976–986. https://doi:10.1016/j.jaad.2015.09.017.
11. Wohlrab J, Lueftl M, Marsch WC. Persistent erythema and edema of the midthird and upper aspect of the face (morbus morbihan): evidence of hidden immunologic contact urticaria and impaired lymphatic drainage. *J Am Acad Dermatol.* 2005;52(4):595–602. https://doi:10.1016/j.jaad.2004.08.061.

Chapter 85

FURTHER READING

Millsop JW, Fazel N. Oral candidiasis. *Clin Dermatol.* 2016;34(4):487–494.

Burns A, Marchitto MC, Jhaveri M, Kang J, Rozati S. Artifactual pseudo-cheilitis: a case series of an underreported condition. *JAAD Case Rep.* 2021;17:111–115.

Cifuentes M, Davari P, Rogers III RS. Contact stomatitis. *Clin Dermatol.* 2017;35(5):435–440.

Trager M, Farmer K, Ulrich C, et al. Actinic cheilitis: a systematic review of treatment options. *J Eur Acad Dermatol Venereol.* 2021;35(4):815–823.

Chapter 86

FURTHER READING

Vachiramon V, McMichael AJ. Approaches to the evaluation of lip hyperpigmentation. *Int J Dermatol.* 2012;51(7):761–770.

Agha-Hosseini F, Sheykhbahaei N. A new approach to the management of caliber-persistent artery: a case report and analysis of previously reported cases. *Int J Dermatol.* 2016;55(1):11–16.

Lee JS, Mun J-H. Dermoscopy of venous lake on the lips: a comparative study with labial melanotic macule. *PLoS One.* 2018;13(10):e0206768.

Trager M, Farmer K, Ulrich C, et al. Actinic cheilitis: a systematic review of treatment options. *J Eur Acad Dermatol Venereol.* 2021;35(4):815–823.

Fatahzadeh M. Kaposi sarcoma: review and medical management update. *Oral Surg Oral Med, Oral Pathol Oral Radiol.* 2012;113(1):2–16.

Chapter 87

FURTHER READING

Billaro V, Miteva M. Traction alopecia: the root of the problem. *Clin Cosmet Investig Dermatol.* 2018;11:149–159.

James GHD, Habif TP. *Hair diseases Habif's Clinical Dermatology: A Color Guide to Diagnosis and Therapy*. 7th ed. Elsevier; 2021:927–960.

McMichael AJ, Hordinsky MK. *Hair and Scalp Disorders: Medical, Surgical, and Cosmetic Treatments*. 2nd ed. CRC Press; 2018.

IMAGE REFERENCES

1. Courtesy Jorge Larrondo, MD, MSc.
2. Courtesy Jorge Larrondo, MD, MSc.
3. Courtesy Jorge Larrondo, MD, MSc.
4. Courtesy Jorge Larrondo, MD, MSc.
5. Courtesy Jorge Larrondo, MD, MSc.
6. Courtesy Jorge Larrondo, MD, MSc.
7. Courtesy Jorge Larrondo, MD, MSc.

Chapter 88

FURTHER READING

Concha JSS, Werth. VP. Alopecias in lupus erythematosus. *Lupus Sci Med.* 2018;5(1):e000291. https://doi.org/10.1136/lupus-2018-000291.

Jain N, Doshi B, Khopkar U. Trichoscopy in alopecias: diagnosis simplified. *Int J Trichology.* 2013;5(4):170–178. https://doi.org/10.4103/0974-7753.130385.

McMichael AJ, Hordinsky MK. *Hair and Scalp Disorders: Medical, Surgical, and Cosmetic Treatments*. 2nd ed. CRC Press; 2018.

Paus Haslam IS, Sharov AA, Botchkarev VA. Pathobiology of chemotherapy-induced hair loss. *Lancet Oncol.* 2013;14(2):e50–e59. https://doi.org/10.1016/S1470-2045(12)70553-3.

IMAGE REFERENCES

1. Courtesy Jorge Larrondo, MD, MSc.
5. Image courtesy Dr. Amy McMicheal.
6. Image courtesy Dr. Amy McMicheal.
7. Image courtesy Dr. Amy McMicheal.
8. Image courtesy Dr. Amy McMicheal.
9. Image courtesy Dr. Amy McMicheal.

Chapter 89

IMAGE REFERENCES

1. Gupta L, Gautam RK, Bharadwaj M. Nevoid Hypertrichosis: Case Report with Review of the Literature. *Int J Trichology.* 2011;3(2):115–117.
2. Tng VE, de Zwaan S, Hypertrichosis cubiti, a case report and literature review. Clinical Case Reports published by John Wiley & Sons Ltd. 2015.
3. Reprinted with permission from Elsevier (Lancet Vol 387, 10032, 2016, Page 2035).

Chapter 90

IMAGE REFERENCES

1. Gacaferri Lumezi B, et al. Mixed form of Hirsutism in an adolescent female and laser therapy. *Iran Red Crescent Med J*. 2014;16(6):E9410.

Chapter 91

FURTHER READING

Walker J, Baran R, Vélez N, Jellinek N. Koilonychia: an update on pathophysiology, differential diagnosis and clinical relevance. *J Eur Acad Dermatol Venereol*. 2016;30(11):1985–1991. https://doi.org/10.1111/jdv.13610.

Spicknall KE, Zirwas MJ, English JC. Clubbing: an update on diagnosis, differential diagnosis, pathophysiology, and clinical relevance. *J Am Acad Dermatol*. 2005;52(6):1020–1028. https://doi.org/10.1016/j.jaad.2005.01.006.

Chen SX, Cohen PR. Parrot beak nails revisited: case series and comprehensive review. *Dermatol Ther*. 2018;8(1):147–155. https://doi.org/10.1007/s13555-017-0217-y. Epub 2017 Dec 19. PMID: 29260428; PMCID: PMC5825322.

Singal A, Arora R. Nail as a window of systemic diseases. *Indian Dermatol Online J*. 2015;6(2):67–74. https://doi.org/10.4103/2229-5178.153002. MID: 25821724; PMCID: PMC4375768.

IMAGE REFERENCES

3. James W, Elston D, Treat J, Rosenbach M, Neuhaus I. *Andrews' Diseases of the Skin*. 13th ed. Elsevier; 2020.
4. Marie I, Gremain V, Nassermadji K, et al. Nail involvement in systemic sclerosis.*J Am Acad Dermatol*. 2017;76(6):1115–1123.
7. James W, Elston D, Treat J, Rosenbach M, Neuhaus I. *Andrews' Diseases of the Skin*. 13th ed. Elsevier; 2020.

Chapter 92

FURTHER READING

Iorizzo M, Starace M, Pasch MC. Leukonychia: what can white nails tell us? *Am J Clin Dermatol*. 2022;23(2):177–193. https://doi.org/10.1007/s40257-022-00671-6.

Thomas L, Azad J, Takwale A. Management of nail psoriasis. *Clin Exp Dermatol*. 2021;46(1):3–8. https://doi.org/10.1111/ced.14314.

Oztas MO. Clinical and dermoscopic progression of subungual hematomas. *Int Surg*. 2010;95(3):239–241. 2010.

Bae Y, Lee GM, Sim JH, Lee S, Lee SY, Park YL. Green nail syndrome treated with the application of tobramycin eye drop. *Ann Dermatol*. 2014;26(4):514–516. https://doi.org/10.5021/ad.2014.26.4.514.

Piraccini BM, Urciuoli B, Starace M, Tosti A, Balestri R. Yellow nail syndrome: clinical experience in a series of 21 patients. *J Dtsch Dermatol Ges*. 2014;12(2):131–137. https://doi.org/10.1111/ddg.12216.

IMAGE REFERENCES

2. Bolognia JL, Schaffer JV, Cerroni L. *Dermatology*. 4th ed. Elsevier; 2018.
7. Courtesy Dr. Nicole Harter.
14. James W, Elston D, Treat J, Rosenbach M, Neuhaus I. *Andrews' Diseases of the Skin*. 13th ed. Elsevier; 2020.
15. Courtesy Adam Rubin, MD.

Chapter 93

FURTHER READING

Zaiac MN, Walker A. Nail abnormalities associated with systemic pathologies. *Clin Dermatol*. 2013;31(5):627–649. https://doi.org/10.1016/j.clindermatol.2013.06.018.

Lee DK, Lipner SR. Optimal diagnosis and management of common nail disorders. *Ann Med*. 2022;54(1):694–712. https://doi.org/10.1080/07853890.2022.2044511.

Schneider SL, Tosti A. Tips to diagnose uncommon nail disorders. *Dermatol Clin*. 2015;33(2):197–205. https://doi.org/10.1016/j.det.2014.12.003.

Robert C, Sibaud V, Mateus C, Verschoore M, Charles C, Lanoy E, Baran R. Nail toxicities induced by systemic anticancer treatments. *Lancet Oncol*. 2015;16(4):e181–e189. https://doi.org/10.1016/S1470-2045(14)71133-7.

Grover C, Singal A, Bhattacharya SN. Pterygium complicating nail psoriasis and trachyonychia: is it rare? *Skin Appendage Disord*. 2021;7(4):298–305. https://doi.org/10.1159/000513455.

IMAGE REFERENCES

1. From James WD et al. *Andrews' Diseases of the Skin*. 12th ed. Elsevier; 2016.
2. Reprinted with permission from Elsevier (The Lancet, 2008;372(9647):1410).
3. Masunaga M, Mizumoto J. Terry's nails due to uncontrolled diabetes mellitus. *Am J Med*. 2021;134(7):e428. https://doi.org/10.1016/j.amjmed.2020.12.016.
4. Huang WT, Wu CC. Half-and-half nail. *CMAJ*. 2009;180(6):687. https://doi.org/10.1503/cmaj.081312.
5. Vélez NF, Jellinek NJ. Simple onycholysis: a diagnosis of exclusion. *J Am Acad Dermatol*. 2014;70(4):793-794. https://doi.org/10.1016/j.jaad.2013.09.061.
6. Goraya JS, Kaur S. Beau lines. *J Pediatr*. 2014;164(1):205. https://doi.org/10.1016/j.jpeds.2013.08.032.
7. Shah RK, Uddin M, Fatunde OJ. Onychomadesis secondary to penicillin allergy in a child. *J Pediatr*. 2012;161(1):166. https://doi.org/10.1016/j.jpeds.2012.01.073.
8. Micheletti RG, James WD, Elston DM, McMahon PJ. *Andrews' Diseases of the Skin Clinical Atlas*. 2nd ed. Elsevier; 2022.
9. Courtesy Steven Binnick, MD.
10. Reprinted with permission from Solomon Geizhals, Christine T. Lauren, Shari R. Lipner, Hydrocolloid dressing application for the treatment of pediatric onychodystrophies, *JAAD*. 2019;80(5): e103–e104.
11. Courtesy Steven Binnick, MD.
12. Harrison S, Bergfeld WF. Diseases of the hair and nails. *Med Clin North Am*. 2009;93(6):1195–1209. https://doi.org/10.1016/j.mcna.2009.08.006. PMID: 19932326.
13. Bolognia, JL., Schaffer, JV., Cerroni, L. *Dermatology*. (4th ed.) Elsevier; 2018.
14. Stern DK, Diamantis S, Smith E, et al. Water content and other aspects of brittle versus normal fingernails. *J Am Acad Dermatol*. 2007;57(1):31–36. https://doi.org/10.1016/j.jaad.2007.02.004.

Chapter 94

FURTHER READING

Bolognia JL, Schaffer JV, Cerroni L. *Dermatology*. 4th ed. Elsevier - OHCE; 2017.

Cohen PR, Scher RK. Geriatric nail disorders: diagnosis and treatment. *J Am Acad Dermatol*. 1992;26(4):521–531. https://doi.org/10.1016/0190-9622(92)70075-q.

Gupta AK, Stec N, Summerbell RC, et al. Onychomycosis: a review. *J Eur Acad Dermatol Venereol*. 2020;34(9):1972–1990. https://doi.org/10.1111/jdv.16394.

Rubin AI, Jellinek NJ, Daniel R, Scher RK. *Scher and Daniel's Nails*. 4th ed. Springer International Publishing; 2018.

Samuelov L, Smith FJD, Hansen CD, Sprecher E. Revisiting pachyonychia congenita: a case-cohort study of 815 patients. *Br J Dermatol*. 2020;182(3):738–746. https://doi.org/10.1111/bjd.18794.

IMAGE REFERENCES

1. Paller AS, Mancini AJ. *Paller and Mancini—Hurwitz Clinical Pediatric Dermatology*. 6th ed. Elsevier; 2022.
2. James WD, Elston DM, Treat JR, Rosenbach MA. *Andrews' Diseases of the Skin*. 13th ed. Elsevier; 2019.
3. Scher RK, Daniel CR. *Nails*. 3rd ed. Elsevier Saunders; 2005.
4. Dinulos JGH. *Habif's Clinical Dermatology*. 7th ed. Elsevier; 2021.
5. Scher RK, Daniel CR. *Nails*. 3rd ed. Elsevier Saunders; 2005.
6. Scher RK, Daniel CR. *Nails*. 3rd ed. Elsevier Saunders; 2005.

Chapter 95

FURTHER READING

Bolognia JL, Jorizzo JJ, Schaffer JV. *Dermatology*. 3rd ed. Elsevier Saunders; 2018.

James WD, Elston DM, Treat JR, et al. *Andrews' Diseases of the Skin: Clinical Dermatology*. 13th ed. Elsevier; 2020.

Rubin AI, Scher RK, Daniel CR, Jellinek NJ, eds. *Scher and Daniel's Nails: Diagnosis, Surgery, Therapy*. 4th ed. Springer Nature; 2019.

van de Kerkhof PCM, Pasch MC, Scher RK, et al. Brittle nail syndrome: a pathogenesis-based approach with a proposed grading system. *J Am Acad Dermatol*. 2005;53(4):644–651. https://doi.org/10.1016/j.jaad.2004.09.002.

IMAGE REFERENCES

1. Courtesy Steven Binnick, MD.
2. James WD, Elston DM, Treat JR, Rosenbach MA, Neuhaus I. *Andrews' Diseases of the Skin Clinical Dermatology*. 13th ed. Elsevier; 2020.
3. van de Kerkhof PCM, Pasch MC, Scher RK, et al. *Brittle nail syndrome: a pathogenesis-based approach with a proposed grading system. J Am Acad Dermatol.* 2005;53(4):644–651. ISSN 0190–9622, https://doi.org/10.1016/j.jaad.2004.09.002.

4. Courtesy Steven Binnick, MD.
5. Bolognia JL, Schaffer JV, Cerroni L, (2018). *Dermatology* (4th ed.) Elsevier. Courtesy of Yale Residents' Slide Collection.
6. Rubin AI, Scher RK, Daniel CR, Jellinek NJ, eds. *Scher and Daniel's Nails: Diagnosis, Surgery, Therapy*. 4th ed. Springer Nature; 2019.
7. Rubin AI, Scher RK, Daniel CR, Jellinek NJ, eds. *Scher and Daniel's Nails: Diagnosis, Surgery, Therapy*. 4th ed. Springer Nature; 2019.
8. James WD, Elston DM, Treat JR, Rosenbach MA, Neuhaus I. *Andrews' Diseases of the Skin Clinical Dermatology*. 13th ed. Elsevier; 2020.

Chapter 96

FURTHER READING

De Das S, Tan KB, Ho S, Athanasian EA, Puhaindran ME. Pigmented nail lesions: when to observe, when to biopsy, when to widely excise, and when to amputate? *J Hand Surg Am*. 2022;47(10):988–997.

Lee DK, Lipner SR. Optimal diagnosis and management of common nail disorders. *Ann Med*. 2022;54(1):694–712.

Iorizzo M, Pasch MC. Bacterial and viral infections of the nail unit. *Dermatol Clin*. 2021;39(2):245–253.

Hare AQ, Rich P. Nail tumors. *Dermatol Clin*. 2021;39(2):281–292.

IMAGE REFERENCES

1. Micali G, Verzì AE, Lacarrubba F. Alternative uses of dermoscopy in daily clinical practice: an update. *J Am Acad Dermatol*. 2018;79(6):1117–1132.e1.
2. Courtesy Dr. Tatiana Andrade.
3. Scher R, Daniel R. *Nails: Diagnosis, Therapy, and Surgery*. 3rd ed. Elsevier; 2005.
4. James WD, Elston DM, Treat JR, Rosenbach MA. *Andrews' Diseases of the Skin*. 13th ed. Elsevier; 2019.
5. Neligan P. *Plastic Surgery: Volume 6: Hand and Upper Extremity*. 5th ed. Elsevier; 2024.
6. James WD, Elston DM, Treat JR, Rosenbach MA. *Andrews' Diseases of the Skin*. 13th ed. Elsevier; 2019.
7. Courtesy of B. Richert, MD, Université de Liège, Belgium.
8. Khanna N. *Illustrated Synopsis of Dermatology & Sexually Transmitted Diseases*. 7th ed. Elsevier; 2024.
9. Paller AS, Mancini AJ. *Hurwitz Clinical Pediatric Dermatology E-Book*. 5th ed. Elsevier; 2015.
10. James WD, Elston DM, Treat JR, Rosenbach MA. *Andrews' Diseases of the Skin*. 13th ed. Elsevier; 2019.

Index

Note: Page numbers followed by *f* indicate figures.

E

T

U

V

W

X

Y

Z